STATISTICS IN MEDICINE

STATISTICS IN MEDICINE

R. H. RIFFENBURGH
Clinical Investigation Department
Naval Medical Center San Diego
San Diego, California

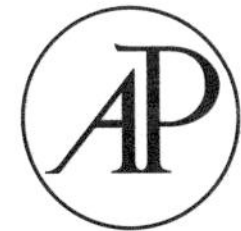

Academic Press
San Diego London Boston New York Sydney Tokyo Toronto

This book is printed on acid-free paper. 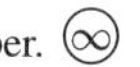

Academic Press
a division of Harcourt Brace & Company
525 B Street, Suite 1900, San Diego, California 92101-4495, USA
http://www.apnet.com

Academic Press
24-28 Oval Road, London NW1 7DX, UK
http://www.hbuk.co.uk/ap/

Library of Congress Catalog Card Number: 98-60460

International Standard Book Number: 0-12-588560-1

PRINTED IN THE UNITED STATES OF AMERICA
99 00 01 02 03 04 QW 9 8 7 6 5 4 3 2 1

This book is dedicated to Gerrye,
my love and best friend for five decades;
Robin and Rick; Scott, Ellen, Alex, and Jasmine;
the memory of Marc; Karen, Matt, and Bryce;
and Doug, Trish and Nichole.

Contents

Chapter 12
Confidence Intervals

Chapter 13
Common Tests on Categorical Data

Chapter 14
Common Tests on Ranked Data

Chapter 18
Sample Size Required in a Study

Chapter 19
Modeling and Clinical Decisions

Chapter 20
Regression and Correlation Methods

Foreword

In my five years as Commander of Naval Medical Center San Diego, which has been termed the world's largest and most technologically advanced military health care complex, I was always humbled by the vast spectrum of clinical challenges successfully met by the staff. In my current position, I have come to realize that all of modern medicine deals with a similar depth and variety of cases as it transitions to a managed-care environment. We have a critical obligation not only to care for our patients, but also to assess thoroughly our decisions on therapy, treatment effects, and outcomes. Scientifically rigorous medical studies including sound statistical analyses are central to this process.

Each year, the demand for sound statistics in medical research is increasing. In recent years, statistical analysis has become the hallmark of studies appearing in the leading journals. It is common for authors to have their manuscripts returned for rework on their statistics. The demand for quality statistics puts intense pressure on medical education to include more statistical training, on practitioners to evaluate critically the medical literature, and on clinical staff to design and analyze their investigations with rigor.

Currently, the field lacks a book that can be used efficiently as both text and reference. Clinical investigators and health care students continuously complain that traditional texts are notoriously difficult for the nonmathematically inclined whose time is saturated with clinical duties. This book addresses that problem. The explanations, step-by-step procedures, and many clinical examples render it a less daunting text than the usual statistics book. This book represents a practical opportunity for health care trainees and staff not only to acquaint themselves with statistics in medicine and understand statistical analysis in the medical literature, but also to be guided in the application of planning and analysis in their own medical studies.

Dr. Riffenburgh, a former professor of statistics, has consulted on medical statistics for decades. He was a linchpin in hundreds of the nearly 1000 studies current at NMCSD during my tenure. Investigators from all disciplines benefited from his collegial advice and rigorous analysis of their projects. His understanding of the unique needs in the training of health care professionals was one motivation for this book. I hope you will find it a valuable addition to your professional library.

Vice Admiral Richard A. Nelson, M.D., USN
Surgeon General of the Navy
Chief, Bureau of Medicine and Surgery

A Navy physician for more than 30 years, Admiral Nelson has served in clinical practice and has directed a number of medical departments and agencies. He has been certified by the American Board of Preventive Medicine and has received numerous medals and awards for his service. In the past decade, he has been Commanding Officer, Naval Hospital Bremerton, WA; Fleet Surgeon, U.S. Atlantic Fleet; Command Surgeon, U.S. Atlantic Command; Medical Advisor, NATO's Supreme Allied Command Atlantic (SACLANT); and Commander, Naval Medical Center San Diego.

Preface: About This Book

A Unique Biostatistics Book Offering Both Text and Reference

This book, in contrast to a traditional university text, is designed to be used as both a textbook and a reference book. Part I: Course of Study serves as a textbook for an introductory course in biostatistics for students in medicine, dentistry, nursing, pharmacy, and other health care fields. Part II: Reference Handbook serves as a reference manual to support practicing clinicians in reading the medical literature or conducting an occasional research study.

Only the More Important Methods and Concepts Are Covered

This book does not attempt to cover all biostatistical methods. It is intended for clinical health care professionals and students rather than for full-time research workers. It might be called a "30/90 book," in that it covers the 30% of statistical methods used for 90% of medical studies. [Emerson and Colditz (1992) [1] analyzed the 301 articles appearing in four volumes of the *New England Journal of Medicine* for statistical content. Part I of this book covers 82% of the biostatistical methods used in these 301 articles and Parts I and II combined cover 90%.]

[1] Emerson, J. D., and Colditz, G. A. (1992). Use of statistical analysis in the New England Journal of Medicine. In *Medical Uses of Statistics* (J. C. Bailar and F. Mosteller, eds.), 2nd ed. pp. 45–57. NEJM Books, Boston.

Using a Few Data Sets Repeatedly Allows the User to Concentrate More on the Method

The book opens with a dozen databases [from screening for prostate cancer (DB1) to risk factors following carinal resection (DB12)] having sample sizes small enough to be given in full. Supplementary examples with larger sample sizes from other medical fields are also included, with summary statistics provided for the user.

PART I: COURSE OF STUDY

The Important Issue Is What the Student Remembers Five Years after the Course, Not What Is Forgotten

It is better for the student to understand and retain some key essentials that to be exposed to a profusion of methods not retained or a depth not understood. Therefore, the textbook part covers only the basic concepts and the most frequently seen methods in biostatistics.

This Book Starts at the Beginning of Mathematics

This book starts at ground zero in mathematics and statistics, but assumes an intelligent, alert, and motivated student with ability in arithmetic. It is designed to be offered without formal university-level prerequisites. It has been honed by use as a text for several lecture series to staff and residents at the Naval Medical Center.

PART II: REFERENCE HANDBOOK

The Reference Part Caters to the Clinician Reading an Article or Doing a Study

Part II forms a "how to" guide to the more common statistical methods in medicine. It does not take the user through derivations or seldom-used details, but sticks to what the clinical investigator needs in order to do the basics of his job; if it's not in the book, see a biostatistician. The reference part is designed to be accessed in two ways. If users see a statistical method in a medical article they are reading, the method and examples of its use may be found through the index. If users have a research plan or actual data and need the appropriate analytic method, they may find it by using a table of study protocol characteristics paired with methods, located in Chapter 10. A detailed table of contents is also available. Part II permits reference use hop-about and avoids an overwhelming deluge of detail. A great effort has been made to make it user friendly.

Part I Provides a Basis for the Reference User Who Needs It

The material found in Part I provides the foundation for the use of Part II as a reference. Users who have learned that material through another medium, such as personal study or an earlier course, need not study Part I, although they might scan it to fill in any knowledge gaps. However, a user who is not familiar with the material of Part I should study it to a reasonable level of understanding. In the same manner that the concepts of addition and multiplication are required to go very far in arithmetic, the concepts of a random variable and its probability distribution are required to do much with statistics.

The Format Is Tailored to the Medical User

Because most statistics users page through a text to find an example first and then read the methodology, each new section starts with an example. Following the example, the method is given step by step. Then an additional example in a different medical specialty is given. Finally, so users can check their understanding of the method, an exercise is posed. The exercise is worked out at the end of chapter. Once users are familiar with the methods of a chapter, they may find summary pages in a section toward the end of the book. These summaries provide quick reference so that users do not have to ferret out formulas and related details from the text.

ACKNOWLEDGMENTS

The author is grateful to VADM Richard Nelson, M.D., Surgeon General of the Navy and Chief, Bureau of Medicine and Surgery, for writing the foreword; to CAPT Bruce Boynton, M.D., Command Surgeon, 1st Marine Expeditionary Force, Camp Pendelton, San Diego; CAPT Brian Nyquist, M.D., Chief of Anesthesiology, Naval Hospital Bremerton; LCDR David Lane, M.D., Bureau of Medicine and Surgery; and Mario Cleves, Ph.D., Lead Statistician, Stata Corporation, for reviewing and evaluating the manuscript; to CAPT Pat Olson, M.D., M.P.H., NEPMU-5, for reviewing and revising the chapter on epidemiology; to CAPT Scott Sageman, M.D., Chief of Pulmonary Medicine, NMCSD, for reviewing some chapters; and to CDR Peter Johnstone, M.D., Chief of Radiation Oncology, NMCSD, for great help on several fronts. Stata, a product of Stata Corporation, College Station, Texas, was used for much of the statistical analysis and figure generation.

Databases

Databases are abbreviated "DB" followed by the database number. A superscript number at end of each title corresponds to References and Data Sources list number.

DB1. INDICATORS OF PROSTATE BIOPSY RESULTS[27]

Purpose for Repeated Use of This Data Set

In this text, these data are used for primary illustration of many of the statistical methods presented, especially those in Part I. Once familiar with this data set, the reader may concentrate on the statistical aspects being discussed rather than focusing on the medical aspects of the data. This data set was selected as much for data reasons as for medical reasons: a mix of data types illustrates different methods, adequate sample size, and the like.

Background

These data were taken from 301 male patients examined in the Urology Department at the Naval Medical Center San Diego who exhibited one of several reasons to suspect the health of their prostate glands. They were recorded in the order they presented. These data have the advantage that they include biopsy outcomes regardless of the results of preliminary examinations. Thus, false negatives (negative biopsy outcomes when a tumor is present) as well as false positives (positive biopsy outcomes when no tumor is present) can be examined.

Data

For each patient, recorded data (units indicated in parentheses) are as follows:

age (years, >0, integers)
digital rectal examination result (DRE) (0 = negative, 1 = positive)
transurethral ultrasound result (TRU) (0 = negative, 1 = positive)
prostate specific antigen level (PSA) (ng/ml, >0, to one decimal place)
volume of prostate (VOL) (ml, >0, to one decimal place)
PSA density level (PSAD) (PSA/VOL, >0, to two decimal places)
biopsy result (BIOP) (0 = negative, 1 = positive)

There are too many data for the reader to do calculations personally. Some summary statistics are given here for the full set of 301 patients and for 296 patients who are at risk of prostate cancer [5 patients with severe benign prostatic hypertrophy (BPH) removed]:

Data set	Age	PSA	Volume	PSAD
301 patients: mean	66.76	8.76	23.47	0.269
standard deviation	8.10	16.91	18.04	0.488
296 patients: mean	66.75	8.79	35.46	0.272
standard deviation	8.13	17.05	16.35	0.491
Patient nos. 11–301: mean	66.82	8.85	36.60	0.270
standard deviation	8.14	17.19	18.12	0.496

Data for the first 10 cases are given in Table DB1.1 for use in calculations. Note that all data are numeric. Most analysis software packages require this, and it is

Table DB1.1
Prostate Test Data from the First 10 of the 301 Patients in the Data Set

Patient no.	Age (years)	Digital rectal exam	Transurethral ultrasound	PSA (ng/ml)	Volume (ml)	PSAD (PSA/volume)	Biopsy result
1	75	0	1	7.6	32.3	0.24	0
2	68	1	0	4.1	27.0	0.15	0
3	54	0	0	5.9	16.2	0.36	1
4	62	1	1	9.0	33.0	0.27	1
5	61	0	0	6.8	30.9	0.22	1
6	61	0	1	8.0	73.7	0.11	0
7	62	0	0	7.7	30.5	0.25	0
8	61	1	1	4.4	30.5	0.14	0
9	73	1	1	6.1	36.8	0.17	0
10	74	1	1	7.9	16.4	0.48	0

much easier to transfer data from one package to another (e.g., from a spreadsheet to a statistical package) with data in numeric form.

DB2. EFFECTIVENESS OF A DRUG IN REDUCING NAUSEA FOLLOWING GALL BLADDER REMOVAL[26]

BACKGROUND

A sample of 81 gall bladder removals by laparoscope were randomized into two groups to receive preoperative ondansetron hydrochloride or a placebo. (Data were edited slightly for the exercise and do not reflect exact original results.) Patients rated their nausea on a scale of 1 (no nausea) to 5 (unbearable nausea) 2 hr after the end of surgery.

DATA

	Nausea scores					
	1	2	3	4	5	Totals
Drug	31	7	2	0	0	40
Placebo	25	6	5	2	3	41
Totals	56	13	7	2	3	81

Rating scores 2–5 may be combined to form a 2 × 2 contingency table of nausea or no nausea:

	No nausea (score 1)	Nausea (score 2–5)	Totals
Drug	34	6	40
Placebo	22	19	41
Totals	56	25	81

DB3. EFFECT OF AZITHROMYCIN ON SERUM THEOPHYLLINE LEVELS OF EMPHYSEMA PATIENTS[10]

BACKGROUND

Theophylline dilates airways in emphysema patients. When azithromycin is indicated for an infection in such a patient, does it alter the serum theophylline level? Serum theophylline levels (mg/dl) were measured in 16 emphysema patients at baseline (just before the start of azithromycin), 5 days (at the end of the course of antibiotics), and 10 days. Clinically, it is anticipated that the antibiotic will raise the theophylline level.

Data

Patient no.	Age	Sex	Baseline	5 days	10 days
1	61	F	14.1	2.3	10.3
2	70	F	7.2	5.4	7.3
3	65	M	14.2	11.9	11.3
4	65	M	10.3	10.7	13.8
5	64	F	15.4	15.2	13.6
6	76	M	5.2	6.8	4.2
7	72	M	10.4	14.6	14.1
8	69	F	10.5	7.2	5.4
9	66	M	5.0	5.0	5.1
10	62	M	8.6	8.1	7.4
11	65	F	16.6	14.9	13.0
12	71	M	16.4	18.6	17.1
13	51	F	12.2	11.0	12.3
14	71	M	6.6	3.7	4.5
15	(Missing)	M	9.9	10.7	11.7
16	50	M	10.2	10.8	11.2

DB4. EFFECT OF PROTEASE INHIBITORS ON PULMONARY ADMISSIONS[61]

Background

Protease inhibitors (PIs) are used in the treatment of infection by human immunodeficiency virus (HIV). A military hospital provides unlimited access to a full spectrum of HIV medications. Has this access reduced admissions due to secondary infections? In particular, has unlimited access to PIs reduced the annual admission rate of patients with pulmonary complications? Numbers of admissions for HIV, separated into patients with pulmonary complications and those without, were obtained for the 4 years (1992–1995) prior to access to PIs and for the 2 years (1996–1997) after PIs became available.

Data

	With pulmonary complications	Without pulmonary complications	Totals
Pre-PIs	194	291	485
Post-PIs	25	67	92
Totals	219	358	577

DB5. EFFECT OF SILICONE IMPLANTS ON PLASMA SILICONE[49]

Background

Silicone implants in women's breasts occasionally rupture, releasing silicone into the body. A large number of women have received silicone breast implants, and some believe that the presence of the implants raises plasma silicone levels, leading to side effects. A study was begun to test this belief. A method was developed for accurately measuring the silicone level in blood. For each of 30 women, plasma silicone levels were taken prior to surgical placement of the implants. A postsurgery washout period was allowed, and plasma silicone levels were retaken.

Data

Patient no.	Pre-op level	Post-op level
1	0.15	0.21
2	0.13	0.24
3	0.39	0.10
4	0.20	0.12
5	0.39	0.28
6	0.42	0.25
7	0.24	0.22
8	0.18	0.21
9	0.26	0.22
10	0.12	0.23
11	0.10	0.22
12	0.11	0.24
13	0.19	0.45
14	0.15	0.38
15	0.27	0.23
16	0.28	0.22
17	0.11	0.18

(Continued)

Patient no.	Pre-op level	Post-op level
18	0.11	0.15
19	0.18	0.04
20	0.18	0.14
21	0.24	0.24
22	0.48	0.20
23	0.27	0.24
24	0.22	0.18
25	0.18	0.19
26	0.19	0.15
27	0.32	0.26
28	0.31	0.30
29	0.19	0.22
30	0.21	0.24

DB6. LASER REMOVAL OF TATTOOS AS RELATED TO TYPE OF INK USED[59]

Background

A frequently used component of tattoo ink is titanium. A dermatologist suspected that tattoos applied with titanium ink are more difficult to remove than those applied with other inks. Fifty patients wanting tattoo removal were tested for ink type, and laser removal was attempted. The numbers responding and not responding to the removal attempt are given here according to the type of ink used.

Data

	Respond	Not respond	Totals
Titanium ink	5	30	35
Nontitanium ink	8	7	15
Totals	13	37	50

DB7. RELATION OF BONE DENSITY TO INCIDENCE OF FEMORAL NECK STRESS FRACTURES[46]

Background

Femoral neck stress fractures occur in young people engaged in sports, combat training, etc. Such fractures have a relatively high rate of poor healing, which in many cases leaves the patient somewhat impaired. Many such events could be avoided if risk factors, i.e., those characteristics that predict a higher probability of fracture, could be identified. One potential risk factor is bone density, measured in milligrams/milliliter. A large database (several thousand) of bone density measures of normal healthy people has been compiled at the University of California—San Francisco (UCSF). Norms were established for age and sex. Do people with femoral neck stress fractures tend to have lower bone density measures than normals? Bone density was measured for 18 young people with femoral neck stress fractures.

DATA

The following data include age, sex, bone density measure, and UCSF norm-value for that age and sex.

Patient no.	Sex	Age	Bone density	UCSF norm
1	F	22	136.9	185
2	F	24	167.2	188
3	F	39	140.1	181
4	M	18	163.6	225
5	M	18	140.0	225
6	M	18	177.4	225
7	M	18	147.0	225
8	M	19	164.9	223
9	M	19	155.8	223
10	M	19	126.0	223
11	M	19	163.4	223
12	M	21	194.9	219
13	M	21	199.0	219
14	M	21	164.6	219
15	M	22	140.8	218
16	M	22	152.4	218
17	M	23	142.0	216
18	M	40	97.3	184

DB8. COMPARING TWO TYPES OF ASSAY ON THE EFFECT OF GAG ON THE BLADDER SURFACE[52]

BACKGROUND

Glycosaminoglycans (GAG) alter the adherence properties of the bladder surface. Four spectrophotometric readings (millimoles/kilogram) on the GAG levels in tissues of normal bladders from cadavers exposed to GAG were taken by each of two types of assay. (Mean instrument error has been established as 0.002.)

Data

Type 1 assay: 0.74, 0.37, 0.26, 0.20
Type 2 assay: 0.51, 0.53, 0.42, 0.29

DB9. PREDICTION OF GROWTH FACTORS BY PLATELET COUNTS[50]

Background

There are two types of platelet gel growth factors: platelet-derived growth factor (PDGF), used primarily in cutaneous wound healing, and transforming growth factor (TGF), used primarily to promote bone healing. Users wish to know the level of a growth factor in platelet gel, but the assay is costly and time-consuming. Can a simple platelet count predict the level of a growth factor in platelet gel? Platelet counts and levels of PDGF and TGF in platelet gel were measured for 20 patients. Because the large numbers in the data are a little tedious to calculate, some data summaries are given to assist the student.

Data

Variable	Mean	Standard deviation
Platelet count	295,000	164,900
Gel PDGF	31,622.9	19,039.7
Gel TGF	31,340.0	16,767.0

Patient no.	Platelet count	Gel PDGF	Gel TGF
1	576,000	61,835	60,736
2	564,000	74,251	61,102
3	507,000	62,022	55,669
4	205,000	10,892	15,366
5	402,000	34,684	41,603
6	516,000	48,689	47,003
7	309,000	26,840	33,400

(Continued)

8	353,000	42,591	36,083
9	65,000	7,970	12,049
10	456,000	49,122	46,575
11	306,000	25,039	35,992
12	281,000	30,810	34,803
13	226,000	19,095	27,304
14	125,000	9,004	10,954
15	213,000	16,398	18,075
16	265,000	25,567	26,695
17	102,000	17,570	13,783
18	159,000	21,813	17,953
19	33,000	16,804	7,732
20	237,000	31,462	23,922

DB10. TESTS OF RECOVERY AFTER SURGERY ON HAMSTRINGS OR QUADRICEPS[2]

BACKGROUND

Tests of strength and control following surgery on hamstring or quadricep muscles or tendons have had varying success in indicating the quality of recovery. Two proposed tests are the time to perform and the distance covered in a triple hop along a marked line, contrasted between the healthy leg and the operated leg. Strength of the operated muscle in the two legs has not been shown to be different for eight post-operative (post-op) patients. The question is whether the proposed tests will detect a difference.

DATA

	Time to perform (sec)		Centimeters covered	
Patient no.	Operated leg	Non-operated leg	Operated leg	Non-operated leg
1	2.00	1.89	569	606
2	2.82	2.49	360	450
3	2.82	2.39	385	481
4	2.97	3.13	436	504
5	2.64	2.86	541	553
6	3.77	3.09	319	424
7	2.35	2.30	489	527
8	2.39	2.13	523	568

DB11. SURVIVAL OF MALARIAL RATS TREATED WITH HEMOGLOBIN, RBCs, OR A PLACEBO[12]

BACKGROUND

The malaria parasite affects the transmission of oxygen to the brain. The infusion of red blood cells (RBCs) in a malaria-infected body slows deterioration, giving the body more time to receive the benefit of antimalarial medication. Does the infusion of hemoglobin provide the same benefit? Three groups of 100 rats each were infected with a rodent malaria. One group was given hemoglobin, a second was given RBCs, and the third was given hetastarch (an IV fluid with protein). Survival numbers (and, coincidentally, percent) at the outset (day 0) and over 10 succeeding days were recorded.

DATA

	Number of rats surviving by treatment type		
Day no.	Hemoglobin	RBCs	Hetastarch
0	100	100	100
1	100	100	100
2	77	92	83
3	77	92	67
4	69	83	58
5	69	83	58
6	62	83	50
7	38	83	33
8	38	75	33
9	31	58	33
10	23	58	33

DB12. IDENTIFICATION OF RISK FACTORS FOR DEATH FOLLOWING CARINAL RESECTION[44]

BACKGROUND

Resection of the tracheal carina is a dangerous procedure. From 134 cases, the following data subset is given from the variables that were recorded: age at surgery (years), prior tracheal surgery (no = 0, yes = 1), extent of the resection (centimeters), intubation required at end of surgery (no = 0, yes = 1), and patient death (no = 0, yes = 1). Because the data set is large for an exercise, some data summaries are given to assist the student.

DATA

Variable	Mean	Standard deviation	Variable	Mean	Standard deviation
Age (years)	47.84	15.78	Extent (sec)	2.96	1.24
Age, died = 0	48.05	16.01	Extent, died = 0	2.82	1.21
Age, died = 1	46.41	14.46	Extent, died = 1	3.96	1.00

Patient no.	Age at surgery	Prior surgery	Extent of resection	Intubated	Died
1	48	0	1	0	0
2	29	0	1	0	0
3	66	0	1	0	0
4	55	1	1	0	0
5	41	0	1	0	0
6	42	0	1	0	0
7	44	0	1	0	0
8	67	1	1	0	0
9	54	1	1	0	0
10	36	0	1.5	0	0
11	63	0	1.5	0	0
12	46	0	1.5	0	0
13	80	0	1.5	0	0
14	47	0	1.5	0	0
15	41	0	1.5	0	0
16	62	1	1.5	0	0
17	53	0	1.5	0	0
18	62	0	1.5	0	0
19	22	0	1.5	0	0
20	65	0	2	0	0
21	73	0	2	0	0
22	38	0	2	0	0
23	55	0	2	0	0
24	56	0	2	0	0
25	66	0	2	0	0
26	36	0	2	0	0
27	48	0	2	0	0
28	49	0	2	0	0
29	29	1	2	0	0
30	14	1	2	0	0
31	52	0	2	1	0
32	39	0	2	0	0
33	27	1	2	0	0
34	55	0	2	0	0
35	62	1	2	0	0
36	37	1	2	0	0
37	26	1	2	0	1
38	57	0	2	0	0

(Continued)

Patient no.	Age at surgery	Prior surgery	Extent of resection	Intubated	Died
39	60	0	2	0	0
40	76	0	2	0	0
41	28	1	2	0	0
42	25	0	2	0	0
43	62	0	2	0	0
44	63	1	2	0	0
45	34	0	2	0	0
46	56	0	2.3	0	0
47	51	0	2.5	0	0
48	42	0	2.5	0	0
49	54	1	2.5	0	0
50	62	0	2.5	0	0
51	47	0	2.5	0	0
52	34	1	2.5	0	0
53	52	0	2.5	1	0
54	49	0	2.5	0	0
55	69	0	2.5	0	0
56	32	0	2.5	0	0
57	19	1	2.5	0	0
58	38	0	2.5	0	0
59	55	0	2.5	0	0
60	40	0	2.5	0	0
61	63	0	2.5	0	0
62	51	0	2.5	0	0
63	8	1	2.5	0	0
64	54	0	2.5	0	0
65	58	1	2.5	1	1
66	48	0	2.5	0	0
67	19	0	2.5	0	0
68	25	0	2.5	1	0
69	49	0	3	0	0
70	27	1	3	0	0
71	47	1	3	1	0
72	58	0	3	0	0
73	8	1	3	0	0
74	41	1	3	0	0
75	18	1	3	0	0
76	31	0	3	0	0
77	52	0	3	0	0
78	72	0	3	0	0
79	62	0	3	0	0
80	38	0	3	0	0
81	59	0	3	0	0
82	62	1	3	0	0
83	33	1	3	1	1
84	62	0	3	0	0
85	25	0	3	1	0
86	46	0	3.2	0	1
87	52	1	3.5	0	0

(*Continued*)

Patient no.	Age at surgery	Prior surgery	Extent of resection	Intubated	Died
88	43	0	3.5	0	0
89	55	0	3.5	0	0
90	66	1	3.5	0	0
91	30	0	3.5	0	0
92	41	0	3.5	0	0
93	53	0	3.5	0	1
94	70	0	3.5	0	0
95	61	1	3.5	1	1
96	28	1	3.6	0	0
97	60	1	4	1	1
98	46	0	4	0	0
99	52	0	4	0	0
100	17	0	4	0	0
101	61	0	4	0	0
102	46	0	4	0	1
103	51	0	4	1	1
104	71	0	4	0	0
105	24	0	4	0	0
106	67	0	4	0	0
107	68	0	4	0	0
108	56	0	4	1	0
109	39	0	4	1	1
110	60	0	4	0	1
111	62	1	4.2	0	0
112	57	1	4.2	0	0
113	60	0	4.5	0	0
114	32	0	4.5	0	0
115	34	0	4.5	0	0
116	48	1	4.5	0	0
117	69	0	4.5	1	0
118	27	1	4.5	1	1
119	66	0	4.5	1	1
120	43	0	4.5	0	1
121	60	0	4.8	0	0
122	66	0	4.8	1	1
123	57	0	5	0	0
124	71	0	5	0	0
125	31	0	5	0	0
126	35	0	5	0	0
127	52	0	5	0	0
128	66	1	5	0	0
129	47	0	5	0	0
130	26	0	5.5	1	1
131	28	0	6	1	1
132	63	0	6	0	0
133	62	0	6	0	0
134	26	0	6	1	0

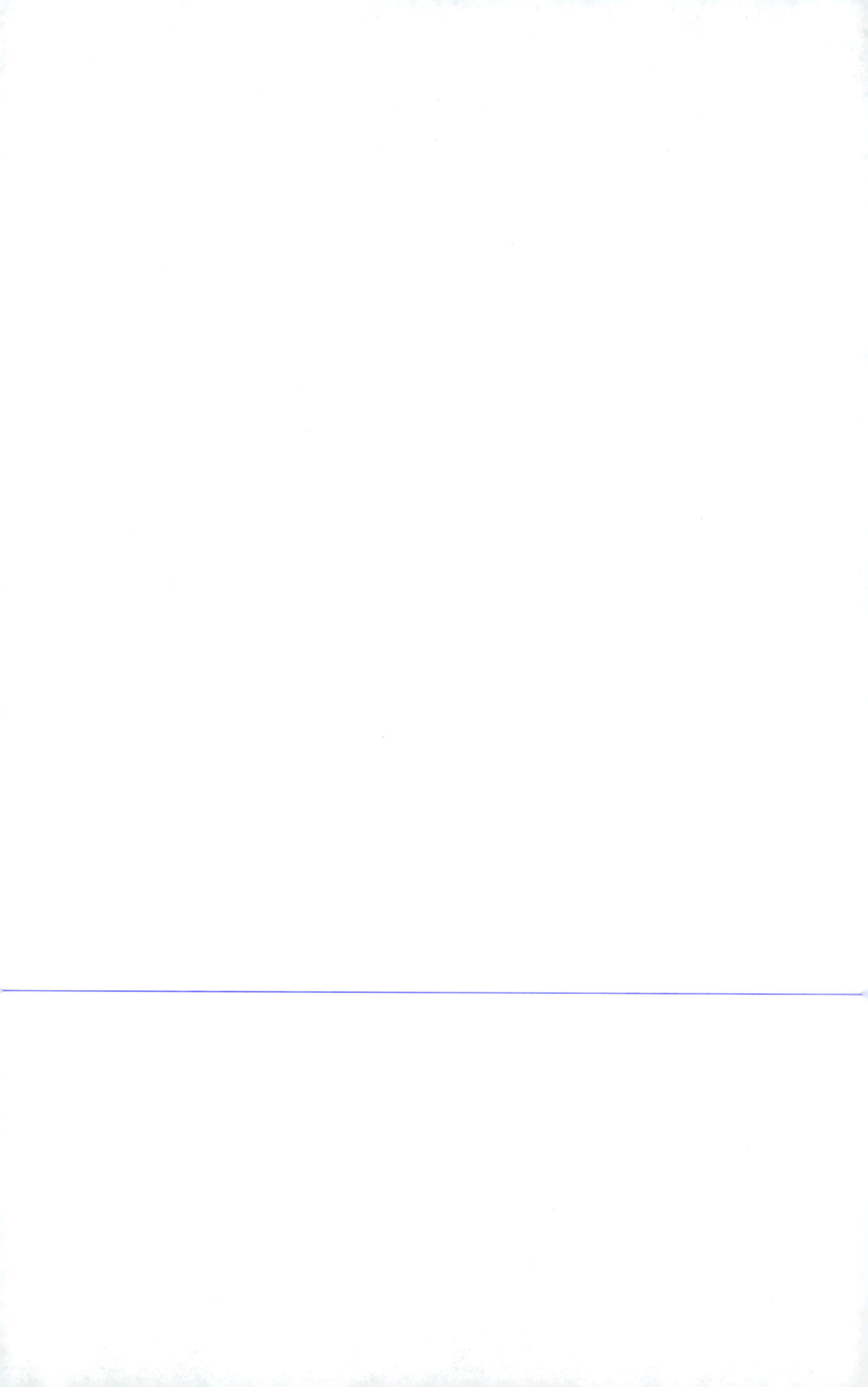

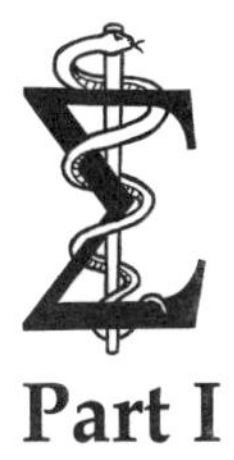

Part I

Course of Study

Chapter 1

Data, Notation, and Some Basic Terms

1.1. STAGES OF SCIENTIFIC KNOWLEDGE

STAGES

We gather data because we want to know something. These data are useful only if they provide information about what we want to know. A scientist usually seeks to develop knowledge in three stages: The first stage is to *describe* a class of events. The second is to *explain* these events. The third is to *predict* the occurrence of these events. The ability to predict an event implies some level of understanding of the rule of nature governing the event. The ability to predict outcomes of actions allows the scientist to make better decisions about such actions. At best, a general scientific rule may be inferred from repeated events of this type.

THE CAUSATIVE PROCESS IS OF INTEREST, NOT THE DATA

A process, or set of forces, generates data related to an event. It is this process, not the data per se, that interests us.

(1) *Description*: The stage in which we seek to describe the data-generating process for cases for which we have data from that process. Description would answer questions such as: What is the range of prostate volumes for a sample of urology patients? What is the difference in average volume between the patients having negative biopsies and those having positive ones?

(2) *Explanation*: The stage in which we seek to infer characteristics of the (overall) data-generating process when we have only part (usually a small part) of

the possible data. Inference would answer questions such as: On the basis of a sample of patients presenting with prostate problems, can we expect the average volumes of patients with positive biopsies to be lower than those of patients with negative biopsies, for all American men presenting with prostate problems? Inferences usually take the form of tests of hypotheses.

(3) *Prediction*: The stage in which we seek to make predictions about a characteristic of the data-generating process on the basis of newly taken related observations. Such a prediction would answer questions such as: On the basis of a patient's negative digital rectal exam (DRE), prostate specific antigen (PSA) value of 9, and prostate volume of 30 ml, what is the probability that he has cancer? Such predictions allow us to make decisions on how to treat our patients to change the chances of an event, for example: Should I biopsy my patient? Predictions usually take the form of a mathematical model of the relationship between the predicted (dependent) variable and the predictor (independent) variables.

Phase I–IV Studies

Stages representing increasing knowledge in medical investigations often are categorized by *phases*. A *Phase I* investigation is devoted to discovering whether a treatment is safe and gaining enough understanding of the treatment to design formal studies. For example, a new drug is assessed to learn the level of dosage to study and whether this level is safe in its main and side effects. A *Phase II* investigation is a preliminary investigation of the effectiveness of treatment. Is this drug more effective than existing drugs? Is the evidence of effectiveness strong enough to justify further study? *Phase III* is a large-scale verification of the early findings, the step from "some evidence" to "proof." The drug was shown to be more effective on several Phase II studies of 20 or 30 patients each over a scatter of subpopulations; now it must be shown to be more effective on, perhaps, 10,000 patients in a sample comprehensively representing the entire population. In *Phase IV*, an established treatment is monitored to detect any changes in the treatment or population of patients that would affect its use. Long-term toxicities must be detected. It must be determined whether a microorganism being killed by a drug can evolve to become partially immune to it.

1.2. QUANTIFICATION AND ACCURACY

Concept of Statistics

Knowledge gained from data usually is more informative and more accurate if the data are *quantitative*. Whereas certain quantities, such as the acceleration of an object in a vacuum, may be expressed with certainty and therefore lie in the realm of (deterministic) mathematics, most quantities that we deal with in life, and particularly in medicine, exhibit some uncertainty and lie in the realm of probability. *Statistics* deals with the development of probabilistic knowledge using observed quantities. These quantities may be as simple as counting the number of patients with flu symptoms or measuring the blood pressure of patients with heart disease, but they should be quantities that shed light on what we want to learn. Statistics as a discipline is interested not in the data themselves, but rather in the process that has generated these data.

Data Should Be Quantified

Often the information being gathered arises in quantitative form naturally, like the counts or measures just mentioned. In other cases, the information is given in words or pictures (e.g., true–false, "patient is in severe pain," X rays) and must be converted to quantities. A great deal of time and work may be saved, indeed sometimes whole studies salvaged, if the form in which the data are needed is planned in advance and the data are recorded in a form subject to analysis.

Quantifying Data

Quantities should be clearly defined and should arise from a common measurement base. Counts are straightforward. True–false, presence–absence, or male–female may be converted to 0–1. Verbal descriptions and visual images are more difficult. Cancer stages may be rated as A, B, C, or D and in turn converted to 1, 2, 3, or 4, but, in order to be compared among patients or among raters, they must be based on clearly defined clinical findings. On an X ray, the diameter of an arterial stenosis may be measured with a ruler. However, because the scale (enlargement) of X rays may vary and the size of patients may vary, the ruler-measured stenosis is better given in ratio to a nonstenotic diameter of the artery at a standardized location.

Accuracy versus Precision

Quantification per se is not enough; the quantities must be sufficiently accurate and precise. *Accuracy* refers to how well the data-gathering intent is satisfied; in simile, how close the arrow comes to the bullseye. *Precision* refers to the consistency of measurement; in simile, how tightly the arrows cluster together, unrelated to the distance of the cluster from the bullseye.

How Much Precision?

To decide how much precision is enough, identify the smallest unit that provides useful clinical information. (Just to be safe, one unit farther might be recorded and then rounded off after analysis.) Body temperature of a patient recorded in 10-degree units is useless. Tenths-of-a-degree units are most useful. Carrying temperature to hundredths-of-a-degree units adds no clinical benefit, as too many unknown variables influence such minute temperature differences.

1.3. DATA TYPES

Types of Data

Quantitative data may be of three major types: continuous, rank-order (also called ordinal), or categorical (also called nominal).

(1) *Continuous* data are positions on a scale. (A common ruler is such a scale.) In continuous data, these positions may be as close to one another as the user can discern and record. Prostate volumes and PSA level form examples of this type. (See DB1 from the Database collection.) One patient's volume was measured as 32.3 ml. If we needed more accuracy for some reason and had a sufficiently accurate measuring device, we might have recorded it as 32.34 or 32.3387.

Discrete data are a subset of continuous data that are recorded only as distinct values; there is a required distance between adjacent data. Age recorded in integral years is this type. The age could be 62 or 63, but we agree not to record 62.491.

(2) *Rank-order* data are indicators of some ordering characteristic of the subject, as ranking smallest to largest, most likely to least likely to survive, etc. There are two classes of data for which ranks are needed. First, for judgment cases in which the investigator cannot measure the variable but can judge the patients' order, ranking is the only data form available. An example would be triaging the treatment order of injured patients following a disaster or military battle. Second, where the distances between adjacent continuous data are very disparate or carry disparate clinical implications, ranking forces equal distances. An example would be platelet counts in thrombocytopenia; the clinical implication of a difference from 20,000 to 80,000 is far different from that of 220,000 to 280,000. The continuous data average of counts of 30,000, 90,000, and 400,000 for three patients is 170,000, implying that the group is healthy. Ranking of the patients 1, 2, 3 removes the misinformation arising from the first minus second difference being 70,000 and the second minus third difference being 310,000. When continuous data are ranked, ties are given the average of the ranks they would have had had they not been tied. For example, let us rank the first eight pre-operative (pre-op)

plasma silicone levels of DB5, smallest to largest. The ranks would be as follows: 1st, 0.13; 2nd, 0.15; 3rd, 0.18; 4th, 0.20; and 5th, 0.24. The 6th and 7th are tied, both being 0.39; their ranks would be 6.5. Last, the 8th is 0.42. It is important to note that ranking retains some, but not all, of the information of continuous data.

(3) *Categorical* data are indicators of type or category and may be thought of as counts. We often see 0–1 for male–female, false–true, or healthy–diseased. In such cases, the names of the categories may occur in any sequence and are not orderable; nonorderable categorical data sometimes are called *nominal* data. In Table DB1.1, the 0–1 indicators of negative–positive biopsies were categorical data; seven (a proportion of 70%) of the patients had negative biopsies and three (30%) had positive biopsies.

Distinguishing between Types

Sometimes categories fall into a natural order and the distinction between ranked and categorical data is not obvious. PSA values are continuous data. Of course, they may also be ranked: smallest, next smallest, . . . , largest. If PSA is categorized into three groups, <4, 4–10, and >10, the values are still ordered, but we have lost a lot of information. There are so many ties that analysis methods will be sensitive only to three ranks, one for each category. Although we could analyze them as categories A, B, and C, the methods treating them as ranks first, second, and third are still "stronger" methods. When rendering data into categories, one should note whether the categories fall into a natural order. If they do, treat them as ranks. For example, categories of ethnic groups do not fall into a natural order, but the pain categories severe, moderate, small, and absent do.

Note that we can always change data from higher to lower type, that is, continuous to discrete to ranked to categorical, but not the other way. Thus, it is *always preferable to record data as high up on this sequence as possible*; it can always be dropped lower.

Rounding, most often a rather benign convenience, can at times change data type. The continuous observations $\frac{1}{3}$ and $\frac{2}{3}$, if rounded to two decimal places, would become 0.33 and 0.67, now discrete observations. If rounded to integers, they would become 0 and 1, which might be taken as categorical data. We should carry full accuracy in calculations and then round to the accuracy that has clinical relevance. For example, if four readings of intraocular pressure (by an applanation tonometer) were 15.96, 17.32, 22.61, and 19.87, the mean would be 18.94. In clinical use, the portion after the decimal is not used and would only add distracting detail, so the mean would be reported as 19.

Ratings form a class of data all their own, in that they may be any type. There is a great deal of confusion between ratings and rankings in medical literature, even in some published textbooks on biostatistics, and the user must be careful to distinguish between them. In contrast to ranks, which are judgments about one patient or event relative to others, ratings are judgments about a patient or event on that patient's own merits alone, irrespective of others, as in the rating of a tumor as one of four cancer stages. In contrast to ranks, which should all be different except perhaps for occasional ties, ratings quite properly could be all the same. Ratings behave like continuous data if there are many categories and may be analyzed as such if the samples are of fair size. Ratings behave like categorical data if there are few categories. Regardless of the number of categories, ratings may be ranked and rank methods used, but usually there are so many ties as to weaken rank methods.

String (or Alphabetic) Data

This section has addressed quantitative data. In some cases, verbal data, called "strings" in computer terminology, can be analyzed statistically, but require analyses more complicated than are appropriate for this text.

1.4. NOTATION (OR SYMBOLS)

(Any reader at ease with formulas and symbols, for example Σ, may well omit this section.)

Purpose of Symbols

Many people have some difficulty with mathematical symbols. They are, after all, a cross between shorthand and a foreign language. They are awkward to use at first, because users must translate before they get a "gut feel" for the significance of the symbols. After some use, a μ or an s^2 takes on an intuitive meaning to the user and the awkwardness fades. Indeed, symbols are intended to avoid awkwardness, not create it. If we were to write out concepts and their relationships in words, we soon would be so overcome by the verbosity that we would lose track of what we were trying to do.

Categories of Symbols

Most symbols arise from one of three categories: names, operators, or relationships.

(1) *Name symbols*, like x or μ, may be thought of as families. x may denote prostate volume measures all taken together as a family; x is the "family name." μ

may denote the mean prostate volume for a population of men. If we need to refer to members of the family, we can affix a "first name" to the family name, usually (but not always) in the form of a *subscript*. x_1 is the name of the first prostate volume listed, x_2 the second, etc. μ_1 may denote the mean of the population of American men, μ_2 that of Japanese men, etc. If we think of name symbols in this fashion, y_7 denoting the seventh member of the y family, the mystique of symbols reduces. Most symbols are name symbols.

(2) *Operator* (or *command*) *symbols* represent an act rather than a thing. There are not very many. Operator symbols, like $\div$ or Σ, say "do this thing." $\div$ says "divide the quantity before me by the quantity after me." Σ says "add together all members of the family that follow me." There is no indicator of which symbols are name and which are operator, in the same way that there is none in grammar that distinguishes nouns from verbs. They become clear by context after a bit of use.

(3) *Relationship symbols*, such as $=$ or $>$, express some relation between two families or two members of a family. We are all familiar with statements such as $2 + 2 = 4$ or $6 > 5$. 2, 4, 5, and 6 are name symbols for members of the family of integers, $+$ is an operator symbol, and $=$ and $>$ are relationship symbols.

Formulas

Putting these ideas together, we can see the meaning of the "formula" for a sample mean, in which we add together all n values of observations named x in the sample and divide by n: $(\Sigma x)/n$. The operator symbol Σ says "add together what follows." The name symbol of what follows is x, the members of the sample of prostate volumes. Thus, we add together all the members of the sample, that is, all prostate volumes. The parentheses say "we do what is indicated within before taking the next action." The operator symbol / (or $\div$) says "we divide what comes before (Σx) by what comes after (n)."

Becoming Familiar with Symbols

The foregoing statement is a tortuously long expression of a simple idea. However, the user having difficulty with symbols and formulas who goes through such a mental process on each formula for *only a few times* will soon find that formulas become a natural way to express relationships much more easily than trying to put them into words. The advantage of symbols over words increases as the relationship becomes more complicated.

Our First Formula

Now we can express symbolically the definition of a mean m: $m = (\Sigma x)/n$.

Indicator Symbols

If we want to indicate a member of a family, but not which member at the moment, we can use what might be called an *indicator symbol*. Any symbol can be used to indicate, but the most common ones in statistics are i, j, and k. If $x_1, x_2, \ldots, x_5$ are the members of the x family of prostate volumes put in order from smallest to largest, we can say $x_i < x_{i+1}$, which is shorthand for the following relationship: any member of the x family (any prostate volume) is smaller than the member (volume) to its right.

Symbols for Ranks

We need a way to differentiate ranked data from unranked. In Table DB1.1, x_1 was 32.3; when ranked, the first x is 16.2, the old x_3. A prime ($'$) is a common way to indicate an observation after it has been ranked. Thus, x'_1 would be the smallest, x'_2 the next to smallest, and x'_n the largest. In Table DB1.1, the first three volumes are $x_1 = 32.3$, $x_2 = 27.0$, and $x_3 = 16.2$. If we ranked the 10 values from smallest to largest, we would have $x'_1 = 16.2$, $x'_2 = 16.4$, and $x'_3 = 27.0$.

1.5. SAMPLES, POPULATIONS, AND RANDOMNESS

Samples and Populations

By the word *population*, we denote the entire set of subjects about whom we want information. If we were to take our measurements on all patients in the population, descriptive statistics would give us exact information about the population and our analysis would be finished. As this generally is not possible, we gather information on a portion of the population, known as a *sample*. We use descriptive statistics from the sample to *estimate* the characteristics of the population, and we generalize conclusions about the population on the basis of the sample, a process known as *statistical inference*.

Example

As an example, patients in a hospital would constitute the entire population for a study of infection control in that hospital. However, for a study of infected patients in the nation's hospitals, the same group of patients would be but a tiny sample. The same group can be a sample for one question about its characteristics and a population for another question.

Representativeness and Bias

To make a dependable generalization about certain characteristics, the sample must *represent* the population in those characteristics. For example, men tend to be heavier than women because they tend to be bigger. We could be led into making wrong decisions on the basis of weight if we generalized about people from a sample containing only men. We would say this sample is *biased*. To avoid bias, our sample should contain the same proportion of men as the human population contains men.

A Pictorial Example

Let us, for a moment, take the patients in a certain hospital as the population. Suppose we have 250 inpatients during an influenza epidemic. We measure the white blood count (WBC in 10^9) of all inpatients and note which arose from 30 patients in the infectious disease wards. Figure 1.1 shows the frequencies of WBCs for the hospital with those from the infectious disease wards shown darker. It is clear that the distribution of readings from the infectious disease wards, i.e., the sample, is biased and does not represent the distribution for the population, i.e., the entire hospital. If we needed to learn about the characteristics of white counts in this hospital, we should insure a representative sample.

Increasing Representativeness by Random Samples

The attempt to ensure representative samples is a study in itself. One important approach is to choose the sample randomly. A *random sample* is a *sample of elements chosen such that any member of the population is as likely to be drawn as any other*. A sample is not random if we have any advance knowledge at all of what value an element will have. If the effectiveness of two drugs is being compared, the drug allocated to give to the next arriving patient should be chosen

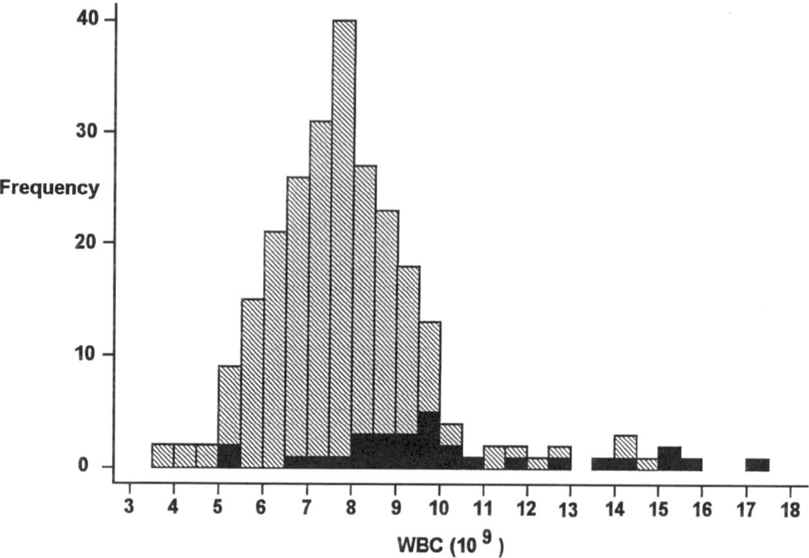

Figure 1.1 Distribution of WBC readings from a 250-inpatient hospital showing an unrepresentative sample from the 30-patient infectious disease wards (black).

by chance alone, perhaps by the roll of a die or flip of a coin or perhaps by using a table of random numbers or a computer-generated random number.

Convergence with Sample Size

Another requirement for a dependable generalization about certain characteristics is that the sample must *converge* to the population in the relevant characteristics. Suppose for a moment we thought of our 301 prostate patients as a population. From the data of DB1, we can see that mean PSA is about 8.8, but the mean of the first 10 is about 6.8. Table 1.1 shows the mean PSA as the sample size increases. The mean of the first 10 readings is below the overall mean. By 50 readings, it has risen and continues to rise until 100, after which it drops, approaching closer and closer to the overall mean. We notice that the pattern of sample values gets closer in nature to the pattern of population values as the sample size gets closer to the population size.

Now think of populations of any size. At some point, enough data are accumulated that the pattern of sample values differs from the pattern of population values only negligibly, and we can treat the results as if they had come from the population; the sample is said to converge to the population. Say the population on

Table 1.1

Mean PSA and Its Difference from the Group Mean as Sample Size Grows

Sample size	Mean PSA level	Deviation from group mean
Entire group = 301	8.8	–
10	6.8	−2.0
50	10.7	1.9
100	11.7	2.9
150	10.0	1.2
200	9.5	0.7
250	9.4	0.6
260	9.2	0.4
280	9.0	0.2
290	8.9	0.1

which we are measuring PSA representatively is the population of American men. As the (random) sample grows to hundreds and then to thousands, the pattern of PSA values in the sample will differ very little from that of the population.

Methods of Sampling

Methods of sampling are myriad, but most relate to unusual designs, such as complicated mixtures of variables or designs with missing data. Four of the most basic methods, used with rather ordinary designs, are sketched here.

Simple Random Sampling

If a sample is drawn from the entire population so that any member of the population is as likely to be drawn as any other, that is, drawn at random, the sampling scheme is termed simple random sampling. This form of sampling was introduced earlier.

Systematic Sampling

Sometimes we are not confident that the members sampled will be drawn truly equilikely. We need to sophisticate our sampling scheme to reduce the risk of bias. In some cases, we may draw a sample of size n by dividing the population into k equal portions and drawing n/k members equilikely from each division. For example, suppose we want 50 measurements of the heart's electrical conductivity amplitude over a 10-sec period, where recordings are available each millisecond (msec).

We could divide the 10,000 msec into 50 equal segments of 200 msec each and sample one member equilikely from each segment. This scheme is termed systematic sampling.

Caution

The term systematic sampling sometimes is used to refer to sampling at equal intervals, as every third patient. In this case, the position of the patient chosen in each portion is fixed rather than random. For example, the third, sixth, etc. patients would be chosen rather than one equilikely from the first triplet, another equilikely from the second triplet, etc. This is not true systematic sampling and may very well introduce bias.

Stratified Sampling

Suppose a cusp exists (sharp peak), say 100 msec in duration, occurring with each of 12 heart beats, and it is essential to obtain samples from the cusp area. The investigator could divide the region into the 1200 msec of cusp and 8800 msec of noncusp, drawing 12% of his members from the first portion and 88% from the second. Division of the population into not-necessarily-equal subpopulations and sampling proportionally and equilikely from each is termed stratified sampling. As another example, consider a sports medicine sample of size 50 from Olympic contenders where sex, an influential variable, is split 80% male to 20% female. We would select 40 sample members randomly from males and 10 randomly from females.

Cluster Sampling

A compromise with sampling costs, sometimes useful in epidemiology, is *cluster sampling*. In this case, larger components of the population are chosen equilikely (e.g., a family, a hospital ward), and then every member of each component is sampled. A larger sample to offset the reduced accuracy usually is required.

Bias Is Not Unusual

Whereas true randomness is a sampling goal, too often it is not achievable. In the spirit of "some information is better than none," many studies are carried out on convenience samples, which include biases of one sort or another. These studies cannot be considered conclusive and must be interpreted in the spirit in which they were sampled.

Sources of Bias

The sources of bias in a study are myriad and no list of possible biases can be complete. Some of the more common sampling biases to be alert to are given in the following list. In the end, only experience and clear thought, subjected when possible to the judgment of colleagues, can provide adequate freedom from bias.

(a) *Bias due to method of selection*. Included would be, for example, patients referred from primary health care sources, advertising for patients (biased by patient awareness or interest), patients who gravitate to care facilities that have certain reputations, and assignment to clinical procedures according to therapy risks.

(b) *Bias due to membership* in certain groups. Included would be, for example, patients in a certain geographical region, in certain cultural groups, in certain economic groups, in certain job-category groups, and in certain age groups.

(c) *Bias due to missing data*. Included would be patients whose data are missing due to, for example, dropping out of the study because they got well or nonresponding to a survey because they were too ill, too busy, or illiterate.

(d) *State-of-health bias* (Berkson's bias). Included would be patients selected from a biased pool, i.e., people with atypical health.

(e) *Prevalence–incidence bias* (Neyman's bias). Included would be patients selected from a short subperiod for having a disease with an irregular pattern of occurrence.

(f) *Comorbidity bias*. Included would be patients selected for study who have concurrent diseases affecting their health.

(g) *Reporting bias*. Some socially unacceptable diseases are under-reported.

1.6. SCIENTIFIC DESIGN OF MEDICAL STUDIES

Steps in Study Design

Our goal is to conduct a valid investigation that adds knowledge to the field of medicine. The design of such investigations sometimes appears involved, even approaching the arcane. However, most design problems can be avoided by rigorous adherence to the principle of scientific inference coupled with good clear thinking. Many of the ideas of scientific inference have been met in this chapter and are supplemented in Sections 2.7, 5.1, and 5.2. The basic trick is to sample without bias.

(1) We specify, clearly and unequivocally, a question to be answered about an explicitly defined population.
(2) We identify a measurable variable capable of answering the question.

(3) We obtain observations on this variable from a sample that represents the population.
(4) We analyze the data with methods that provide an answer to the question.
(5) We generalize this answer to the population, limiting the generalization by the measured probability of being correct.
(6) As evidence accrues from similar investigations, confidence in the correctness of the answer increases.

Experimental Design Can Reduce Bias

The crucial step giving rise to most of the design aspects lies in the phrase "a sample that represents the population." Sampling bias can arise in many ways. Clear thinking about this step avoids most of the problems. Let us consider some common design characteristics that can diminish biases. The terms used here appear in the most common usage, although nuances occur and different investigators sometimes use the terms slightly differently. The reader–investigator should identify just what is meant when such a term is encountered.

Control Group and Placebo

One mode of reducing bias is to include a control group, which is a group having all the characteristics of the experimental group except the treatment under study. For example, in an animal experiment on the removal of a generated tumor, the control animals would be surgically opened and closed without removing the tumor, so that the surgery itself will not influence the effect of the tumor becoming absent. In the case of a drug efficacy study, a control group may be provided by introducing a *placebo*, a capsule identical to that being given the experimental group except lacking the drug being studied.

A *variable* is just a term for an observation or reading giving information on the study question to be answered. Blood pressure is a variable giving information on hypertension. Blood uric acid is a variable giving information on gout. The term variable may also refer to the symbol denoting this observation or reading.

In designing a study, it is essential to differentiate between independent and dependent variables. Let us define these terms.

Independent versus Dependent Variables

An *independent* variable is a variable that, for the purposes of the study question to be answered, occurs independently of other influences. A *dependent* variable is a variable that depends on, or more exactly is influenced by, the independent variable. In a study on gout, we ask whether blood uric acid is a factor in causing pain. We record blood uric acid as a measurable variable that occurs in the patient. Then we record pain as reported by the patient. We believe that blood uric acid is predictive of pain. In this relationship, the blood uric acid is the independent variable and pain is the dependent variable.

A *registry* is an accumulation of data from an uncontrolled sample. It usually is not considered to be a "study." It may start with data from past files or with newly gathered data. It is useful in planning a formal study to get a rough idea of the nature of the data: typical values to be encountered, the most effective variables to measure, the problems in sampling that may be encountered, and the sample sizes required. It does not, however, provide definitive answers, as it is subject to many forms of bias. The very fact of needing information about the nature of the data and about sampling problems implies the inability to assure freedom from unrepresentative sampling and unwanted influences on the question being posed.

A *case–control study* is a study in which an experimental group of patients is chosen for being characterized by some outcome factor, such as having acquired a disease, and a control group lacking the factor is matched patient-for-patient. Control is exerted over the selection of cases but not over the acquisition of data within these cases. Sampling bias is reduced by choosing sample cases using factors that are independent of the factors influencing the variables under study. It still lacks evidence that chance alone selects the patients and, therefore, lacks assurance that the sample properly represents the population. There still is no control over how the data were acquired and how carefully recorded. Often, but not always, a case–control study is based on prior records and therefore sometimes is loosely termed a *retrospective study*. (With proper design and given the right records, it is possible for a study based on records to be prospective.) Case–control studies are useful in situations in which the outcomes being studied have a very small incidence, which would require a vast sample, are very long developing, which would require a prohibitively long time to gain a study result; or cannot be conducted for ethical reasons.

A *cohort study* starts by choosing groups that have already been assigned to study categories, such as diseases or treatments, and follows these groups forward in time to assess the outcomes. To try to insure that the groups arose from the same population and differ only in the study category, their characteristics, both medical and demographic, must be recorded and compared. This type of study is risky, because only the judgment of what characteristics are included guards against the influence of spurious causal factors. Cohort studies are useful in situations in which the proportion in one of the study categories (not in an outcome as in the case–control study) is small, which would require a prohibitively large sample size.

Cohort contrasted with case–control studies. The key determinant is the sequence of the risk factor (or characteristic) to the disease (or condition). In a cohort study, experimental subjects are selected for the risk factor and are examined (followed) for the disease; in a case–control study, experimental subjects are selected for the disease and are examined for the risk factor.

Clinical trials; prospective study, blinding. The soundest type of study is the *randomized controlled trial* (or RCT), often called a *clinical trial*. An RCT is a true experiment in which patients are assigned randomly to a study category, such as clinical treatment, and are then followed forward in time (making it a *prospective study*) and the outcome assessed. (A fine distinction is that, in occasional situations, the data can have been previously recorded, and it is the selection of the existing record that is prospective rather than the selection of the not-yet-measured patient.) An RCT is *randomized*, meaning that the sample members are allocated to treatment groups by chance alone, so that the choice reduces the risk of possibly biasing factors. In a randomized study, the probability of influence by unanticipated biases diminishes as the sample size grows larger. An RCT should be *masked* or *blinded* when practical, meaning that the humans involved in the study do not know the allocation of the sample members, so they cannot influence measurements. Thus, the investigator cannot judge greater improvement in a patient receiving the treatment that the investigator prefers. Often both the investigator and the patient are able to influence measurements, in which case both might be masked; such a study is termed *double-masked* or *double-blinded*.

Paired designs. Some studies permit a design in which the patients serve as their own controls, as in a "before-and-after" study or a comparison of two treatments in which the patient receives both in sequence. For example, to test the efficacy of drugs A and B to reduce intraocular pressure, each patient may be given one for a period of time and then (after a "washout" period) the other. A *crossover* design would give half the patients drug A followed by B and the other half B followed by A, so that any effect of the first treatment carrying over into the second does not contaminate the contrast between A and B.

CHAPTER EXERCISES

1.1. Give an example of a question from DB1 whose answer would fall into (a) the description stage, (b) the explanation stage, and (c) the prediction stage.

1.2. Into what Phase type would the question of drug effectiveness based on DB2 data fall?

1.3. How could the variable sex in DB3 be quantified?

1.4. For the platelet counts of DB9, "normal" often is taken as lying in the range

150,000–400,000. How accurately should platelet counts be recorded to avoid interfering with clinical decisions?

1.5. In the femoral neck fracture database (DB7), which variables are (a) categorical and (b) continuous? (c) Can bone density be ranked?

1.6. Which database contains ratings that could be treated as categorical, ranked, or continuous data?

1.7. In DB6, to what population would the dermatologist like to generalize results? From the information given, would such generalization be justified?

1.8. Is the study represented by DB6 an RCT? Why or why not?

Chapter 2

Distributions

2.1. FREQUENCY DISTRIBUTIONS

The frequency distribution is a concept through which most of the essential elements of medical statistics can be accessed. It is nothing more than the way the data are distributed along the scale (or axis) of the variable of interest. Let us look at the prostate volumes in Table DB1.1. The variable of interest is volume in milliliters (ml). We scan the (entire set of) data to ascertain the range of volumes, which extends from about 3 to about 114 ml. We list 5-ml intervals (choosing intervals is discussed later), starting with 0 to <5 (expressed this way to indicate "up to but not including 5" and done to avoid a possible overlap) and ending with 110 to <115. We go through the data sequentially, making a tick mark for each datum. A space or a crossover or some other indicator might be placed every five tick marks to facilitate counting. Such a tally sheet for the 10 data from Table DB1.1 is shown as Fig. 2.1A. If we rotate Fig. 2.1A one-quarter turn counterclockwise and enclose the tick marks in boxes, towers or bars are formed, as shown in Fig. 2.1B. Continuing this procedure for the first 50 data, we produce Fig 2.1C. The pattern of the distribution is beginning to emerge. Figure 2.1D represents the distribution of 100 data, Fig. 2.1E that for 200, and Fig. 2.1F that for all 301 data. Figure 2.1F is the frequency distribution for the volume data.

FREQUENCIES EXPRESSED AS A BAR CHART

A certain number of values has fallen into each defined interval or bin. This is the *frequency* for that bin. There are 40 patients with volumes between 20 and 25 ml.

Bins may be combined: the frequency for volumes less than 30 ml is 122. This type of chart, representing frequencies by the heights of bars, is called a *bar chart*.

Relative Frequencies

The frequency itself does not always tell us what we want to know. Often of more interest is the *relative frequency*, which is the proportion of the sample in a bin. The proportion of patients with volumes between 20 and 25 is $40/301 = 0.133$. The proportion of patients with volumes less than 30 is $122/301 = 0.405$. We have

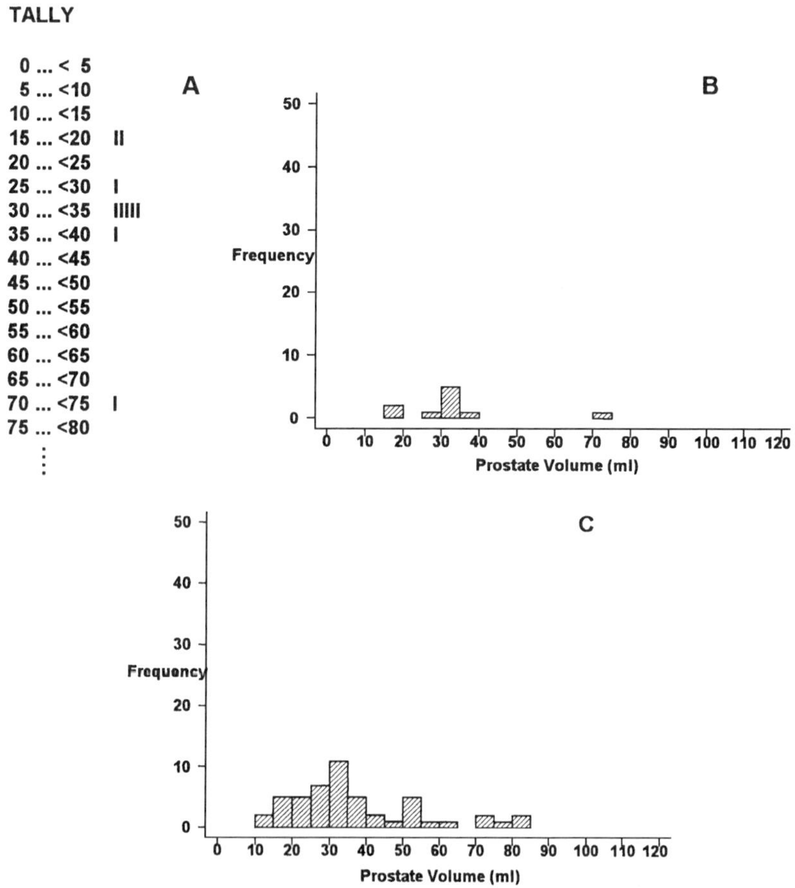

Figure 2.1 Evolution of a bar chart showing the frequency distribution of prostate volume on 301 patients: (A) tally; (B) first 10 data; (C) 50 data; (D) 100 data; (E) 200 data; and (F) 301 data.

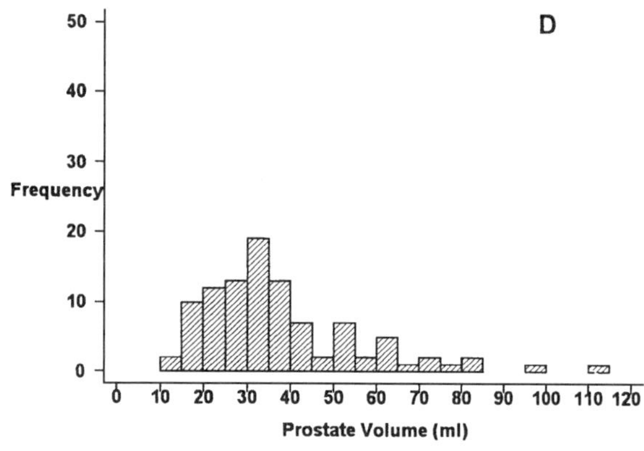

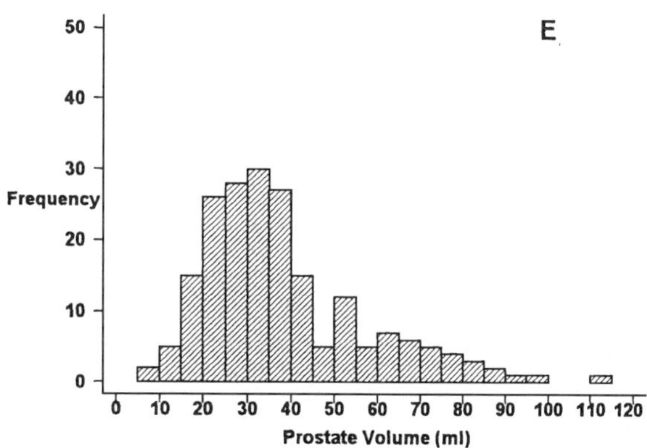

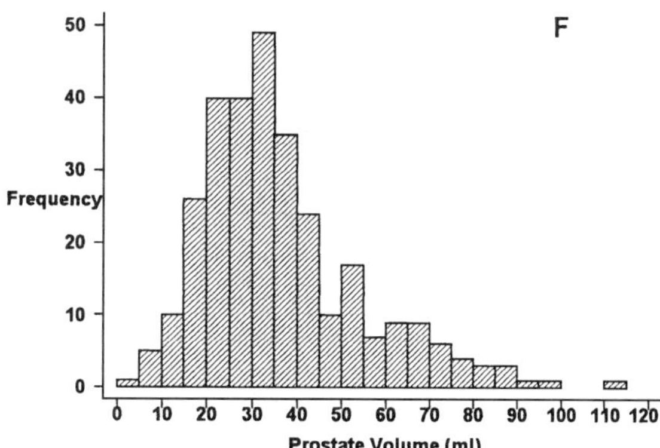

Figure 2.1 *(Continued)*

been trained by news reports and such sources to think in terms of parts per hundred, or *percent*, the proportion multiplied by 100. In the preceding sample, 40.5% of the prostate volumes are less than 30 ml.

EFFECT OF INCREASING SAMPLE SIZE

We can observe an interesting phenomenon by comparing Figs. 2.1B–F. The distribution patterns are rather different for the earlier figures, but become increasingly stable as we add more and more data. The *increasing stability of statistical behavior with increasing sample size* is a very important property of sampling, about which more will be seen later.

Example

Consider the PSA data of Table DB1.1 as a sample. What is the range, i.e., largest minus smallest values? The smallest value is 4.1 and the largest 9.0. The range is $9.0 - 4.1 = 4.9$. What intervals should we choose for a tally? With only 10 observations, a small number of intervals is appropriate. Interval widths easy to plot and easy to interpret are sensible, such as a width of 1.0 here. With a range of about 5, we are led to five intervals. If we had had a large number of data, we might have chosen 10 or even 15 intervals. Our intervals become >4 to 5, >5 to 6, . . . , >8 to 9. The reader can construct the tally and the bar chart.

2.2. RELATIVE FREQUENCIES AND PROBABILITIES

FREQUENCY DISTRIBUTION VERSUS PROBABILITY DISTRIBUTION

Suppose a prostate volume ≥65 ml is taken as suggestive of benign prostatic hypertrophy (BPH). From our sample of 301 prostates, 28 readings equal or exceed 65 ml; the proportion $28/301 = 0.093$ shows evidence of BPH. This is the *relative frequency* of BPH suspects in our sample. If r patients out of n show a certain characteristic, r/n is the relative frequency of that characteristic. However, we are less interested in the characteristics of the sample of older male patients at our hospital than those of the population of older male patients in America: we want to know what proportion of the population is suspect for BPH. If we could measure the prostate volume of every older male in America, we would be able to find the frequency distribution for the population, which we would name the *probability distribution*. We could then find the *probability* that any randomly chosen older male in America shows indications of BPH. This probability would be represented as the area under the probability distribution ≥65 ml divided by the total area. This calculation is similar to measuring the area under the bars in the sample distribution $\geq$65 ml and dividing by the area under all the bars, yielding 9.3%.

Estimated Probability; the Term "Parameter"

Because we cannot measure prostate volume for the entire population, we use what information we can obtain from the sample. The 9.3% relative frequency does not tell us the exact probability of equaling or exceeding 65 ml in the population, but it *estimates* this probability. If we took a similar sample from another hospital, the relative frequency of that sample would be different, but we would expect it to be somewhere in the same vicinity. The term *parameter* is used to distinguish an unchanging characteristic of a population from an equivalent characteristic of a sample, an estimate of this parameter, which varies from sample to sample. How well does the estimate approximate the parameter? We are able to measure the confidence in this estimate by methods to be discussed later.

2.3. CHARACTERISTICS OF A DISTRIBUTION

The fundamental piece of statistical information is the distribution of data, as it contains all the information we need for our statistical methods. From distributions, we can learn what sample proportion of individuals falls in an interval of interest, or the population probability of a randomly chosen individual falling in that interval. We can learn what is typical or characteristic of a distribution and how closely the distribution clusters about this typical value. We can learn about the regularity or "bumpiness" of a distribution and about its symmetry. We can learn about classes or types of distributions. In the next few sections, these characteristics of distributions are addressed conceptually; formulas are given in Chapter 3 on summary statistics.

2.4. WHAT IS TYPICAL

Averages

If we could have only one quantity to give us information about a distribution, it would be the typical, central, or "average" value. There are several averages, three of which will be mentioned here.

The *mean* is the average used most often. The population mean is denoted μ, and we will denote the sample mean m for reasons explained in the next section, although some books denote it by the letter representing the variable being averaged with a bar over it. To obtain the sample mean, we add all values and divide by the number of observations added. The mean prostate volume from Table DB1.1 is 32.73 ml. The mean of a probability distribution is the "center of gravity" of that distribution. If the picture of the distribution were cut from a material of uniform density, say wood, the mean would be the position on the horizontal axis at which the distribution would balance. Thus, values far from the center carry more influence, or "moment," than values near the center.

If we are sampling from two populations, say x and y, we can use subscripts, which as previously mentioned is the "member-of-the-family" indicator, to keep them straight, such as μ_x and μ_y for the population means, respectively, and m_x and m_y for the sample means, respectively.

The *median* of a sample is the position on the horizontal axis at which one-half the observations fall on either side. If we order the prostate volumes in Table DB1.1, that is, put them in increasing sequence, the median would be the midpoint between the fifth and sixth volumes. The fifth is 30.5 ml and the sixth is 30.9 ml, so that the median is 30.7 ml. For a distribution with some extreme observations, e.g., income of HMO executives in the distribution of HMO employee incomes or unusually long-lived patients in the distribution of survival times of cancer patients, the median is a better descriptor of the typical than is the mean. For a probability distribution, the population median is the position on the horizontal axis at which one-half the area under the curve falls on either side.

The *mode* of a sample is the most frequently occurring value, which is the position on the horizontal axis centered under the tallest bar. The mode of the prostate volumes in Table DB1.1 can be seen in Fig. 2.1B as 32.5 ml. The mode is not very dependable for small samples and should be used only for large samples. The position of the mode depends on the bar width and starting position. Also, the mode is not necessarily unique. An example of a distribution with two modes might be the heights of a mixed sample of men and women, because men tend to be taller on average than women. For a probability distribution, the mode is the horizontal axis value under the highest point on the curve. For a multimodal probability distribution, the position of each height on the curve having a lesser height to both left and right is a mode.

Convergence with Increasing Sample Size

In Section 2.1, the increasing stability of a sample with increasing sample size was mentioned. The mean of a sample gets closer to, that is, it *converges on*, the population mean as the sample size grows larger. This property is known as the Weak Law of Large Numbers or as the Bienaymé–Tchebycheff inequality (also Tchebycheff alone, and using various spellings). Although we need not remember the name, this relationship is essential to expressing confidence in our sample estimates of population means and to finding the sample size required for studies and experiments. To illustrate this convergence, mean prostate volumes were calculated for the first 5 and then the first 10, 15, 20, and 30 patients as estimates of the mean of all 301 patients. Figure 2.2 shows the convergence of these means on the 36.47-ml overall mean as sample size increases. Estimates are under, under, over, under, and under, respectively, but the size of error diminishes with each sample size increase.

2.5. THE SPREAD ABOUT THE TYPICAL

Types of Spread Indicators

After we know the typical value of a distribution, naturally it follows to want to know how closely the values cluster about this average. The *range* (highest minus lowest values) gives us a hint, but it uses the information from only two of our observations, and those are the two most unstable values in the sample. As with the average, there are different measures of variability, but the variance and its square root, the standard deviation, are used primarily.

The *variance* of a set of values is the *average of squared deviations from the mean.* Just for computational illustration, consider a population composed of the

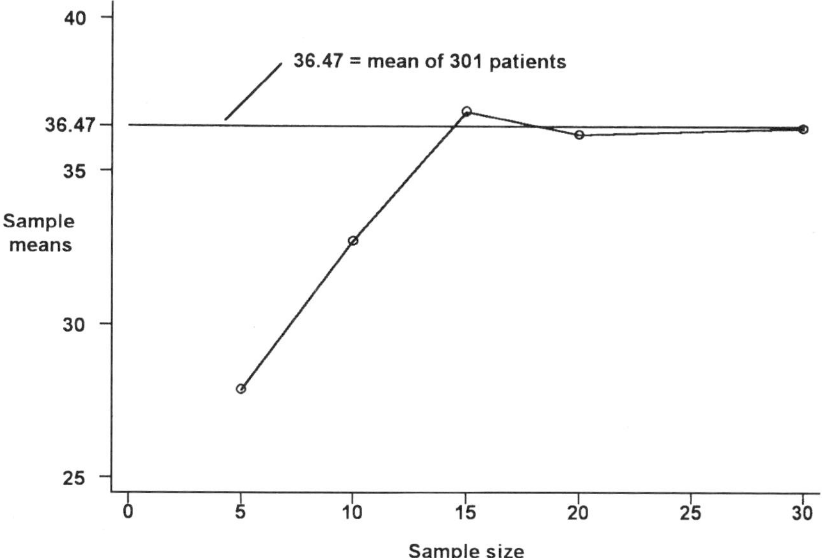

Figure 2.2 Sample prostate volume means of the first 5, 10, 15, 20, and 30 patients seen (they are listed in the order they presented) can be seen to converge on the 36.47-ml mean of all 301 patients as the sample size increases.

values 1, 2, and 3, which have the mean 2. First, the mean is subtracted from each observation and each difference is squared, yielding $(1-2)^2$, $(2-2)^2$, and $(3-2)^2$. The squaring makes all values positive so that they do not cancel each other out, and it allows the more deviant observations to carry more weight. Then these squared differences are averaged, that is, added and divided by their number, resulting in the population variance: $(1+0+1)/3 = 0.666\ldots$. The population variance is denoted σ^2. A sample variance, commonly denoted s^2, is calculated in the same way if μ is known. However, if μ is estimated by m, it has been found that the divisor must be the sample size less one (as $n-1$) in order to converge on the population variance properly.

The standard deviation is the square root of the variance, denoted by σ for populations and s for samples. The variance often is used in statistical methods because square roots are difficult to work with mathematically. On the other hand, the standard deviation usually is used in describing and interpreting results because it can represent distances along the axis of the variable of interest, whereas the variance is expressed in squared units. The meaning of squared volumes of the prostate would be somewhat obscure.

Example

Let us calculate the variance and standard deviation of prostate volumes from Table DB1.1. By using the sample mean $m = 32.73$ ml from the last section, the observations minus m are $-0.43, -5.73, \ldots, 4.07, -16.33$. Their squares are $0.1849, 32.8329, \ldots, 16.5649, 266.6689$. The sum of these squares is 2281.401. Division of the sum of squares by 9 gives the variance, often called the *mean square*, as $s^2 = 253.409$. The standard deviation is just the square root of the variance or $s = 15.92$. Engineers often call the standard deviation the *root-mean-square*, which may help keep its meaning in mind. The computation used here follows the conceptual method of calculation. A simpler computational formula, plus examples, will be given in the next chapter on summary statistics.

Greek versus Roman Letters

The beginnings of a commonly used pattern in statistics starts to emerge. It is common among statisticians to use Greek letters to represent population names and Roman letters to represent sample names. Thus, to represent a mean and variance, we use μ and σ^2 for the population and m and s^2 for the sample. Some users of statistics have not adopted this convention, but it helps keep the important distinction between population and sample straight and will be used in this text. In the author's view, the use of $\bar{x}$ to denote the mean is an inconsistent historical remnant.

2.6. THE SHAPE

A distribution may have almost any shape (provided it has areas only above the horizontal axis). Fortunately, only a few shapes are common, especially for large samples and populations where the laws of large numbers hold. Sample distributions, although different from sample to sample, often approximate probability distributions. When they do, this correspondence allows more informative conclusions about the population to be inferred from a sample.

Most Common Shapes

The two most famous distributions are the uniform and the normal curve, sometimes loosely termed a "bell" curve. The uniform distribution is an equal likelihood case, in which all events (such as choosing patients for a certain treatment in a study) have an equal chance of occurring, so that all probabilities achieve the same height on the graph of the distribution. The bell curve has a graph showing a central hump (mode) with observations tailing off symmetrically, or approximately so, on either side. The normal is a bell curve with certain additional characteristics to be noted in Section 2.8 and Chapter 4.

In describing the shape of a distribution, we look first for the number of modes and what might be called smoothness. A "well-behaved" distribution has a clearly seen mode, tails off in not too jagged a fashion on either side, and relates in a meaningful way to the variable of interest. Then we look for symmetry. If one tail is "dragged out" more than the other, we say that the distribution is *skewed* in that direction. We look for the approximate center of the distribution. In a unimodal unskewed curve, the mode, median, and mean will coincide. If it is right skewed, the median is to the right of the mode and the mean to the right of both. And finally, we look to see how much it is spread out about its center, that is, its approximate standard deviation. By examining the distribution in this fashion, we can get a much clearer picture of what forces are at work in the generation of the data than through knowing only the mean and standard deviation.

Example

Figure 2.3 shows the frequency distribution of 301 prostate volumes from Fig. 2.1F with the population probability distribution approximated by a freehand fit. We note that it is skewed to the right. In agreement with this, the mean of 36.5 ml is to the right of both the median (32.4 ml) and the mode (32.5 ml). Before seeing any data, we might have expected a symmetric distribution. Perhaps the skew arises from the presence of BPH, which causes a large increase in prostate

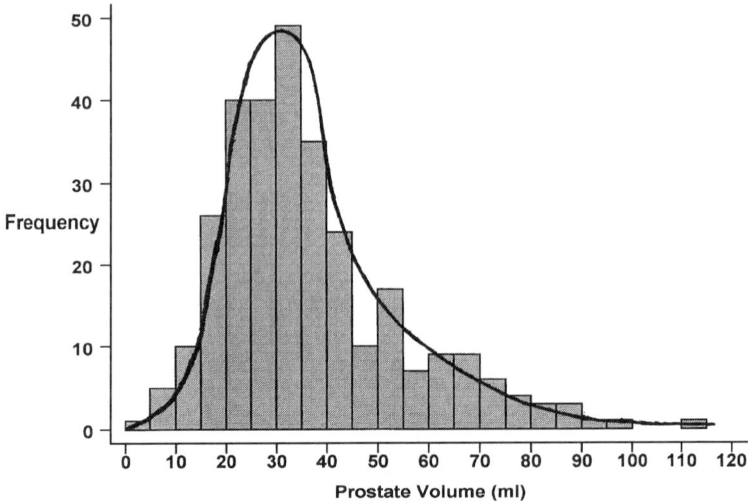

Figure 2.3 The frequency distribution of 301 prostate volumes from Fig. 2.1F, with the population probability distribution approximated by a freehand fit.

volume. The mean ± one standard deviation includes the interval on the volume scale of about 21–52 ml; probabilistic interpretations of this are better discussed later, but it seems safe to say that we would not consider a prostate volume in this interval to be clinically abnormal.

Standardizing a Distribution

Distributions come in various sizes, in particular having various scales on the variable of interest. However, the scale differences can be overcome by standardizing the distribution. A distribution is *standardized* by subtracting the mean from every observation and dividing the result by the standard deviation. This forces the distribution to have a mean of 0, a standard deviation of 1, and a scale measured in standard deviations. This transformation allows shapes of different distributions to be compared uncluttered by scale differences, and it allows a single table of areas under a curve of a particular type to be made rather than a new table for every scale. The *sample distribution* of a variable, say x, is standardized when x is transformed into y by using

$$y = \frac{x - m}{s}$$

and the *probability distribution* of x is transformed by using

$$y = \frac{x - \mu}{\sigma}$$

Probability distributions are transformed further so that their total area under the curve is always 1.

2.7. STATISTICAL INFERENCE

Making inferences about a population on the basis of a sample from that population is a major task in statistics.

INFERRING A CONFIDENCE INTERVAL

One important application of such inferences is to generate confidence intervals. Given a sample mean on some variable x, for example, what can be said about the mean of the population? m mathematically has been shown to be the best estimate of μ, but how good is it in a particular case? By following a number of steps, we can place a confidence interval about this mean to say "We are 95% confident that this interval encloses the population mean." (For medical purposes, 95% confidence is used most often, more by habit than because a 5% risk is better than some other risk. We can never be 100% sure.) This procedure *infers* that an interval is likely to contain the mean, reserving a 5% chance that it does not. This chance (5% risk of error) usually is designated as α in statistics.

INFERRING A DIFFERENCE

Another important application of inference is to make a decision about a characteristic, such as a mean, estimated from a sample relative to another such characteristic, such as either the population mean or the mean of another sample. We state that these two means are the same by means of a "null hypothesis," so termed because it postulates a null difference between the means. Then we specify the probability that this hypothesis will be wrong, i.e., the chance that we conclude that there is no difference when in fact there is. This is may be thought of as the probability of a false positive, the same α, frequently taken as 5%. Finally, by using this α, we reject or accept the null hypothesis, which is equivalent to inferring that there is or is not, respectively, a difference between the means.

Steps in Inference

In making statistical inferences about a sample estimate, we follow these steps: (1) We assume the nature of the probability distribution of this estimate on the basis of the data from which it is drawn, e.g., "The distribution of the sample mean is normal (a particular type of bell shape)." (2) We arbitrarily choose the probability, often but not necessarily 5%, that the statement to be investigated (confidence interval or null hypothesis about the relationship between this estimate and another value) is wrong. (3) We find an interval about our sample estimate on the x-axis designated by those values outside of which lies 5% (or other risk) of the area under the probability distribution (calculated or looked up in tables). (4) If we want a confidence interval, this interval is it. If we are testing a null hypothesis, we accept the hypothesis if the other value in the statement lies inside this interval and reject the hypothesis if the other value lies outside. The user can see that there is a logical relationship between confidence intervals and hypothesis testing.

The logic in the preceding paragraph does not follow the way we usually think. It will require intense concentration on first exposure. Students seldom comprehend it fully at first. Return to it repeatedly, preferably by using it when working through the methods given in later chapters, and give it time to "sink in."

One admonition should be noted. The assumption in step (1) seldom is actually stated, but it IS MADE whether explicitly or implicitly. Indeed, many statistical inferences are based on *more than one* assumption, for example, that the underlying probability distribution is normal *and* that each sample value drawn cannot be predicted by other sample values (the observations are independent).

Effect of Violated Assumptions; Robustness

What happens when an assumption is violated? The computations can be made in any case and there is no flag to alert the user to the violation. When assumptions presume characteristics of probability distributions, the areas under the curves are computed wrongly and decisions are made with erroneous confidence. For example, in finding a confidence interval, we may believe that α is 5% when in fact it is much greater or smaller. We must give careful attention to assumptions. Fortunately, the commonly used statistical methods often are *robust*, meaning that they are not very sensitive to moderate violations of assumptions.

More details on confidence intervals and hypothesis testing are given in Chapters 4 and 5, respectively, after additional foundation is provided; additional attention to assumptions appears at the end of Section 5.1.

2.8. DISTRIBUTIONS COMMONLY USED IN STATISTICS

In Section 2.1, we saw how frequency distributions arise from sample data. In Section 2.2, we saw that the population distribution, arising from sampling the entire population, becomes the probability distribution. In Section 2.7, we saw that this probability distribution is used in the process of making statistical inferences about population characteristics on the basis of sample information. There are, of course, endless types of probability distributions possible. However, luckily, the great majority of statistical methods use only six probability distributions.

The six distributions commonly used in statistics are the normal, t, χ^2 (chi-square), F, binomial, and Poisson. Continuous data depend mostly on the first four. Rank-order methods depend on distributions of ranks rather than continuous data, but several of them use the normal or chi-square. Categorical data depend mostly on the chi-square, binomial, and Poisson, with larger samples transformed to normal. We need to become familiar with only these six distributions to understand most of the methods given in this text. Figure 2.4 shows examples of these six types of distributions. The following paragraphs describe these distributions and some of their properties needed to use and interpret statistical methods.

Normal Distribution

The normal distribution, called Gaussian by some users, is the perfect case of the famous bell curve. We standardize a normal (Gaussian) variable, transforming it to z by subtracting the mean and dividing by the standard deviation, e.g.,

$$z = \frac{x - \mu}{\sigma}.$$

The normal distribution then becomes the *standard normal*, which has mean 0 and standard deviation 1. This transformation usually is made in practice as the probability tables available usually are of the standard normal curve. The statistical "normal" must not be confused with the medical "normal," meaning nonpathological.

Shorthand for the Normal

The normal distribution is used so much that a shorthand symbol is helpful. The common symbol is N for "normal," with the mean and variance (square of the standard deviation) following in parentheses. Thus, N(5,4) indicates a normal distribution with mean 5 and variance 4 (standard deviation 2). N(0,1) indicates the standard normal with mean 0 and standard deviation 1, used for normal tables.

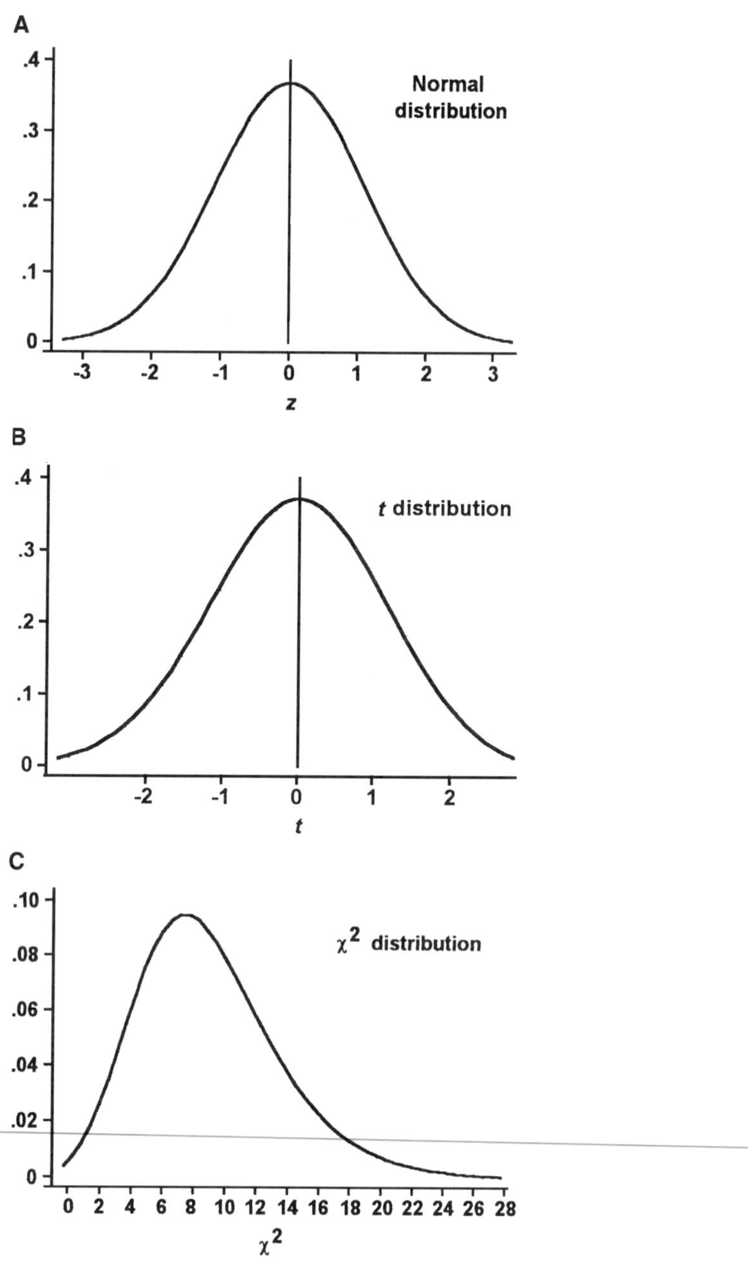

Figure 2.4 The six common probability distributions used in elementary statistical methods. The normal (A) and t (B) are used with inferences about means of continuous data, the χ^2 (C) and F (D) about standard deviations (more exactly, variances) of continuous data, and the binomial (E) about proportions of categorical data. The Poisson (F) and χ^2 are used to approximate the binomial for larger sample sizes.

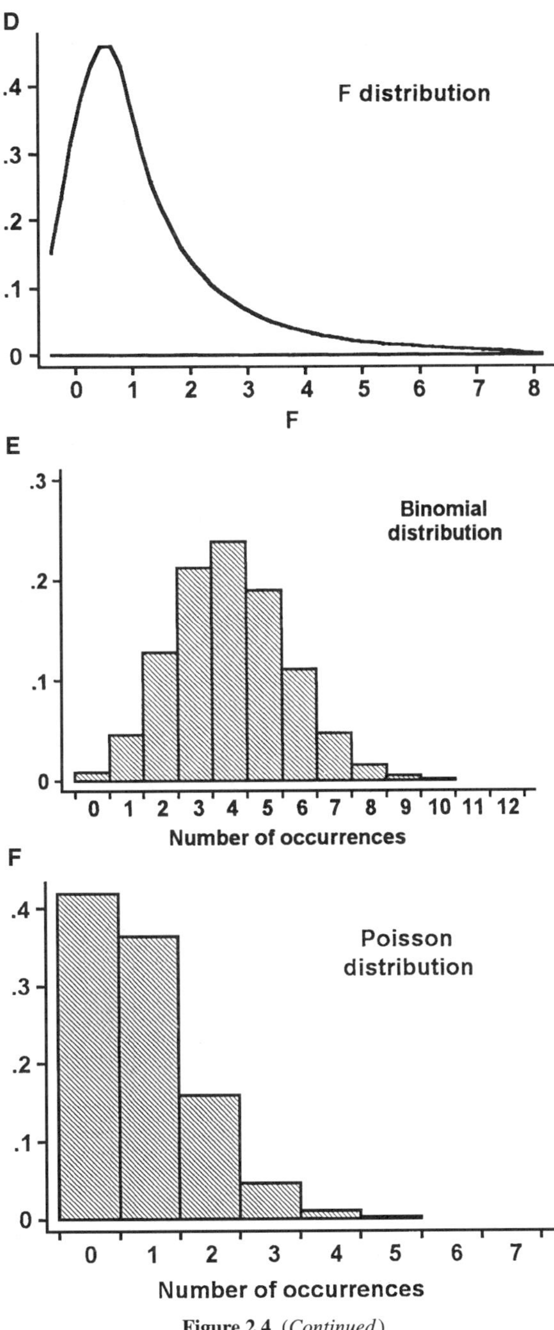

Figure 2.4 *(Continued)*

The Sample Mean Follows Its Own Probability Distribution

Very often we want to make inferences about a population mean based on a sample mean. For example, consider our prostate volume data from 301 patients. Each observation is drawn from a population that has a given probability distribution. If we wanted to make conclusions about a single patient, we would use this distribution. However, suppose we want to use the sample data to make conclusions about the average prostate volume of American men. Because the sample mean is composed of individual volume readings, each of which has a probability distribution, the sample mean also must have a probability distribution, but it will be different.

Sample Means of Continuous Data Are Distributed Normal

If the sample in question is drawn from a normal population (e.g., if prostate volumes were distributed normally), the probability distribution of the sample mean is exactly normal. If the sample is drawn from any other distribution (e.g., the prostate volumes are from a skewed distribution), the probability distribution of the sample mean is still approximately normal and converges on normal as the sample size increases. This remarkable result is due to a famous mathematical relationship, named the *Central Limit Theorem*. Because much of our attention to statistical results is focused on means, this theorem is applied frequently.

The *Central Limit Theorem* is illustrated dramatically in Fig. 2.5. We draw random samples from a far-from-normal distribution and observe how the frequency distribution of means becomes closer to normal as we take means first of 5 observations, then 10, and finally 20. Figure 2.5A shows 117 PSA readings of patients whose PSA leaves little doubt about a biopsy decision, that is, PSA < 4 (no biopsy) or PSA > 10 (definite biopsy). A normal curve with the PSA data's mean and standard deviation is superposed. Figure 2.5B shows the frequency distribution of 200 means of five observations each drawn randomly (using a computer random number generator) from the 117 PSA readings, with a normal curve superposed. Figures 2.5C and 2.5D show the same sort of display for means of samples of 10 and 20, respectively. The convergence to the normal can be seen clearly.

t Distribution

The *t* distribution answers the same sorts of questions about the mean as does the normal distribution. It arises when we must use the sample s to estimate an unknown population σ.

The Standard t

Standardization of the mean includes dividing by the standard deviation. The known σ is a constant, so that the division just changes the scale. However, when σ is unknown, which happens in most cases of clinical studies, we must divide by s. Instead of

$$z = \frac{x - \mu}{\sigma}$$

as in the normal case, we use

$$t = \frac{x - \mu}{s}.$$

s is not a constant like σ, but is composed of observations and therefore follows a probability distribution. This division introduces a new variable: one drawn from a normal distribution divided by a variable drawn from a more difficult distribution, that for the root of a sum of squares of normals. The probability distribution for this variable was published in 1908 by W. S. Gossett,[69] who named it t. (As a historical note, he published under the pseudonym "Student," because the policy of his employer, Guinness Brewery, forbade the publication.)

The t looks like the normal curve, as seen in Fig. 2.4. However, it is a little fatter because it uses s, which is less accurate than σ. Whereas the normal is a single distribution, t is a family of curves. In Fig. 2.6, two standard t distributions are superposed on a standard normal. The particular member of the t family depends on the sample size or, more exactly, on the degrees of freedom.

Degrees of Freedom

Degrees of freedom, often abbreviated *df*, is a concept that may be thought of as *that part of the sample size n not otherwise allocated*. This concept relates to quite a number of aspects of statistical methods, and so *df* may be explained in a number of ways. Some of these aspects are more difficult than others, and even experienced users find some of them very challenging. Do not expect to understand *df* fully at once. Usually comprehension starts at a rudimentary level and sophisticates slowly with use. *df* is related to the sample number, usually to the number of observations for continuous data methods and to the number of categories for categorical data methods. It will be enough for a start to conceive of *df* as such a sample number adjusted for other sources of information, more specifically, the number of unrestricted and independent data entering into a calculated statistic. In the t distribution, we might think very informally of n "pieces" of information available. Once we know m, we have $n-1$ pieces of information remaining that can be selected by the sampling procedure; when we have obtained $n-1$ observations, the nth one may be found by subtraction. (This is, of course, not how the data are obtained, but rather a more abstract mathematical allocation of information.) Because df is tied to n, the sample values converge to the population values as both n and df increase. t converges on the normal as df increases. Figure 2.6 shows the standard normal curve with two t curves superposed, one with 10 df and the other with 5 df. The fewer the df, the less accurate an estimate s is of σ, so the greater the t's standard deviation (the "fatter" the t curve).

Chi-Square (χ^2) Distribution

We often want to make inferences about a standard deviation. For computational ease, we usually make the inference about its square, the variance, because

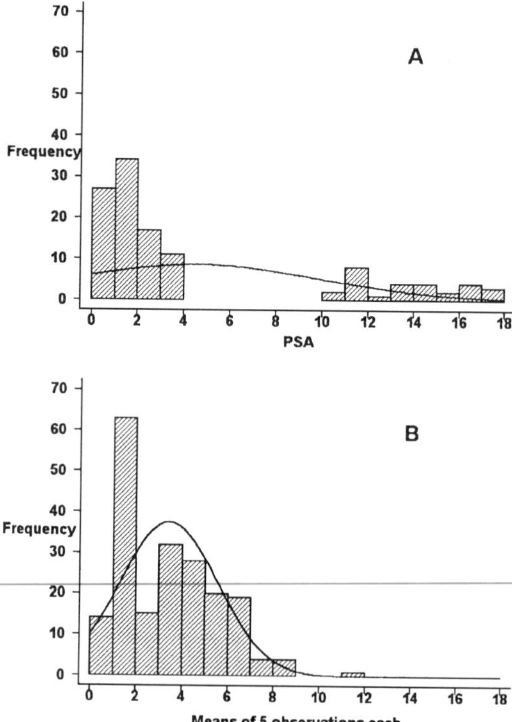

Figure 2.5 Part A shows 117 PSA readings of patients whose PSA < 4 (no biopsy) or PSA >10 (definite biopsy) (excluding a few high PSAs as BPH). Parts B–D show the frequency distribution of 200 means of 5 (B), 10 (C), and 20 (D) observations each drawn randomly from the 117 PSA readings, with a normal curve fitted to the data's mean and standard deviation for each figure. The convergence to normal can be seen clearly.

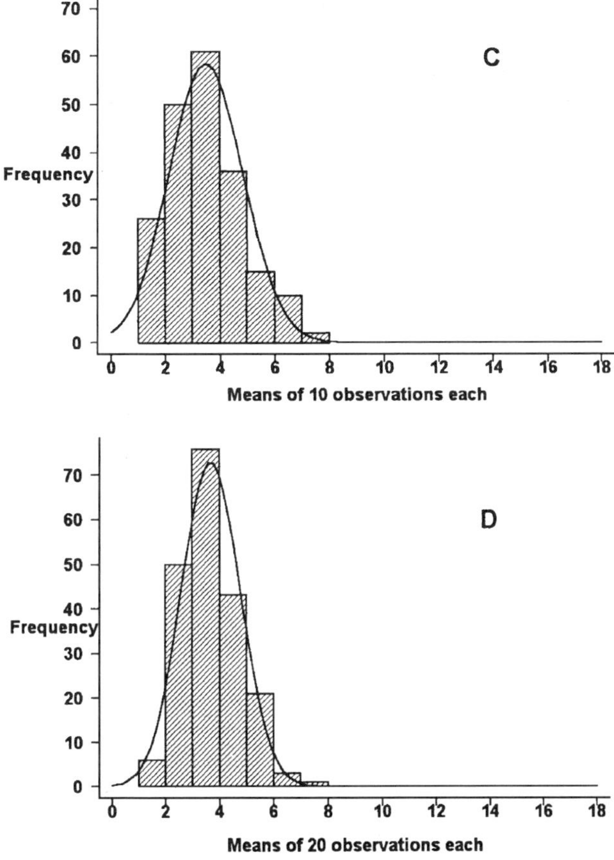

Figure 2.5 *(Continued)*

any inference about one implies the equivalent inference about the other. A variance basically is a sum of squares of values. If each comes from a normal curve, its mathematical pattern has a right-skewed shape like that in Fig. 2.4C. That distribution is called the chi-square distribution ("ch" pronounced like "k"). It is obtained by multiplying the calculated sample variance s^2 by the constant df/σ^2, where $df = n - 1$ and σ^2 is the population variance. Often the Greek symbol for chi-square is used, as χ^2. Because all elements are squares, a chi-square cannot be negative. It rises from 0 to a mode and then tails off in a skew to the right. As in the normal and the t, we use areas under the curve taken from tables or computer calculation routines to make inferences.

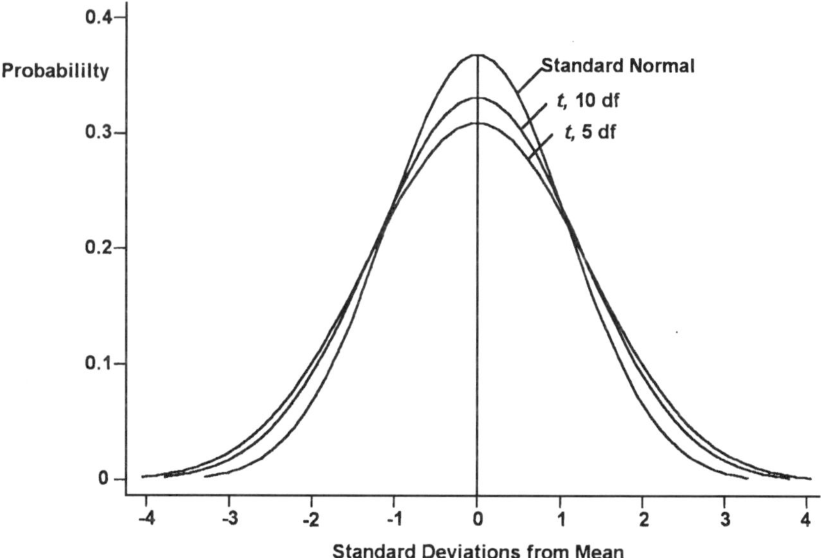

Figure 2.6 A standard normal distribution with two t distributions superposed, one for 10 *df* and one for 20 *df*. The mean of the t is the same as that of the normal. The spread of the t is larger than that of the normal, much larger for small sample sizes and converging on the normal as the sample size grows larger.

Chi-Square in a Hypothesis Test; Critical Value

As a further example of hypothesis testing, introduced in the previous section, consider the days to heal to a certain standard after a new surgical procedure compared to an older established one. Say we know the new one is slightly better on average, but could it be so much more variable as to nullify its advantage? The heal-time variance of the old procedure is known from such a large number of cases that it can be taken as having converged to the population variance σ^2. Our estimate of the heal-time variance of the new procedure from a sample of patients is s^2. We are asking whether s^2 is probably larger than σ^2. We test the null hypothesis that s^2 is no different from σ^2 by using the ratio

$$\frac{s^2 \times df}{\sigma^2},$$

which can be shown to follow the chi-square distribution. If s^2 is much greater than σ^2, the ratio will be large. We choose our α, the risk of being wrong if we say there is a difference when there is not. This α is associated with a certain value of chi-square, which we term the *critical value*, because it is the value that separates the acceptance from the rejection of the null hypothesis. If the calculated value of $s^2 \times df/\sigma^2$ is greater than the critical value, we reject the null hypothesis and conclude that there is statistical evidence that s^2 is larger. Otherwise, we conclude that s^2 has not been shown to be larger.

F Distribution

In the example of the preceding paragraph, suppose we were comparing heal times for two new surgical procedures rather than a new one against an established one. The variances for both are estimated. We test the two sample variances s_1^2 and s_2^2 to determine whether, in the populations being sampled, one is greater in probability. To do this, we use their ratio, dividing the bigger by the smaller. (Again, the result also may be extended to standard deviations: Is one standard deviation greater in probability than the other?) The probability distribution for this ratio is called F, named (by George Snedecor) after Sir Ronald Fisher, the greatest producer of practical theories in the field of statistics. The F distribution looks very much like the chi-square (indeed it is the ratio of two independent chi-square-distributed variables), as can be seen in Fig. 2.4D. F has one more complication than χ^2: because it involves two samples, the degrees of freedom for each sample must be used, making table reference a bit more involved.

Rank-Order Methods

If we ask statistical questions about data recorded as ranks rather than measurements on intervals, we are dealing with fewer assumptions about the distributions of the data being measured. Statistical methods have been developed for rank-type data, very often called *nonparametric* methods. In addition, continuous-type data can always be ranked. The advantage of using rank-order methods for continuous data is that we do not need to consider their sampling distributions. In the case of data following well-defined distributions, such as the normal, rank-order methods are not as "powerful" as methods assuming distributions. However, if the sampling distributions of continuous data are "poorly behaved," assumptions are violated and results of statistical methods can be very wrong. In such cases, rank-order methods give more dependable results and are preferred.

Binomial Distribution

When using *categorical data*, we usually are asking questions about counts or proportions, which are based on the same theory, because one can be converted into the other. The binomial distribution has a proportion as its parameter. This proportion, π for a population and p for a sample, and the number in the count, n, fully characterize the binomial. The binomial shown in Fig. 2.4E is the distribution for $\pi = 1/3$ and $n = 12$. If our population were split evenly by sex, the probability that a randomly selected patient is male is 0.5, the binomial parameter. Suppose we treated 20 patients for some disease and found that 15 were male. Is the disease sex-related? If not, this mix of male and female would have arisen by chance alone from our binomial with parameter 0.5. We can calculate this probability and find that the chance of 15 or more males from an equal population is only 2% (0.0207). We have strong evidence that the disease is more prevalent in males.

Large-Sample Approximations to the Binomial

When we have more than a few observations, the binomial becomes difficult to calculate. Fortunately, the binomial can be approximated fairly well by one of two distributions, the normal or the Poisson. If the population proportion (the binomial parameter) is toward the middle of its 0–1 range, say, between 0.1 and 0.9, the normal distribution approximates large-sample binomials fairly well. In this case, the mean of the population being sampled is π and the variance is $\pi(1-\pi)/n$ (with its square root being the standard deviation). As the population proportion moves toward either 0 or 1, the binomial becomes too skewed to use the normal. The binomial distribution pictured in Fig. 2.4E has a parameter of $1/3$, and already we can see its skew.

Poisson Distribution

In the case of a population parameter very near 0 or 1, the large-sample binomial can be approximated adequately by the Poisson distribution, named after the French mathematician, Siméon Denis Poisson, who published a theory on it in 1837. The Poisson distribution arises in cases in which there are many opportunities for an event to occur, but a very small chance of occurrence on any one trial. Exposure to a common but not very infectious virus should result in an incidence of illness that follows the Poisson. For large samples, again a normal approximation exists. In this case, the mean of the population being sampled remains π, but the variance becomes π/n (with its square root being the standard deviation).

2.9. STANDARD ERROR OF THE MEAN

Measure of Variability in the Sample Mean

Before we meet the concepts of hypothesis testing, it will be convenient to become familiar with the *standard deviation of the sample mean*. This quantity measures the variability of the sample mean m. It has been called the standard error of the mean (SEM) for historical reasons that do not have much meaning today.

Population SEM

Let us consider our 301 prostate volumes as a population. The mean of the 301 volumes becomes the population mean $\mu = 36.47$ ml and the standard deviation $\sigma = 18.04$ ml. If we randomly draw prostate volumes, they generally will be somewhat different and these differences will follow some frequency distribution; σ is the standard deviation of this distribution. Similarly, if we calculate means $m_1, m_2, \ldots,$ from repeated samples, they generally will be somewhat different and will follow some frequency distribution; the SEM is the standard deviation of this distribution. It often is symbolized σ_m. It will be smaller than σ, because it reflects the behavior of 301 observations rather than 1. It turns out that

$$\sigma_m = \sigma \big/ \sqrt{n},$$

the population standard deviation divided by the square root of the population size. In the case of the 301 volumes, $\sigma_m = 18.04/\sqrt{301} = 1.0398$ ml. Because we know from the Central Limit Theorem that the probability distribution of m is normal, we have the distribution of m as $\mathrm{N}(\mu, \sigma_m^2) = \mathrm{N}(36.47, 1.0812)$ (because the notation uses σ^2 rather than σ).

Sample SEM

In the same way that we can estimate σ by s when we do not know σ, we can estimate σ_m by s_m using the standard deviation of a sample. The estimated SEM, s_m, is the sample standard deviation divided by the square root of the sample size, or

$$s_m = s \big/ \sqrt{n}.$$

Let us take the 10 prostate volumes given in Table DB1.1 as our sample. We can calculate $m = 32.73$ ml and $s = 15.92$ ml. Then $s_m = 15.92/\sqrt{10} = 5.3067$ ml.

2.10. JOINT DISTRIBUTIONS OF TWO VARIABLES

Example

Suppose we had platelet counts, say x, on patients with ideopathic thrombocytopenic purpura (ITP) prior to treatment and then a second count, say y, 24 hr after administering immunoglobulin (Ig). We wonder whether there is any relationship between x and y, i.e., might it be that the lower the pretreatment level, the less effect there is from the Ig, or vice versa? If so, a study might be carried out to learn whether we can predict the dosage of Ig on the basis of the pretreatment platelet count. Or is there no relation?

Joint Frequency Distribution

If we plot the two measures, x on one axis and y on the other, we are likely to find points more concentrated in some areas than others. Imagine drawing a grid on the plot, which is lying flat on a table, and making vertical columns proportional in height to the number of points in each grid square. This *joint frequency distribution* is a three-dimensional analogue to a two-dimensional bar chart. Where the points are concentrated, we would find a "hill," sloping off to areas in which the points are sparse. If the hill is symmetrically round (or elliptical with the long axis of the ellipse parallel to one of the axes), any value of x would lead to the same y as the best prediction, i.e., the value of y at the top of the hill for that x. We would think that there is no predictive capability. On the other hand, if the hill is a ridge with a peak extended from the lower left to the upper right of the graph, the peak y associated with a value of x would be different for each x, and we would think that some predictive relationship exists; y increases as x increases.

Relationship between Two Variables

There are statistical methods to assess the relationship between two variables, mostly falling under the topics *correlation* (Chapters 3 and 20) and *regression* (Chapters 8 and 20).

The concept of covariance is fundamental to all treatments of the relation between two variables. It is an extension of the ideas of variance and standard deviation. Let us think of sampling from the two variables x and y; we might keep their standard deviations straight by suffixing an indicator name on the appropriate σ or s, for example σ_x or s_x. The covariance of two variables measures *how they jointly vary, one with respect to the other*. The common symbol is similar to the standard deviation symbol, but with two subscripts indicating which variables are being included. Thus, the population and sample covariances would be σ_{xy} and s_{xy}, respectively. Formulas for these concepts and examples appear in Section 3.1.

CHAPTER EXERCISES

2.1. For the extent of carinal resection in DB12, (a) select intervals for a tally, (b) tally the data, (c) find the median, and (d) convert the tally into a relative frequency distribution. (e) Comment on whether the distribution appears by eye to be near normal. If not, in what characteristics does it differ? (f) Give a visual estimate (without calculation) of the mean and mode. How do these compare with the median found in (c)?

2.2. For patient age in DB12, (a) select intervals for a tally and (b) tally the data. In tallying, (c) record the median when 25, 50, 75, and 100 data have been tallied and at the end. Plot the median depending on the number of data sampled, similar to the plot of Fig. 2.2. Does the median converge to the final median? (d) Convert the tally into a relative frequency distribution. (e) Comment on whether the distribution appears by eye to be near normal. If not, in what characteristics does it differ? (f) Give a visual estimate (without calculation) of the mean and mode. How do these compare with the final median found in (c)?

2.3. For computational ease, use the glycosaminoglycan (GAG) levels for Type 1 assay in DB8 rounded to 1 decimal place: 0.7, 0.4, 0.3, 0.2. Calculate (a) the variance and (b) the standard deviation.

2.4. As an investigator, you want to make an inference from DB3 about whether or not the drug affects serum theophylline level (5 days). From Section 2.7, what steps would you go through?

2.5. The squares of the 60 plasma silicone levels in DB5 are ($\times 10^4$) 225, 169, 1521, 400, 1521, 1764, 576, 324, 144, 676, 100, 121, 225, 361, 729, 784, 121, 121, 324, 324, 576, 2304, 484, 729, 361, 324, 1024, 961, 361, 441, 441, 576, 100, 144, 784, 625, 484, 441, 529, 484, 484, 576, 1444, 2025, 529, 484, 324, 225, 16, 196, 576, 400, 324, 576, 225, 361, 676, 900, 484, and 576. Plot a relative frequency distribution of these squares using the intervals 0–0.02, 0.02–0.04, ..., 0.22–0.24. Does it appear more similar to the normal or the chi-square probability distribution in Section 2.8? Why?

2.6. If we were to make an inference about the mean of differences between pre-operative and post-operative plasma silicone levels in DB5, what would be the *df*? To make this mean into a *t* statistic, we subtract what value and then divide by what statistic? To decide whether *t* is significantly larger than 0, we choose a "cut point" greater than which *t* is significant and smaller than which it is not. What do we call this cut point?

2.7. Assign ranks (small to large) to the platelet counts in DB9.

2.8. If we wanted to make an inference about the proportion of patients experiencing any nausea in DB2, what distribution would we be using in this inference?

2.9. If we wanted to make an inference about the proportion of patients in DB12 who die after $\leq$2 cm of carinal resection, what distribution would we be using?

2.10. Calculate the sample SEM of the rounded GAG levels (0.7, 0.4, 0.3, 0.2) for Type 1 assay in DB8.

2.11. In DB3, the two related variables baseline and 5-day theophylline levels vary jointly. If we were to calculate a measure of how one varies relative to the other, what would it be named?

Chapter 3

Summary Statistics

3.1. NUMERICAL SUMMARIES

Section Format

Concepts for numerical summary statistics were given in Chapter 2. In this section, formulas for these summary statistics are given so that the user will know just how they are calculated and will have a convenient reference to verify the calculation method used. The symbol representing a concept will be given, followed by the formula.

When the number n of observations is indicated, n refers to the sample size when the formula is calculated from a sample and refers to the population size when the formula is calculated from a population. The distinction between samples and populations usually is clear from the context and will be stated if not.

Quantiles

We are all familiar with percentiles. A set of values is divided into 100 parts; the 90th percentile, for example, is the value below which 90% of the data fall. Other quantile types are deciles, in which the set of values is divided into 10 parts, and quartiles, four parts. Quantiles are useful descriptors of how a data distribution is shaped. For example, suppose Q_1, Q_2, and Q_3 are the first, second, and third quartiles (one-quarter, one-half, and three-quarters of the data fall below). It can be seen that, if $Q_2 - Q_1 \approx Q_3 - Q_2$ ("$\approx$" means "approximately equal to"), the distribution is approximately symmetric; if $Q_2 - Q_1$ and $Q_3 - Q_2$ are quite different, the distribution is skewed.

MEAN

μ denotes a population's arithmetic mean, and m denotes a sample's arithmetic mean. The two have the same calculation, so that the difference is whether n represents the size of a population or a sample. The sample mean m sometimes is seen in the literature represented by the variable with an overbar, as $\bar{x}$. Recall that Σ means "add together all data elements whose symbol follows me." Thus, if the variable x contains the three data elements 1, 2, and 4, Σx implies $1+2+4$.

$$\mu = \frac{\sum x}{n} \quad \text{or} \quad m = \frac{\sum x}{n}, \tag{3.1}$$

depending on whether n denotes the number in a population or a sample, respectively. (The usual mean is called arithmetic because the values are added, in contrast to the geometric mean, a form used only in some special cases, in which they are multiplied.)

Example

Consider the mean PSA value from Table DB1.1.

$$m = (7.6 + 4.1 + \cdots + 7.9)/10 = 67.5/10 = 6.75.$$

MEDIAN

The median, having no standard symbol (sometimes *md* is used and, rarely, m with a wiggle over it), may be found for either a population or a sample. The following formula is an algorithm in words rather than in symbols:

Put the n observations in order of size.
Median is the middle observation if n is odd.
Median is halfway between the two middle observations if n is even.

It will be apparent that the median is also the 2nd quartile (Q_2) and the 50th percentile. The median frequently is used to represent the average of survival data, where occasional long survivors skew the data, rendering the mean not very descriptive of the typical patient.

Example

Let us put the 10 PSA observations from Table DB1.1 in order of size: 4.1, 4.4, 5.9, 6.1, 6.8, 7.6, 7.7, 7.9, 8.0, 9.0. n is even. The two middle observations are 6.8 and 7.6. The median is halfway between them, 7.2.

Mode

The *mode*, also having no standard symbol (sometimes *mo* is used), may be found for either a population or a sample, provided that n is large. The mode can be read from a bar chart, but will be approximate, depending on the choice of the bar chart's interval widths and start point.

Make a bar chart of the data.
Mode is the center value of the highest bar.

Example

We can again use PSA values from Table DB1.1 as an example, although a mode from 10 observations would not be used in practice. The mode requires a large number of observations to have any accuracy and is not used very often in clinical studies. A bar chart of the observations with a bin width of 1 would appear as in Fig. 3.1. The mode is the center of the tallest bar, 7.5.

Variance

The variance of a population is denoted σ^2. Conceptually, it is the average of the squares of differences between the observations and their mean: $\sigma^2 = \sum(x-\mu)^2/n$.

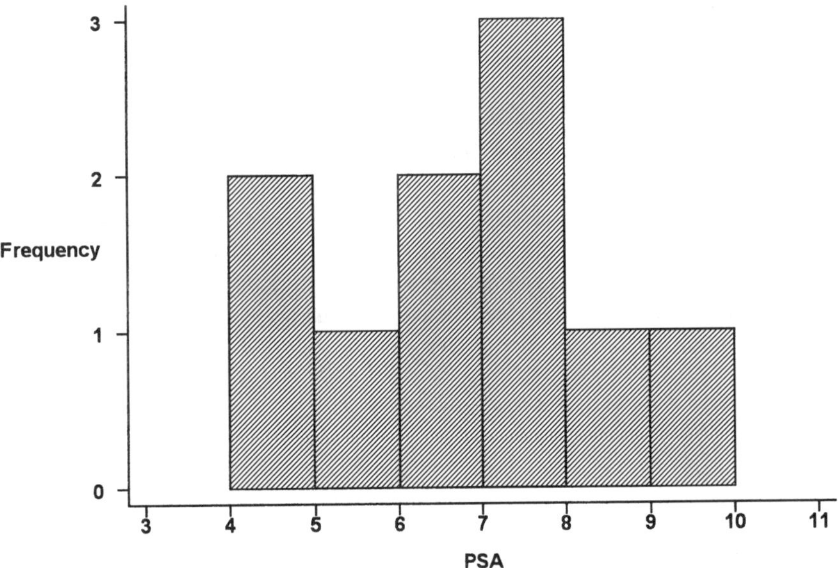

Figure 3.1 Bar chart of PSA values from Table DB1.1. The *mode* is 7.5, the center of the tallest bar.

It may be calculated more easily by the equivalent form

$$\sigma^2 = \frac{\sum x^2 - n\mu^2}{n}. \tag{3.2}$$

The variance of a sample is denoted s^2. It is similar, with m replacing μ and $n-1$ in place of n to avoid a theoretical bias. The form equivalent to Eq. (3.2) is

$$s^2 = \frac{\sum x^2 - nm^2}{n-1}. \tag{3.3}$$

The *standard deviations* σ and s are just the square roots of the respective variances.

Example

The mean of the PSA values from Table DB1.1 was $m = 6.75$. The variance may be found by

$$\begin{aligned} s^2 &= (7.6^2 + 4.1^2 + \cdots + 7.9^2 - 10 \times 6.75^2)/9 \\ &= (57.76 + 16.82 + \cdots 62.41 - 10 \times 45.5625)/9 \\ &= (478.890 - 455.625)/9 = 23.265/9 = 2.585. \end{aligned}$$

The standard deviation is just the square root of the variance or

$$s = \sqrt{2.585} = 1.6078.$$

Standard Error of the Mean (SEM)

The standard error of the mean was introduced in Section 2.9. It is simply the standard deviation of the value m, the mean of n observations. If n is the *population* size, the SEM is symbolized σ_m; if n is the *sample* size, the (estimated) SEM is symbolized s_m. They are calculated by using the standard deviations of the observations, σ or s, as appropriate:

$$\sigma_m = \frac{\sigma}{\sqrt{n}} \quad \text{or} \quad s_m = \frac{s}{\sqrt{n}}. \tag{3.4}$$

Example

From the 10 PSA values of Table DB1.1, s was found to be 1.6078. The estimated SEM is $1.6078/\sqrt{10} = 1.6078/3.1623 = 0.5084$.

Covariance

The *covariance* was introduced in Section 2.10, in the context of joint frequency distributions. This statistic is a measure of how two paired variables, say x and y, vary jointly, one with respect to the other. The calculation of the covariance is similar to that of the variance, except that instead of squaring the x term, we use the x term multiplied by its paired y term, as $\sigma_{xy} = \sum(x - \mu_x) \times (y - \mu_y)/n$. The calculational forms for the population and sample covariances, respectively, become

$$\sigma_{xy} = \frac{\sum xy - n\mu_x\mu_y}{n} \tag{3.5}$$

and

$$s_{xy} = \frac{\sum xy - nm_x m_y}{n - 1}. \tag{3.6}$$

Example

Let age from Table DB1.1 take the x position in Eq. (3.6) and prostate volume take the y position.

$$\begin{aligned} s_{xy} &= (75 \times 32.3 + 68 \times 27.0 + \cdots + 74 \times 16.4 - 10 \times 65.1 \times 32.73)/9 \\ &= (2422.50 + 1836.00 + \cdots + 1213.60 - 10 \times 2130.723)/9 \\ &= (21211.40 - 21307.23)/9 = -95.83/9 = -10.6478. \end{aligned}$$

Interpretation

If one variable tends to increase as the other increases, such as systolic and diastolic blood pressure, the covariance is positive and large; large values of one are multiplied by large negative values of the other, which makes a very large sum. If one tends to decrease as the other increases, as with PSA and prostate density, the covariance is negative and large; large positive values of one are multiplied by large negative values of the other. On the other hand, if increases and decreases in one variable are unrelated to those of the other, the covariance tends to be small.

Correlation Coefficient

The covariance could be very useful in indicating a shared behavior or independence between the two variables, but there is no standard for interpreting it. The covariance can be standardized by dividing by the product of standard deviations of the two variables. It is then called the *correlation coefficient*, designated

ρ (Greek rho) for a correlation between two populations and r for a correlation between two samples. Thus, the formulas for calculating correlation coefficients ρ (population) or r (sample), respectively, are

$$\rho_{xy} = \frac{\sigma_{xy}}{\sigma_x \sigma_y} \quad \text{or} \quad r_{xy} = \frac{s_{xy}}{s_x s_y}. \tag{3.7}$$

Interpretation

This standardized covariance, the correlation coefficient, may be interpreted easily. If either variable is perfectly predictable from the other, the correlation coefficient is 1.00 when they both increase together and -1.00 when one increases as the other decreases. If the two variables are independent, i.e., a value of one provides no information about the value of the other, the correlation coefficient is 0. A correlation coefficient of 0.10 is rather low, showing little predictable relationship, and one of 0.90 is rather high, showing that one increases rather predictably as the other increases.

Example

Continuing with the age and volume example from before, we note that the standard deviation of age is $s_x = 6.9992$ and that of volume is $s_y = 15.9351$. The covariance was calculated as $s_{xy} = -10.6478$. Then

$$r_{xy} = -10.6478/(6.9992 \times 15.9351) = -0.09556.$$

This result would tell us that, for our 10 patients in Table DB1.1, volume tends to decrease as age increases, but not in a very strong relationship. We should note that $n = 10$ is too small a sample to provide us with much statistical confidence in our result.

CAUTION

We must remember that correlation methods measure relationship only along a straight line. If one variable increases when the other increases but not in a straight line, for example, as when weight is predicted by height (weight is a power of height) or when teenage growth depends on time (growth is a logarithm of time), the correlation may not be high despite good predictability. More sophisticated prediction methods are needed for curvilinear relationships. Elementary information on this topic appears in Chapter 8.

Furthermore, this linear correlation measures only the pattern of data behavior, not the interchangeability of data. For example, temperature measured in the same patients using one thermometer in degrees Celcius and another in degrees Fahrenheit would have an almost perfect correlation of 1.0, but the readings could not be intermingled.

Standard Error of the Mean (SEM) for Two Samples

In many cases, we are faced with two samples that may be drawn from the same population, and we want to know whether their means are different. To assess this, we need to use the standard deviation of the mean (SEM) using the information from both samples. If the standard deviation of observations from that population is known, say σ, the SEM is simply that σ divided by a sample size term, namely,

$$\sigma_m = \sigma\sqrt{\frac{1}{n_1} + \frac{1}{n_2}}. \tag{3.8}$$

If, however, as is usually the case, we do not know the population standard deviation, we must estimate it from s_1 and s_2, the sample standard deviations calculated from the two sets of observations. This requires two steps: first, use s_1 and s_2 to find the standard deviation of the pooled observations, say s_{p}, and then find the SEM, say s_m, in a form similar to Eq. (3.8). The algebra is worked backward from the formulas for the two sample standard deviations to find s_{p}, as we would have calculated it had we pooled all the observations at the outset. It turns out to be

$$s_{\text{p}} = \sqrt{\frac{(n_1 - 1)s_1^2 + (n_2 - 1)s_2^2}{n_1 + n_2 - 2}}. \tag{3.9}$$

Then s_m is

$$s_m = s_{\text{p}}\sqrt{\frac{1}{n_1} + \frac{1}{n_2}}. \tag{3.10}$$

Example

Consider again the PSA values from Table DB1.1. Suppose we had taken two samples, the first four observations ($n_1 = 4$) and the remaining six ($n_2 = 6$). Their standard deviations are $s_1 = 2.1205$ and $s_2 = 1.3934$. By substituting these values into Eq. (3.9), we obtain

$$s_{\text{p}} = \sqrt{\frac{3 \times 2.1205^2 + 5 \times 1.3934^2}{8}} = \sqrt{2.8997} = 1.7029.$$

The 1.7029 estimate is slightly larger than the 1.6078 we obtained from the original 10 observations because we had to allocate a degree of freedom for each of two means (one appearing in s_1 and the other in s_2) and had to divide by $n-2$ rather than $n-1$. $s_m = 1.7029 \times 0.6455 = 1.0992$.

3.2. PICTORIAL SUMMARIES

Common Types

Graphs and charts allow us to visualize distributions and other properties of data. From a chart, we often can get a rough idea of a mean, a standard deviation, or a proportion. Although there are several types of charts, the most common are the bar chart (which was introduced in Chapter 2 and can be seen again in Fig. 3.1), histogram, pie chart, line chart, and scattergram. Nowadays the mean-and-standard-error chart and box-and-whisker chart also are being seen frequently in medical literature.

Making a Bar Chart

When forming a bar chart, the choice of intervals is important. It is, to some extent, an art. An unfortunate choice of intervals can change the apparent pattern of the distribution. Enough intervals should be used so that the pattern will be little affected by altering their beginning and ending positions. The beginning and ending positions should be chosen to be convenient in reading the bar chart and should relate to the meaning of the variable being charted. Let us recall the prostate volume data depicted in Fig. 2.1F. Figure 3.2A shows the prostate volume data allocated to 6 intervals rather than the 24 of Fig. 2.1F; useful information is obscured by the lack of detail. Figure 3.2B shows the data allocated to 48 intervals; the viewer is distracted by too much detail. Furthermore, if we had fewer data, say only 50 or so, the excess number of intervals would obscure the distribution pattern as badly as too few. The choices of number, width, and starting points of intervals arise from the user's judgment. They should be considered carefully before forming a bar chart.

Histogram

The histogram appears much like the bar chart, but differs in that the number of observations lying in an interval is represented by the *area* of a rectangle (or bar) rather than its height. If all intervals are of equal width, the histogram is no different from the bar chart (except perhaps cosmetically). However, if one interval had been chosen to be twice the width of the others, the rectangle height over that interval must be one-half the height it would be in a bar chart. This area-in-lieu-of-height

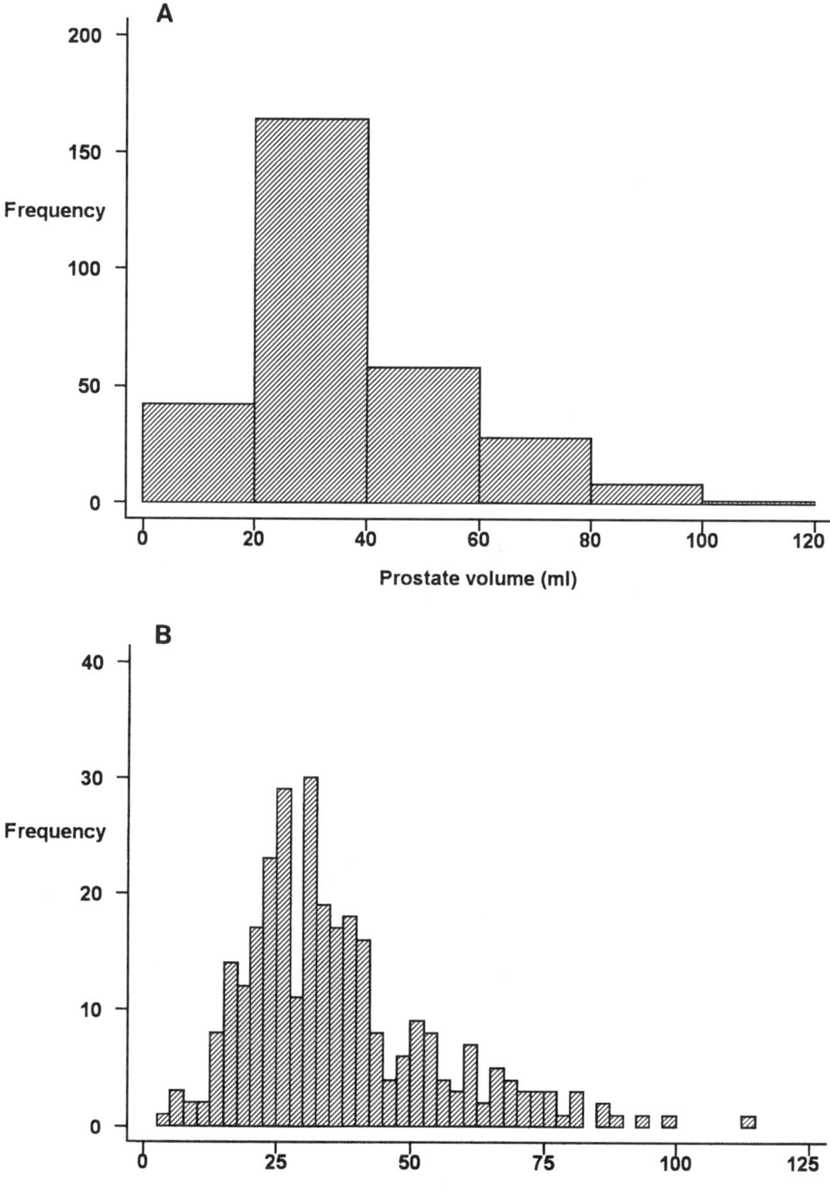

Figure 3.2 The effects on a bar chart displaying a frequency distribution of too few intervals (A) and too many intervals (B).

presentation avoids a possible misinterpretation by the viewer. For example, if the prevalence of a disease in an epidemic is displayed monthly for several months, but the last rectangle represents only 15 days, its height per infected patient would be doubled in a histogram in order to convey the true pattern of prevalence.

Example

Figure 3.3 illustrates the requirement for using areas in lieu of heights for unequal intervals. Suppose in recording prostate volumes the intervals had been organized by 5-ml increments until 65 ml, and a final interval of 65–115 ml was used. Then the bar chart of volumes (Fig. 2.1F) would be amended so that the last bar would have height 28, as in Fig. 3.3A. If we adjust by converting the height to area, we obtain Fig. 3.3B, which gives a more accurate depiction.

Pie Chart

A pie chart represents proportions rather than amounts. Its main use is to visualize the *relative* prevalence of a phenomenon rather than its absolute prevalence. It also has the advantage of avoiding the illusion of sequence that sometimes is implied by the order of bars in a bar chart, intended or not. To draw a pie chart, the user must allocate the 360° of a circle to the components in proportion to their prevalence. A prevalence of 20% is shown by a $0.2 \times 360° = 72°$ angle about the center of the circle.

Example

Let us look at the prediction of biopsy result by DRE from Table DB1.1. There are 30% true negatives (DRE−, BIOP−), 20% false negatives (DRE−, BIOP+), 10% true positives (DRE+, BIOP+), and 40% false positives (DRE+, BIOP−). Figure 3.4 visually conveys these percentages of results in a pie chart. The first piece of pie includes 30% of $360° = 108°$.

Line Chart

If, in a bar chart, we connected the center of the bar tops by line segments and then erased the bars, we would have a form of line chart. The main use of a line chart is to convey information similar to a bar chart, but for cases in which the intervals form a sequence of time or order of events from left to right. In Fig. 2.1F, we intend no progression of frequency in logical sequence as prostate volumes increase. In contrast, the frequencies of patients per age follow an interesting pattern as age progresses.

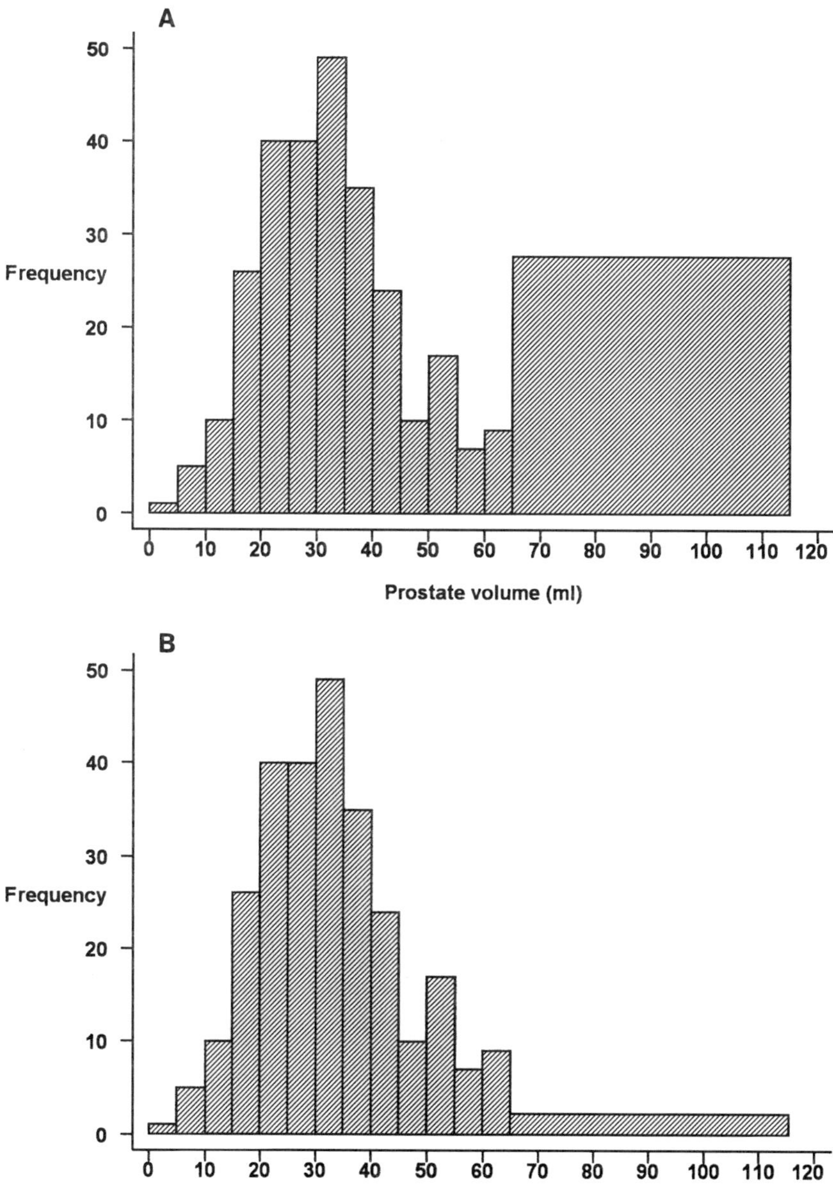

Figure 3.3 The effect, when intervals are unequal, of representing frequency in an interval by height (using a bar chart) (A) as opposed to representing that frequency by area (using a histogram) (B).

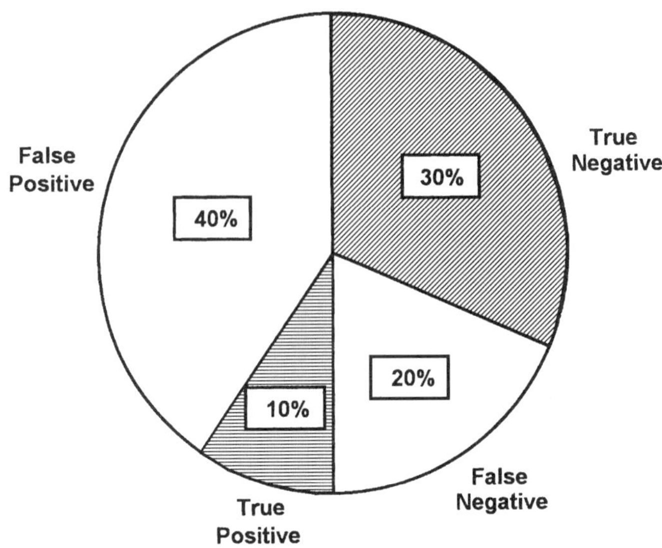

Figure 3.4 A pie chart representing proportions of biopsy results as predicted by the DRE.

Example

Figure 3.5 depicts frequencies for our 301 patients for 5-year age intervals. We note that the frequencies increase successively to about the mid-60s and then decrease successively thereafter. It is not difficult to conjecture the forces causing this data pattern in these patients who have presented for possible prostate problems. Prostate problems are rare in young men and increase in frequency with age. However, starting in the late 60s, men are dying in increasing numbers due to other causes, so that the number of survivors available to present decreases with age.

Relation of a Line Chart to a Probability Distribution

Conceptually it is important to observe that, as the sample size increases and the width of the intervals decreases, the line chart of a sample distribution approaches the picture of its probability distribution.

Scattergram

Another view of a distribution is shown by the scattergram, in which the occurrence of each observation on a variable is shown as a tick mark or some other symbol positioned on the axis for that variable. Figure 3.6 shows two scatters: those for prostate volumes of men with negative biopsies and those with positive

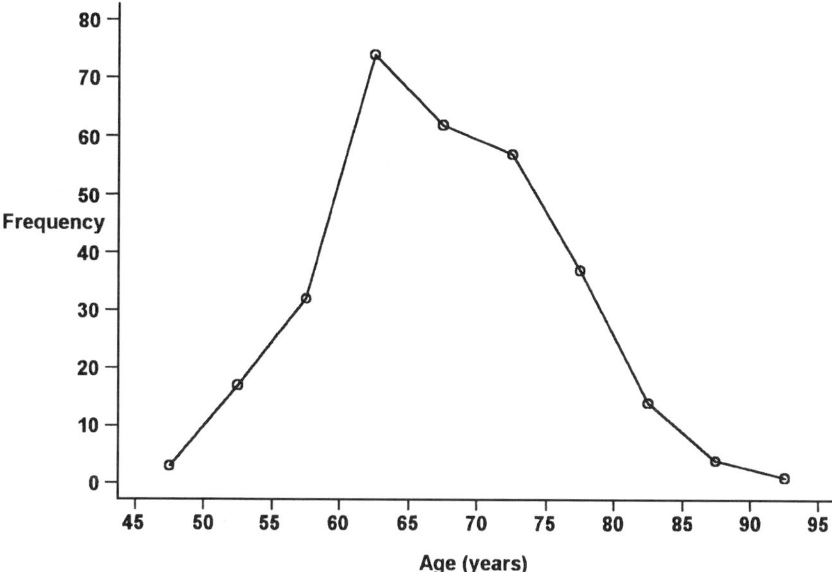

Figure 3.5 A line chart representing frequencies of men presenting with prostate problems according to age. The points (circles) showing frequencies are positioned over the centers of the defined age intervals and are then connected by straight line segments.

biopsies. The distinction between the two distributions is apparent. This sort of scattergram gives much the same information as the bar chart but has a serious disadvantage. The shape of the distribution is more difficult to see, so that the relationship to the parent probability distribution is not as apparent. However, there also are advantages. First, no arbitrary and possibly biasing choice of intervals is necessary. Second, the distributions of various subsamples can be shown as one

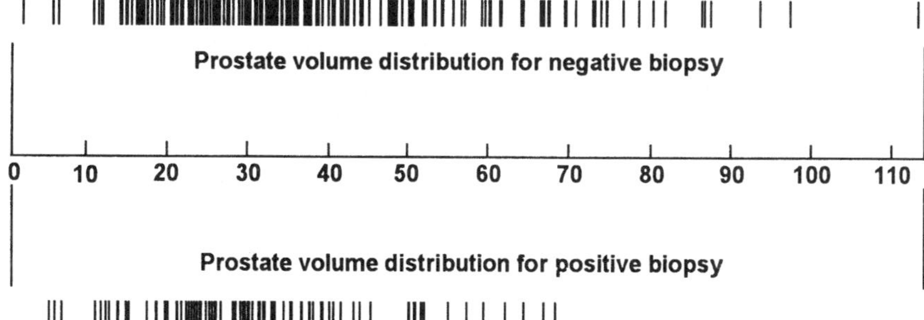

Figure 3.6 Adjacent one-dimensional scattergrams showing prostate volumes for negative and positive biopsies.

superposed on another, as in Fig. 3.6, more easily than on bar charts. In general, when choosing charts, we must consider all options and select that that best conveys the information to be depicted.

Scattergram in Two Dimensions

Scattergrams are not confined to one dimension, but often are used to explore the way data are distributed in two dimensions. Pairs of values are plotted on two perpendicular axes.

Example

The population in which we are interested is composed of prostate volume as a possible indicator of prostate cancer, and patients with benign prostate hypertrophy (BPH) lie in a different population. Thus, we confine ourselves to smaller prostates, namely, those below 65 ml. In Fig. 3.7, those volumes are plotted on the vertical axis and age on the horizontal axis. A pattern of some sort, for example, if prostate volumes tended to reduce with age, might have suggested a relationship. However, no obvious pattern appears. If you were given an age, would this plot allow you to suggest an average volume different from the overall average? No. We would say the two variables appear independent.

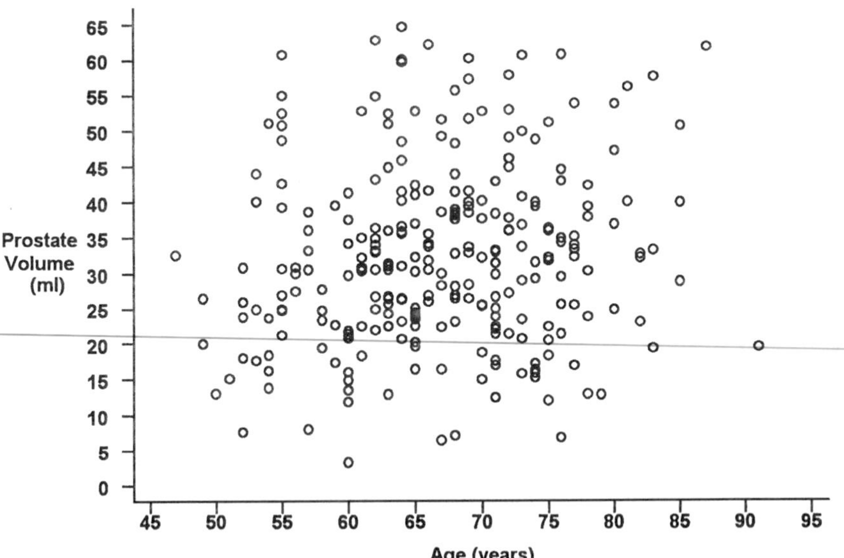

Figure 3.7 A two-dimensional scattergram depicting prostate volumes below 65 ml as related to age of patient.

Scattergram in Three or More Dimensions

Scattergrams can be extended, with varying degrees of success, to additional dimensions. Showing different subsamples with contrasting data symbols or colors is one way. In some cases, a three-dimensional picture may be shown as projected on a two-dimensional surface, perhaps with data circles decreasing in size in proportion to the distance away from the viewer, but care must be taken to organize angles and scales so that the information being presented is perceptible and so that background data are not obscured by foreground data.

Mean-and-Standard-Error Chart

A diagram showing a set of means to be compared, augmented by an indication of the size of uncertainty associated with each mean, is being seen more and more frequently in medical articles.

Showing the Means

When a relationship among several groups is of interest, a lot of information is given by a plot in which groups are given positions on the horizontal axis and means are shown by vertical height above each position. Increasing time or increasing amount of a drug might appear on the horizontal axis. The clinical response to this sequence is shown by the mean. For example, post-operative pain rated by patients on a visual analogue scale may be related to the amount of pain-relieving drug used. Four standard levels of drug dose, starting with 0, could be positioned on the horizontal scale, and mean pain rating could be shown vertically over each respective dose. In this case, we would expect the means to be decreasing with increasing dose. In other cases, they could be increasing or going up then down or even scattered in no perceptible pattern. We can tell a great deal about the process occurring from the pattern.

Showing the Variability about the Means

We must ask whether, for example, the downward pattern of pain with increasing drug is meaningful, because we can make it look huge or minuscule by altering the vertical scale. A crucial part of the information is how different the means are relative to the variability in the data. The means may be decreasing, but with such small decrements relative to the data variability that it might have happened by chance and we do not accept the decreasing pattern as shown to be real. A useful solution is to show the associated uncertainty as "whiskers" on the means, that is, as lines up and down from the mean, indicating variability by their lengths. This variability depicted may be standard deviation, standard error, or some related measure.

Example

Figure 3.8 shows prostate volume between 0 and 50 ml for 291 patients in the 50- to 89-year age range separated into decades of age: 50s, 60s, 70s, and 80s. The means are shown by solid circles. The whiskers indicate about 2 standard errors above and below the mean, which includes 95% of the data on an idealized distribution. (More about this can be found in Chapter 4.) We can see by inspection that the mean volumes seem to increase somewhat by age, but that there is so much overlap in the variability that we are not sure this increase is a dependably real phenomenon from decade to decade. However, we would take a small risk in being wrong by concluding that the increase from the youngest (50s) to the oldest (80s) is a real change.

Effect of Irregular Data

Does this chart tell the full story? If the data per group are distributed in a fairly symmetrical and smooth bell-type curve, most of the relevant pattern may be

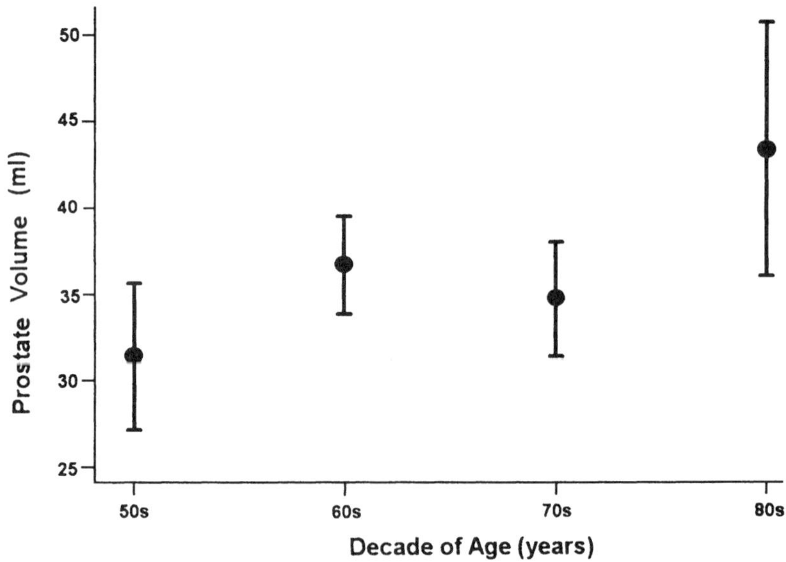

Figure 3.8 Prostate volume (milliliters) means (symbols) for 297 men allocated to their decades of age, with attached whiskers representing about 2 standard deviations (exactly 1.96) above and below the respective means.

discerned. However, if the data are distributed irregularly and/or asymmetrically, this chart actually covers up important relationships and may lead to false conclusions. That is because the assumptions of regularity and symmetry are made for this chart, and, as usual, relationships are distorted when assumptions are violated. Charts that are "data-dependent" rather "assumption-dependent," such as the box-and-whisker charts discussed next, often will provide a better understanding of the data.

Box-and-Whisker Charts

A practical way to explore and understand data we may have in hand is to diagram it such that it displays not only the typical aspects, e.g., distribution center and spread, but also atypical characteristics, e.g., asymmetry, data clumps, and outlying values. The box-and-whisker chart does this rather well, although no technique displays all the vagaries of data. Figure 3.9 shows such a diagram, representing aspects of the distribution of age for the 301 urological patients. As indicated in the diagram, the box includes the 25th to the 75th percentiles of data, with the median (the 50th percentile) as an intermediate line. If the median is in the center of the box, the middle half of the data is nearly symmetric, with the median not far different from the mean. An off-center median indicates asymmetry. The whiskers extend the plot out to the last datum reached before $\frac{3}{2}$ the box height. (In a large normal sample, the box and whiskers would include about 90% of the

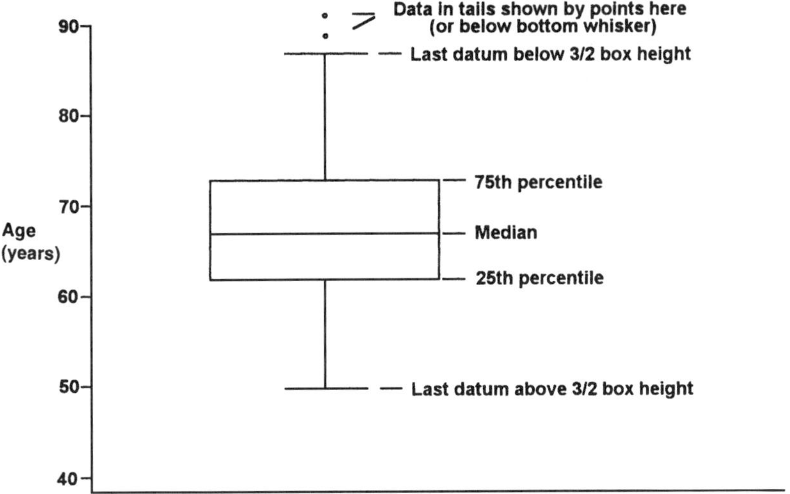

Figure 3.9 Representative box-and-whisker plot showing component definitions.

data.) Whisker lengths that are similar and are about half again the box height are further evidence of symmetry and a near-normal distribution. Unequal whisker lengths indicate asymmetry in the outer parts of the data distribution. Whisker lengths shorter or longer than $3/2$ the box height indicate tendency toward a "flat-topped" or "peaky" distribution. A short whisker attached to a long box portion or vice versa shows evidence of "lumpy" data. Finally, the presence of data far out in the tails as well as their distance out is shown by dots above and below the whisker ends. Other characteristics can be detected with a little experience using the box-and-whisker chart.

Effect of No Assumptions

Charts like the box-and-whisker with no distributional assumptions, such as was used in the mean-and-standard-error chart, suffer from being completely dependent on the data in hand at the moment, and general distributional characteristics cannot be easily inferred; they are designed to describe the sample, not the population. This is at once their great strength and their great weakness. They must be used with care.

Example

Consider the sample of 291 urological patients with PSA not over 50 ng/ml included in the 50- to 89-year age range separated into decades of age: 50s, 60s, 70s, and 80s. Figure 3.10 shows a box-and-whisker chart of PSA level by age decade. Immediately obvious are the many high values stretching out above the whiskers, with none symmetrically below. That plus the longer whisker on the upper side indicates a strong skewness. The data suggest that PSA has a narrower distribution in the 50s, becoming worse with age. However, by the time the 80s are reached, the worst cases appear to have died, so that the distribution narrows again, except for a couple of extreme cases. It should be apparent that a mean-and-standard error chart would not be appropriate for these data.

Showing Sample Size

One piece of information lacking from the chart in Fig. 3.10 is sample size. Might some of the differences be due to a small number of patients in the group? A variation on the box-and-whisker chart is to draw the width of the box proportional to sample size so that relative sample sizes (not actual numbers) can be compared. Figure 3.11 is a redrawing of Fig. 3.10 with box widths proportional to sample size. The smaller sizes in the 50s and especially in the 80s lend less credence to the results for these age decades.

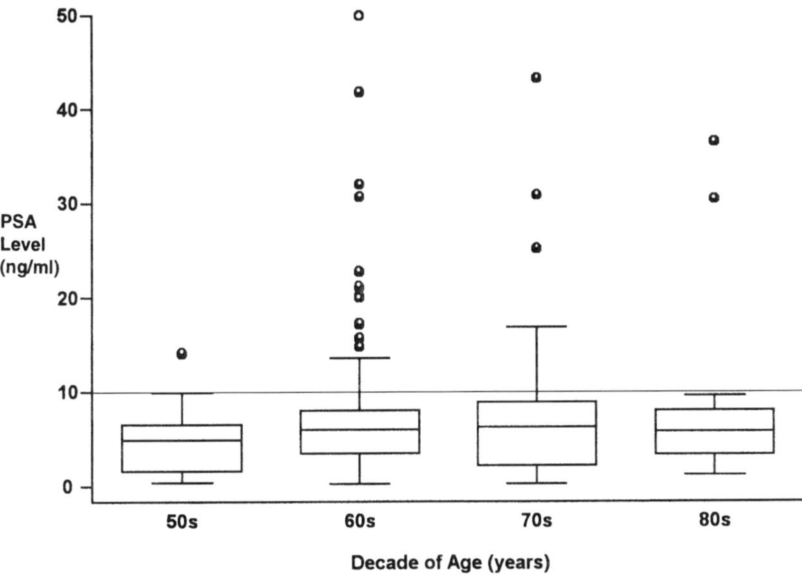

Figure 3.10 A box-and-whisker chart of PSA level for 291 urological patients in the 50- to 89-year age range separated into decades of age: 50s, 60s, 70s, and 80s. Readings above the line drawn at PSA level of 10 ng/ml show a high risk of prostate cancer.

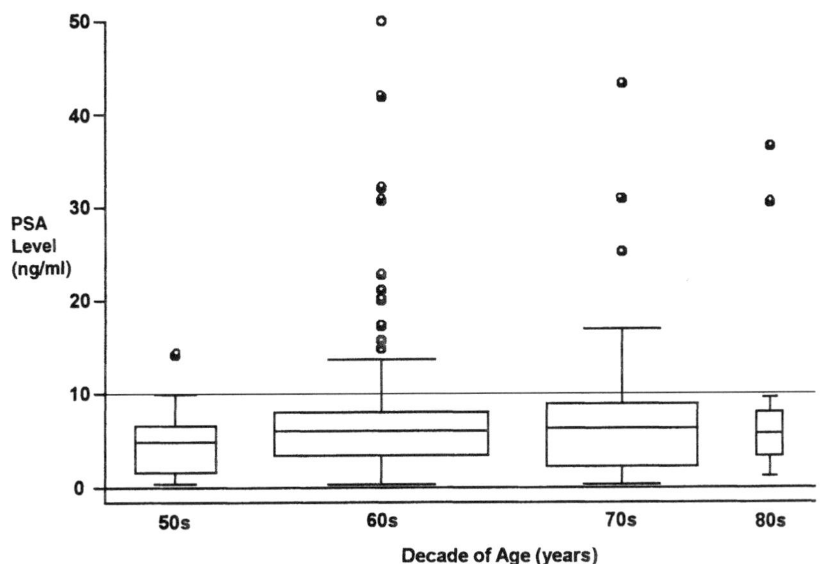

Figure 3.11 A redrawing of Fig. 3.10 with widths of the boxes proportional to the number of data in the respective age decade.

Conclusions on Statistical Graphs

The use of pictorial summaries has two main purposes. First, as descriptive statistics, they present a visual image of the data all at once, which often is the most helpful way to describe the interrelationship among the data. Second, as was conjectured in the text about Fig. 3.7, they suggest the forces giving rise to patterns of data. These perceived patterns are not sufficient evidence in themselves for scientific conclusions, but they suggest hypotheses to be posed that can then be tested with quantitative results. Graphs and charts are formidable tools in *data exploration*.

CHAPTER EXERCISES

3.1. From DB7, find the (a) mean, (b) median, (c) variance, (d) standard deviation, (e) 1st quartile, (f) 3rd quartile, and (g) SEM of the bone density. Round all answers to one decimal place after calculation.

3.2. From DB10, find the (a) mean, (b) median, (c) variance, (d) standard deviation, (e) 1st quartile, (f) 3rd quartile, and (g) SEM of the distance covered in a triple hop on the operated leg.

3.3. From DB12, find the mode age.

3.4. From DB10, find the two-sample SEM of distance covered using the operated leg and nonoperated leg samples.

3.5. From DB10, find the (a) covariance and (b) correlation coefficient of distance covered between the operated and nonoperated legs.

3.6. From DB10, find the (a) covariance and (b) correlation coefficient of seconds to perform the hops between the operated and nonoperated legs.

3.7. From DB7, construct a bar chart of patient ages.

3.8. From DB7, construct a histogram of bone density in the intervals 80 to <140, 140 to <160, 160 to <180, and 180 to <200.

3.9. From DB7, construct pie charts of patient (a) sexes and (b) ages (grouped 17–19, 20–22, 23–25, and >25).

3.10. From DB11, construct a line chart of the number of rats surviving malaria by day number for the three treatments.

3.11. From DB3, construct a scattergram of serum theophylline level at 10 days, depending on level at baseline.

3.12. From DB3, construct a (a) mean-and-standard-error chart ($\pm$1.96 SEM) and (b) box-and-whisker chart for serum theophylline level at baseline, 5 days, and 10 days.

Chapter 4

Confidence Intervals and Probability

4.1. OVERVIEW

BASIS OF A CONFIDENCE INTERVAL

We have all observed that hematocrit (Hct) values (measured in percent) for healthy patients are not all the same; they range over an interval. What is this interval? We know that extreme values occasionally arise in healthy patients. We cannot specify an interval that will always include only healthy patients and exclude only unhealthy patients. The best we can do is to find an interval that most frequently includes healthy patients and excludes unhealthy patients. This is an expression of relative frequency or likelihood. We might say that the interval should include 95% of the healthy population, which is to say that a randomly chosen healthy patient has a 0.95 probability of falling in the interval. This leads to the term *confidence interval*, because we are 95% confident that a healthy patient will fall in the interval.

ERROR RATE

We let the symbol α represent the probability that a healthy patient's Hct will fall outside the healthy interval; in this case, $\alpha = 5\%$. When a patient's Hct does fall outside the healthy interval, we think, "It is likely that the patient has arisen from an unhealthy population, but not certain. We must compare the Hct with other indicators to derive a total picture."

Estimating the Interval

In Section 2.7, it was pointed out that probabilities of occurrences correspond to areas under portions of probability distributions. Thus, if we know the distribution of Hcts, we can find the Hct values outside of which 5% of the area (2.5% in each tail) will fall. The mechanism for this will be seen in the following sections.

A General Statement of Confidence

The confidence interval need not be constrained to 95% probability, and it may apply to any distribution. A general statement for a confidence interval on an individual observation drawn randomly from a population, for any probability distribution and any desired interval, may be stated as follows (with indentations designed to help identify subconcepts):

The probability
  that a randomly drawn observation
    from a given probability distribution
  is contained in a specified interval
is given by
  the area of the distribution under the curve over that interval. (4.1)

Other Uses for Probabilities

The use of probabilities is by no means limited to confidence intervals. Suppose we needed to know the chance of encountering a healthy patient with a Hct < 0.30. If we knew the Hct probability distribution, we could calculate this chance as the area under that distribution to the left of the horizontal axis value of 0.30. Rarely must we calculate such probability values directly, because we may use computers and/or tables to find them. Sections in this chapter and Chapter 11 describe the methods for finding probabilities from the distributions commonly met in statistics, introduced in Section 2.8.

Use of the Normal Distribution

The most frequently used distribution in biostatistics is the normal one, for both biological and mathematical reasons. In biology, a great many data sets naturally follow the normal distribution, at least approximately. In mathematics, due to the

Central Limit Theorem introduced in Chapter 2, any mean of a data set follows the normal, at least approximately. Thus, our look at probability will begin with the normal distribution.

4.2. THE NORMAL DISTRIBUTION

THE STANDARD NORMAL

Recall from Section 2.8 that the normal distribution is a perfect case of the famous bell curve. Although an infinite number of cases of the normal exist, we need deal with only one, the standard normal. Any normally distributed variable or sample of observations becomes a standard normal variable, symbolized z, by subtracting the mean from each value and dividing by the standard deviation. Thus, *z represents the number of standard deviations away from the mean*, positive for above the mean and negative for below the mean. Figure 4.1 shows a standard normal distribution with $z = 1.96$ (frequently seen in practice) and the corresponding area $\alpha = 2.5\%$ under the curve to the right of that z. (Addition of a similar area in the left tail would provide $\alpha = 5\%$ in total.)

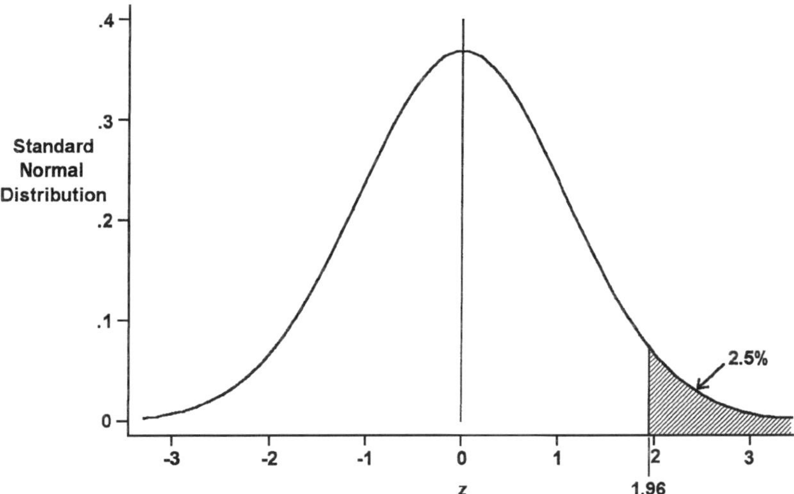

Figure 4.1 A standard normal distribution shown with a 2.5% α and its corresponding $z = 1.96$. The α shown is the area under the curve to the right of a given or calculated z. For a two-tailed computation, α is doubled in order to include the symmetric opposite tail. A two-tailed $\alpha = 5\%$ lies outside the ± 1.96 interval, leaving 95% of the area under the curve between the tails.

Table 4.1
Segment of Normal Distribution Table A[a]

z (no. std. deviations to right of mean)	One-tailed applications		Two-tailed applications	
	One-tailed α (area in right tail)	$1-\alpha$ (area except right tail)	Two-tailed α (area in both tails)	$1-\alpha$ (area except both tails)
0	0.500	0.500	1.000	0.000
0.50	0.308	0.692	0.619	0.381
1.00	0.159	0.841	0.318	0.682
1.281	*0.100*	*0.900*	*0.200*	*0.800*
1.50	0.067	0.933	0.134	0.866
1.645	*0.050*	*0.950*	*0.100*	*0.900*
1.960	*0.025*	*0.975*	*0.050*	*0.950*
2.00	0.023	0.977	0.046	0.934
2.326	*0.010*	*0.990*	*0.020*	*0.980*
2.50	0.006	0.994	0.012	0.088
3.00	0.0013	0.9987	0.0026	0.9974

[a] For selected distances (z) to the right of the mean, given are (a) one-tailed α, the area under the curve in the positive tail; (b) one-tailed $1-\alpha$, the area under all except the tail; (c) two-tailed α, the areas combined for both positive and negative tails; and (d) two-tailed $1-\alpha$, the area under all except the two tails. Entries for the most commonly used areas are italicized.

Table of the Standard Normal

Table A, in the back of the book, contains selected values of z with four areas that often are used: (a) the area under the curve in the positive tail for the given z, i.e., one-tailed α; (b) the area under all except that tail, i.e., $1-\alpha$; (c) the areas combined for both positive and negative tails, i.e., two-tailed α; and (d) the area under all except the two tails, i.e., $1-\alpha$. Table 4.1 shows a segment of Table A.

Probability of Certain Ranges Occurring

Prostate volume has been posed as a possible indicator of prostate cancer. Because the population we want to examine is composed of patients with possible prostate cancer, we omit five patients with known benign prostate hypertrophy (BPH), as they lie in a different population. The remaining prostate volumes, shown in Fig. 2.1F, are distributed approximately normally. These remaining 296 volumes have mean = 35.46 ml and standard deviation = 16.35 ml. Let us round them to 35 and 16 ml to make the arithmetic easy in this illustration. Two patients present to you, one with volume 59 ml and one with volume 83 ml. How typical are they? They are 1.5 and 3 standard deviations above the mean, respectively. By looking in Table 4.1 under a z of 1.5, we find a one-tailed $\alpha = 0.067$ and a two-tailed $\alpha = 0.134$. Approximately 6.7% of the area under the curve lies to the right of the z-value. This tells us that 6.7% of normal patients have prostate volumes at least this much greater than the mean, and similarly 13.4% have volumes this deviant from (larger or smaller than) the mean. This indicates a large prostate, but not an obviously atypical one. On the other hand, the second patient's z of 3 yields a one-tailed α of 0.0013; only about 1 in 1000 normal patients would have a prostate so large by chance alone. We are led to conclude that this patient is unlikely to have arisen from the clinically normal population; he more likely arose from a population with atypically large prostates.

Using the Standard Normal

Another way to look at the same information is to transform the data to the standard normal by the relationship $z = (x - \mu)/\sigma$. Because $\mu = 35$ ml and $\sigma = 16$ ml, our prostate with volume 59 ml becomes $z = (59 - 35)/16 = 1.5$, which refers to the same position in the table. Similarly, the volume 83 ml becomes $z = (83 - 35)/16 = 3$. A standard normal z-value just represents the number of standard deviations from the mean.

Critical Value

If we wanted to select out as abnormal all patients with prostate volumes in the 1% upper tail, that is, to identify the upper 1%, what would be our *critical*, or separating, value? By looking in Table A, we find that $\alpha = 0.01$ is paired with $z = 2.326$. This indicates that all patients with volumes more than about 2.3 standard deviations greater than the mean would be classified as abnormal. The actual critical volume will be $x = \mu + 2.3\sigma = 35 + 2.3 \times 16 = 71.8$ ml.

4.3. Confidence Interval on an Observation from an Individual Patient

Example

Now we can look at a confidence interval on Hct with actual numbers. Suppose, for example, we should find that healthy Hcts arise from a $N(47,3.6^2)$ probability distribution. [Recall that $N(47,3.6^2) = N(47,12.96)$ symbolizes a normal distribution with mean $\mu = 47$ and standard deviation $\sigma = 3.6$.] In Table 4.1, we see that, when $1 - \alpha$ (the area except for both tails) is 95%, the area is enclosed by

1.96 standard deviations above and below the mean. This implies that the upper limit of the healthy interval lies at $\mu + 1.96\sigma = 47 + 1.96 \times 3.6 = 54$. Similarly, the lower limit lies at $\mu - 1.96\sigma = 47 - 1.96 \times 3.6 = 40$. Our healthy interval is 40–54%. If we have a healthy patient, we would bet 95 to 5 (or 19 to 1) that his Hct will fall in the interval, which is to say we are 95% confident that it will include a healthy patient.

We can restate the form Eq. (4.1) for the Hct case as follows:

The probability
  that a randomly drawn Hct
    from $N(47,3.6^2)$
  is contained in the interval (40,54)
= 95%.

A briefer and easier way to say the same thing would be

$$P[40 < \text{Hct} < 54] = 0.95.$$

Caution

An important caveat is implicit in the preceding method, but it is so often overlooked that we should note it explicitly. If the frequency distribution involved is other than a normal curve, the so-often-seen "95% confidence contained in ±2 standard deviations" statement does NOT apply; the limits must be found from the appropriate distribution for that case.

4.4. CONCEPT OF A CONFIDENCE INTERVAL ON A DESCRIPTIVE STATISTIC

The Most Frequent Use of a Confidence Interval Is on a Mean

In the preceding section, we used a distribution of patients to obtain a confidence interval, in relation to which we interpreted an observation from a single patient. This observation may be thought of as a sample of size 1 from a population with known μ and σ. Although this often is useful in clinical practice, in research we are interested in the confidence interval on the estimate of a population statistic, most often a mean or a standard deviation.

Confidence Interval Defined

A random sample is a set of observations drawn from a population, in which the method of drawing is random. When we calculate a descriptive statistic from a random sample, we obtain an estimate of the equivalent population statistic. m and s are our best estimates of μ and σ, respectively. But what is the accuracy of these estimates? How much confidence do we have that the estimate is "on target?" We want an interval about an estimate that will tell us the width of the target. *A confidence interval is an interval about an estimate, based on its probability distribution, that expresses the confidence, or probability, that that interval contains the population statistic being estimated.*

General Form for a Confidence Interval on a Statistic

A general form may be given in the same pattern as Eq. (4.1):

The probability
  that a population statistic
    from a distribution of estimates of that statistic
  is contained in a specified interval
is given by
  the area of the distribution over that interval. (4.2)

Common Form for a Confidence Interval on a Statistic

Any estimate of a statistic from a random sample follows a probability distribution. We have already noted that a sample mean follows a normal distribution, and a sample variance follows a chi-square distribution. The estimate usually will be toward the center of the distribution, with only the rare cases lying in the tails. To express the confidence, we find the critical values that separate the tails from the main body of the distribution; we are confident that the interval between these critical values contains the population statistic to the extent of the proportion of the curve contained in the main body between the tail areas. The concept in Eq. (4.2) usually is written in the following format:

$$\text{P[lower critical value} < \text{population statistic} < \text{upper critical value]} = 1 - \alpha, \tag{4.3}$$

which implies that the interval defined by the critical values, excluding α proportion of the curve, will enclose the population statistic with probability $1 - \alpha$.

One Tail Is Sometimes Used

Whereas most confidence intervals are formed as intervals excluding both tails, an occasional case occurs in which we want to exclude only one tail. This option is examined further in Chapter 12.

4.5. CONFIDENCE INTERVAL ON A MEAN, KNOWN STANDARD DEVIATION

Confidence Interval Example

In Section 4.2, we took the 296 non-BPH prostate volumes as a population with $\mu = 35$ ml and $\alpha = 16$ ml. We also know from Sections 2.8 and 2.9 that a sample mean m is distributed normal and that the population standard deviation of the sample mean of m (SEM), σ_m, is $\sigma/\sqrt{n}$.

Suppose we did not know μ, but wanted to describe it as well as possible from the sample of 10 volumes in Table DB1.1. We would estimate μ by calculating m (=32.73 ml), we would find σ_m ($=16/\sqrt{10} = 5.06$ ml), and then we would use these calculations to put a confidence interval on μ.

To find a 95% confidence interval with 2.5% of unusual cases in each tail, we find the end points of the interval as $m \pm 1.96\sigma_m = 32.73 \pm 1.96 \times 5.06 = 22.81$ and 42.65 ml. In the format of Eq. (4.3),

$$\text{P}[22.81 < \mu < 42.65] = 0.95.$$

We are 95% confident that the population mean is included in the interval 22.81–42.65 ml; and, indeed, the population mean of 36.47 ml is so included.

Method for 95% Confidence Interval

If we want 95% confidence, we look in Table A (or Table 4.1) for 0.950 under "two-tailed $1-\alpha$ (area except both tails)." To its left in the first column, i.e., under "z (no. std. deviations to right of mean)," we find 1.960. Thus, our critical values that include 95% of the curve are the sample mean m plus and minus 1.96 times σ_m, the standard deviation of m. (Recall that σ_m also is called the population standard error of the mean or SEM.) In symbols,

$$\text{P}[m - 1.96 \times \sigma_m < \mu < m + 1.96 \times \sigma_m] = 0.95. \tag{4.4}$$

Method for Other Confidence Levels

For any other level of confidence, e.g., 90% or 99%, for a sample mean with a known population standard deviation, we follow the same pattern, just looking in the 0.90 or 0.99 row in Table A (or Table 4.1). We may express this in general terms by denoting the confidence as $1 - \alpha$, so that $\alpha/2$ denotes the area in each tail. By substituting $1 - \alpha$ for 95% and $z_{1-\alpha/2}$ for 1.96 in Eq. (4.4), we obtain the more general confidence statement:

$$P[m - z_{1-\alpha/2}\sigma_m < \mu < m + z_{1-\alpha/2}\sigma_m] = 1 - \alpha \qquad (4.5)$$

Additional Example

An orthopedist is experimenting with the use of nitronox as an anesthetic in the treatment of children's arm fractures.[21,22] He anticipates that it may provide an attractively short procedure. He treats $n = 50$ children and records the treatment time in minutes. He finds $m = 26.26$ min and $\sigma = 7.13$ min. (The sample size is large enough to use the calculated standard deviation as σ.) He wants a 95% confidence interval on mean treatment time. He will require $\sigma_m = \sigma/\sqrt{n} = 7.13/\sqrt{50} = 1.008$ min. From Eq. (4.4),

$$\begin{aligned} &P[m - 1.96 \times \sigma_m < \mu < m + 1.96 \times \sigma_m] \\ &\quad = P[26.26 - 1.96 \times 1.008 < \mu < 26.26 + 1.96 \times 1.008] \\ &\quad = P[24.28 < \mu < 28.24] = 0.95. \end{aligned}$$

He is 95% confident that the mean time to treat lies between about 24 and 28 min.

4.6. The *t* Distribution

Why We Need *t*

Often we need to look at a confidence interval on a mean when we do not know the population standard deviation and must estimate it from a small sample. In this case, the normal distribution does not apply. We need the *t* distribution, introduced in Section 2.8. This is a distribution similar in appearance to the normal, but giving a slightly wider confidence interval to compensate for lack of accuracy in the standard deviation. Recall that the smaller the sample, the wider the distribution, so that the particular member of the family of *t* distributions to be used depends on the sample size or a variation of it, the degrees of freedom (*df*). Let us examine the *t* distribution in more detail.

The Nature of t

The t distribution is a symmetric, bell-shaped distribution very much like the standard normal distribution but with a larger standard deviation. As in the standard normal, t is given by the deviation of the observation from the mean divided by the standard deviation. As the t is used for smaller samples in which the mean and standard deviation are estimated, $t = (x - m)/s$. In methods of inference using t involving one sample, the number of degrees of freedom (df) equals the sample size (n) less one, or $df = n - 1$. In inferences involving two samples, $df = n - 2$. When the number of degrees of freedom is infinite, the t *is* the standard normal. As the number of degrees of freedom grows smaller, the t distribution grows wider. Because the t distribution is similar to the normal distribution except for an adjustment for *df*, methods of inference for small samples using small sample standard deviations follow logic identical to the normal case, except that we remember to look up the areas under the tail for the appropriate *df*.

The t Pictured

Figure 4.2 shows a t distribution for 9 *df* with 2.5% of the area under the curve's right tail shaded. Note that it is similar in appearance to the normal distribution depicted in Fig. 4.1, except that the 2.5% critical value lies $2.262s$ (sample standard deviations) to the right of the mean rather than 1.96σ (population standard deviations).

Table of t Probabilities

Table B, in the back of the book, contains selected distances (t) away from the mean for the most commonly used one- and two-tailed α and $1 - \alpha$ areas under the curve for various *df*. These t-values correspond to italicized z-values in Table A. Table 4.2 shows a portion of Table B, which may be used to follow the examples.

Example of Confidence Interval for an Individual Patient Using t

Let us follow the prostate volume example as in the preceding section on the standard normal distribution, except that we shall use m and s from the small sample of Table DB1.1 rather than μ and σ. (Actually, a small skewed sample like this would better be treated by the rank-order methods of Chapter 14, but

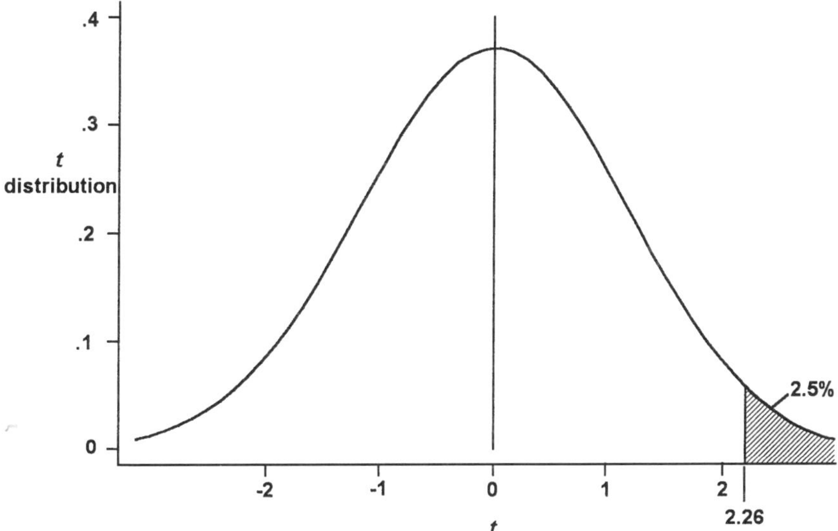

Figure 4.2 A t distribution shown with $\alpha = 2.5\%$ and its corresponding t for 9 *df*. The α shown is the area under the curve to the right of a given or calculated t. For a two-tailed computation, α is doubled in order to include the symmetric opposite tail. As pictured for 9 *df*, 2.5% of the area lies to the right of $t = 2.26$. For a two-tailed use, the frequently used $\alpha = 5\%$ lies outside the interval $\pm t$, leaving 95% of the area under the curve between the tails.

the example will serve to illustrate t.) For the 10 volumes, $m = 32.7$ ml and $s = 15.9$ ml. Because we are dealing with only one sample, $df = n - 1 = 9$. We need look only at the $df = 9$ row in Table 4.2. The prostate volume 59 ml yields $t = (59 - 32.7)/15.9 = 1.65$, which places it 1.65 standard deviations above the mean. This lies between 1.38, which falls under $\alpha = 0.10$ on the 9 *df* row, and 1.83, which falls under $\alpha = 0.05$. We can say that between 5% and 10% of patients will have volumes greater than this patient. Similarly, the 83-ml prostate yields $t = 3.16$, which falls between $\alpha = 0.01$ and $\alpha = 0.005$; less than 1% of patients will have volumes this large. We do not tabulate t for as many possible values as we do the standard normal, because a full table would be required for every possible *df*. We can calculate on a computer $\alpha = 0.067$ for $t = 1.65$ and $\alpha = 0.006$ for $t = 3.16$ if we need them.

Critical Value for t

The critical value above which 1% of prostate volumes occur is found by using the 9 *df* t-value in the one-tailed $\alpha = 0.01$ column, viz., $t = 2.82$. We calculate the

Table 4.2

Segment of *t* Distribution Table B[a]

One-tailed α (right tail area)	0.10	0.05	0.025	0.01	0.005	0.001	0.0005
One-tailed $1-\alpha$ (except right tail)	0.90	0.95	0.975	0.99	0.995	0.999	0.9995
Two-tailed α (area both tails)	0.20	0.10	0.05	0.02	0.01	0.002	0.001
Two-tailed $1-\alpha$ (except both tails)	0.80	0.90	0.95	0.98	0.99	0.998	0.999
$df = 5$	1.476	2.015	2.571	3.365	4.032	5.893	6.859
9	1.383	1.833	2.262	2.281	3.250	4.297	4.781
10	1.372	1.812	2.228	2.764	3.169	4.144	4.587
14	1.345	1.761	2.145	2.624	2.977	3.787	4.140
20	1.325	1.725	2.086	2.528	2.845	3.552	3.850
30	1.310	1.697	2.042	2.457	2.750	3.385	3.646
40	1.303	1.684	2.021	2.423	2.704	3.307	3.551
60	1.296	1.671	2.000	2.390	2.660	3.232	3.460
100	1.290	1.660	1.984	2.364	2.626	3.174	3.390
∞	1.282	1.645	1.960	2.326	2.576	3.090	3.291

[a] Selected distances (t) to the right of the mean are given for various degrees of freedom (df) and for (a) one-tailed α, area under the curve in the positive tail; (b) one-tailed $1-\alpha$, area under all except the positive tail; (c) two-tailed α, areas combined for both positive and negative tails; and (d) two-tailed $1-\alpha$, area under all except the two tails.

volume at 2.82 standard deviations above the mean, i.e., $m + 2.82s = 32.7 + 2.82 \times 15.9 = 77.54$ ml. We expect that no more than 1% of volumes will exceed 77.5 ml.

4.7. CONFIDENCE INTERVAL ON A MEAN, ESTIMATED STANDARD DEVIATION

Example

Suppose we wanted to use the 10 data from Table DB1.1 to put a 95% confidence interval on the population mean prostate volume. We have found that the 10 prostate volumes in Table DB1.1 have $m = 32.73$ ml and $s = 15.92$ ml. We calculate $s_m = s/\sqrt{n} = 15.92/3.16 = 1.87$. To find the t value for 95% confidence, we look under 0.95 for "two-tailed $1-\alpha$ (except both tails)" in Table 4.2 for 9 *df* to find $t_{1-\alpha} = 2.262$. Because we had to use a sample SEM rather than that for the population, the confidence interval based on the t distribution extends more than two (exactly 1.96) SEMs above and below the mean, as in the interval based on the normal distribution. By substituting for m and s_m in the formula introduced in the next paragraph,

$$\begin{aligned} &\mathrm{P}[m - t_{1-\alpha/2}s_m < \mu < m + t_{1-\alpha/2}s_m] \\ &\quad = \mathrm{P}[32.73 - 2.262 \times 1.87 < \mu < 32.73 + 2.262 \times 1.87] \\ &\quad = \mathrm{P}[28.50 < \mu < 36.96] = 0.95. \end{aligned}$$

We note from the first table in DB1 that $\mu = 36.47$ ml, which the interval includes.

Method

More often than not in medical applications we do not know σ and must estimate it by a small sample s. Finding a confidence interval on μ using m and s follows the same logic as using m and σ, except that we use a t table rather than a normal table. Because the t distribution has a greater spread than the normal, the confidence interval will be slightly wider. If we want 95% confidence, we look under 0.95 for "two-tailed $1 - \alpha$ (except both tails)" in Table B for the appropriate *df*. By replacing the σ and z symbols in Eq. (4.5) with the equivalent s and t symbols, we obtain

$$\mathrm{P}[m - t_{1-\alpha/2}s_m < \mu < m + t_{1-\alpha/2}s_m] = 1 - \alpha. \tag{4.6}$$

(We know from Sections 2.8 and 4.6 that m follows a t distribution when we use s instead of σ and from Section 2.9 that the sample standard deviation of m, s_m, is $s/\sqrt{n}$. Recall that s_m also is called the sample standard error of the mean or sample SEM.) A treatment of one-sided confidence statements may be found in Chapter 12.

Additional Example

A dermatologist is studying the efficacy of tretinoin in treating $n = 15$ women's post partum abdominal stretch marks.[68] Tretinoin was used on a randomly chosen side of the abdomen and a placebo on the other. Neither patient nor investigator knew which side was medicated. The patient rated the improvement on each side on a 10-cm-long visual analogue scale (VAS), and ratings were recorded as a reading between 0 and 10. The difference, treated-side rating minus untreated-side rating, indicating the excess improvement due to tretinoin over the placebo, was calculated. $m = -0.33$ and $s = 2.46$. $s_m = s/\sqrt{n} = 2.46/\sqrt{15} = 0.64$. From Table B or 4.2, the 95% t-value for 14 *df* is 2.145. When these values are substituted in Eq. (4.6), the confidence interval evolves as

$$\begin{aligned} &\mathrm{P}[m - t_{1-\alpha/2}s_m < \mu < m + t_{1-\alpha/2}s_m] \\ &\quad = \mathrm{P}[-0.33 - 2.145 \times 0.64 < \mu < -0.33 + 2.145 \times 0.64] \\ &\quad = \mathrm{P}[-1.70 < \mu < 1.04] = 1 - \alpha. \end{aligned}$$

The dermatologist is 95% confident that the mean stretch-mark improvement lies between -1.7 and $+1.0$. The sample average is negative (untreated side better), the confidence interval includes 0, and the upper confidence bound of 1 is not very important clinically; evidence is insufficient to conclude a benefit from tretinoin in this particular medical application.

4.8. THE CHI-SQUARE DISTRIBUTION

Why We Need Chi-Square

Although the mean is the statistic upon which we most frequently focus, we sometimes do focus on measures of variability. Suppose the amount of active ingredient in a medicinal capsule is crucial: less than $\mu - c$ mg fails to work and more than $\mu + c$ mg damages the patient. We need a confidence interval on c, a multiple of the standard deviation, to be confident that the probable variability in content is not too large. Because the standard deviation is a square root, which is difficult to work with mathematically, confidence intervals on variability are found on the variance s^2 and afterward converted to standard deviation units. As noted in Section 2.8, the sample variance s^2, drawn randomly from a normal population, when multiplied by the constant df/σ^2 follows a chi-square distribution, so that we need chi-square to find confidence intervals on the variance. (*df* for simple confidence intervals will be $n - 1$.)

Chi-Square Pictured

Remember that the chi-square, being composed of squares, cannot be negative, but can grow to any large size. Thus, it is like a lop-sided bell curve with the right tail stretched out (right-skewed). Figure 4.3 shows the chi-square distribution for 9 *df*.

Tables of Chi-Square

Table C, in the back of the book, provides the chi-square values that yield commonly used values of α, i.e., the probability that a randomly drawn value from the distribution lies in the tail demarked by the tabulated chi-square value. Table 4.3 shows a segment of Table C, which may be used to follow the examples. Because the chi-square distribution is asymmetric, we cannot take an area in one tail and expect the other tail to be the same. Finding areas in a tail is much the same as in the t: the desired area in the tail specifies the column, the *df* specifies

Table 4.3
Segment of Chi-Square Distribution, Right Tail, Table C[a]

α (area in right tail)	0.10	0.05	0.025	0.01	0.005	0.001	0.0005
$1-\alpha$ (except right tail)	0.90	0.95	0.975	0.99	0.995	0.999	0.9995
$df = 1$	2.71	3.84	5.02	6.63	7.88	10.81	12.13
3	6.25	7.81	9.35	11.34	12.84	16.26	17.75
5	9.24	11.07	12.83	15.08	16.75	20.52	22.15
7	12.02	14.07	16.01	18.47	20.28	24.35	26.02
9	14.68	16.92	19.02	21.67	23.59	27.86	29.71
10	15.99	18.31	20.48	23.21	25.19	29.58	31.46
15	22.31	25.00	27.49	30.57	32.81	37.71	39.73
20	28.41	31.41	34.17	37.57	39.99	45.31	47.46
25	34.38	37.65	40.65	44.31	46.93	52.65	51.93
30	40.26	43.77	46.98	50.89	53.68	59.68	62.23
40	51.80	55.76	59.34	63.69	66.76	73.39	76.11
50	63.17	67.51	71.42	76.16	79.50	86.66	89.56
60	74.40	79.08	83.30	88.38	91.96	99.58	102.66
100	118.50	124.34	129.56	135.81	140.16	149.41	153.11

[a] Selected χ^2 values (distances above zero) are given for various degrees of freedom and for (a) α, the right tail area under the curve, and (b) $1-\alpha$, the area under all except the right tail.

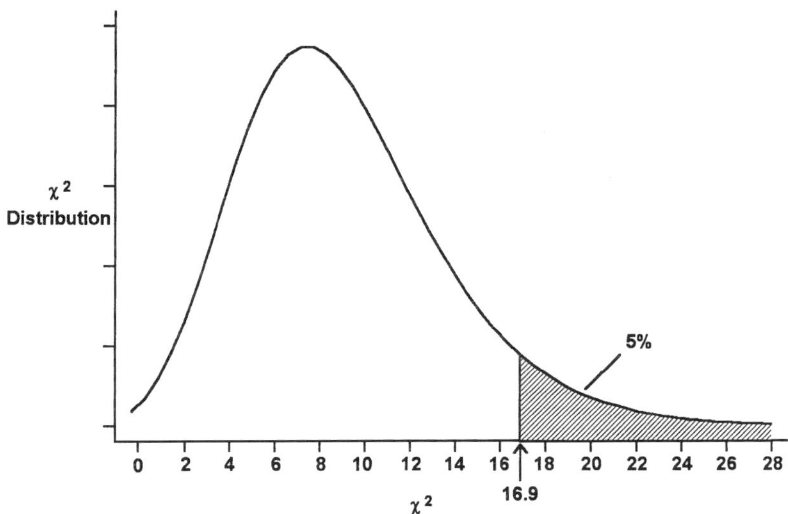

Figure 4.3 The χ^2 (chi-square) distribution for 9 *df* with a 5% α and its corresponding chi-square value of 16.9. The α probability is shown as the shaded area under the curve to the right of a critical chi-square, in this case representing a 5% probability that a value drawn randomly from the distribution will exceed a critical chi-square of 16.9.

the row, and the *critical* chi-square value (the value demarking the tail area) lies at the row–column intersection. Table C provides chi-square values for the more commonly used right tail, Table D, the left tail.

Example

We saw that $\sigma = 16.35$ ml for the population of prostate volumes (excluding known BPH). How large a standard deviation s would we have to observe in a sample of size 10 to have a 5% or less probability that it could have been so large by chance alone? From either Table 4.3 or Fig. 4.3, the critical chi-square value (the value demarking the tail area) for a 5% tail for $n - 1 = 9$ *df* is $\chi^2 = 16.9$. That is to say,

$$\chi^2 = df \times s^2/\sigma^2 \quad \text{or} \quad 16.9 = 9s^2/16.35^2 = 0.033667s^2.$$

We solve to find $s^2 = 501.98$ or $s = 22.40$. A sample standard deviation exceeding 22.4 ml would have less than 5% probability of occurring by chance alone.

4.9. CONFIDENCE INTERVAL ON A VARIANCE OR STANDARD DEVIATION

Example

Using the 10 prostate volumes from Table DB1.1, what is a 95% confidence interval on the population standard deviation, σ? We have calculated $s = 15.92$ ml which has $n - 1 = 9$ *df*. We know the probability distribution of s^2 but not of s, so we shall find the interval on the population variance, σ^2, and take the square root. $s^2 = 15.92^2 = 253.4464$. By looking in Table C or Table 4.3 under the right tail area $= 0.025$ for 9 *df*, we find 19.02. Similarly, in Table D, under left tail area $= 0.025$ for 9 *df*, we find 2.70. By substituting these values in the formula for confidence limits on a variance, Eq. (4.7), we find

$$\begin{aligned} &\mathrm{P}\left[s^2 \times df/\chi^2_R < \sigma^2 < s^2 \times df/\chi^2_L\right] \\ &= \mathrm{P}[253.45 \times 9/19.02 < \sigma^2 < 253.45 \times 9/2.70] \\ &= \mathrm{P}[119.92 < \sigma^2 < 844.83] = 0.95. \end{aligned}$$

By taking the square root within the brackets, we obtain

$$\mathrm{P}[10.95 < \sigma < 29.07] = 0.95.$$

We note from the first table of DB1 that the population standard deviation (excluding known BPH to make the distribution more symmetric) is 16.35 ml, falling well within the confidence interval.

Method

We know (from Section 2.8) that sample variance s^2 drawn randomly from a normal population is distributed as chi-square (multiplied by the constant σ^2/df). We make a confidencc-type statement on s^2 from this relationship, excluding 2.5% in each tail as usual, and use some algebra to put it in the form of a statement on σ^2, arriving at the following expression:

$$\mathrm{P}\left[s^2 \times df/\chi^2_{\mathrm{R}} < \sigma^2 < s^2 \times df/\chi^2_{\mathrm{L}}\right] = 0.95, \tag{4.7}$$

where χ^2_{R} is the critical value for the right tail found from Table C and χ^2_{L} is that for the left found from Table D. We have to calculate separately a critical value for each tail of the chi-square distribution (using both Tables C and D) because the distribution is not symmetric like the normal or t. For an exact chi-square, the sample must be taken from a normal distribution. However, if the population is at all close to normal, even roughly bell-shaped, the approximation is close enough to use this confidence method.

Confidence on σ

To find the confidence on σ rather than σ^2, we just take the square root of the components within the brackets.

Confidence Other Than 95%

We are not confined to 95% confidence, of course. For any general $1 - \alpha$ confidence, we find the two critical chi-square values that cut off $\alpha/2$ in each tail, χ^2_{L} for the left and χ^2_{R} for the right.

Additional Example

We are investigating the reliability of a certain brand of tympanic thermometer (temperature measured by a sensor inserted into the patient's ear).[55] The standard deviation will give us an indication of its precision. We want an upper 95% confidence limit on this precision, that is, a value of the standard deviation that would be exceeded no more than 5 times in 100. Sixteen readings (°F) were taken on a healthy patient at intervals of 1 min. Data were 95.8, 97.4, 99.3, 97.1, ..., yielding $s = 1.23$. $s^2 = 1.23^2 = 1.51$. We use the right side of Eq. (4.7), i.e., $\mathrm{P}[\sigma^2 < s^2 \times df/\chi^2_{\mathrm{L}}] = 0.95$. The chi-square value from Table D for 95% area except the left tail for 15 *df* is $\chi^2_L = 7.26$. We find

$$P[\sigma^2 < s^2 \times df/\chi^2_L] = P[\sigma^2 < 1.51 \times 15/7.26] = P[\sigma^2 < 3.12] = 0.95.$$

By taking the square root within the bracket, we obtain

$$P[\sigma < 1.77] = 0.95.$$

We are 95% sure that the standard deviation of this thermometer will not exceed 1.8°F.

4.10. OTHER FREQUENTLY SEEN CONFIDENCE INTERVALS AND PROBABILITIES

WHAT PROBABILITIES ARE POSSIBLE?

Any datum that has a component of chance in its selection follows some probability distribution or another, although very often we do not know what it is. The number and forms of probability distributions are unlimited. Fortunately, in the common medical applications of statistics, we meet only a few of these distributions. In this book, we need only six, which were introduced in Section 2.8. The normal, t, and χ^2 have been examined in this chapter, and the other three, F, binomial, and Poisson, are treated in Chapter 11.

WHAT CONFIDENCE INTERVALS ARE POSSIBLE?

A confidence interval may be placed on any statistic for which the probability distribution is known. Fortunately there are only a few statistics of frequent interest in medical statistics. Confidence intervals on an observation from an individual patient, on μ using σ, on μ using s, and on σ itself, have been examined in this chapter. Others used very commonly are confidence intervals on proportions and on correlation coefficients, which are treated in Chapter 12.

CHAPTER EXERCISES

4.1. In DB12, the age distribution of patients undergoing carinal resections is approximately normal, with mean = 47.8 years and standard deviation = 14.8 years. The sample is large enough to take the standard deviation as if it were the population σ. You have a 12-year-old patient whose tracheal carina requires resection. Does this patient fall within a 95% confidence limit of age for individual patients, or is this patient improbably young?

4.2. The orthopedist in the nitronox example at the end of Section 4.5 also is interested in the patients' pain, which he has measured using the CHEOPS rating form. For his $n = 50$ patients, $m = 9.16$ and $\sigma = 2.04$. Find the (a) 95%, (b) 99%, and (c) 90% confidence interval on mean pain rating.

4.3. Among the indicators of patient condition following pyloromyotomy (correction of stenotic pylorus) in neonates is time (hours) to full feeding.[16] A surgeon wants to place a 95% confidence interval on mean time to full feeding. He has readings from $n = 20$ infants. Some of his data are 3.50, 4.52, 3.03, 14.53, ... He calculates $m = 6.56$ hr and $s = 4.57$ hr. What is his 95% confidence interval?

4.4. An emergency medicine physician samples the heart rate of $n = 8$ patients following a particular type of trauma. She finds the mean $m = 67.75$ bpm and the standard deviation $s = 9.04$ bpm. What is her 95% confidence interval on the mean?

4.5. The surgeon referenced in Exercise 4.3 is concerned about the variability of time to full feeding in neonates. Even if the mean is satisfactory, if the variability is too large, the outlying neonates on the longer side of the scale would be at risk. Recall that $n = 20$, $m = 6.56$ hr, and $s = 4.57$. Establish 95% confidence intervals on (a) the variance and (b) the standard deviation.

4.6. The ED physician of Exercise 4.4 is concerned not only about the average heart rate of the trauma patients, but also about the variability. Even if the mean is satisfactory, if the standard deviation is too large, outlying patients would be at risk. Recall that $n = 8, m = 67.75$ bpm, and $s = 9.04$ bpm. Establish 95% confidence intervals on (a) the variance and (b) the standard deviation.

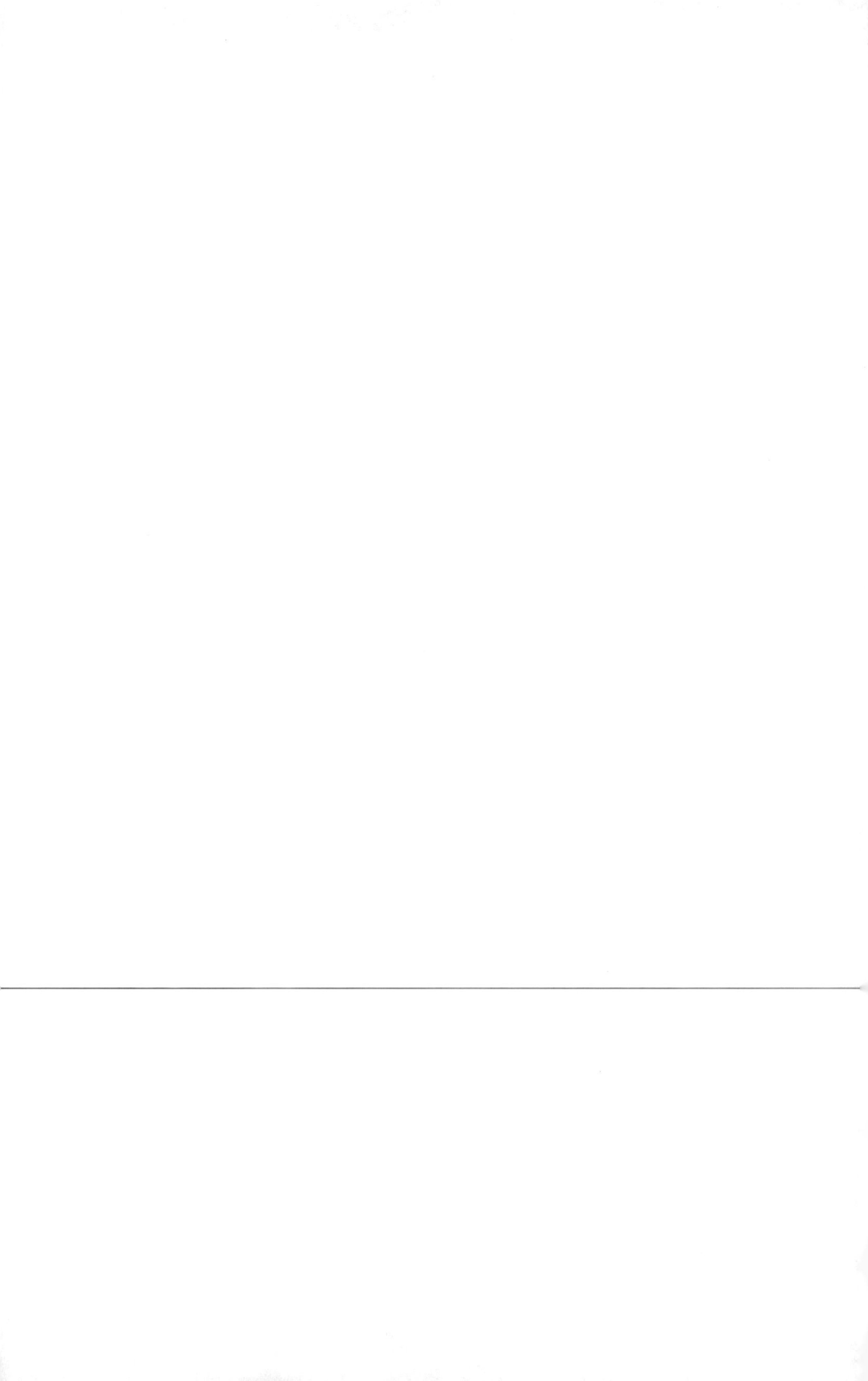

Chapter 5

Concept and Practice in Hypothesis Testing

5.1. HYPOTHESES IN INFERENCE

A Clinical Hypothesis

Suppose we want to know whether a new antibiotic reduces the time for a particular type of lesion to heal. We already know the mean time μ to heal in the population, i.e., the general public, without an antibiotic. We take a sample of lesion patients from the same population, randomizing the selection to assure representativeness (Section 1.6), and measure the time to heal when treated with the antibiotic. We compare our sample mean time to heal, say m_a (a for antibiotic), with μ. Our *clinical hypothesis* (not statistical hypothesis) is that the antibiotic helps, i.e., $m_a < \mu$. To be sure that our comparison gives us a believable answer, we go through the formal sequence of steps that composes the scientific method.

Decision Theory Introduced

In very general terms, the decision theory portion of the scientific method uses a decision function (mathematically expressed strategy), which includes explicit costs (not just monetary costs) of observation and losses due to less-than-optimum decisions, to reach a conclusion. In most cases, the decision problem is expressed as a strategy to select one of a number of options on the basis of a criterion of minimum loss. The loss might include risk of making a wrong decision, loss to the patient (financial cost as well as cost in pain, lowered quality of life, or even death), and/or financial or time cost to the investigator–institution. In the industrial, business, and military fields, applied decision theory most often has come under the heading of operations research (British: operational analysis). In medicine, some forms of applied decision theory using multiple sources of loss in the decision strategy are appearing under the heading of outcomes analysis, which will be introduced in Chapter 8.

Decision Making by Testing a Statistical Hypothesis

We noted in Chapter 1 that medicine's major use of statistical inference is in making conclusions about a population on the basis of a sample from that population. Most often, we form statistical hypotheses, usually in a form different from the clinical hypothesis, about the population. We use sample data to test these hypotheses. This procedure is a special case of two-option decision theory in which the decision strategy uses only one loss, that of the risk (probability) of making an erroneous decision. More specifically, the cost is measured as the known controlled probability of each of two possible errors: choosing the first hypothesis when the second is true and choosing the second when the first is true.

How We Get from Observed Data to a Test

From the data, we calculate a value, called a *statistic*, that will answer the statistical question implied by the hypothesis. For example, to answer the time-to-heal question, we compare the statistic m_{a} (mean time to heal using the antibiotic) with the parameter μ (mean time to heal for the population). Such *statistics* are calculated from data that follow probability distributions, and therefore the statistics themselves will follow a probability distribution. We noted in Section 2.8 that a mean, the time-to-heal statistic here, is distributed (at least approximately) normal. Areas under the tails of such distributions provide probabilities, or risks, of error associated with "yes" or "no" answers to the question asked. Estimation of these error probabilities from the sample data constitutes the test.

The Null Hypothesis

The question to be answered must be asked in the form of a hypothesis. This *statistical hypothesis*, which is different from the clinical hypothesis, must be stated carefully in order to relate to a statistic, especially so because the statistic must have a known or derivable probability distribution. In most cases, we start with a *null hypothesis*, which says that our sample is no different (hence, "null") from known information. (The hypothesis to be tested must be based on the known distribution, in this case that of the established healing time, as it cannot be based on the unknown antibiotic healing time. This is explained further later.) We hypothesize that the population mean time to heal with an antibiotic, μ_a (which we estimate by our sample mean, m_a), is no different from the mean time to heal without the antibiotic.

The Alternate Hypothesis

After forming the null hypothesis, we form an *alternate hypothesis* stating the nature of the difference if it should appear. Hypotheses in words may be long and subject to misunderstanding. For clarity, they usually are expressed in symbols, where the symbols are carefully defined. The null hypothesis usually is symbolized H_0 and the alternate, H_1.

Forms the Hypotheses Can Take

To answer the time-to-heal question, we hypothesized that the population mean μ_a from which our sample is drawn is no different from μ. Our alternative hypothesis is formed logically as *not* H_0. In this case, we truly believe that the antibiotic *cannot lengthen* the healing, so that the alternative to no difference is shortened healing. Thus, our statistical hypotheses are

$$H_0\colon \mu_a = \mu \quad \text{and} \quad H_1\colon \mu_a < \mu. \tag{5.1}$$

The alternative here is known as a *one-sided* hypothesis. If we believed that the antibiotic could either lengthen *or* shorten the healing, we would have used a *two-sided* hypothesis, $H_1\colon \mu_a \neq \mu$. More generally, when a decision is made about using or not using a medical treatment, the sidedness is chosen from the decision possibilities, not physical possibilities. If we will alter treatment only for significance in the positive tail and not in the negative tail, a one-tailed test is appropriate.

Why the Null Hypothesis Is Null

It may seem a bit strange at first that our primary statistical hypothesis says that there is no difference, even when, according to our clinical hypothesis, we believe there is a difference and might even prefer to see one. The reason lies in the ability to calculate errors in decision making. When the hypothesis says that our sample is no different from known information, we have available a known probability distribution and therefore can calculate the area under the distribution associated with the erroneous decision: a difference is concluded when in truth there is no difference.

This area under the probability curve provides us with the risk of a false positive. The alternative hypothesis, on the other hand, says just that our known distribution is not the correct distribution, not what that alternative distribution is. Without sufficient information about the distribution associated with the alternative hypothesis, we cannot calculate the area under the distribution associated with the erroneous decision: no difference exists when there is one, i.e., the risk of a false negative.

A Numerical Example

As a numerical example, consider the sample of 10 Table DB1.1 prostate volumes. Suppose we want to decide whether the population mean μ_v from which the sample was drawn is the same as the mean of the population of 291 remaining volumes. Because the mean of sample volumes may be either larger or smaller than the population mean, the alternative is a two-sided hypothesis. Our hypotheses are

$$H_0: \mu_v = \mu \quad \text{and} \quad H_1: \mu_v \neq \mu. \tag{5.2}$$

m estimates the unknown μ_v, and, if H_0 is true, m is distributed $N(\mu, \sigma_m^2)$. [μ is the mean and σ the standard deviation of the 291 volumes, and σ_m is the SEM $\sigma/\sqrt{n}$ (Section 2.9).] Standardization of m provides a statistic z, which we know to be distributed N(0,1), that is,

$$z = \frac{m - \mu}{\sigma_m} = \frac{m - \mu}{\sigma/\sqrt{n}}. \tag{5.3}$$

We know that $m = 32.73$ ml, $\mu = 36.60$ ml, and $\sigma = 18.12$ ml; $n = 10$ is the size of the sample we are testing. By substituting in Eq. (5.3), we find $z = -0.675$, i.e., the sample mean is about two-thirds of a (population) standard deviation below the population mean. The following small excerpt from Table A shows the two-tailed probabilities for the 0.60 and 0.70 standard deviations.

z (no. std. deviations to right of mean)	Two-tailed α (area in both tails)
0.60	0.548
0.70	0.484

The calculated z lying between these two values tells us that the probability of finding a randomly drawn normal observation more than 0.675σ away from the mean is a little more than 0.484, or about 0.5. We conclude that we have a 50% chance of being wrong if we decide that the sample mean did not arise from this distribution. There is not enough evidence to conclude a difference. This result may be visualized on a standard normal distribution as in Fig. 5.1.

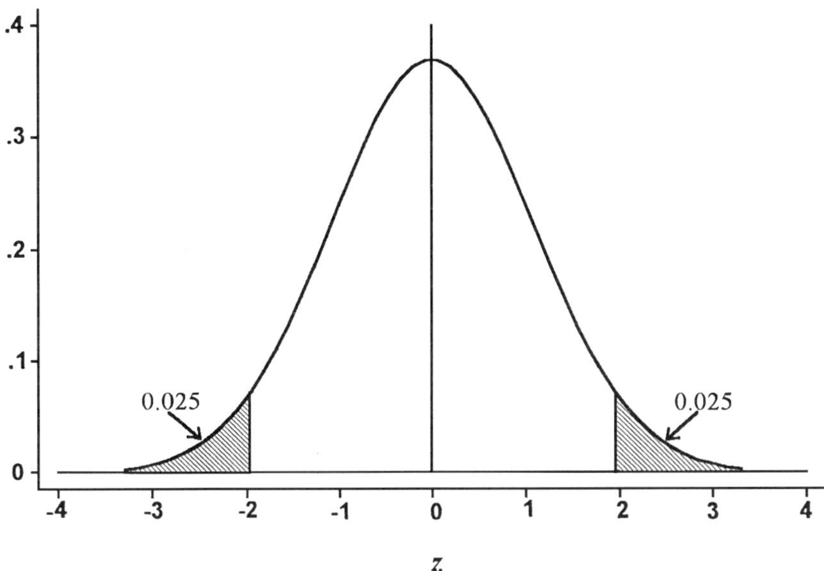

Figure 5.1 A standard normal distribution showing 2.5% tail areas adding to 5% risk of error from concluding that a random value did not arise from this distribution (risk of a false positive). The 0.025 area under the right tail represents the probability that a value drawn randomly from this distribution will be 1.96σ or farther above the mean.

The Most Common Types of Statistic Being Tested and Their Associated Probability Distributions

We have just seen how a hypothesis having a general pattern of a sample mean divided by a known population SEM follows a standard normal distribution. In the same fashion, a hypothesis about a mean when the standard deviation must be estimated (the population standard deviation is not known) has the general pattern, namely, a sample mean divided by a *sample* SEM, so that it follows a *t* distribution. A hypothesis about a standard deviation uses a variance, which follows a chi-square distribution. And finally, a hypothesis comparing two standard deviations uses a ratio of two variances, which follows an F distribution. Thus, a very large number of statistical questions can be tested using just these four well-documented probability distributions.

Confidence Intervals Are Closely Related

Confidence intervals procedurally are closely related to hypothesis tests, in that null and alternate hypotheses could state that the interval does and does not, respectively, enclose the population mean. However, the use differs: a confidence interval is used to estimate, not to test.

Assumptions in Hypothesis Testing

In Section 2.7, it was shown that various assumptions underlie hypothesis testing and that the result of a test is not correct when these assumptions are violated. Furthermore, the methods do not tell the user when a violation occurs or by how much the results are affected. Results appear regardless. It is up to the user to verify that the assumptions are satisfied. The assumptions required vary from test to test, and which apply are noted along with each test methodology. The most common assumptions are that errors are normal and independent one from another and, for multiple samples, that variances are equal.

The Meaning of "Error"

An "error" in an observation does not refer to an error in the sense of a mistake, but rather to the deviation of the individual observation from the typical. The term error, and sometimes the term residual, is used for historical reasons; if you find the term "error" in referring to observations confusing in your reading, read "deviation from typical" instead.

The Assumption of Independence of Errors

When a set of observations is taken, we assume that knowledge of the error on one tells us nothing about the error on another, i.e., that *the errors are independent one from another*. Suppose we take temperature readings on a ward of patients with bacterial infections. We expect them to be in the 38–40°C region, averaging, say, 39°C. We assume that finding a 39.5°C reading on one patient, i.e., an error of 0.5°C above average, tells us nothing about the deviation from average we will find on the patient in the next bed. How might such an assumption be violated? If the ward had been filled starting from the far end and working nearer as patients arrived, the patients at the far end might be improving and have lower fever, so that knowledge of the temperature error of a particular patient might indeed give us a clue about the temperature error in the patient in the next bed. The assured independence of errors is a major reason for incorporating randomness in sampling. This assumption is made in almost all statistical tests.

The Assumption of Normality of Errors

Second, many, but not all, tests also assume that *these errors are drawn from a normal distribution*. A major exception is rank-order (or nonparametric) tests. Indeed, the avoidance of this assumption is one of the primary reasons to use rank-order tests.

The Assumption of Equality of Standard Deviations

The third frequently made assumption occurs when the means of two or more samples are tested. It is assumed that *the standard deviations of the errors are the same*. This assumption is stated more often as requiring equality of variances rather than of standard deviations.

5.2. ERROR PROBABILITIES

Posing an Example

We have a mean of PSA readings from a patient group, and we want to compare it to the mean of healthy patients to predict the presence or absence of prostate cancer. The null hypothesis, H_0, states that cancer is absent, i.e., our new sample mean is no different from the healthy mean.

Type I (α) Error

The null hypothesis may be rejected when it should have been accepted; we conclude that our patients are not healthy when they are. Such an error is denoted a *Type I error*. Its probability of occurring by chance alone is denoted α. Formally, $\alpha = \text{Prob}[\text{rejecting } H_0 | H_0 \text{ true}]$ (read: "probability of rejecting H_0 given H_0 is true"). The conclusion of a difference when there is none is similar to the *false positive* of a clinical test. Properly, α is chosen before data are gathered so that the choice of critical value cannot be influenced by study results.

Type II (β) Error; Power of a Test

Alternatively, the null hypothesis may be accepted when it should have been rejected; we conclude that our patients are healthy when they are not. Such an error is denoted a *Type II error*. Its probability of occurring by chance alone is denoted β. Formally, $\beta = \text{Prob}[\text{accepting } H_0 | H_0 \text{ false}]$. The conclusion of no difference when there is one is similar to the *false negative* of a clinical test. $1 - \beta$ is the *power* of the test, which is referred to often in medical literature and is used especially when assessing the sample size required in a clinical study (introduced in Chapter 7).

p-Value

After the data have been gathered, new information is available: the value of the decision statistic, for example, the (standardized) difference between control and experimental means. The error of rejecting the null hypothesis when it is true that can now be estimated using sample data is termed the *p-value*. If the p-value is smaller than α, we reject the null hypothesis; otherwise, we do not have enough evidence to reject it. The size of the p-value can give a clue about the relationship of the null hypothesis to the data. A p-value near 0 or 1 leaves little doubt as to the conclusion to be drawn from the study, but a p-value close to α may suggest that further study is warranted. A listing of the actual p-value in a study result often adds information beyond just indicating a value greater or lesser than α. This issue is addressed further in the next section.

Relation among Truth, Decision, and Errors

Type of error depends on the relationship between decision and truth, as is depicted in Table 5.1.

Logical Steps in a Statistical Test

The logic of a statistical test used historically is the following: (a) We choose an α, the risk of Type I error, that we are willing to accept. (b) Because we know the distribution of the statistic we are using, e.g., z or t, we use a probability table

Table 5.1

Relationships among Types of Error and Their Probabilities as Dependent on the Decision and the Truth

		Decision	
		H_0 true	H_0 false
Truth	H_0 true	Correct decision True negative (Probability $1 - \alpha$)	Type I error False positive (Probability α)
	H_0 false	Type II error False negative (Probability β)	Correct decision True positive (Probability $1 - \beta$)

to find the value of the statistic greater than which would yield such an error, i.e., its *critical value*. (c) We take our sample and calculate the value of the statistic arising from it. (d) If our statistic falls on one side of the critical value, we do not have the evidence to reject H_0; on the other side, we do reject H_0.

The Critical Value and the Errors Illustrated

Illustrative null and alternate distributions and their α and β values are shown in Fig. 5.2.

A Reality in Testing

We usually know or have reason to assume the nature of the null distribution, but we seldom know or have enough information to assume that of the alternate distribution. Thus, instead of minimizing both risks, as we would wish to do, we fix a small α and try to make β small by taking as large a sample size as we can. In medical applications, the choice of $\alpha = 5\%$ has become commonplace, but 5% is by no means required. Other risks, perhaps 1% or 10%, may be chosen so long as they are stated and justified.

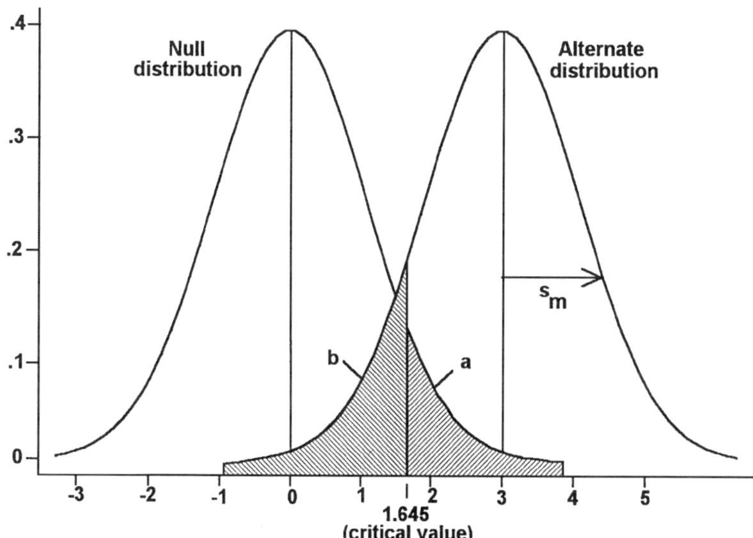

Figure 5.2 Depiction of null and alternate distributions along with the error probabilities arising from selecting a particular critical value. To the left of the critical value is the rejection region, to the right, the acceptance region.

Accepting H_0 versus Failing to Reject H_0

It is common in the medical literature to speak of accepting H_0 if the satistic falls on the "null side" of the critical value (see Fig. 5.2). Users often then are mystified to see that a larger sample leads to contradiction of a conclusion already made. The issue is one of evidence. The conclusion is based on probabilities, which arise from the evidence given by the data. The more accurate statement about H_0 is the following: The data provide inadequate evidence to infer that H_0 probably is false. With additional evidence, H_0 may be properly rejected. The interpretation is that our data-based evidence gives inadequate cause to say that it is untrue, and therefore we act in clinical decision making as if it were true. The reader encountering the "accept H_0" statement should recall this admonition.

5.3. TWO POLICIES OF TESTING

A Bit of History

During the early development of statistics, calculation was a major problem. It was done by pen in the western cultures and by abacus (7-bead rows) or soriban (5-bead rows) in eastern cultures. Later, hand-crank calculators and then electric ones were used. Probability tables were produced for selected values with great effort, the bulk being done in the 1930s by the U.S. Government's Works Project Administration (WPA) by hundreds of women given work during the economic depression. It was not practical for a statistician to calculate a p-value for each test, so the philosophy became to make the decision of acceptance or rejection of the null hypothesis on the basis of whether the p-value was bigger or smaller than the chosen α ($p \geq 0.05$ versus $p < 0.05$, for example) without evaluating the p-value itself. The investigator (and reader of published studies) then had to not reject H_0 if p was not less than α (result not statistically significant) and reject it if p was less (result statistically significant).

Calculation by Computer Provides a New Option

With the advent of computers, calculation of even very involved probabilities became fast and accurate. It is now possible to calculate the exact p-value, for example, $p = 0.12$ or $p = 0.02$. Users now have the option to make a decision on the risk they are willing to take.

Contrasting Two Approaches

The later philosophy has not necessarily become dominant, especially in medicine. The two philosophies have generated some dissension among statisticians. Advocates of the older approach hold that sample distributions only approximate the probability distributions and that exactly calculated p-values are not accurate anyway; the best we can do is select a "significant" or "not significant" choice. Advocates of the newer approach hold that the inaccuracy limitation is outweighed by the advantages of knowing the p-value. A difference in our action may be based on whether a not significant result suggests a most unlikely difference (perhaps $p = 0.80$) or is borderline and suggests further investigation (perhaps $p = 0.08$) and, similarly, whether a significant result is close to the decision of having happened by chance (perhaps $p = 0.04$) or leaves little doubt in the reader's mind (perhaps $p = 0.004$).

Other Factors Must Be Considered

The preceding comments are not meant to imply that decisions based on test results depend solely on p-values. Certainly the sample size and the clinical difference being tested must enter into the interpretation. Indeed, the clinical difference often is the most influential of values used in a test equation. The comments on the interpretation of p-values relative to one another do hold for adequate sample sizes and realistic clinical differences.

Select What Seems Most Sensible to You

Inasmuch as the controversy is not yet settled, users may select the philosophy they prefer. The author tends toward the newer approach.

5.4. ORGANIZING DATA FOR INFERENCE

The First Step: Identify the Type of Data

After the raw data are obtained, they must be organized into a form amenable to analysis by the chosen statistical test. We often have data in patient charts, instrument printouts, or observation sheets and want to set them up so that we can conduct inferential logic. The first step is to identify the type of data to be tested. We saw in Section 1.3 that most data could be typed as categorical (we count

Table 5.2
Format for Recording Joint Occurrences of Two Binary Data Sets

		DRE result		
		0	1	Totals
Biopsy result	0			
	1			
	Totals			

the patients in a disease category, for example), rank-order (we rank the patients in numerical order), or continuous (we record the patient's position on a scale). Although there is no comprehensive rule for organizing data, an example of each type will help the user become familiar with the terminology and concepts of data types.

Categorical Data

In the data of Table DB1.1, consider the association of a DRE result with a biopsy result. We ask the following question: "Does DRE result give some indication of biopsy result, or are the two events independent?" Both results are either positive or negative by nature. We can count the number of positive results for either, so they are nominal data. For statistical analysis, we almost always want our data quantified. Each of these results may be quantified as 0 (negative result) or 1 (positive result). Thus, our variables in this question are the numerical values (0 or 1) of DRE and the numerical values (0 or 1) of biopsy. The possible combinations of results are 0,0 (0 DRE and 0 biopsy), 0,1, 1,0, and 1,1. We could set up a 2×2 table (Table 5.2) in the format of Table 5.1.

Entering the Data

After setting up the format, we go to the data (from Table DB1.1) and count the number of times each event and joint event occur and enter the counts into the table. It is possible to count only some of the entries and obtain the rest by subtraction, but it is much safer to count the entry for every cell and use subtraction to check the arithmetic. The few extra seconds are a negligible loss compared to the risk of publishing erroneous data or conclusions. After the data are entered, we obtain Table 5.3. Our data table is complete and we are ready to perform a categorical test.

Table 5.3
Format of Table 5.2 with Table DB1.1 Data Entered

		DRE result		
		0	1	Totals
Biopsy result	0	3	4	7
	1	2	1	3
	Totals	5	5	10

Rank Data

Remaining with Table DB1.1, suppose we ask whether average PSAD is different for positive versus negative biopsy. PSAD is a continuous-type measure, i.e., each value represents a point on a scale from 0 to a large number, which ordinarily would imply using a test of averages with continuous data. However, PSAD values come from a very right-skewed distribution. (The mean of the 301 patients' PSADs is 0.27, which lies very far from the center of the range 0–4.55.) The assumption of normality is violated; it is appropriate to use rank methods.

Converting Continuous Data to Rank Data

Sometimes ranks arise naturally, as in ranking patients' severity during triage. In other cases, such as the one we are addressing now, we must convert continuous data to rank data. To rank the PSAD values, we write them down and assign rank 1 to the smallest, rank 2 to the next smallest, etc. We associate the biopsy results and sort out the ranks for biopsy 0 and biopsy 1. These entries appear here. Our data entry is complete and we are ready to perform a rank test.

PSAD	PSAD ranks	Biopsy results	Ranks for biopsy = 0	Ranks for biopsy = 1
0.24	6	0	6	
0.15	3	0	3	
0.36	9	1		9
0.27	8	1		8
0.22	5	1		5
0.11	1	0	1	
0.25	7	0	7	
0.14	2	0	2	
0.17	4	0	4	
0.48	10	0	10	

Continuous Measurement Data

Suppose we ask whether average PSA is different for positive versus negative biopsy. For each patient, we would record the PSA level and a 0 or 1 for biopsy result, ending with data as in columns 5 and 8 of Table DB1.1. PSA is a continuous measurement, i.e., each value represents a point on a scale from 0 to a large number. We noted in Section 4.2 that PSA is not too far from normal when patients with BPH are excluded. Thus, a continuous-data-type test of averages would be appropriate. We would need means and standard deviations. One way to display our data in a form convenient to use is shown here. Our data entry and setup are complete and we are ready to perform a means test.

PSA	Biopsy result	PSA for biopsy = 0	PSA for biopsy = 1
7.6	0	7.6	
4.1	0	4.1	
5.9	1		5.9
9.0	1		9.0
6.8	1		6.8
8.0	0	8.0	
7.7	0	7.7	
4.4	0	4.4	
6.1	0	6.1	
7.9	0	7.9	
		$m = 6.54$, $s = 1.69$	$m = 7.23$, $s = 1.59$

5.5. EVOLVING A WAY TO ANSWER YOUR DATA QUESTION

Fundamentally, a Study Is Asking a Question

Clinical studies ask questions about variables that describe patient populations. A physician may ask about the PSA of a population of patients with prostate cancer. Most of these questions are about the characteristics of the probability distribution of those variables, primarily its mean, standard deviation, and shape. Of most interest in the prostate cancer population is the average PSA. Three stages in the evolution of scientific knowledge about the population in question were discussed in Section 1.1: description (the physician wants to know the average PSA of the cancerous population), explanation (the physician wants to know if and why it is different from the healthy population), and prediction (the physician wants to use PSA to predict which patients have cancer).

DESCRIPTION AND PREDICTION

When we know little about a distribution in question, the first step is to describe it. We take a representative sample from the population and use the statistical summarizing methods of Chapter 3 to describe the sample. These sample summaries estimate the characteristics of the population. We can even express our confidence in the accuracy of these sample summaries by the confidence methods of Chapter 4. The description step will not be pursued again in this chapter. Prediction combines the result of the inference with a cause–explanatory model to predict results for cases not currently in evidence. This is a more sophisticated stage in the evolution of knowledge that will be treated in Chapter 8. The current chapter addresses statistical testing, which leads to the inference from sample to population.

TESTING

We often want to decide (a) whether our patient sample arose from an established population (Does a sample of patients who had an infection have the same average white blood count (WBC) after treatment with antibiotics as the healthy population?) or (b) whether the populations from which two samples arose are the same or different (Does a sample of patients treated for infection with antibiotics have the same average white count as a sample treated with a placebo?). In these examples, the variable being used to contrast the differences is mean WBC. Let us subscript the means with h for healthy patients, a for patients treated with antibiotics, and p for patients treated with a placebo. Recall that μ represents a population mean and m a sample mean. Then question (a) contrasts m_a with μ_h and question (b) contrasts m_a with m_p.

STEPS IN SETTING UP A TEST

These contrasts are carried out by statistical tests following the logic of inference (Section 5.1) with measured risks of error (Section 5.2). The step-by-step logic is as follows (assuming the simplest case of one question to be answered using one variable):

(1) Write down the question you will ask of your data. (Does treating my infected patients with a particular antibiotic make them healthy again?)

(2) Select the variable on which you can obtain data that you believe to best highlight the contrasts in the question. (I think WBC will best show the state of health.)

(3) Select the descriptor of the distribution of the variable that will furnish the contrast, e.g., mean, standard deviation. (Mean WBC will furnish the most telling contrast.)

(4) Write down the null and alternate hypotheses indicated by the contrast. (H_0: $\mu_a = \mu_h$; H_1: $\mu_a \neq \mu_h$.)

(5) Write down a detailed, comprehensive sentence describing the population(s) measured by the variable involved in that question. (The healthy population is the set of people who have no current or chronic infections affecting their WBC. The treated population is the set of people who have the infection being treated and no other current or chronic infection affecting their WBC.)

(6) Write down a detailed, comprehensive sentence describing the sample(s) from which your data on the variable will be drawn. [My sample is selected randomly from patients presenting to my clinic who pass my exclusion screen (other infections, etc.).]

(7) Ask yourself what biases might emerge from any distinctions between the makeup of the sample(s) and the population(s). Could this infection be worse for one age, sex, cultural origin, etc. of patient than another? Are the samples representative of the populations with respect to the variable being recorded? [I have searched and found studies that show that mortality and recovery rates, and therefore probably WBC, are the same for different sexes and cultural groups. One might suspect that the elderly have begun to compromise their immune systems, so I will stratify my sample (Section 1.5) to assure that it reflects the age distribution at large.]

(8) Recycle 1–7 until you are satisfied that all steps are fully consistent with each other.

(9) In terms of the variable descriptors and hypotheses being used, choose the most appropriate statistical test (more in Section 10.2) and select the α level you will accept.

(10) If your sample size is not preordained by availability and/or economics, satisfy yourself that you have an adequate sample size to answer the question (more in Chapter 7).

At this point, you are ready to obtain your data (which might take hours or years).

Additional Example

We want to test (and lay to rest) the assertion: "People who do not see a physician for a cold get well faster than people who do."

(1) Question being asked: Does seeing a physician for a cold retard the time to heal?

(2) Variable to use: Length of time (days) for symptoms (nasal congestion, etc.) to disappear.

(3) Descriptor of variable that will provide contrast between patients who see a physician (group 1) and those who do not (group 2): Mean number of days μ_1 (estimated by m_1) and μ_2 (estimated by m_2).

(4) Hypotheses: $H_0: \mu_1 = \mu_2; H_1: \mu_1 \neq \mu_2$.

(5) Populations: Populations are the sets of people in this nation who have cold symptoms but are otherwise healthy and who see a physician for their condition (population 1) and those who do not (population 2).

(6) Samples: For sample 1, 50 patients will be chosen randomly from those who present at the walk-in clinic of a general hospital with cold symptoms but evince no other signs of illness. Sample 2 is more difficult. A random sample of five pharmacies in the area is taken and each is monitored for customers who have signs of a cold. Of these customers, a random sample of 10 from each pharmacy is taken, with the customers agreeing to be included and being followed by telephone.

(7) Biases and steps to prevent them: There are several possible sources of bias, as there are in most medical studies. However, the major questions of bias are the following: (a) Are patients and customers at and in the vicinity of our general hospital representative of those in general? (b) Are customers who buy cold medicines at a pharmacy representative of cold sufferers who do not see physicians? We can answer question (a) by analyzing the demographics statistically after our study is complete; question (b) requires a leap of faith.

(8) Recycle: These steps seem to be adequately consistent as they are.

(9) Statistical test and α: Two-sample t test with $\alpha = 0.05$.

(10) Sample size: From Chapter 7, we will learn that we need not only (a) α (=0.05), but also (b) the power ($1 - \beta$, which we take to be power $= 0.80$), (c) the difference between means that we believe to be clinically meaningful (which we choose as 2 days), and (d) σ_1 and σ_2. We estimate σ_1 from a pilot survey of patients presenting with cold symptoms and followed by telephone to be 3 and assume that σ_2 is the same. From Section 7.4, we will find that we need at least 36 in each sample; our planned 50 per group is a large enough sample.

Now we may begin to collect our data.

CHAPTER EXERCISES

5.1. In DB4, a hypothesis to be investigated is that protease inhibitors reduce pulmonary admissions. Is this a clinical or a statistical hypothesis? What would be a statement of the other type of hypothesis?

5.2. A clinical hypothesis arising from DB3 might be the following: The mean serum theophylline level is greater at the end of the antibiotic course than at baseline. (a) What probability distribution is associated with this hypothesis? (b) What assumptions about the data would be required to investigate this hypothesis? (c) State in words the Type I and Type II errors associated with this hypothesis. (d) How would the probability (risk) of these errors be designated? How would the power of the test be designated?

5.3. A clinical hypothesis arising from DB9 might be the following: The standard deviation of platelet counts is 60,000 [which gives about 95% confidence (mean $\pm 2 \times 60{,}000$) coverage of the normal range of 240,000]; this hypothesis is equivalent to supposing that the variance is $60{,}000^2 = 3{,}600{,}000{,}000$. (a) What probability distribution is associated with this hypothesis? (b) What assumptions about the data would be required to investigate this hypothesis? (c) State in words the Type I and Type II errors associated with this hypothesis. (d) How would the probability (risk) of these errors be designated?

5.4. A clinical hypothesis arising from DB5 might be the following: The variances (or standard deviations) of plasma silicone before and after implant are different. (a) What probability distribution is associated with this hypothesis? (b) What assumptions about the data would be required to investigate this hypothesis? (c) State in words the Type I and Type II errors associated with this hypothesis. (d) How would the probability (risk) of these errors be designated?

5.5. Of what data type are the following: (a) The variable "respond" versus "not respond" in DB6? (b) The variable "nausea score" in DB2? (c) The variable "platelet count" in DB9?

5.6. In DB10, rank the seconds to perform the triple hop with the operated leg, small to large.

5.7. Using the 2×2 table in DB2, follow the first nine steps of Section 5.5 in setting up a test to learn whether the drug reduces nausea score.

Chapter 6

Medical Decisions: Statistical Testing, Risks, and Odds

6.1. OVERVIEW

Each Data Type Has a Different Form of Test

We have noted repeatedly that there are three types of data: categorical, rank-order, and continuous. Each requires its own form of statistical testing. In this chapter, the unique character of each data type is introduced, and the statistical test used for that type most frequently in medical studies is then explained and exemplified.

Categorical Form

To compare two variables using categorical data, we form two-way tables of counts with one variable representing rows and the other representing columns. We test the proposition that knowledge of the counts in one variable's categories tells us something about the counts in the other variable's categories, i.e., that the two variables are not independent. Furthermore, if one variable represents a proposed event (diagnosis, acquiring a disease) and the other the known outcome of this event ("truth"), the table becomes a truth table allowing risks and odds to be calculated, such as sensitivity, specificity, etc.

Rank-Order Form

To compare two groups that are in rank order, we attach ranks to the data combined over the two groups and then add the rank values for each group separately, forming rank sums. If the group rankings are not much different, the rankings from the two groups will be interleaved and the rank sums will not be much different. If one group has most of its members preceding the other in rank, one rank sum will be large and the other small. Probabilities of rank sums have been tabulated, so that the associated p-value can be looked up in the table and the decision about the group difference made.

Continuous Form

Whether a difference between means exists most often is the focus in comparing two groups with data in continuous form. Our first inclination is to look at the difference between means. However, this difference depends on the scale. The offset distance of a broken femur appears larger if measured in centimeters than in inches. The distance must be standardized into units of data variability. We divide the distance between means by a measure of variability and achieve a statistic (z if the population variability is known or closely estimated; t if it is estimated by small samples). The risk of concluding a difference when there is none (the p-value) is looked up in a table and the decision about the group difference is made.

6.2. CATEGORICAL DATA: BASICS

Nominal Data: Categories and Counts

In Table DB1.1, the variables DRE, TRU, and BIOP can be quantified by associating their outcomes with 0 or 1. If we had recorded patient job occupation, say construction worker, secretary, professional, cook, etc., we could categorize "job" as A, B, C, D, etc. or 0, 1, 2, 3, etc. Data of this sort that are placed into named categories (as opposed to being measured as a point on a scale or ranked in order) usually are referred to as *categorical* or *nominal* data (see the discussion of data types in Section 1.3). When dealing with categorical data, the basic statistic, the *count*, is obtained by counting the number of events per category. In the Table DB1.1 data, there are five positive DREs and three positive BIOPs. The symbol for number of "successes" used in calculational formulas is n with the appropriate subscript. Unsubscripted n represents the total number summed over all categories.

Proportions and Percents

Another important statistic obtained from categorical data is the *proportion* of data in that category, which is the count in a category divided by the total number in the variable. The proportion of positive DREs is $5/10 = 0.50$ and that of positive BIOPs is $3/10 = 0.30$. Multiplication by 100 yields percent (denoted %), which in the case of BIOP is 30%. Percent is useful in that most of the public is used to thinking in terms of percent, but statistical methods have been developed for proportions. A symbol for a sample proportion could be p. To use the binomial in a medical application, we need a theoretical or population proportion to specify the member of the family of binomials with which we are dealing. This theoretical proportion is symbolized π, in keeping with the convention of using Greek letters for population values and Roman letters for sample values.

Choosing Counts versus Proportions

When should tables of counts be tested and when should proportions? When all cells of the table of counts can be filled in, use the methods for counts. Interestingly, the number of degrees of freedom (*df*) for tests of these tables is the minimum number of cells that must be filled to be able to calculate the remainder of cell entries using the totals at the side and bottom. For example, for a 2×2 table with the sums at the side and bottom, only one cell need be filled and the others can be found by subtraction; it has 1 *df*. Tests of proportions are appropriate for cases in which certain table totals are missing, but for which proportions can still be calculated.

Categories versus Ranks

Consider cases for which counts or proportions are obtained for each sample group. If the order in which these groups are written down can be swapped without affecting the interpretation, for example, Group 1, high hematocrit (Hct), Group 2, high white blood cell count, and Group 3, high platelet count, then analysis is constrained to categorical methods. If, on the other hand, sample groups fall into a natural order in which the logical implication would change by altering this order, such as Group 1, low Hct, Group 2, normal Hct, and Group 3, high Hct, rank methods are appropriate. Categorical groups may be formed by dividing the scale upon which continuous data occur. If we were to categorize age by decade (50–59, 60–69, and 70–79 years), we would have age groupings, which we could name 1, 2, and 3. These groups could be considered as categories and categorical methods used. However, they fall into a natural rank order, as group 1 clearly comes before group 2, etc. Rank methods give better results than categorical methods. Although rank methods lose power when there are a large number of ties, they are still more powerful than categorical methods, which are not very powerful. *When ranking is a natural option, rank methods should be used.*

Table 6.1

Contingency Table of Simultaneous Biopsy and DRE Results from Table DB1.1 Data

		DRE		
		1	0	Totals
BIOP	1	1	2	3
	0	4	3	7
	Totals	5	5	10

Organizing Data for Categorical Methods

If the relationship between two variables is at question, such as, are they independent or associated, the number of observations falling simultaneously into the categories of two variables is counted. For example, the categories of the variables DRE and BIOP may be counted at the same time. This gives rise to the four possible categories: both positive, both negative, and two counts of one positive, one negative. These counts may be organized as shown in Table 6.1 with the counts from data Table DB1.1 filled in, where the DRE result is thought of as predicting the biopsy result. We can see that 3 is the number of negative DREs, contingent upon also being a negative biopsy. Such tables are called *contingency tables*, because the count in each cell is the number in that category of that variable contingent upon also lying in a particular category of the other variable.

Symbols Are Needed for Contingency Table Computations

Symbols to represent the numbers in tables like Table 6.1 are needed for formulas, and they must be capable of being used in tables with more than four categories. For example, if we tried to predict BIOP by PSA categories <4, 4–10, and >10, we would have a 2×3 table. To be general, r could denote the number of rows and c the number of columns; we would have an $r \times c$ table. Because we do not know the values of r and c until we specify a particular case, we need to symbolize the cell numbers and the marginal (row and column) totals in a way that can apply to a table of any size.

Symbols Used in Contingency Tables

The symbolism biostatisticians have been almost forced into over the decades by practicality is n (for "number") with two subscripts: the first to indicate the

Table 6.2

Contingency Table of Simultaneous Biopsy and DRE Results from Table DB1.1 Data[a]

		DRE		
		1	0	Totals
BIOP	1	$n_{11} = 1$	$n_{12} = 2$	$n_{1\cdot} = 3$
	0	$n_{21} = 4$	$n_{22} = 3$	$n_{2\cdot} = 7$
	Totals	$n_{\cdot 1} = 5$	$n_{\cdot 2} = 5$	$n = 10$

[a] n symbols are included to illustrate cell counts, marginal totals, and grand total.

row and the second the column. Thus, the number of cases observed in row 1, column 2 is n_{12}. The row and column totals are denoted by placing a dot in place of the numbers we summed to get the total. Thus, the total of the first row would be $n_{1\cdot}$ and the total of the second column would be $n_{\cdot 2}$. The grand total can be denoted just n; sometimes $n_{\cdot\cdot}$ is used. Table 6.2 repeats Table 6.1 with the various n symbols attached for illustration.

6.3. CATEGORICAL DATA: TESTS ON 2 × 2 TABLES

Testing a Contingency Table Will Answer the Question: Are the Row Categories Independent of the Column Categories?

Less technically, does knowledge of the outcome of one of the variables give us any information about the associated outcome of the other variable? Another way to express the question would be to ask, are the data homogeneous?

Is Prediction (Diagnosis) of Prostate Cancer by DRE Better Than Chance?

Table 6.3 shows a contingency table in a format similar to that of Table 6.2 in which all 301 data have been tabulated. Does knowledge of a patient's DRE give us any help in predicting whether he will have a positive biopsy, or would we do just as well to choose randomly? Let us conceive of a spinner in the center of a circle with circumference divided into 301 equal parts. We color a sector (slice of pie) of 95 parts red, to match the 95 positive biopsies. To predict a patient's biopsy

Table 6.3

Contingency Table of Simultaneous Biopsy and DRE Results from 301 Patients[a]

		DRE		
		1	0	Totals
BIOP	1	$n_{11} = 68$	$n_{12} = 27$	$n_{1.} = 95$
	0	$n_{21} = 117$	$n_{22} = 89$	$n_{2.} = 206$
	Totals	$n_{.1} = 185$	$n_{.2} = 116$	$n = 301$

[a] *n* symbols are included to illustrate cell counts, marginal totals, and grand total.

result randomly, we spin. If the spinner stops on red, we choose positive, otherwise, negative. If the DRE adds no information, the ratio of positive biopsy prediction to total for a positive DRE should be about the same as the 95/301 ratio our spinner would give. We would say that biopsy result is independent of DRE outcome.

The Chi-Square Test of Contingency Is a Common Way to Test Independence

Different tests exist to answer the question of independence of the two variables. The time-honored test and the one seen most frequently in the medical literature is the *chi-square test of contingency*.

We Should Understand Where the Method Comes From

We can better understand the chi-square method if we survey the ideas underlying it. For the data of Table 6.3, the question may be expressed statistically as follows: Are the numbers of DRE positive predictions and negative predictions, contingent upon actual outcome, distributed the same as they would be without the outcome information, that is, as the right-hand column (the right margin)?

Expected Values

This last question gives rise to what is termed an *expected value*. If the occurrence of predicted positive cases is unrelated to biopsy outcome, the number of correct positive predictions we would *expect* to occur (call it e_{11} to match n_{11}) in ratio to all positive predictions ($e_{11}/n_{.1}$) would be the same as the number of either prediction for positive biopsy in ratio to total cases ($n_{1.}/n$), or $e_{11}/n_{.1} = n_{1.}/n$.

By multiplying both sides by $n_{\cdot 1}$, we find the *expected number* of correct positive predictions to be *its row sum multiplied by its column sum, divided by the total sum.* In general, for row i and column j, the expected value of the ijth entry is given by

$$e_{ij} = \frac{n_{i\cdot} n_{\cdot j}}{n}. \quad (6.1)$$

For example, the expected value for the upper left position in Table 6.3 is $95 \times 185/301 = 58.4$, in contrast to the observed value of 68. The expected values e_{12}, e_{21}, and e_{22}, respectively, are 36.6, 126.6, and 79.4.

The Basis of the Chi-Square Test of Contingency

The chi-square test of contingency is based on the differences between the observed values and those that would be expected if the variables were independent. If these differences are small, there is little dependence between the variables; large differences indicate a dependence. The actual chi-square statistic is the sum of these differences squared in ratio to the expected value. A small chi-square statistic arises if the observed values are close to the values we would expect if the two variables were unrelated. A large chi-square statistic arises if the observed values are rather different from those we would expect from unrelated variables. If the chi-square statistic is large enough that it is unlikely to have occurred by chance, we say that it is significant and conclude that the rows variable is not totally independent of the columns variable. However, it does *not* follow that one can be well predicted by the other.

We Would Hope That DRE Is Not Independent of the Biopsy Outcome

This chi-square test should tell us whether the digital rectal exam result is independent of the biopsy outcome. We would hope not; the two should be closely related if we are to detect prostate cancer using the DRE. Let us detail the calculations in the test so that we can answer this question.

Calculation for the Chi-Square Test of Contingency

The chi-square calculation is based on the difference between the observed cell count and the cell count that would be expected if the rows and columns were independent. The expected count for a cell is its row total multiplied by its column total, divided by the grand total, as given in Eq. (6.1). After the four e_{ij} are determined, the chi-square is found using the following simple pattern: sum of [(|observed − expected| − 0.5)^2/expected], where the 0.5 term is a correction to adjust for the counts being restricted to integers. The symbolic form of this pattern is given in

$$\chi^2 = \sum_i^2 \sum_j^2 \frac{(|n_{ij} - e_{ij}| - 0.5)^2}{e_{ij}}. \tag{6.2}$$

One Σ symbol tells us to add across the two rows and the other tells us to add over the two columns. The p-value can be found by calculation or from tables of chi-square probabilities.

The Chi-Square Test for the DRE versus Biopsy Data

Let us test the null hypothesis that DRE result and biopsy result are independent, i.e., knowledge of the DRE result tells us nothing about the biopsy result. The expected values, e_{ij}, were noted just following Eq. (6.1). The chi-square statistic is calculated $\chi^2 = [(|68 - 58.4| - 0.5)^2/58.4] + \cdots + [(|89 - 79.4| - 0.5)^2/79.4] = 6.62$. Table C (right tail of the chi-square distribution) will tell us whether this chi-square value is significant. A fragment of Table C is shown as Table 6.4. The statistic 6.62 lies just below 6.63, associated with $\alpha = 0.01$, so that the p-value is about 0.01, which clearly is a statistically significant result. (Exact calculation on a computer tells us it is $p = 0.010$.) We reject the null hypothesis of independence and conclude that the DRE result does indeed give us some information about the presence of prostate cancer. Note the wording: it gives us some information, but it does not tell us how good this information is.

Assumption Required for the Chi-Square Test of Contingency

The chi-square method should not be used for extremely small samples. It really is an approximation to more exact methods (which can be found in Chapter 13), and the approximation is not dependable for small samples. In particular, it is valid

Table 6.4

Fragment of Table C, the Right Tail of the Chi-Square Distribution[a]

α (area in right tail)	0.10	0.05	0.025	0.01
$df = 1$	2.71	3.84	5.02	6.63

[a] χ^2 values (distances to the right of 0 on a χ^2 curve) are tabulated for 1 *df* for four values of α.

Table 6.5

Contingency Table of Simultaneous Biopsy and DRE Results with Each Cell Showing One-Fifth the Count Arising from the 301 Patients[a]

		DRE		
		1	0	Totals
BIOP	1	$n_{11} = 14$	$n_{12} = 5$	$n_{1\cdot} = 19$
	0	$n_{21} = 23$	$n_{22} = 18$	$n_{2\cdot} = 41$
	Totals	$n_{\cdot 1} = 37$	$n_{\cdot 2} = 23$	$n = 60$

[a] New cell counts are rounded to integers. The pattern of proportions is approximately maintained, but the p-value loses its significance due to the smaller sample size.

only if the expected value (row sum × column sum ÷ total sum) of every cell is at least 1 and a minimum count of 5 appears in every cell.

The Effect of Sample Size on Contingency Tests

A significant chi-square result indicates that the types of category are not independent, but does not indicate how closely they are associated, because the significance is influenced by both sample size and association. To illustrate this, Table 6.5 has each cell count in Table 6.3 replaced by one-fifth of its value, rounding to maintain integers. We have approximately the same pattern of proportions, which gives about the same level of association (37% correct positive prediction for the full sample and 38% correct positive prediction for the smaller one). However, now the chi-square has shrunk from 6.62 to 2.55. From Table 6.4, we can see that $\chi^2 = 2.71$ is associated with $\alpha = 0.10$, so that the p-value for 2.55 will be greater than 0.10. (Direct calculation yields $p = 0.110$.) Reduction of the sample size while keeping the same general pattern of relationship between the variables has caused the p-value to grow from a significant 0.010 to a nonsignificant 0.110. Contingency test results must be interpreted with care.

What Do We Do if We Have the Percentages but Not the Counts?

Just note that tests of proportions exist, which are just percent with the decimal point moved two places. We can test a sample proportion against either a known population proportion or another sample proportion. For example, suppose we are concerned with the efficacy of an antibiotic in treating pediatric otitis media accompanied by fever. We know that, say, 85% of patients get well within 7 days without treatment. We learn that of 100 such patients, 95% of those treated with the antibiotic got well within 7 days. Is this improvement statistically significant? Note that we cannot fill in a contingency table because we do not have the number of untreated patients nor the total number of patients. However, we do have the theoretical proportion and so can answer the question using a test of proportions. (More details can be found in Chapter 13.)

6.4. CATEGORICAL DATA: RISKS AND ODDS

True and False Positive and Negative Events

A special case of the contingency table is the case in which one variable represents a prediction that a condition will occur and the other represents the outcome, i.e., "truth." Suppose we are predicting the occurrence of a disease among a sample of patients by means of a clinical test (or, alternatively, from the fact of exposure or nonexposure to a disease). If we also know the outcomes of the test (or occurrence of the disease), we can count the possible relations between predictions and outcomes and array them as n_{11} through n_{22} in a 2×2 *truth table*, as illustrated in Table 6.6. Four possible situations are named in the table: (1) *true positive*, the event of a predicted disease being present; (2) *false negative*, the event of predicting no disease when disease is present; (3) *false positive*, the event of a predicted disease being absent; and (4) *true negative*, the event of predicting no disease when disease is absent. These four concepts are used a great deal in several fields of clinical medicine and should be noted well. The n values are the counts of these

Table 6.6

Truth Table Showing Counts of the Prediction of Presence or Absence of a Malady as Related to the Truth of That Presence or Absence

		Prediction (Exposure or test result)		
		Have disease	Do not have	
	Have disease	n_{11} True positive	n_{12} False negative	$n_{1\cdot}$ (Yes)
TRUTH	Do not have	n_{21} False positive	n_{22} True negative	$n_{2\cdot}$ (No)
		$n_{\cdot 1}$ (Predict yes)	$n_{\cdot 2}$ (Predict no)	n (or $n_{\cdot\cdot}$)

Table 6.7

Table of Biopsy Results Predicted by DRE and by PSAD > 0.14 as Related to the True Outcomes of the Biopsies for 301 Patients

		Predicted by DRE			Predicted by PSAD > 0.14		
		+	−		+	−	
	+	68 (n_{11})	27 (n_{12})	95	75 (n_{11})	20 (n_{12})	95
Truth (biopsy)	−	117 (n_{21})	89 (n_{22})	206	88 (n_{21})	118 (n_{22})	206
		185	116	301	163	138	301

events' occurrences and will be considered extensively in the remainder of this section.

Example Data

In Table 6.7, the format of Table 6.6 is used to show DRE and PSAD values of the 301 prostate patients in predicting biopsy results. The DREs are symbolized as + for predicted positive biopsy and − for predicted negative biopsy. By using a PSAD value of 0.14 as the critical value (decision criterion), PSAD > 0.14 predicts a positive biopsy and PSAD ≤ 0.14 predicts a negative biopsy.

Probability and Odds Defined

The probability (defined in Section 2.2) of an event is estimated by the number of ways the event in question can occur in ratio to the number of ways any event can occur. If r out of n patients have a disease, the chance that one of those patients chosen randomly has the disease is r/n. The *odds* that the randomly chosen patient has the disease is the number of ways the event can occur in ratio to the number of ways it does not occur, $r/(n-r)$. For example, the probability of a one-spot on the roll of a die is $1/6$; the odds are 1 to 5.

Sensitivity, Specificity, Accuracy, and Odds Ratio

Definitions of a number of concepts related to estimates of correct and erroneous predictions from the sample truth table are given in Table 6.8. Column 1 gives the names of the concepts, and column 2 gives the formulas for computing them from the sample truth table. Columns 3 and 4 give population definitions and the

Table 6.8

Concepts of False Positive and Negative, Sensitivity, Specificity, Accuracy, and Odds Ratio Based on Sample Error Rates Arising from the Format of Table 6.6[a]

Values found from a sample truth table		Population definitions of probabilities and odds of values being estimated		Examples of prediction	
Names of estimates	Sample computing formulas	Definitions	Relationships	By DRE	By PSAD
False positive sample rate (p-value)	$n_{21}/n_{2\cdot}$	Probability of a false positive (α)	P(predict yes|no)	0.568	0.427
False negative sample rate	$n_{12}/n_{1\cdot}$	Probability of a false negative (β)	P(predict no|yes)	0.284	0.210
Sensitivity	$n_{11}/n_{1\cdot}$	Probability of a true positive: *power* $(1-\beta)$	P(predict yes|yes)	0.716	0.790
Specificity	$n_{22}/n_{2\cdot}$	Probability of a true negative $(1-\alpha)$	P(predict no|no)	0.433	0.573
Accuracy	$(n_{11}+n_{22})/n_{\cdot\cdot}$	Overall probability of a correct decision	P(predict no|no or yes|yes)	0.522	0.641
Odds ratio (OR)	$\frac{n_{11}/n_{21}}{n_{12}/n_{22}}$ or $n_{11}n_{22}/n_{12}n_{21}$	Odds of a disease when predicted in ratio to odds of the disease when not predicted	$\frac{\text{Ratio(yes/no\|predicted yes)}}{\text{Ratio(yes/no\|predicted no)}}$	1.916	5.028

[a] The third and fourth columns show the population entities these values are estimating. The rightmost two columns show biopsy outcome predictions of these values from the data of Table 6.7.

relationships these concepts are estimating, i.e., what they would be if all data in the population were available. These are the values that relate to error probabilities in statistical inference, as discussed in Sections 2.1 and 2.2. As before, a vertical line, |, is read "given." Columns 5 and 6 show numerical estimates of the probabilities and odds in predicting biopsy results from DRE and PSAD values calculated from the counts displayed in Table 6.7. Interpretations of these outcomes appear later. (A number of other related concepts, e.g., positive and negative predictive values, appear in Chapter 13.)

False Positive Rate and False Negative Rate

The false positive rate is the relative frequency of not cancer when cancer is predicted. This value is the p-value of the test, the post-test estimate of α. The

DRE estimates this chance as $117/206 = 57\%$ and PSAD as $88/206 = 43\%$. The false negative rate is the relative frequency of cancer when not cancer is predicted, estimated as $27/95 = 28\%$ by DRE and $20/95 = 21\%$ by PSAD. It is the post-test estimate of β.

Sensitivity

The sensitivity, $1 -$ (false negative rate), is the sample estimate of the chance of detecting cancer when it is present. Sensitivity is the sample estimate of the frequently met *power* of the decision and is related to power in the same way that the p-value is related to α. The sensitivity of DRE is $68/95 = 72\%$ and that of PSAD is $75/95 = 79\%$.

Specificity

The specificity, $1 -$ (false positive rate), is the post-test estimate of the chance of correctly classifying the patient as free of cancer, i.e., ruling out cancer when it is absent. The specificity of DRE is $89/206 = 43\%$ and that of PSAD is $118/206 = 57\%$. From the results so far, we see that PSAD has both a higher sensitivity and a higher specificity than DRE.

Accuracy

Sometimes the interest is in the rate of overall accuracy, combining the true positives and true negatives. Accuracy is calculated as true positive plus true negative counts, divided by the total count. The accuracy of DRE is $(68 + 89)/301 = 52\%$ and that of PSAD is $(75 + 118)/301 = 64\%$. However, this definition of accuracy assumes the errors of a false positive and a false negative have the same weight, i.e., the same importance in the decision process, which they often do not. For example, a false negative in a test of carcinoma implies a missed cancer, whereas a false positive implies an unnecessary biopsy; clearly the two errors are not equal in severity. Accuracy must be used judiciously and interpreted carefully.

Odds Ratio

The odds ratio (OR) gives the odds of cancer when predicted in ratio to the odds of cancer when not predicted, indicating the usefulness of the prediction method. The PSAD OR of $(75 \times 118) \div (20 \times 88) = 5.03$ indicates that PSAD's odds of cancer when predicted is 5 times its odds when not predicted. The PSAD OR is more than 2.5 times the DRE OR of $(68 \times 89) \div (27 \times 117) = 1.92$, indicating that, for these data, PSAD is a much better predictor of prostate cancer than DRE. The OR gives us some indication of level of association between the two variables; tests of association exist but are not addressed in this section. (The curious may see Chapter 13.)

6.5. RANK DATA: BASICS

WHAT ARE RANKS?

Ranked data are data entries put in order according to some criterion: smallest to largest, worst to best, cheapest to costliest. Such rank-order data may arise from ranking events directly, such as a surgeon ranking in order of difficulty the five types of surgery he or she performs most often. Alternatively, rank-order data may arise from putting already recorded continuous-type quantities in order, such as ordering the PSA of Table DB1.1 from smallest to largest. These latter ranks would appear as follows:

Patient number	1	2	3	4	5	6	7	8	9	10
PSA	7.6	4.1	5.9	9.0	6.8	8.0	7.7	4.4	6.1	7.9
PSA rank	6	1	3	10	5	9	7	2	4	8

RANKING CATEGORIZED DATA THAT FALL INTO A NATURAL ORDER

Note that if PSA were categorized into A, PSA < 4, B, PSA 4–10, and C, PSA > 10, the data could still be ranked and analyzed using rank-order methods, although there would be so many ties that the analysis would be much less sensitive.

WHEN DO WE USE RANKS?

Continuous measurements contain more information than ranks, and ranks contain more than counts. When the user can rank events but cannot measure them, it is obvious that rank-order statistical methods are to be used. The question of when and why to use ranks arises primarily with using rank-order methods for data on which continuous measurements are available.

Why Do We Use Ranks?

Statistical methods using continuous measurements on variables depend on the probability distributions of those variables. We assume certain properties of those probability distributions, such as that we are sampling from a normal distribution. When we have small sample sizes, our sample frequency distributions are insufficient to tell us whether the assumptions are justified. Rank-order methods do not require the same assumptions about the underlying distributions. Further, even when we have larger samples, we may have evidence that the assumptions are not satisfied. Recall that the distribution of prostate volumes (cf. Fig. 2.1) is skewed to the right. The use of methods that assume a normal distribution would violate this assumption, because the sample distribution is not the same shape as the assumed distribution, causing the probability calculations to be wrong. Rank-order methods, which are not subject to the skew, would not violate the assumption.

Summary of When to Use Rank-Order Methods

Rank-order methods should be used (1) when the primary data consist of ranks, (2) when samples are too small to form conclusions about the underlying probability distributions, or (3) when data indicate that necessary assumptions about the distributions are violated.

Ties in Ranked Data

If ranks are tied, the usual procedure is to average the tied ranks. For example, a sample of heart rates in increasing order is 64, 67, 67, 71, 72, 76, 78, 89. We have the ranks 1–8 to assign. However, the 2nd and 3rd heart rates are the same. We average 2 and 3 to assign 2.5 to each. The ranks are 1, 2.5, 2.5, 4, 5, 6, 7, 8. Some statisticians prefer to assign the potential ranks to tied values randomly to avoid ties, but this technique introduces a bit of false information. Ties disturb the theory of rank methods somewhat, but they still are approximately correct.

6.6. RANK DATA: THE RANK-SUM TEST TO COMPARE TWO SAMPLES

What Is Being Tested

Given two samples, the hypothesis being tested is whether the value for a randomly chosen member of the first sample probably is smaller than one of the second sample, a slightly technical concept. For practical purposes, the user may think of it informally as testing whether the two distributions have the same median.

Steps in Conducting the Test

Steps for conducting the rank-sum test are given in the left-hand column that follows. In the parallel position in the right-hand column, a numerical example is given.

Example

Returning to Table DB1.1, we ask, are the PSA levels different for the $n_1 = 3$ positive biopsy results and the $n_2 = 7$ negative results? (In this test, the symbol n_1 is always assigned the smaller of the two n's.) The PSA levels, their ranks (small to large), and the biopsy results are as follows:

PSA	7.6	4.1	5.9	9.0	6.8	8.0	7.7	4.4	6.1	7.9
Ranks	6	1	3	10	5	9	7	2	4	8
Biopsy	0	0	1	1	1	0	0	0	0	0

Steps in method:	*Steps in example:*
(1) Satisfy yourself that the sample has been drawn such that it represents the population and such that observations are independent from each other. This step is pure judgment based on the way the data have been collected. If these requirements are violated, statistics will not help.	(1) We ask whether PSA is a risk factor for prostate cancer. Do our urological patients with cancer have PSA different from those without? We judge that the data are independent and that the sample is adequately representative.
(2) Specify α and hypotheses, which usually are null, distributions are not different, and alternate, distributions are different.	(2) $\alpha = 0.05$. Hypotheses are as at left.
(3) Name the sample sizes n_1 and n_2; n_1 is the smaller.	(3) $n_1 = 3; n_2 = 7$.
(4) Combine the data, keeping track of the sample from which each datum arose.	(4) First and third rows in preceding data display.
(5) Rank the data.	(5) Second row in preceding data display.
(6) Add up the ranks of the data from the smaller sample and name it T.	(6) The rank sum T for positive biopsies is $3 + 10 + 5 = 18$.

Table 6.9

Portion of Table I, Rank-Sum U Two-Tailed Probabilities[a]

	n_2:	6						7						
	n_1:	1	2	3	4	5	6	1	2	3	4	5	6	7
U	7			0.714	0.352	0.178	0.094			0.516	0.230	0.106	0.052	0.026
	8			0.904	0.476	0.246	0.132			0.666	0.316	0.148	0.074	0.038
	9				0.610	0.330	0.180			0.834	0.412	0.202	0.102	0.054
	10				0.762	0.428	0.240			1.00	0.528	0.268	0.138	0.072
	11				0.914	0.536	0.310				0.648	0.344	0.180	0.098

[a] For two samples of size n_1 and n_2 ($n_2 > n_1$) and the value of U, the entry gives the p-value.

(7) If $n_2 \leq 8$, calculate $U = n_1 n_2 + n_1(n_1 + 1)/2 - T$. If $n_2 > 8$, calculate $\mu = n_1(n_1+n_2+1)/2$, $\sigma^2 = n_1 n_2(n_1 + n_2 + 1)/12$, and $z = (T - \mu)/\sigma$.

(7) $n_2 = 7$; find $U = 3(7) + 3(4)/2 - 18 = 9$.

(8) Look up p-value from the appropriate table: Table I for U or Table A for z.

(8) Table 6.9 gives the portion of Table I including $n_2 = 7$, $n_1 = 3$, and U varying from 7 to 11. The p-value for $U = 9$ is 0.834.

(9) Accept the null hypothesis if $p \geq \alpha$; do not accept the null hypothesis if $p < \alpha$.

(9) p is much greater than α. We have no significant evidence that the PSA distributions are different for positive and negative biopsy results.

Why U Is Calculated from T

The Mann–Whitney U is tabulated in this book rather than the rank-sum T, as U requires a much smaller table size.

A One-Tailed Test

If we have some sound nonstatistical reason why the result of the test must lie in only one tail, such as a physiological limit preventing the other tail (a knee does not bend forward), we can halve the tabulated value to obtain a one-tailed p-value.

The Name of This Test

This test may be referred to in the literature as the rank-sum test, Mann–Whitney U test, Wilcoxon rank-sum test, or Wilcoxon–Mann–Whitney test. Mann and

Whitney published what was thought to be one test and Wilcoxon another. Eventually they were seen to be only different forms of the same test.

6.7. CONTINUOUS DATA: BASICS OF MEANS

The Mean Is Studied More Than Other Characteristics

The mean is the most important characteristic of a population, but certainly not the only one. The standard deviation and various aspects of the shape often are crucial for reasons discussed later.

The Most Frequent Question: Are Two Means the Same?

The basic question asked is whether a sample mean is the same as a population mean or whether two samples have the same mean. The question is answered by testing the null hypothesis that the means are equal and then accepting or rejecting this hypothesis. The concept was discussed in Sections 5.1 and 5.2.

The Robustness Concept

Tests of means were developed under the assumption that the sample was drawn from a normal distribution. Whereas usually not truly normal, a distribution that is roughly normal in shape is adequate for a valid test. That is because the test is moderately *robust*. Robustness is an important concept. A robust test is one that is affected little by deviations from the underlying assumptions. If a small-to-moderate sample is too far from normal in shape, the calculation of error probabilities, based on the assumed distribution, will lead to erroneous decisions; use rank-order methods. If a large sample is too far from normal, a statistician may be able to find a suitable data transformation to reshape the distribution, such as a logarithmic, square, square root, or other transformation. In particular, tests of means are only moderately robust and are especially sensitive to outliers, whereas tests of variance are much more robust.

Other Assumptions: Independently Sampled Data and Equal Variability

A normal shape to the frequency distributions is not the only assumption made in tests of means. Along with most other tests of hypotheses, means tests assume that the data being used are independent of each other and that the standard deviations are the same. Independence implies that knowledge of the value of one datum will provide no clue about the value of the next to be drawn. An example of violating this assumption would be pooling repeated blood pressure measurements on several hypertensive patients. Knowledge of a pressure for one patient would give some information about what pressure would be expected from the next reading if it arose from the same patient, but would give no information if the patient were different; thus, the readings are not all independent. An example of different standard deviations might arise upon comparing WBCs from a sample of healthy patients with those from a sample of patients having bacterial infections. The infected sample might be much more variable than the healthy sample. Techniques exist to adjust for unequal standard deviations, but not much can be done to salvage data with dependencies. In the remainder of this chapter, independent data and equal standard deviations will be assumed.

The Alternate Hypothesis Must Specify a One- or Two-Tailed Test

The null hypothesis states that the mean of the population from which the sample is drawn is not different from a theorized mean or from the population mean of another sample. We also must choose the alternate hypothesis, which will select a two-tailed or a one-tailed test. We should decide this before seeing the data so that our choice will not be influenced by the outcome. We often *expect* the result to lie toward one tail, but expectation is not enough. If we are sure the other tail is impossible, such as for physical or physiological reasons, we unquestionably use a one-tailed test. Surgery to sever adhesions and return motion to a joint frozen by long casting will allow only a positive increase in angle of motion; a negative angle physically is not possible. A one-tailed test is appropriate. There are cases in which an outcome in either tail is possible, but a one-tailed test is appropriate. When making a decision about a medical treatment, i.e., whether we will alter treatment depending on the outcome of the test, the possibility requirement applies to the alteration in treatment, not the physical outcome. If we will alter treatment only for significance in the positive tail and it will in no way be altered for significance in the negative tail, a one-tailed test is appropriate.

6.8. Continuous Data: Normal (*z*) and *t* Tests to Compare Two Sample Means

The Normal Test and the *t* Test Are Two Forms of the Two-Sample-Means Test

We will concentrate on the type of means test most frequently seen in the medical literature: the test for a difference between two means. We will look at two subclasses: the case of known population standard deviations, or samples large enough that the sample standard deviations are not practically different from known, and the case of small-sample estimated standard deviations. The means test uses a standard normal distribution (z distribution) in the first case and a t distribution in the second, for reasons discussed in Section 2.8. (Review: The means are assumed normal. Standardization places a standard deviation in the denominator. If the standard deviation is known, it behaves as a constant and the normal distribution remains. If the standard deviation is estimated from the sample, it follows a probability distribution and the ratio of the numerator's normal distribution to this distribution turns out to be t.)

The Steps to Follow; Example of z Test

The steps to follow for either the z or the t test are rather straightforward. They are given below on the left with an example to the right.

Steps in method:

(1) Satisfy yourself that the sample has been drawn such that it represents the population and such that observations are independent from each other. This step is pure judgment based on the way the data have been collected. If these requirements are violated, statistics will not help very much.

(2) Make quick frequency plots of the two samples' basic data to check the normality and equal standard deviation assumptions. If one or both are violated, use rank-order methods.

(3) Choose the z test or t test as appropriate. You have n data split between two samples of size n_1 and n_2. If σ (the population standard deviation under the null hypothesis) is known or if n is large (greater than 50 or 100), use z. If σ is not known and n is small, use t.

(4) Specify null and alternate hypotheses. The null hypothesis usually will be H_0: $\mu_1 = \mu_2$. Select the alternate as

Steps in example, normal (z) test:

(1) We ask whether age is a risk factor for prostate cancer. Are our urological patients with cancer older than those without? We judge that the data are independent and the sample is adequately representative.

(2) Figure 6.1 shows a plot of the two frequency distributions. They appear adequately normal in shape, with equivalent standard deviations.

(3) Of $n = 301$, $n_1 = 206$ biopsies were negative and $n_2 = 95$ were positive. The samples are large enough to use the z test. From the data, we calculate $m_1 =$ 66.59 years, $s_1 = 8.21$ years, $m_2 = 67.14$ years, and $s_2 = 7.88$ years.

(4) H_0: $\mu_1 = \mu_2$. Because it is possible for positive biopsy patients to be either older or younger (although we might

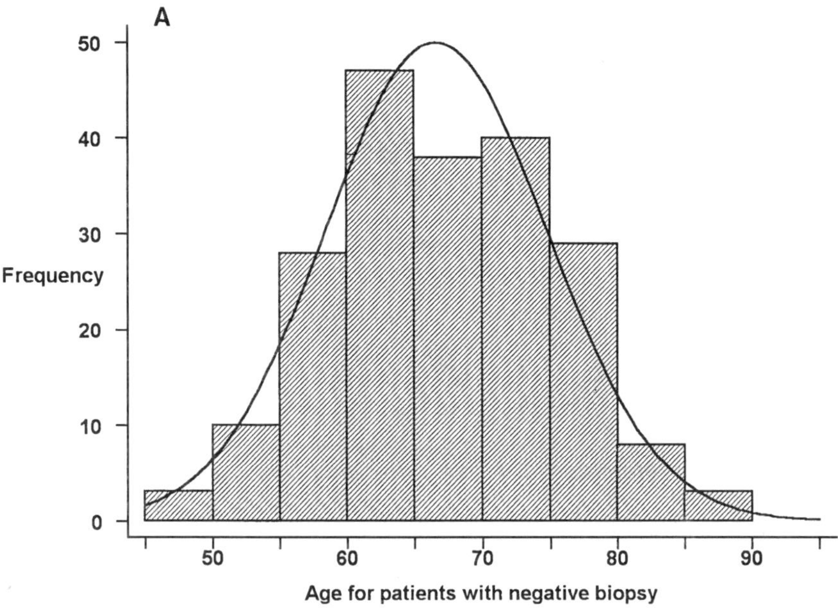

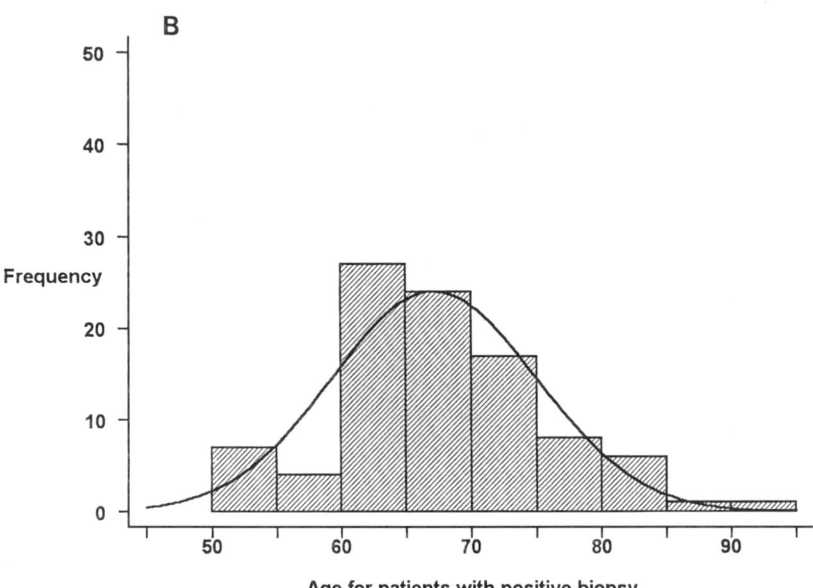

Figure 6.1 A plot of age distributions by biopsy result for 301 patients: (A) negative biopsy; (B) positive biopsy.

Table 6.10
Fragment of Table A, Normal Distribution

	One-tailed applications		Two-tailed applications	
z (no. std. deviations to right of mean)	One-tailed α (area in right tail)	$1-\alpha$ (area except right tail)	Two-tailed α (area in both tails)	$1-\alpha$ (area except both tails)
1.90	0.029	0.971	0.054	0.946
1.96	*0.025*	*0.975*	*0.050*	*0.950*
2.00	0.023	0.977	0.046	0.934

H_1: $\mu_1 \neq \mu_2$ for a two-sided test, or H_1: $\mu_1 < \mu_2$ or H_1: $\mu_1 > \mu_2$ for a one-sided test.

not expect younger), we choose a two-sided alternative, H_1: $\mu_1 \neq \mu_2$.

(5) Choose an appropriate α and look up the associated critical value from Table A (z) or Table B (t) with n_1+n_2-2 degrees of freedom. For a two-sided test, use the "two-tailed α" heading. For a one-sided test, use "one-tailed α."

(5) We choose $\alpha = 0.05$. Table 6.10 shows a fragment of Table A, the normal distribution. Under "Two-tailed applications," for $\alpha = 0.05$, we find the critical $z = 1.96$.

(6) Calculate as appropriate the z or t statistic. The test is in the form of a standardized difference between means, i.e., the difference $m_1 - m_2$ divided by the standard error σ_d or s_d. Calculate z by

$$z = (m_1 - m_2)/\sigma_d, \qquad (6.4)$$

where

$$\sigma_d = \sigma\sqrt{\frac{1}{n_1} + \frac{1}{n_2}}, \qquad (6.5)$$

or t by

$$t = (m_1 - m_2)/s_d, \qquad (6.6)$$

where

$$s_d = \sqrt{\left(\frac{1}{n_1} + \frac{1}{n_2}\right)\left[\frac{(n-1)s_1^2 + (n_2-1)s_2^2}{n_1+n_2-2}\right]}. \qquad (6.7)$$

(6) We want to use the z form. From the data set statistics in the first table of DB1, the standard deviation for the 301 ages is 8.10; we take it as σ. Then, from Eq. (6.5), $\sigma_d = 8.10 \times \sqrt{1/206 + 1/95} = 1.00$, and from Eq. (6.4), $z = (m_1 - m_2)/\sigma_d = (66.59 - 67.14)/1 = -0.55$.

(7) Accept or reject the null hypothesis, depending on where the statistic lies relative to the critical value.

(7) The statistic $z = -0.55$ is well within the null hypothesis acceptance bounds of ± 1.96. We accept the null hypothesis.

(8) If a statistical software package is available, the actual p-value may be calculated to facilitate further interpretation of the decision (as in Section 5.2).

(8) $p = 0.582$. We would be more likely wrong than not to conclude a difference. We feel justified in dismissing this question and not revisiting it with larger samples.

Could the *t* Test Have Been Used Instead of the *z* Test?

What would have been the effect of using the t test instead of the normal test of means in examining the age difference between positive and negative biopsy patients? Is the t test appropriate? It is. The normal test assumes that the variances are obtained from the entire population, which often is an infinite number, so that the t really is an approximation to the normal. Upon comparison of Tables A and B, we can see that the critical t values for ∞ df are the same as the normal values. Let us compare the critical values for a two-tailed α of 5%. The normal critical value is 1.96. With samples of 206 negative biopsies and 95 positive ones, $df = (206 - 1) + (95 - 1) = 299$. We want to use Table B, t distribution, a fragment of which is shown as Table 6.11. Probabilities for 299 df will lie between the rows for 100 df and an unmeasurably large number of df (symbolized by infinity, ∞). Under the column for two-tailed $\alpha = 0.05$, the t critical value will lie between 1.98 and 1.96, or about 1.97, which is quite similar to the 1.96 critical value for the normal. Let us illustrate the steps in performing the two-sample t test for these data.

Following the Steps for the *t* Test

The first four steps and the choice of α are identical to the z test for these data. Determination of the critical value in the fifth step was addressed in the preceding

Table 6.11

Fragment of Table B, *t* Distribution

One-tailed α (right tail area)	0.10	0.05	0.025	0.01	0.005	0.001	0.0005
Two-tailed α (area both tails)	0.20	0.10	0.05	0.02	0.01	0.002	0.001
$df = 40$	1.303	1.684	2.021	2.423	2.704	3.307	3.551
60	1.296	1.671	2.000	2.390	2.660	3.232	3.460
100	1.290	1.660	1.984	2.364	2.626	3.174	3.390
∞	1.282	1.645	1.960	2.326	2.576	3.090	3.291

paragraph, our critical value is 1.97. Step six is actual calculation. The formula in Eq. (6.7) for the standard error of the mean in the case of small samples gives

$$s_d = \sqrt{\left(\frac{1}{n_1} + \frac{1}{n_2}\right)\left[\frac{(n_1 - 1)s_1^2 + (n_2 - 1)s_2^2}{n_1 + n_2 - 2}\right]}$$

$$= \sqrt{\left(\frac{1}{206} + \frac{1}{95}\right)\left[\frac{205 \times 8.21^2 + 94 \times 7.88^2}{206 + 95 - 2}\right]} = 1.01.$$

t then is the simple calculation of Eq. (6.6):

$$t = (m_1 - m_2)/s_d = (66.59 - 67.14)/1.01 = -0.54.$$

For the z test, the z statistic was -0.55, falling well within the H_0 acceptance region of ± 1.96. Similarly, to follow step seven for the t test, the t statistic falls well within the H_0 acceptance region of ± 1.97. We note that, for samples of over 100, the difference between the methods is negligible. Indeed, upon calculating the exact p-value, we find it to be 0.582, which is identical with that for the z test.

6.9. OTHER TESTS OF HYPOTHESES

TESTS OF HYPOTHESES EXIST FOR MANY OTHER RESEARCH QUESTIONS

In this chapter, an understanding of the concepts of testing is at issue, not use of the right method for the reader's specific problem. A wide variety of tests exists for various types of data (counts, ranks, measurements), various sample groupings (paired versus unpaired data, groups of one, two, and more than two), and various distributional characteristics at question (proportions, order precedence, means, variability, shape). The reader who completes Part I of this book and seeks to find the appropriate test for a particular question will find some guidance in Chapter 10 and be taken through a number of specific methods in Chapters 13–17.

CHAPTER EXERCISES

6.1. In DB4, test the contingency table using chi-square to decide whether access to protease inhibitors has reduced the rate of pulmonary admissions.

6.2. In DB6, test the contingency table using chi-square to decide whether titanium-containing tattoo ink is harder to remove than other inks.

6.3. In DB2, test the 2×2 contingency table using chi-square to decide whether nausea score is reduced by the drug.

6.4. A general surgeon noted a number of errors in his hospital's diagnosis of appendicitis. Of the next 200 abdominal pain patients, 104 turned out to have appendicitis and 96 turned out not to have appendicitis. Of those with appendicitis, 82 were correctly diagnosed, and of those without, 73 were correctly diagnosed. (a) Form a truth table. Calculate and state the interpretation of (b) the false positive rate, (c) the false negative rate, (d) sensitivity, (e) specificity, (f) accuracy, and (g) the odds ratio (OR) for this hospital's clinical diagnosis of appendicitis.

6.5. In DB3, calculate the difference: serum theophylline level at baseline minus that at 5 days; assign ranks to this new variable and perform the rank-sum test to learn whether there is evidence that the reduction in level due to the drug differs between men and women.

6.6. In DB7, rank bone density and perform the rank-sum test to learn whether there is evidence that the bone density is different between men and women.

6.7. In DB12, the sample is large enough to take the sample standard deviation as if it were a population standard deviation σ. For convenience, carry the calculations to only two decimal places. Perform a normal (z) test to learn whether there is evidence that (a) mean age and (b) extent of carinal resection is different for the patients who survived versus those who died.

6.8. In DB3, use the difference between theophylline level at baseline minus that at 5 days and perform a t test to learn whether there is evidence that the mean reduction in level due to the drug differs between men and women. Compare the result with the result of Exercise 6.5.

6.9. In DB7, perform a t test to learn whether there is evidence that the mean bone density is different between men and women. Compare the result with the result of Exercise 6.6.

Chapter 7

Sample Size Required for a Study

7.1. OVERVIEW

The Bigger the Sample, the Stronger the Statistical Conclusions

How large a sample do we need? Speaking statistically, *the larger the better.* Larger samples provide better estimates, more confidence, and smaller test errors. The best way to choose a sample size is to take *all the data* our time, money, support facilities (hospital, animal lab), and ethics of patient use will permit. Then why all the attention to methods for estimating the minimum sample size required? The purpose is to *verify that we will have enough* data to make the study worthwhile. If we can manage only 50 subjects and the sample size requirement methods show we need 200, we should not undertake the study.

Concept

Estimation of the minimum sample size required for a decision is not a single unique method, but the concepts underlying most methods are similar. Figure 7.1 shows distributions for null and alternate hypotheses in a test of means for samples of size n (A) and size $4n$ (B). The size of the difference between treatment outcomes that will answer the clinical question being posed often is termed clinical significance or, better, *clinical relevance*. For such a clinically important difference between means, the sizes of error probabilities (α and β) are illustrated by the shaded areas. When the sample is quadrupled, the curves become more slender,

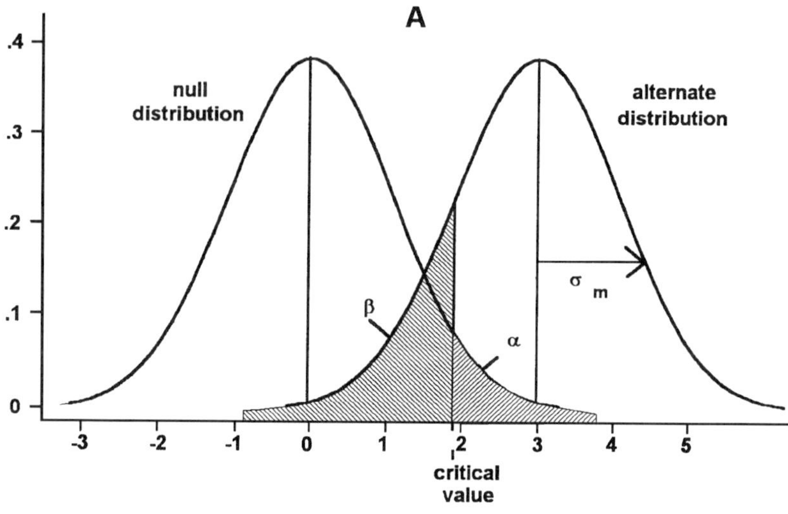

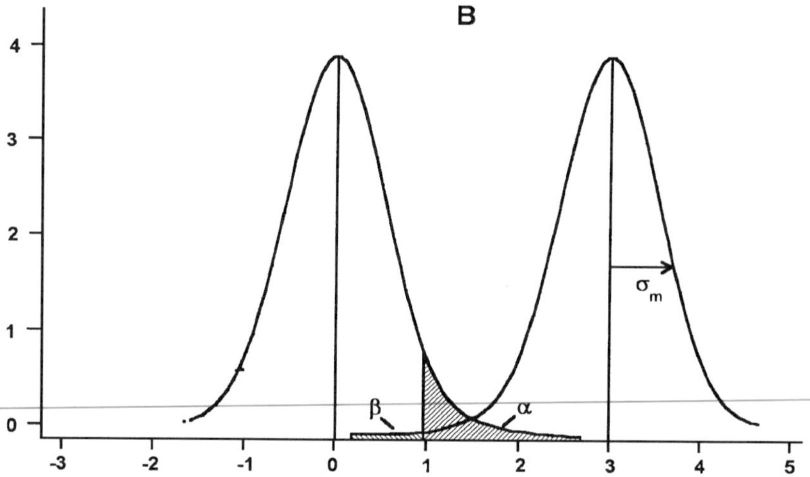

Figure 7.1 Distributions for null and alternate hypotheses in a test of means (A) with sizes of associated error probabilities indicated by shaded areas (see Section 5.2). If the sample size is quadrupled, $\sigma_m = \sigma/\sqrt{n}$ shrinks to half the size, yielding an equivalent diagram (B) with more slender curves. Note how much β has shrunk for a fixed α. The method of estimating a minimum sample size to yield specified error sizes for detecting a given distance between means is to start with those error sizes and that distance and "back-solve" the relationships to find the associated n.

overlapping less, and consequently yield smaller error probabilities. The method of estimating a minimum sample size is to specify the difference between means and the required chances of error and then to find the n that satisfies these specifications.

The Term Power Analysis

A note on terminology: $1 - \beta$ is called "power." As β is the chance of falsely accepting the null hypothesis, power is the chance of correctly accepting the alternate hypothesis. This approach to estimating the minimum sample size required often is termed *power analysis* because it depends on α (the chance of erroneously accepting the alternate hypothesis) and β ($1 -$ power).

Value of Very Small Samples

Much is said about small samples in medicine. Although derision directed toward generalizing from "samples of size one" (i.e., anecdotal data) is just, nevertheless the first datum encountered in a situation of complete ignorance provides the greatest amount of information from any one datum an investigator will encounter. Consider the appearance of a new disease for which there is no knowledge whatsoever about the incubation period. The first patient for whom we know the time of exposure and the time of appearance of the disease syndrome provides a great deal of useful information. This first incubation period datum gives us an order of magnitude, improves our study planning, and suggests many hypotheses about disease patterns such as infectious sources.

Effect of Increasing the Sample Size

Let us see what happens in estimating the minimum sample size as we gradually increase our sample size from 1 to its final n. Intuitively we observe that the informative value per datum decreases as the number of data increase. Consider how much more is learned from data 1–5 than from data 101–105. There are, in fact, theoretical reasons we will not pursue to say that the amount of information increases as the square root of the sample size, i.e., $\sqrt{n}$. That is to say, to double the information about an event, we must quadruple the data.

Convergence

At some point, enough data are accumulated that the sample distribution only negligibly differs from the population distribution, and we can treat the results as if they came from the population; the sample is said to *converge* to the population.

Choosing Test Sidedness

We should note that sample size estimation may be based on a one- or two-sided alternate hypothesis, just as is the test for which the sample size is being estimated. In the methods of this chapter, the more commonly used two-sided form of the normal tail area ($z_{1-\alpha/2}$) is given. For one-sided cases, just replace $z_{1-\alpha/2}$ with $z_{1-\alpha}$ wherever it appears. For example, replace the two-tailed 5% α's $z = 1.96$ with the one-tailed 5% α's $z = 1.645$. The effect on the patient should be considered in selecting sidedness. When a two-sided test is appropriate, a one-sided test doubles the error rate assigned to the chosen tail, in which case too large a number of healthy patients will be treated as ill and too small a number of ill patients will not be treated. Choice of a two-sided test when a one-sided one is appropriate creates the opposite errors.

Choosing Test Parameters

Although $\alpha = 5\%$ and power $= 80\%$ ($\beta = 20\%$) have been the most commonly selected error sizes in the medical literature, a 20% β is larger than is appropriate in most cases. Furthermore, a β/α ratio of 4/1 may affect the patient. When the false positive is worse for the patient than the false negative, as in a case of testing a drug used for a non-life-threatening disease but that has severe side effects, the common choices of $\alpha = 5\%$ and $\beta = 20\%$ are not unreasonable. On the other hand, in testing treatments for cancer, the rate of false negatives (failing to treat cancer) is worse and the ratio β/α should decreased.

Clinical Relevance and Patient Care

The clinical relevance, often denoted d or δ, usually is the statistical parameter that most influences the sample size. It also may affect patient care. Because a larger difference will require a smaller n, the temptation exists to maximize the difference to allow for a small enrollment with subsequent early closure. This clearly is statistical tampering, as the choice is made on statistical rather than clinical grounds and begs an ethical question: If the proposed new therapy really is *so much* better than the current one, how may the researcher in good faith not offer the patient the superior course? The difference should be chosen with patient care as part of the consideration.

7.2. IS THE ESTIMATE OF MINIMUM REQUIRED SAMPLE SIZE ADEQUATE?

A "SAFETY FACTOR" IS ADVISABLE

Whatever method we use to estimate the sample size required for a study, this sample size ideally should be estimated on the basis of the *results* of that study. Thus, we cannot know the sample size until we do the study, and we do not want to do the study until we know the sample size. The usual solution to this "Catch 22" is to estimate the sample size required for our study from the results of other sources, such as a pilot study or results quoted in the literature. Because these are not the actual data from our study, there is a *wrong data* source of possible error in our estimate. Furthermore, sample size is estimated on the basis of data that are subject to randomness, so that there is also a *randomness* source of possible error in the estimate. Due to these errors from different data or chance, the α and β errors upon which we based our sample size estimate may be larger than we anticipated. Because the estimated sample size represents the *very minimum allowable*, whatever the method used, *we should add a "safety factor" to the estimated required sample size* to account for these two sources of possible error. The size of this safety factor is an educated guess. The more uneasy we are about how well the data used in the sample size estimate will agree with the ultimate study data, the larger the safety factor we should allow. The resulting estimate of sample size is a mixture of guess and statistics, a number that may be taken only as a rough indicator.

7.3. SAMPLE SIZE IN MEANS TESTING

WHAT INPUTS ARE NEEDED

In Section 5.8, we introduced a test for the difference between the means of samples from two normal distributions. If we are planning a study that will require such a test, we want to estimate how much data we will need. To follow the development of a method of such estimation, let us look at the simpler case of testing a sample mean against a known population mean. Values used in minimum sample size estimation are the error risks (α and β), the standard deviation of the population data (σ), and the difference we want to detect between the two means being tested. This difference, often denoted d or δ, is the clinical relevance, the difference clinically important to detect. The minimum sample size depends more on this difference than on the other inputs. The sample size grows large quickly as this difference grows small.

The Logic behind the Method

An emergency medicine physician knows from large-sample historical evidence that mean heart rate (HR) from a particular healthy population is $\mu = 72$ bpm (beats per minute) with standard deviation $\sigma = 9.1$ bpm. She wants to know whether mean HR from a population of patients who have just been exposed to a particular type of toxin is the same or greater. She plans to collect data from the next sample of patients who present with that toxic exposure and test the sample mean against the population mean. She needs to estimate the minimum sample size she will need. She designates the unknown population mean μ_s (subscript s for "sample's distribution"). The hypotheses tested will be

$$\mathrm{H}_0 : \mu_s = \mu \quad \text{versus} \quad \mathrm{H}_1 : \mu_s > \mu.$$

From the data that will be forthcoming, the value of μ_s will be estimated by the sample mean m. Thus, to decide whether $\mu_s = \mu$, we test m against μ. Figure 7.2 shows the two distributions involved; as they are standardized, the HR numbers must be adjusted to match the figure. The first is the null, with its mean μ standardized to 0 indicated by a vertical line. The second is a possible alternate, with its

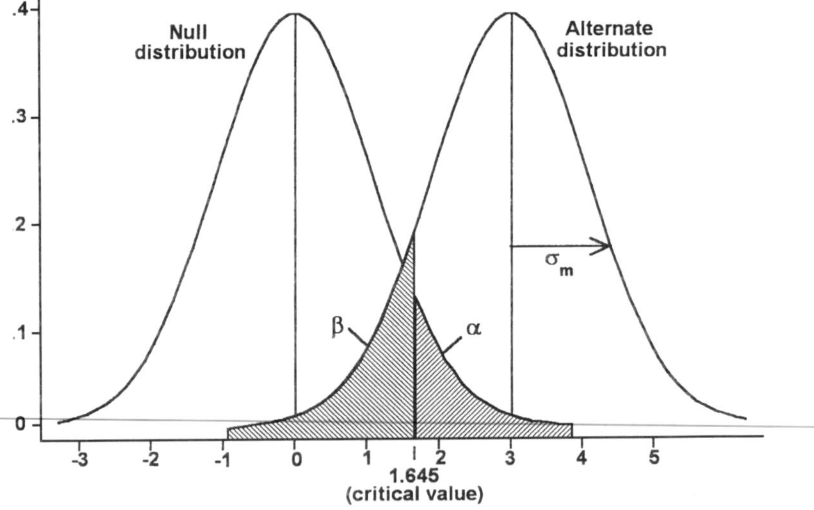

Figure 7.2 Distributions of null and alternate hypotheses showing Type I and Type II errors separated by the critical value, chosen as 1.645 (standard normal value) to provide $\alpha = 5\%$. We specify the difference in standard errors between the means (here about 3) that we want the test to detect. The error probabilities are dictated by the overlap of distributions, which in turn is dictated by the standard error $\sigma_m = \sigma/\sqrt{n}$. As we increase n, σ_m and, therefore, the areas under the overlap giving the error sizes shrink until the specified error probabilities are reached. The resulting n is the minimum sample size required to detect the specified difference in means.

mean μ_s, estimated by m, indicated by a vertical line at about 3. σ is the standard deviation of the population data, so σ_m, the standard error of the mean (the standard deviation of distribution shown in the figure), is $\sigma/\sqrt{n}$, where n is the sample size we seek. We use a form very much like a test for a significant difference between means, $m - \mu$, except the error risks are inputs and the n is output. For this discussion, we will use $\alpha = 5\%$ and $\beta = 20\%$ (power $= 1 - \beta = 80\%$). The critical value (here $\mu + 1.645\sigma_m$) is the position separating the two types of error, shown in Fig. 7.2 as the number of standard errors above μ that yields a 5% α (area under a tail of the null distribution; 1.645 is the value from the normal table for $\alpha = 5\%$). Similarly, β is the area under a tail of the alternate distribution and is specified by the number of standard errors below m that the critical value lies, or $m - 0.84\sigma_m$ (0.84 is the value from the normal table for 20% in the tail area). Because these two expressions both equal the critical value, we set them equal to each other, or $\mu + 1.645\sigma/\sqrt{n} = m - 0.84\sigma/\sqrt{n}$. Solution of the equation for n yields

$$n = \frac{(z_{1-\alpha/2} + z_{1-\beta})^2\sigma^2}{d^2} = \frac{(1.645 + 0.84)^2\sigma^2}{(m - \mu)^2}. \tag{7.1}$$

Other formulas for minimum required sample size follow equivalent logic. In particular, the formula for the case of two means, which will be introduced next, uses a formula recognizably similar to Eq. (7.1).

What if σ Is Not Known?

Note that the methods given here primarily use normal distribution theory and the population or large-sample σ, rather than a small-sample s. If s is all we have, we just use it in place of σ. The reason for this is two-fold. First, if n is unknown, we have no df to use in finding the appropriate t-values to use in the calculation. Second, the nicety of using t would be lost in the grossness of the approximation, because the process depends on pilot data or results from other studies and not the data to be used in the actual analysis.

7.4. MINIMUM SAMPLE SIZE ESTIMATION FOR A TEST OF TWO MEANS

Example from Orthopedics

Two types of artificial knee are to be compared for range of motion (measured in degrees). Theoretically, either could give a greater range, so a two-sided alternative hypothesis is appropriate. The hypotheses to be tested become $H_0: \mu_1 = \mu_2$ versus $H_1: \mu_1 \neq \mu_2$. A journal article on the first type of knee gave $m_1 = 112°$ with

$s_1 = 13°$, and an article on the second gave $m_2 = 118°$ with $s_2 = 11°$. If we want to carry out a prospective randomized clinical trial to decide whether a 6° difference is statistically significant, what is the minimum number of patients receiving each knee we must record?

The Method in General

We ask whether μ_1 (estimated by m_1) is different from μ_2 (estimated by m_2). Choose the smallest distance d (clinically relevant difference) between m_1 and m_2, i.e., $d = m_1 - m_2$, to be detected with statistical significance. From the medical literature or pilot data, find σ_1^2 and σ_2^2, estimated by s_1^2 and s_2^2, if necessary. Choose the risk required of an erroneous rejection of H_0 (α) and an erroneous acceptance of H_0 (β, or 1 − power). Look up the z-values in Table A, $z_{1-\alpha/2}$ and $z_{1-\beta}$, for these two risks. Substitute the z-values and d along with the standard deviations in Eq. (7.2) to find n_1 ($=n_2$), the minimum sample size required in *each* sample. [Note how similar Eq. (7.2) is to Eq. (7.1).] For a one-sided test, substitute $z_{1-\alpha}$ for $z_{1-\alpha/2}$.

$$n_1 = n_2 = \frac{(z_{1-\alpha/2} + z_{1-\beta})^2(\sigma_1^2 + \sigma_2^2)}{d^2}. \tag{7.2}$$

The Orthopedic Example Using the Method

We chose $d = m_1 - m_2 = -6°$ and found the values $\sigma_1^2 = 169$ and $\sigma_2^2 = 121$ from the literature. We choose α as 5% and $1 - \beta$ (the power) as 80%. From Table A (with interpolation), $z_{1-\alpha/2} = 1.95$ and $z_{1-\beta} = 0.84$. Substitution in Eq. (7.2) yields

$$n_1 = n_2 = \frac{(z_{1-\alpha/2} + z_{1-\beta})^2(\sigma_1^2 + \sigma_2^2)}{d^2} = \frac{2.8^2 \times 290}{6^2} = 63.16.$$

The required minimum sample size is 64. For the reasons of given in Section 7.2, a few more would be advisable.

7.5. OTHER SITUATIONS IN WHICH MINIMUM SAMPLE SIZE ESTIMATION IS USED

Sample Size Methods Exist for Confidence Limits and Statistical Tests

Two basic uses for minimum sample size estimation are in confidence limits and statistical tests. In confidence limits, we estimate a parameter, for example, m

estimating μ, and we want some idea of how large a sample we need to find 95% (or other) confidence limits on the parameter. In testing, we pose a clinically relevant effect, for example, difference between two means, and we want some idea of how large a sample we need to detect this difference with statistical significance.

Sample Size Methods Have Been Developed for Some but Not All Requirements

Methods for minimum sample size estimation have been developed for some of the most frequently used statistical techniques, but not for the majority of techniques. In the reference part of this book, specifically Chapter 18, minimum sample size methods may be found for the following statistical techniques:

- Categorical data
  - Confidence interval on a proportion
  - Test of a sample proportion against a theoretical proportion
  - Test of two sample proportions (equivalent to use for a 2×2 contingency table)
- Continuous data
  - Confidence interval on a mean
  - Confidence interval on a correlation coefficient
  - Test on one mean (normal distribution)
  - Test on two means (normal distributions)
  - Test on means from poorly behaved distributions
  - Test on means in the presence of clinical experience but no prior objective data

Minimum sample size estimation methods for other statistical techniques exist, some developed with considerable thoroughness and rigor and others not. To list them all would be misleading, because new approaches appear in the statistical literature from time to time. Some of the more common statistical techniques for which sample size methods exist are tests on $r \times c$ contingency tables, tests on variances (standard deviations), one-way analysis of variance (a test on three or more means), and tests on regression models.

CHAPTER EXERCISES

7.1. Should minimum sample size estimation be based on a one-sided or a two-sided test, assuming the underlying distributions are normal, of (a) a difference in nausea scores between ondansetron hydrochloride and placebo in DB2 and (b) the difference between assay types in DB8?

7.2. Assess the clinical effects of false positive and false negative outcomes and specify whether β should be the usual 4α in estimating minimum sample size for a test of (a) the effect of ondansetron hydrochloride on nausea following gall bladder surgery in DB2 and (b) a change in plasma silicone following implant in DB5.

7.3. DB7 contains very small samples of bone density measures for men and women. On the basis of the standard deviations of those samples, estimate the minimum sample size required to detect a difference of 10 units of bone density between the means for men and women with $\alpha = 0.05$ and power = 0.80 ($\beta = 0.20$).

7.4. In DB12, the extent (centimeters) of the carinal resection appears to affect survival. By using the standard deviations given for surviving (Died = 0) and dying (Died = 1) patients, estimate the minimum sample size required for a test between means of resection extent for those two groups with $\alpha = 0.05$ and power = 0.80 ($\beta = 0.20$).

7.5. In DB3, the mean for the 16 patients' differences between baseline and 5-day serum theophylline level is 0.993, with standard deviation 3.485. For such a difference to be significant with $\alpha = 0.05$ and power = 0.80, $n = 50$ pairs would be required [using a formula slightly different from Eq. (7.2) that can be found in Chapter 18]. By generating three random samples of 50 on a computer from a normal distribution with the same mean and standard deviation, we find t tests yielding p-values of 0.040, 0.042, and 0.072. Comment on the adequacy of the estimated minimum sample size.

Chapter 8

Statistical Prediction

8.1. WHAT IS A "MODEL?"

Patterns in Diagnosis, Etiology, and Outcomes

In medicine, we need to recognize the *pattern* of a malady (diagnosis), we need to understand its *pattern* of development (etiology), and we need to be able to predict its *pattern* of response to treatment (outcome). These patterns, which underlie every stage of medical practice, historically have been only implicit. They were developed intuitively through experience and not recognized formally even by the practitioner in earlier days. They represented the *art* of medicine. As medicine evolves from art more and more toward science, these patterns are beginning to be recognized and formalized. When a pattern is formalized into word-based logic, it often is termed a *paradigm*. When a pattern is formalized into quantitative logic, it often is termed a *model*. (These terms are used differently by different people. The reader must ascertain how a writer is using them, and the writer should define clearly the terms being used.)

Definition of Model

In the context of this book, a *model* is a *quantitative representation of a relationship or process*. A patient's white blood count at a fixed interval of time after infection depends on the dose level of infecting bacteria. The white count and the density of infecting organisms are both quantities. The relationship can be represented by a rising curve. We might conjecture, as a starting point, that it looks

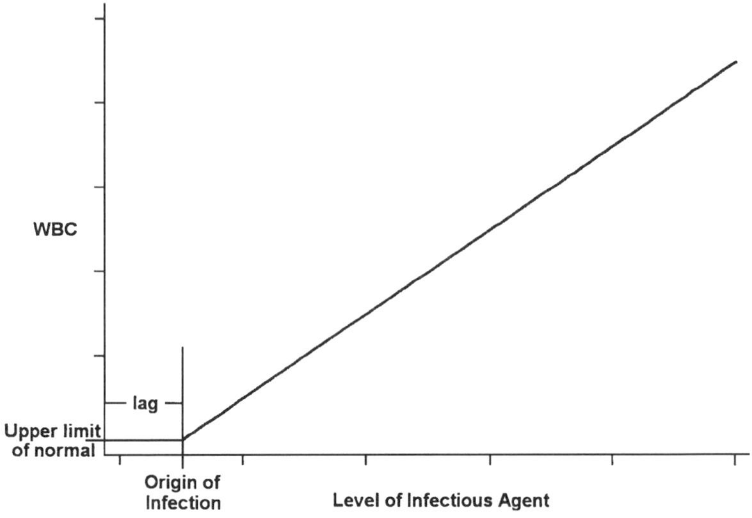

Figure 8.1 A symbolic relationship between WBC and an infectious agent.

something like Fig. 8.1. At this point, we are conjecturing only about the pattern or shape of the relationship, so values are not yet assigned to the axes. This would be a *model*, not of real data but as a conceptual preliminary step. In the next section, we will refine our model and make it more realistic with the acquisition of data.

A Model Is a Limited Tool

A model expresses some important aspect between two (or more) variables. It does not purport to express all the subtleties. The model may say that WBC tends to increase with dose level of a certain bacterium. It may not take into account the time since initial exposure or the state of the patient's immune system. The model is a tool, a window through which we can see the aspect of the relationship we are questioning.

What We Need to Know to Form the WBC Model

Suppose we have data on infection dosages and the related WBC at various points in time. Some questions we might ask are the following:

1. How big an initial dose is required to cause a WBC response?
2. Does WBC increase as a straight line with dose of infection?
3. What is the gradient of this line, i.e., how steep is it?

In the next section, we will see that the dose requiring WBC to begin to rise is the point at which the WBC exceeds normal, that a straight line fit might be appropriate if the data do not curve as they increase (there are tests for this fit), and that the gradient is given by the amount of rise in WBC per unit increase in infection level. In later sections, we will look at curved models and the use of more than one indicator at a time.

8.2. STRAIGHT LINE MODELS

A LINE IS DETERMINED BY TWO DATA

A mathematical straight line on a graph with x (horizontal) and y (vertical) axes is defined by two pieces of information, for example, a point and a slope. If we think of a straight line segment as a piece of straight wire, we can anchor it at a point about which it can rotate. Then we can specify its slope leading out of that point, and the wire is fixed. The point is the location of a known x, y pair. The slope is given by the amount of rise the line makes in the y direction for each unit of movement in the x direction. We can see this fixing occurring in Fig. 8.1. The point occurs where the dose of infection begins to affect the upper limit of normal WBC. If we then specify the rate of increase of WBC as caused by the dose of infection, we have the slope, or gradient. The line will be determined. Similarly, two points will specify a line.

FITTING A LINE

Note that this line is a mathematical certainty and is not subject to statistical variation. When we are subject to real data, we must use these data to *estimate* rather than to determine the two pieces of information that specify the line. Estimation of a point and a slope from data subject to variability is termed *fitting* the line to the data.

CHOOSING THE FORM FOR THE WBC EXAMPLE

To exemplify this process of data and estimation, let us look at some leukocyte counts as related to counts of a specific bacterium resulting from a culture. Figure 8.2 shows 30 data of this sort. (Both x and y are counts $\times 10^9$.) A straight line fit is a reasonable model. Most statistical fits use one of two forms: intercept and slope or mean and slope. (Simple algebra can change any one form to any other.) The intercept is the point, say β_0, at which the line crosses the y-axis, i.e., the (x, y) point $(0, \beta_0)$. If we denote the slope by β_1, the intercept-and-slope form would be $y = \beta_0 + \beta_1 x$. In the current example, a zero value of culture count is

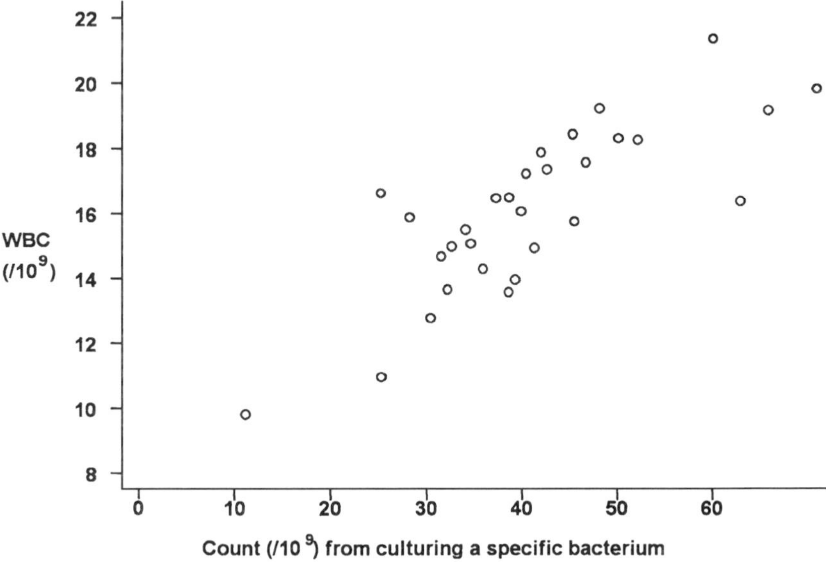

Figure 8.2 WBC data as dependent on culture count of initial infectious agent at a fixed period of time after exposure.

out of the realm of reality, because all of the data come from infected patients. We would do better to choose the defining point as the mean (m_x, m_y), because it lies amid the data. In this case, the mean-and-slope form would be

$$y - m_y = \beta_1(x - m_x). \tag{8.1}$$

We understand that m_x is the sample mean of the culture count and m_y is the sample mean WBC. We are left with the manner of estimating the slope, which will be considered in the next two sections.

8.3. WHAT IS "REGRESSION" (AND ITS RELATION TO CORRELATION)?

PREDICTION

A frequent use of a straight line fit is to predict a dependent variable on the y-axis by an independent variable on the x-axis. In the leukocyte example, WBC can be predicted by the infection culture count. Of course, because the fit is estimated from variable statistical data rather than exact mathematical data, the prediction also will be an estimate, subject to probability and susceptible to confidence interval statements.

How to Calculate a Fit

It seems intuitively obvious that a fit should use all the data and satisfy the most important mathematical criteria of a good fit. The simplest and most commonly used fitting technique of this sort is named *least squares*. The name comes from minimizing the squared vertical distances from the data points to the proposed line. A primitive mechanical way of thinking about it would be to imagine the points as tacks, each holding a rubber band. A thin steel bar representing the line segment is threaded through all the rubber bands. The tension on each rubber band is the square of the distance stretched. The bar is shifted about until it reaches the position at which the total tension (sum of tensions of each rubber band) is a minimum. In the form of Eq. (8.1), the point in the point-slope fit is given by the sample means of x and y, and the slope can be shown mathematically to be estimated by the sample estimates of the x, y covariance divided by the x variance, or s_{xy}/s_x^2. Let us denote by b's the estimates of the β's, to conform with the convention of Greek letters for population (or theoretical) values and Roman letters for sample values. Then $b_1 = s_{xy}/s_x s_y$, yielding

$$y - m_y = b_1(x - m_x) = \frac{s_{xy}}{s_x s_y}(x - m_x). \tag{8.2}$$

For the data plotted in Fig. 8.2, $m_x = 16.09, m_y = 40.96, s_x^2 = 163.07$ ($s_x = 12.77$), and $s_{xy} = 25.86$. By substituting these quantities in Eq. (8.2), we obtain Eq. (8.3) as the fit:

$$y - 40.96 = 0.1585(x - 16.09). \tag{8.3}$$

Figure 8.3 shows the data with the fit superposed.

The Term Regression

The term "regression" has a historical origin unnecessary to remember. It may well be thought of as just a name for fitting a model to data by least squares methods. In case the reader is interested, the name arose from a genetic observation. Evidence that certain characteristics of outstanding people were genetic anomalies rather than evolutionary changes was given by fitting the characteristics of the children of outstanding people to those of their parents and grandparents. As the children's characteristics could be better predicted by their grandparents' characteristics than their parents', the children were said to have "regressed" to the more normal grandparent state.

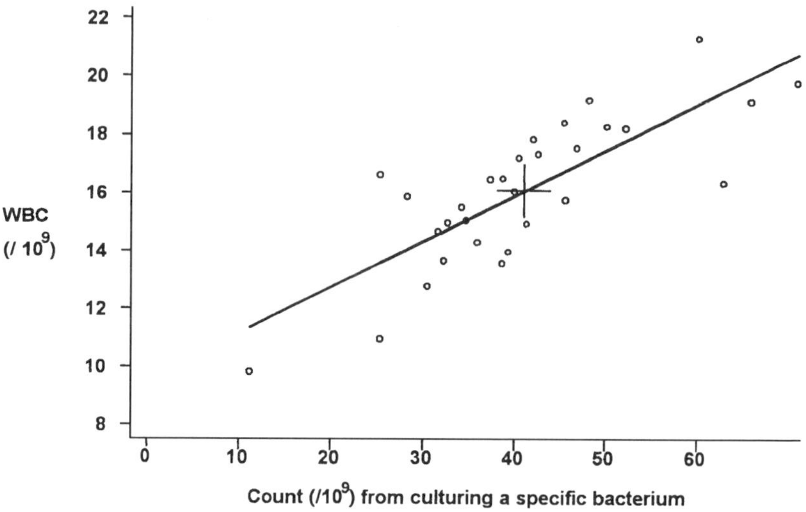

Figure 8.3 WBC data as dependent on culture count with the least squares (regression) fit superposed. Crosshairs show the point composed of means, about (41,16). Note that the line rises about 1.6 units for each horizontal advance of 10 units.

Correlation as Related to Regression

Correlation was introduced in Section 3.1. Clearly both correlation and the straight line regression slope express information about the relationship between x and y. However, they clearly are not exactly the same because the sample correlation r, by Eq. (3.7), is

$$r = \frac{s_{xy}}{s_x s_y} = \frac{\mathrm{cov}(x, y)}{sd(x)sd(y)} \tag{8.4}$$

and the sample slope b_1, from Eq. (8.2), is

$$b_1 = \frac{s_{xy}}{s_x^2} = \frac{\mathrm{cov}(x, y)}{sd(x)sd(x)}. \tag{8.5}$$

Simple algebra will verify that

$$r = b\frac{s_x}{s_y}. \tag{8.6}$$

What does this difference imply? In correlation, the fit arises from simultaneously minimizing the distances from each point perpendicular to the proposed line. In regression, the fit arises from simultaneously minimizing the vertical (y) distances from each point to the proposed line. Thus, regression makes the assumption that *the x measurements are made without random error*. Another difference is that regression may be generalized to curved models, whereas correlation is restricted to straight lines only. A difference in interpretation is that correlation primarily is used to express how closely two variables agree (the width of an envelope enclosing all the points), whereas regression can indicate this (the amount of slope in the fit) plus provide a prediction of the most likely y-value, and a confidence interval on it, for a given x-value. Both can be subjected to hypothesis tests, but tests on regression are more incisive, can be generalized to curved models, and often can be related to other statistical methods (such as analysis of variance).

Assumptions

As in most of statistics, certain assumptions underlie the development of the method. If these assumptions are violated, we can no longer be sure of our conclusions arising from the results. In the case of least squares regression fits, we assume not only that x-values are measured without error, but also that, for each x, the distribution of data vertically about the regression line is approximately normal and that the variability of data vertically about the regression line is the same from one end of the line segment to the other.

8.4. ASSESSING AND PREDICTING RELATIONSHIPS BY REGRESSION

Does Hospital Stay for Mental Patients Relate to IQ?

At a mental hospital, a psychologist's clinical experience suggests to him that brighter patients seem to stay in the hospital longer. If true, such a finding might result from brighter patients being harder to treat. He collects intelligence quotient (IQ) measurements (x) and days in the hospital (y) for the next 50 patients he treats.[17] By using Eqs. (3.1), (3.3), and (3.6) to calculate means, variances, and the covariance, he finds $m_x = 100$, $m_y = 10.5$ days, $s_x = 10$, $s_y = 11.2$ days, and $s_{xy} = 39.43$, from which he uses Eq. (8.4) to find

$$r_{xy} = 39.43/(10 \times 11.2) = 0.35.$$

The correlation coefficient of 0.35 is not decisive, but is large enough to believe that some relationship exists. (Tests of significance on correlation coefficients are treated in Chapter 20.) He wants to regress days in the hospital on IQ, test his ability to predict, and assess how much of the causal forces that decide days in the hospital may be attributed to IQ.

Regression and Prediction

By using Eq. (8.2), he finds that the regression line follows the equation

$$y - 10.5 = 0.3943(x - 100).$$

The data from the 50 patients with the regression line superposed are shown in Fig. 8.4. What would be his best prediction of days in the hospital for a patient with a 90 IQ? With 110 IQ? By substituting 90 for x in Eq. (8.4), he finds about 6.6 days to be the expected stay for a patient with 90 IQ. Similarly, about 14.4 days is the best prediction of hospital stay for a patient with 110 IQ.

Assessment of the Regression Model

How much of the possible causal influence on hospital stay does IQ represent? A good indication of this is given by a statistic named the *coefficient of determination*, designated R^2, which is nothing more than the square of the correlation coefficient when only one predictor is used. In this case, $r = 0.35$, so $R^2 = 0.12$, implying that IQ represents only about 12% of the causal influence. Our psychologist would be inclined to conclude that IQ is a real but rather minor influence on length of hospital stay. Would he be justified? We have not yet considered the satisfaction of the assumptions upon which this regression analysis was based. Let us consider the

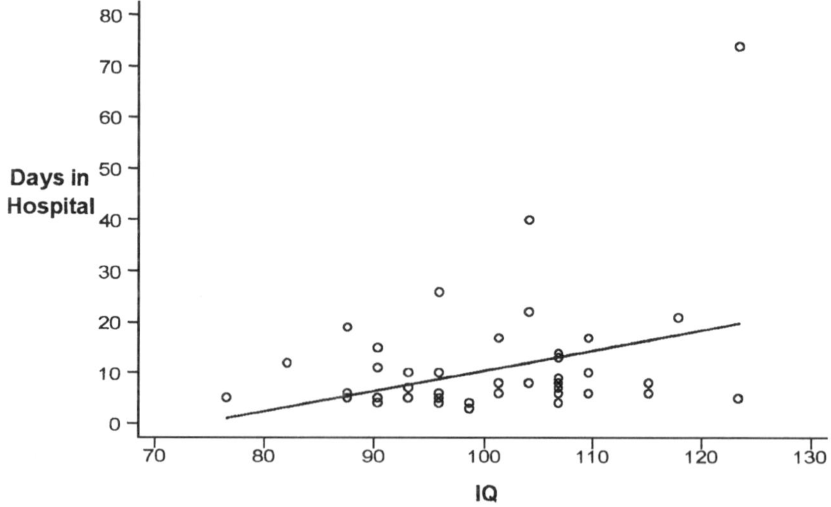

Figure 8.4 Regression of days in the hospital on IQ for 50 mental patients.

three assumptions, assisted by the graph in Fig. 8.4. (Actual tests of assumptions can be made and are considered further in Chapter 20.) Is the assumption that the x-values are measured without error satisfied? The patient's true IQ is a fixed but unknown value. The measured IQ is an effort to estimate the true IQ, but its accuracy certainly is recognized as less than perfect. In addition to accuracy missing the mark, measured IQ varies from time to time in a patient and varies from type to type of IQ test. No, the assumption of exact x-values is not well-satisfied. Is the assumption of normal shape about the line for each x satisfied? There are too few data to be very sure. From the appearance in Fig. 8.4, a case might be made toward the center, but data in the tails appear to be rather skewed. Satisfaction of this assumption is questionable. Finally, is the assumption of equal variability for each x-value satisfied? A glance at Fig. 8.4 will show that the data spread out more and more as we move to the right along the regression line. This assumption seems violated. So where does violation of the assumptions underlying the method leave the investigator? It is possible to adjust for some of the violations by using more sophisticated statistics, but the sample size per IQ value still is too small. He cannot trust his flawed results. About all he can say is that he has some informal pilot results suggesting a small influence by IQ on the length of hospital stay, on the basis of which he will carry out a more carefully designed study with a much larger sample and seek the assistance of a biostatistician at both planning and analysis time.

8.5. OTHER QUESTIONS THAT CAN BE ANSWERED BY REGRESSION

Curved Line Models

Just as a model can be a segment of a straight line, a segment of a curved line can be used as well if the data are better fit by it or, preferably, if known physiologic or medical relationships follow a curve. The curve may be a segment of a parabola (number of cells of a foetus or cancer may increase as the square of time units) a logarithmic form [number of bacteria surviving an antibiotic may decrease as constant $-$ $\log(x)$], or even a cyclic pattern (aspergillosis is seen in Chapter 19 to follow a sine wave over the seasons).

Multiple Variables Simultaneously

Furthermore, multiple variables may be used as predictors. Number of days a patient must be retained in the hospital may be predicted by body temperature, bacterial count, presence–absence of emesis, presence–absence of neurologic signs, etc. No one may be very useful as a predictor, but several in consort may provide sufficient accuracy to assist in hospital bed planning.

Predicting One of Two States

The regression described earlier assumes the y variable is a continuous-type variable. Suppose we want to predict outcome as one of two states, e.g., survival or not, cure or not, disease type A or another. There is a technique termed *logistic regression* in which a transformation can "spread" the two states onto an interval on the y-axis, after which ordinary regression methods may be used on the transformed data. As the transformation is logarithmic in nature, the technique is a log-istic regression. It has come to be mispronounced logistic, although it has nothing to do with the logistics of material. (The transformation is defined in Section 20.8.)

Implication of This Section for the Reader

The cases curvilinear regression, multiple regression, and logistic regression introduced in this section are pursued a little further in Chapter 20. The reader at this stage should remember their names and what sorts of problems they treat, so as to recognize the names or the classes of analysis when meeting them.

8.6. CLINICAL DECISION AND OUTCOMES ANALYSIS

Measures of Effectiveness and Outcomes Analysis

Clinical decisions usually are made on the basis of a *measure of effectiveness (MOE)*, or often more than one. There is no unique MOE. The effectiveness of a treatment may be measured in terms of the probability of cure, the probability of cure relative to other treatments, the risk of debilitating side effects, the cost of treatment relative to other treatments, etc. What might be best under one MOE may not be under another. When quantified MOEs first began to be used, measures easy to quantify were used, e.g., the reduction in number of days for a patient to achieve a certain level of improvement. However, these simple measures usually omitted other important considerations, such as those just mentioned. Investigators began to be dissatisfied with settling for measurably reduced edema following a knee injury when the really important issue was whether the patient could walk again. MOEs of this sort represent the eventual "outcome" of the treatment rather than an interim indicator of progress. Their use therefore has come to be termed *outcomes analysis*. Certainly outcomes often are more difficult to quantify and take much longer to obtain, but without doubt are better indicators of the patient's general health and satisfaction.

A Combination MOE

How should a surgeon's effectiveness be measured? Some possible MOEs are time in surgery, time to heal, patient survival rate, or a hatfull of others. Most of us would say that some combination of measures would be best, i.e., wisely chosen indicators are combined in a balanced way to form a resultant MOE. However, there is no formula to build MOEs. Like so many aspects of medicine, it is a matter of thoughtful judgment. We must start with the question, *What are we really trying to accomplish?* Is our goal a perfect surgery? Patient survival rate? Minimum pain? Minimum cost? We might think of adding several measures together, but we must remember that most are in different units of measurement and represent different levels of relative importance. We must weight each component to adjust for units and importance. A serious question is how relative importances are rated. Indeed, there is controversy about weighing the cost of treatment against the chance of it being effective. The best an investigator can do is set forth a best judgment and allow readers to accept or reject it for themselves.

Example Posed

A dramatic illustration is the issue of quality of life for a terminal patient. Consider an elderly stroke patient. He suffered a cerebral embolism followed by cerebral hemorrhage. He is severely hemiplegic with aphasia. Consciousness and dysphagia are sporadic. At present his airway is intubated and he is fed by IV infusion. Brain edema contraindicates corticosteriods and anticoagulant drugs, but he is receiving a diuretic. Furthermore, he is uninsured, with costs being paid by his adult children, who have marginal incomes. Let us attempt to build an MOE for him.

Example Formed

An overly simple illustration might be to maximize days of survival in which the patient would rather live than die: n_g for number of good days minus n_b for bad days, or MOE $= n_g - n_b$. If the patient has more good than bad days, we keep him alive. If he stops having good days, our MOE grows smaller each day and we would maximize the remaining value of the MOE by immediately ceasing life support. But there are other relevant indicators. Our MOE might contain p, the probability of (partial) recovery. These are medical judgments suggested by the percentages reported in epidemiological studies tempered by the characteristics of this case. Earlier, we used MOE $= n_g - n_b$. By including p, it becomes MOE $= pn_g - (1 - p)n_b$, where we interpret n_g as the total number of good days if he recovers plus those if he does not recover and n_b as the total number of bad days if he recovers plus those if he does not recover. Suppose we judge p to be 0.30. We judge his life expectancy, given recovery, to be a little over 4 years or about 1500 days and, given no recovery, 30 days. We judge that if he recovers, he will have 60% good days. If he does not, he will have 100% bad days. Then $n_g = 60\%(1500) + 0\%(30) = 900$ and $n_b = 40\%(1500) + 100\%(30) = 630$. MOE $= pn_g - (1 - p)n_b = 0.3(900) - 0.7(630) = 270 - 441 = -171$. On average, our patient will live a life of poor quality in which he would rather be dead. We have not yet factored in cost. We do not want to destroy his family's financial future. (The effects of this decision may ripple through two or three generations, such as costing his grandchildren a college education.) Our MOE must add together quality of life levels plus money. To do this, we would have to judge the relative importance of a good day in terms of money units, say \$1000, of cost to the family, and this would stretch our judgment rather far. In this case, we do not have to, as we have already seen that life-sustaining medical intervention will generate primarily misery for the patient.

Different MOEs

This MOE certainly could be built in a different way, which is quite acceptable if it serves the same purpose, just as houses built in different ways may acceptably keep the inhabitant warm, dry, and safe. Every practitioner would find it helpful to try building some MOEs. It makes us think through the issues involved and rank them in importance. It gives us a basis for a decision in those tortured cases in which we are just not sure. Perhaps most important, it reduces our number of erroneous decisions.

CHAPTER EXERCISES

8.1. It is believed that respiration rate in infants decreases with age. To examine that belief, respiration rate was recorded for 232 infants from 0 to 24 months.[42] The scatter diagram of respiration rate against age is shown. Form a conceptual model.

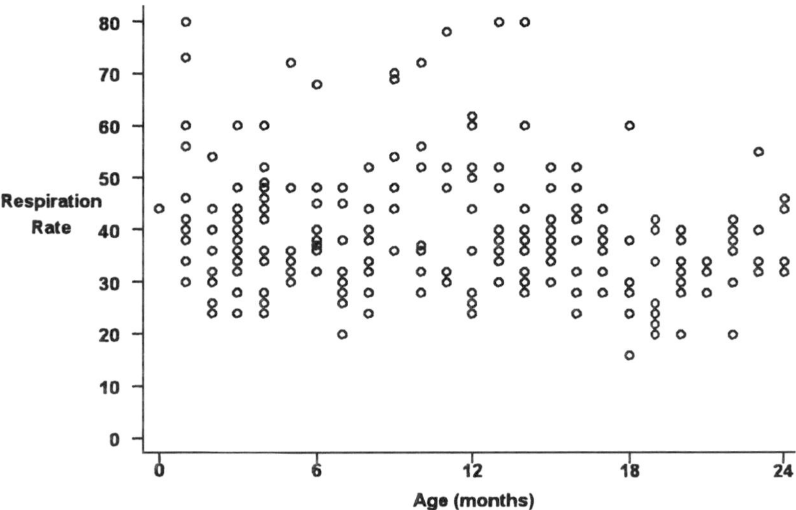

8.2. Summary statistics for the data in Exercise 8.1 (where subscripts a and r represent age and respiration rate, respectively) are $m_a = 10.9$, $m_r = 39.0$, $s_a = 6.7$, $s_r = 11.8$, $s_{ar} = -15.42$. What is the correlation coefficient between age and respiration rate? How is this correlation coefficient interpreted?

8.3. What is the equation for the straight line regression of r on a for Exercies 8.1? Lay a thin paper over the scattergram of respiration rate by age and sketch in this line.

8.4. What is the coefficient of determination? How is this coefficient of determination interpreted?

8.5. Two types of medication exist to treat a certain medical condition. Medicine A costs x dollars for a course of treatment and has always been successful. Medicine B costs y dollars, but fails in 1 out of 10 cases. When failure occurs, medicine A must be used. (There is no contagion or deterioration in medical condition due to the delay.) The question is which medicine should be used, inconvenience to the patient aside. (a) What is the MOE? (b) Set up a relationship between the two medicines such that when the relationship holds true, medicine B should be used. (c) If $x = \$100$ and $y = \$75$, what is the gain per patient by using medicine B?

Chapter 9

Epidemiology

9.1. THE NATURE OF EPIDEMIOLOGY

DEFINITIONS

An *epidemic* is the occurrence in a community or region of cases of an illness, specific health-related behavior, or other health-related events clearly in excess of normal expectancy.[33] *Epidemiology* is the study of the occurrence of illness in populations. To the epidemiologist comparing the rate of occurrence with expectancy, two cases of plague in a city of 6 million people may constitute an epidemic, whereas 10,000 cases of influenza may not. Epidemiology started with the analysis of mortality recordings, from which surprising insights into the patterns of public disease and health events immediately demonstrated its importance. It long concentrated on mortality from infectious diseases (e.g., smallpox), then evolved to include any disease (e.g., cardiovascular disease, cancer) and morbidity of diseases, and finally broadened to include any condition threatening public health (e.g., smoking, mercury in a water or food supply).

EPIDEMIOLOGY COMPARED WITH OTHER BRANCHES OF MEDICINE

Epidemiology, like all of medicine, seeks to understand and control illness. The main conceptual difference between epidemiology and other branches of medicine is its primary focus on health in the group rather than in the individual, from which arises the concept of *public health*. The main methodological difference between epidemiology and other branches of medicine is its attention to rates and distributions. Basic to epidemiology is thinking probabilistically rather than in mutually exclusive categories. The epidemiologist is concerned not with a patient who is sick or well, but rather with the proportion ill from a catchment of patients and the probability that the proportion will grow. To have a baseline for estimating these proportions and probabilities, the epidemiologist continually is concerned with *denominator data*.

Stages of Scientific Knowledge in Epidemiology

The accrual of knowledge in epidemiology follows the same stages as in other fields of medicine, first described in the beginning words of this book: description, explanation, and prediction. Let us consider these stages in sequence. In *description*, the etiology of a public health disease or condition is documented. This stage generates basic epidemiological data and the scientific hypotheses to be tested. In *explanation*, the epidemiological data are assessed in order to explain the outbreak of public disease. The scientific hypotheses are tested. The next stage is *prediction*, which integrates the test results and provides a model of the course of an epidemic, which can be used in the prevention or control of the outbreak and even to assess the efficacy of potential treatments or measures of prevention and control.

Epidemiology Is an Eclectic Science

Epidemiology must interact with many fields of study to isolate causal factors: human and veterinary clinical medicine in their various specialties; biological, biochemical, and genetics investigations; social, economic, and demographic factors; geographic and historic patterns; and the personal habits of individuals. The epidemiologist must be a very general health scientist.

9.2. SOME KEY STAGES IN THE HISTORY OF EPIDEMIOLOGY

The respective beginnings of the descriptive, explanatory, and predictive stages in epidemiology may be followed over three centuries. Quantified description in epidemiology began in 1662 when John Graunt in Great Britain published a tabular analysis of mortality records. In 1747, James Lind in Great Britain pioneered isolating causes by experimentation, finding the nutritional rather than infectious basis of scurvy. Although epidemiology was to wait a century for formal predictive modeling, the theory of contagion allowed the predictive stage of epidemiological science to begin on an informal basis in the 1800s. An example is the 1847 work of

Ignaz Semelweiss in Austria (see also the example of Section 13.6, which recounts his origin of antiseptic surgery), who traced the source of the highly fatal disease puerperal fever by epidemiological methods and showed how to control it.

9.3. CONCEPT OF DISEASE TRANSMISSION

Spectrum of Disease

The sequence of events from exposure to a disease to resolution, often death, is termed the spectrum of disease. It arises from the interaction among three main factors: the host, the agent, and the environment. The *host* includes primary hosts in which a parasite develops, for example, intermediary hosts in which the host is a component in the disease cycle and carrier hosts, which only transport the disease in space or time. The host as a member of the epidemiological catchment is characterized by the susceptibility to acquiring the disease, which includes behavior leading to exposure, immunization or resistance, and the like. The *agent* is not necessarily an infectious agent. It may simply consist of the deficiency of a necessary nutrient (vitamin C in the case of scurvy), the excess of a deleterious substance (tobacco smoke), or a metabolic condition (metabolic acidosis). More dramatically, it may consist of microbes (the bacterium *Yersinia pestis* in the case of plague) or toxins (mercury poisoning, or *yusho*, the name arising from the classic episode at Minamata, Japan). The *environment* as a component in the spectrum is characterized not only by the physical and biological properties (in malaria, still water to breed mosquitoes, access by the mosquitoes to previously infected hosts, exposure of the catchment member to the infected mosquito) that affect disease transmission but also the social properties (as in sexually transmitted diseases).

Modes of Transmission

The classic book by Lilienfeld[37] classifies two modes of transmission: common-vehicle epidemics, in which the vehicle is water, food, air, etc. and serial transfer epidemics, in which the vehicle is a host-to-host transfer, such as infectious transmission by touching, coughing, etc.

Herd Immunity

Rates of infectious disease transmission are not constant. The pattern of an epidemic (depending considerably on incubation period) usually is an initial surge of infected patients, continuing until a substantial number of the epidemiological catchment is immune. At this point, the rate slows, the return cycle to the infectious agent is interrupted, and the epidemic wanes. This high proportion of immunity within a demographic catchment has been termed *herd immunity*. When the herd immunity reaches a critical level, the rate of change of new infection changes from positive to negative and the epidemic starts to decline. The susceptibility of a population to epidemic may be reduced by increasing the herd immunity, for example, by vaccination. It should be noted that herd immunity is by no means the only mechanism to alter the rate of new infection. Many occurrences may alter it. For example, it was noted as early as the 1700s that a yellow fever epidemic often was terminated by a change in the weather.[38]

9.4. DESCRIPTIVE MEASURES

Incidence and Prevalence

Incidence and prevalence have been used in prior chapters, informally although not incorrectly, assuming that the student is familiar with the everyday connotations of the terms. In epidemiology, the terms are used with technical precision, as indeed they should be in all fields of medicine. The incidence rate of a disease is the rate at which new cases of the disease occur in the epidemiological population. The prevalence rate of the disease is the proportion of the epidemiological population having that disease at a point in time. Thus, during an influenza epidemic in a certain city in November, the prevalence rate indicates how much of the population is sick and the incidence rate indicates how rapidly the epidemic is increasing. Incidence and prevalence rates usually are given per 1000 members of the population, unless otherwise indicated.

Mortality Rate

Very similar to incidence rate is mortality rate, the rate at which the population is dying rather than becoming ill. For a disease leading to certain death, the mortality rate at the end of the duration period of the disease would be the same as the incidence rate at the beginning of the period.

Formulas

Incidence rate must be expressed in relation to an interval in time, as "2000 new cases of illness per month." This is because the number of new cases will be zero at a point in time, i.e., when the interval goes to zero. Prevalence rate, on the other hand, can be measured at a point in time, although sometimes a short interval must be used to allow for the time to obtain the prevalence data. Let us denote the number of individuals in the epidemiological population as n, the number of new cases in a specified interval as n_{new}, and the number of cases present at any one point in time by n_{present}. Then incidence rate I is given by

$$I = 1000 \times \frac{n_{\text{new}}}{n}, \tag{9.1}$$

and the prevalence rate P is

$$P = 1000 \times \frac{n_{\text{present}}}{n}. \tag{9.2}$$

If we denote by n_{dying} the number dying during the specified interval, the mortality rate M becomes

$$M = 1000 \times \frac{n_{\text{dying}}}{n}. \tag{9.3}$$

In the remainder of this chapter, the terms incidence and prevalence will be used when incidence rate and prevalence rate are actually intended, because that is the general custom in medical articles, at least outside strict technical usage in epidemiological articles.

Cervical Cancer in the Acornhoek Region of the Transvaal[70]

The population served is given as 56,000. From diagrams of sex ratios and assumptions about the child/adult ratio, we take the adult female population served to be 13,000. (A further subtraction should be made for adult women who never present to medical services, but this unknown number will be ignored for this illustration.) The study covered the 9 years from 1957 to 1968. Cervical cancer was seen in 53 cases, or about 9 per year. Substitution in Eq. (9.1) yields $I = 1000 \times 9/13{,}000 = 0.692$. The yearly incidence of cancer of the cervix is about 0.7. These women's cancer rarely goes into remission. To find prevalence, let us assume, quite arbitrarily, that a woman survives on average 2 years after diagnosis. Then there will be about 18 women with cancer of the cervix surviving at any one time, and Eq. (9.2) yields $P = 1000 \times 18/13{,}000 = 1.384$, or about 1.4. After the first 2 years, M, from Eq. (9.3), is the same as I.

The Odds Ratio (OR)

The OR that we introduced in Section 6.4 also is used in epidemiology. Let us examine an epidemiological study of the interrelation between occurrences of cervical cancer and schistosomiasis.[58] (Schistosomiasis is a parasitic infection

Table 9.1

Frequencies of Occurrence of *S. haematobium* Cervicitis, Cervical Cancer, Both, and Neither Pooled from Two Similar Studies in Africa

Observed frequencies:	With schistosomiasis	Without schistosomiasis	Totals
With cervical cancer	101	5212	5313
Without cervical cancer	165	2604	2769
Totals	266	7816	8082

common in parts of the Third World contracted during immersion in river or stream water.) Table 9.1 reproduces Table 1 from reference 58. Some clinicians in Africa have suggested a protective effect against cancer of the cervix by schistosomiasis. Do the figures support this? Let us calculate the cervical cancer OR for schistosomiasis. Odds of cervical cancer given schistosomiasis, $101/165 = 0.6121$, in ratio to odds of cervical cancer given not schistosomiasis, $5212/2604 = 2.0015$, provides OR $= 0.3058$. These figures say that a woman is more than 3 times as likely ($1/0.3058 = 3.27$) to have cervical cancer if she does not have schistosomiasis! The figures appear to support the claim of a protective effect. However, the epidemiological OR has been derived from biased sampling. The rate of schistosomiasis *without* cervical cancer is markedly *over*reported. The often overwhelmed, undertrained African clinician who finds the presence of *S. haematobium* often ceases to look further; the patient's complaints have been explained adequately and the cervical cancer is not detected. Thus, we could expect that many of the patients reported in the lower left cell of the table should be moved to the cell above it. Furthermore, the rate of cervical cancer *with* schistosomiasis is markedly *under*reported for an entirely different reason: schistosomiasis tends to be acquired at an earlier age (mean = 30 years), and these patients are less likely to live to the age at which cervical cancer tends to appear (mean = 45 years). If these two reportings were corrected, the OR would be changed considerably. It should be clear to the student that high-quality data are crucial prerequisites to meaningful epidemiological results.

9.5. TYPES OF EPIDEMIOLOGIC STUDIES

Basic Variables

All epidemiologic studies are framed in terms of *exposures* and *outcomes*. In simplest terms, the exposure is the putative cause under study, and the outcome is the disease or other event that may result from the exposure.

Experimental Studies and Intervention Trials

The investigator assigns exposure (or nonexposure) according to a plan. The concept of an experimental *control*, introduced in Section 1.6, is used for non-exposed subjects in experimental studies. In *clinical trials*, patients already with disease are subjects; an example would be James Lind's study of scurvy. In *field trials*, patients without disease are subjects; an example would be a vaccine trial in a population. *Community intervention trials* are field trials that are conducted on a community-wide basis.

Nonexperimental or Observational Studies

In these studies, the investigator has no influence over who is exposed. Two types of such study are cohort studies and case–control studies, both discussed in the context of clinical research in Section 1.6. Each study design has inherent strengths and weaknesses.

Cohort Studies

These also are termed *follow-up* or *incidence* studies. In cohort studies, outcomes among two or more groups initially free of that outcome are compared. Subjects may be selected randomly or according to exposure. Indeed, if outcome comparison is the purpose, the study by definition is a cohort study. Cohort studies may be prospective (if exposed and unexposed subjects are enrolled before outcome is apparent) or retrospective (if subjects are assembled according to exposure after the outcome is known). Cohort studies are particularly well-suited to evaluating a variety of outcomes from a single exposure (e.g., smoking). Population-based rates or proportions, or relative risk, that will be discussed in Section 13.4 may be computed.

Case–Control Studies

These also are termed case–referent studies or, loosely and confusingly, sometimes retrospective studies. In case–control studies, the cases and noncases of the outcome in question are compared for their antecedent exposures. If exposure comparison is the purpose, the study by definition is a case–control study. The investigator generally has no influence over these antecedent exposures. The appropriate measure of risk in these studies is the exposure odds ratio (OR), discussed in Sections 6.4 and 13.4.

Prevalence or Cross-Sectional Studies

These are studies of an entire population enrolled, irrespective of exposure and outcome, with exposure and outcome ascertained at the same time. Effectively these are "snapshots" of a population, where analysis may be performed as a cohort study or a case–control study.

Inferring Causation

Identifying causal relationships in observational studies can be difficult. If neither chance nor bias is determined to be a likely explanation of a study's findings, a valid statistical association may be said to exist between an exposure and an outcome. Statistical association between two variables does not establish a cause-and-effect relationship. The next step of inferring a cause follows a set of logical criteria by which associations could be judged for possible causality, which was first described by Sir Bradford Hill in 1965.

Evidence Supporting Causality

Seven criteria now in widespread use facilitate logical analysis and interpretation of epidemiologic data.

(1) *Size of effect.* The difference between outcomes given exposure and given nonexposure is termed *effect*. Large effects are more likely to be causal than small effects. Effect size is estimated by the relative risk (RR). (Relative risk is the probability of having a disease when it is predicted in ratio to the probability of having the disease when the prediction is not having it; see Section 13.4 for further details.) As a rule of thumb, a RR > 2.0 in a well-designed study may be added to the accumulating evidence of causation.

(2) *Strength of association.* Strength of association is based on the p-value, the estimate of the probability of rejecting the null hypothesis. A weak association is more easily dismissed as resulting from random or systematic error. By convention, a p-value of less than 0.05 is accepted as evidence of association.

(3) *Consistency of association.* A particular effect should be reproducible in different settings and populations.

(4) *Specificity of association.* Specificity indicates how exclusively a particular effect can be predicted by the occurrence of potential cause. Specificity is complete where one manifestation follows from only one cause.

(5) *Temporality.* Putative cause must precede putative effect.

(6) *Biologic gradient.* There should be evidence of a cause-to-outcome process, which frequently is expressed as a dose–response effect, the term being carried over from clinical usage.

(7) *Biologic plausibility*. There should be a reasonable biologic model to explain the apparent association.

Further information on the evidence list can be found in refs 20, 39, and 60.

9.6. AN INFORMAL APPROACH TO PUBLIC HEALTH PROBLEMS

Gathering and Assessing Epidemiological Information

The essence of epidemiologic methodology can be expressed informally rather simply and briefly, encapsulating it in the classic journalistic guideline: answer the questions what, who, where, when, and how. Let us examine these steps through the example of discovery of a smallpox vaccine. Suppose you are working with Edward Jenner in the 1790s encountering smallpox.

What

The first step is to characterize a *case definition*. We must describe the disease with all the signs, symptoms, and other properties that characterize it in minute detail. We do not know which variable or combination of variables will relate to others. In this example, smallpox is characterized by chills, high fever, backache, headache, and sometimes convulsions, vomiting, delirium, and rapid heart rate (HR); after a few days, these symptoms retreat and papules erupt, becoming pustules that leave deep pock marks. Complications include blindness, pneumonia, and kidney damage. The mortality rate approaches 250 per 1000. (We have no means to assess its viral origin; we do not even know viruses exist.)

Where

We investigate the incidence by geographical area. The disease never appears in the absence of an infected patient. By investigating in greater detail where the disease occurs, i.e., at the household level, we find that no one contracts the disease without having been in proximity to an infected patient. It appears that the infection passes only person to person. However, it seems to pass with *any* type of contact: airborne vaporized fluids, touch, or second-level touch (touch of things touched).

When

We record the times an infected patient had contact with a previously infected patient. The period from contact to the origin of symptoms is identified as between

1 and 2 weeks, implying a 10 ± 3-day incubation period. Infectious contact may be from the very beginning to the very end of symptoms.

Who

Only humans are affected. We gather demographic data, estimating the incidence of smallpox among all sorts of groups. We compare incidence by sex, age groupings, ethnic origin, socioeconomic level, and occupation. We gather biological, physical, and genetic data and estimate incidences among groupings within these variables. We gather personal data, estimating incidences by cleanliness habits, diet, food and drink types, food and water sources, and how bodily and food waste products are disposed of. We find little difference among groupings. We are beginning to think that we must experiment with controlling food, water, waste, etc. when a secondary occupational analysis turns up a surprising result: dairymaids do not contract smallpox!

How

We now further isolate the events and characteristics. We examine what is different about dairymaids that leads to immunity. We find that they differ little in any respect from the usual smallpox victim, except in socioeconomic level and disease history. Socioeconomic level already has been ruled out. In the disease history, we find that most dairymaids have undergone a course of cowpox, a mild form of pox that has some similarities. Exposure to cowpox conveys immunity! We are well on the way to a control for this heinous disease.

Isolating the Cause

The key to epidemiological detective work is isolating the cause, or at least a variable associated with the cause, which can start a fruitful chain of reasoning. If we understand the biology of the disease, we can pose hypotheses to test experimentally. However, we seldom understand the biology without clues leading to theory. To isolate a causal clue, sampling must be undertaken and done with great care and in great detail. A strategy should be planned, trading off ease, cost, and speed of sampling the potential variables with the likelihood that each is a causal clue. Sometimes factors can be isolated physically, sometimes by data analysis, comparing counts by groupings, and sometimes only statistically, inferring relationships probabilistically from odds ratios. At times, variables may be introduced experimentally that provide contrasts not available by sampling. Representativeness in sampling (first discussed in Section 1.5) is crucial. The effect of a sampling bias is illustrated dramatically in the schistosomiasis and cervical cancer example in Section 9.4.

9.7. THE ANALYSIS OF SURVIVAL AND CAUSAL FACTORS

LIFE TABLES LIST SURVIVAL THROUGH TIME

The life table is historic, having been used for survival analysis during the 1700s by Daniel Bernoulli in Switzerland. A life table gives the proportion of a demographic group surviving to the end of each time interval. If no patients are lost to follow-up, the proportion simply is surviving number divided by initial number. When a patient is lost to follow-up before dying, we face a dilemma: we do not know if or when that patient died, but we have useful information on a period during which we know he lived and we do not want to jettison that information. In consequence, we include him in the base number to calculate survival up to the point at which he was lost, but afterward we drop him from the base number in calculating survival. Patients removed from the database without knowledge of their survival status are termed *censored*.

SURVIVAL CAN BE USED TO SEE PATTERNS OF EVENTS OTHER THAN LIFE AND DEATH THROUGH TIME

In this treatment, survival is discussed as representing a patient's remaining alive. However, replacement of "time to death" by "time to onset of illness" provides a window on morbidity rather than mortality. Replacement of "time to death" by "time to fail" provides a window on the reliability of medical instruments.

DATA AND CALCULATIONS REQUIRED FOR A LIFE TABLE

Basic data for a life table on a number of n patients are (1) time intervals, (2) *begin*, the number at the beginning of each time interval, (3) *died*, the number dying in each time interval, and (4) *lost*, the number lost to follow-up in each time interval. Each time interval may be of any length, perhaps 2 weeks or perhaps 6 months. The rest of the table arises from calculations. Calculations are more exact when the precise time of death or loss to follow-up occurs, but, to be practical, we often know only at the end point of an interval of time that the death or loss occurred during the interval. Epidemiologists often make sophisticated adjustments for the unknown point of time in the interval, but this text will take the simplest form in which death or loss is taken as occurring at the end of the interval. Survival may be calculated by formulas. Perhaps the easiest is as follows. When loss to follow-up occurs, we will enter a second line for that time interval to list it. The remaining calculations are as follows: (5) We fill in a column for *end*, the number at the end of each time interval, which is *begin* − *died* − *lost*. Either *died* or *lost* (or both) will be 0. (6) The proportion surviving, say S, is the proportion surviving up to the current period multiplied by the proportion surviving that period, i.e., S for last period × (*end* for this period ÷ *end* for last period).

Life Table for Infant Malaria

Table 9.2 provides basic and calculated data for a life table on the malarial morbidity of 155 infants in Cameroon[34] (born of mothers without malarial infection of their placentas). Note that survival in this example is not thought of as remaining alive but as remaining disease-free. S for the first period is $1.00 \times (141/155) = 0.9097$. In the second period (>13–26 weeks), 23 died and 3 were lost to follow-up, which were separated on two lines, with died first. S for that period is $0.9097 \times (118/141) = 0.7613$. At the end of that period, we subtracted the 3 *lost*, leaving 115. Because we assumed that they remained alive to the end of the period they did not reduce the survival rate, but they are removed for calculating survival rate in the next period. For the third period (>26–39 weeks), the end is divided by the end just above it, which has had the 3 lost removed. S for the third period is $0.7613 \times (98/115) = 0.6488$. Calculations are continued in this fashion. At the end of the first year, 58% of the infants remain free of malaria. This also may be interpreted as the probability that an infant randomly chosen at the outset will remain disease-free longer than 1 year is estimated to be 0.58.

Table 9.2
Life Table on Malaria (*Plasmodium falciparum*) Morbidity of 155 Infants Born in Cameroon 1993–1995

Interval (weeks)	*begin*	*died*	*lost*	*end*	S (survival rate)
0 (outset)	155	0	0	155	1.0000
>0–13	155	14	0	141	0.9097
>13–26	141	23	0	118	0.7613
	118	0	3	115	
>26–39	115	17	0	98	0.6488
>39–52	98	11	0	87	0.5760
	87	0	4	83	
>52–65	83	14	0	69	0.4788
>65–78	69	24	0	45	0.3123
	45	0	2	43	
>78–91	43	17	0	26	0.1888
>91–104	26	4	0	22	0.1598

Graphing Survival Information

The graphical display of survival data was developed by E. L. Kaplan and P. Meier in 1958. One mode of display just is to graph the survival data from the life table against the time intervals. A survival datum stays the same for the period of an interval, so the graph is a horizontal line over that interval. At the interval's end, a vertical drop shows the reduction in survival to the next interval. Thus, the survival curve has a stepped pattern. The survival curve for Table 9.2 is shown in Figure 9.1. Note that the number lost to follow-up (censored) is shown as a small integer over the line for the period in which they were lost, distinguishing between those lost and those dying.

Kaplan–Meier Curves

Kaplan and Meier developed this form of survival graph in connection with a nonparametric estimate of the survival function at each death or censoring time. For small samples, this Kaplan–Meier product limit method provides a more accurate representation of the survival pattern than does the life table, and a statistical software package with Kaplan–Meier capability should be used when actual death and censoring times are available. If computer software is used, it will provide a Kaplan–Meier survival graph. For large samples in which the number of losses per time interval is large and the width of the interval is small, the graph of the

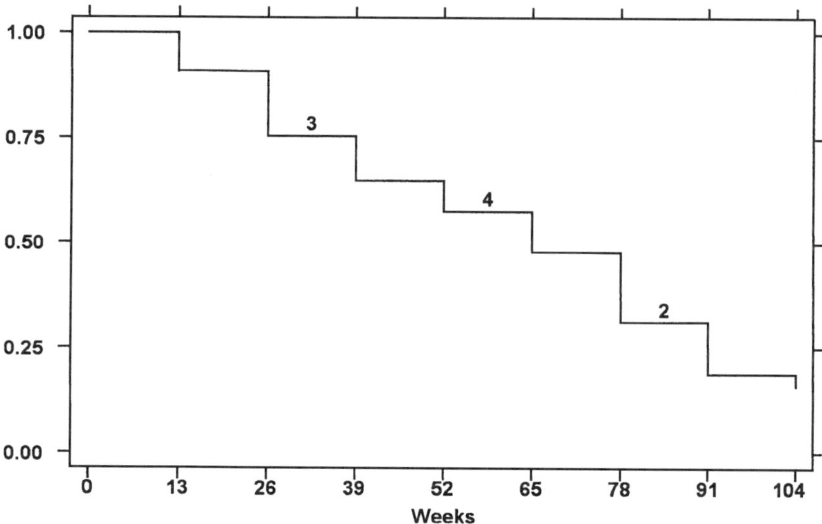

Figure 9.1 A survival curve for the infant malaria morbidity data of Table 9.2.

life table data is approximately the same. Survival graphs based on life tables are much simpler to understand and so will be used here and in Chapter 21.

Confidence Intervals

A method exists to find a confidence interval for a Kaplan–Meier survival curve. It appears as two similar stepped patterns enclosing the survival curve. The calculation of confidence intervals on survival curves is addressed further in Chapter 21.

Additional Concepts

Two additional statistical methods useful in epidemiology should be noted: the log-rank test and correlation through time.

The Log-Rank Test Compares Two Survival Curves

If we also had examined the data of malaria morbidity of infants whose placentas had been infected with malaria, we might ask whether the two curves are in probability the same or different. If they are different, we would conclude that placental infection in the mother affects the morbidity of the child. The log-rank test, a form of chi-square, is calculated in much the same way as the χ^2 statistic in Eq. (17.2) of Section 17.2. The difference between survival number expected if the two curves are the same and survival number observed is squared, divided by expected, and added. A critical value for the resulting χ^2 statistic is found from Table C. The log-rank test is addressed further in Chapter 21.

Serial Correlation

Recall from Chapter 3 that a correlation coefficient is the adjusted covariance between two matching data sets. (Covariance is the sum of cross products of the deviation of observations from their means.) If the matching data sets are observations not taken at a point in time but taken sequentially through time, the correlation between them is termed serial correlation. A serial correlation in which the second of the matching sets is a repeat of the first is designated an *autocorrelation*; if the second is a different variable, the serial correlation is a *cross correlation.*

Cross Correlation

The correlation of infant malarial morbidity between malaria-free mothers and infected mothers through the 104 weeks is a cross correlation. It tells us how closely related the two variables are through time. The correlation is based on the difference between them, not on their individual behavior through time. Thus, if they both rise and fall together, the correlation is high even though the pattern may not be simple. Serial correlation also can be calculated with one of the sets lagged behind the other. For example, the appearance of symptoms of a disease having a 2-week incubation period can be correlated with exposure to the disease, where exposure observations are paired with the symptom observations that occurred 2 weeks later. By varying the lag, we may be able to find the incubation period. Alternatively, by knowing the incubation period, finding lagged cross correlations with several potential exposure candidates may help identify how the exposure occurred.

Autocorrelation

Observations through time may be correlated with themselves. A set of observations through time is taken as the first set, and the same set is taken as the second, except lagged. If the autocorrelation coefficient retreats from 1.00 as the lag increases and then returns to nearly 1.00, we know that we have a periodically recurring disease. If that lag is 12 months, the disease is seasonal. A plot of autocorrelation depending on lag is termed a *correlogram*. Periodicities in a time series can be seen easily in a correlogram as the time values at which the autocorrelation coefficient reapproaches 1.00.

CHAPTER EXERCISES

9.1. How is epidemiology similar to clinical diagnosis? How is it different?

9.2. From Section 9.2, extract and list the major steps in the evolution of epidemiological methodology.

9.3. Name two diseases in which there can be no herd immunity.

9.4. In a Canadian study including the effect of caffeine consumption on fecundability,[8] 2355 women drank caffeine-containing drinks and 89 did not. Of those who consumed caffeine, 236 conceived within 6 months of beginning pregnancy attempts. Of those who did not consume caffeine, 13 became pregnant. Calculate the 6-month incidence of pregnancy for the two groups. Note carefully that the population being considered is women attempting pregnancy, not the general population. Among this group, prevalence might be thought of as the rate at which pregnancy occurs at all, where the population attempting it is equivalent to the population at risk in morbidity studies. A total of 1277 couples attempting pregnancy was followed for an extensive period of time and 575 succeeded. Of these, 304 of the women consumed caffeine. Calculate the prevalence of caffeine consumption among women

Table 9.3

Survival Data of 370 Women in Rochester, Minnesota, Having Adult-Onset Diabetes Mellitus Who Were Older Than 45 Years at Onset during 1980–1990

Interval (years)	*begin*	*died*	*lost*	*end*	*S* (survival rate)
0 (outset)	370	0	0	370	1.0000
>0–2		33	0		
>2–4		20	0		
		0	3		
>4–6		18	0		
>6–8		22	0		
		0	2		
>8–10		20	0		

who became pregnant. Further, calculate the odds ratio (fecundity ratio) of a caffeine-consuming woman becoming pregnant.

9.5. Suppose you are working with James Lind in 1747, attempting to isolate the cause of scurvy. *What*: After a long period at sea, a number of crew members are suffering from scurvy, characterized by weakness, fatigue, listlessness, bleeding gums, loose teeth, and subcutaneous bleeding. *Where*: You note that scurvy most often occurs aboard ship, never in a fertile countryside. Although the hold is stuffy, sailors get considerable fresh air working topside. Food and human waste are emptied over the side daily, not remaining to decay. Water and food are stored and are the same for all, except that the officers eat better. Bathing is available frequently, but in sea water, not fresh. *When*: Scurvy never occurs at the beginning of a voyage, but always after a lengthy time without landfall. Once begun, scurvy only worsens aboard ship and improves only upon return to shore. *Who*: Anyone aboard ship is susceptible, but the incidence rate for officers is much lower. Crew members are in very close contact over extended periods. Some contract it, but not others. Therefore, you conclude that it is not contagious. (You have no knowledge of other limits to contagion such as immunization.) *How*: How do you further your investigation?

9.6. Table 9.3 gives the basic life table data[35] for the survival of 370 women with diabetes mellitus. Complete the table. What is the estimate of probability that a diabetic woman survives more than 10 years?

9.7. Sketch a rough survival graph from the life table survival results of Exercise 9.6.

9.8. Give one example each of a medical phenomenon that could be detected using serial correlation, lagged cross correlation, and (lagged) autocorrelation.

Answers to Problems from Part I

CHAPTER 1

1.1. Many such questions are possible. Some examples follow. (a) What is the average PSA for the 301 patients? The sample frequency distribution? What is the correlation coefficient between age and PSA? (b) Is the average PSA different for patients with positive and negative biopsy results? Is the correlation coefficient between age and PSA statistically significant or could it have happened by chance alone? (c) Can PSA predict (within limits) biopsy outcome and therefore serve as a risk factor? Can age predict (within limits) a patient's PSA and therefore serve as a risk factor?

1.2. Phase II.

1.3. $m = 0$, $f = 1$ (or vice versa).

1.4. Recording to the nearest 10,000 would be adequate; to the nearest 25,000 would not. The clinical decision for a range of 156,000–164,000 recorded as 160,000 would not be affected, but the clinical decision for a range of 135,000–185,000 recorded as 160,000 might be.

1.5. (a) Sex. (b) Age, bone density, UCSF norm. (c) Yes.

1.6. DB2: nausea scores.

1.7. He wants to generalize to humankind as a whole, or at least to humankind in the U.S. He is not justified in doing so based on the information given, because there is no indication of how the sample was drawn. (For example, it might have been drawn from deck sailors who are constantly in the sun and wind and have developed different skin properties, which would form a sampling bias.)

1.8. No. Among the reasons why not are the following. Rather than being a prospective study, the sample is a "convenience sample," i.e., drawn from patients presenting already tattooed and decided on removal. There is no control group for comparison. The investigator is not masked from the decision about "response" to the treatment.

CHAPTER 2

2.1. (a) 1 to <1.5, 1.5 to <2, 2 to <2.5, . . . , 5 to <5.5, 5.5–6.

(b) Tally can be verified by comparing frequencies with plot in (d).

(c) Median = 2.5.

(d)

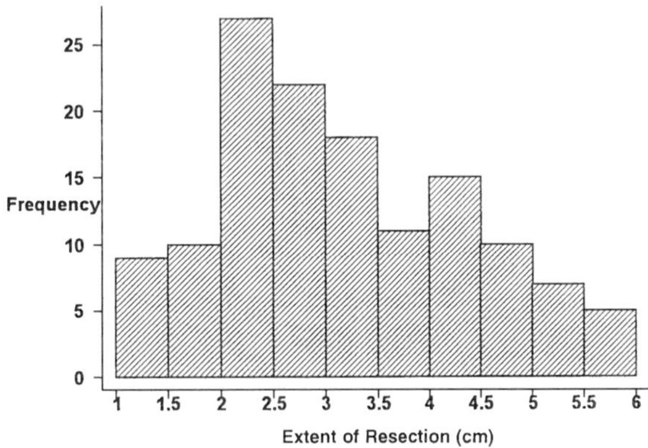

(e) Distribution is skewed to the right and does not grow negligible in the tails, but is not dramatically abnormal.

(f) Mean appears to be about 3. Mode is 2.25. Mode < median < mean, as expected in a right-skewed distribution.

2.2. (a) 6–10, 11–15, 16–20, . . . , 76–80.

(b) Tally can be verified by comparing frequencies with the plot in (d).

(c) Yes, median of accumulating data converges to final median of 51.

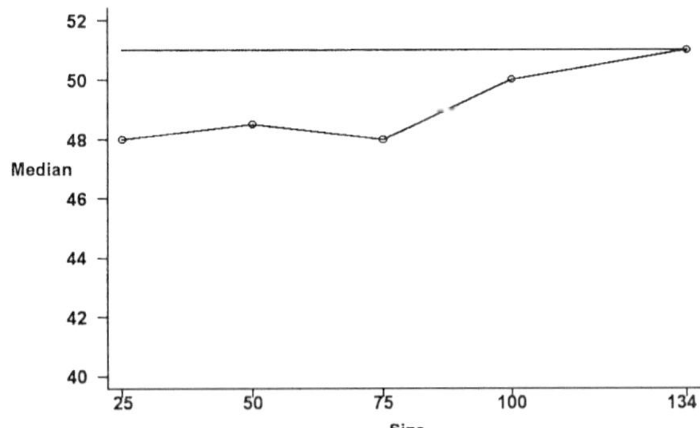

(d)

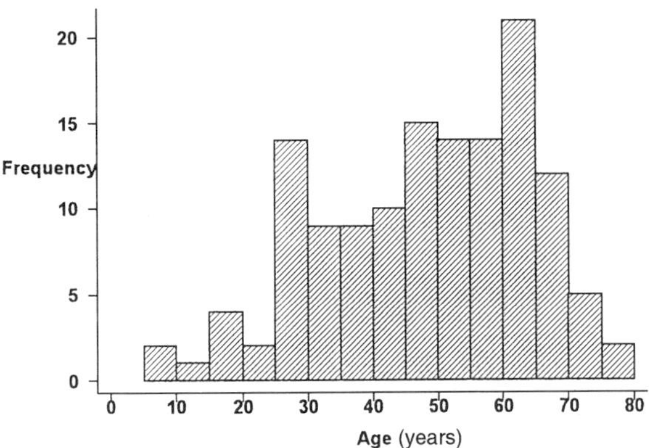

(e) Distribution is skewed a little to the left, is a little too "bulky" in the center, but is not dramatically abnormal.

(f) The mean appears to lie in the 46–50 interval. The mode is 62.5. The mean < median < mode, as expected in a left-skewed distribution.

2.3. (a) variance = 0.0467. (b) standard deviation = 0.2160.

2.4. The sample estimate we would use is the mean (averaged over patients) of changes in serum theophylline level from baseline to 5 days. We assume that this mean is drawn from a normal distribution. We choose the probability of a false positive (concluding there is a real change when there is not), usually (but not always) 0.05. We use the t probability table (for this small sample of size 16) to establish an interval about the theoretical mean of 0 (no difference) within which there probably is no difference. We reject the hypothesis of no difference if the calculated t falls outside this interval or conclude that no difference was shown if t falls in the interval.

2.5. Chi-square. Because chi-square is based on squared data. (Thus, variances, for example, are distributed as chi-square.)

2.6. $df = n - 1 = 29$. Subtract 0, the theoretical mean difference if pre-op and post-op arise from identical distributions; divide by the standard deviation of the sample mean (see SEM in Section 2.9). The cut point is named the *critical value*.

2.7. In the order appearing in the database, ranks are 20, 19, 17, 6, 15, 18, 13, 14, 2, 16, 12, 11, 8, 4, 7, 10, 3, 5, 1, 9.

2.8. Proportion is not close to 0: Binomial.

2.9. Proportion is very close to 0: Poisson.

2.10. $\text{SEM} = 0.2160/\sqrt{4} = 0.1080$.

2.11. Covariance.

CHAPTER 3

3.1. (a) 154.2, (b) 154.1, (c) 576.4, (d) 24.0, (e) 140.1, (f) 164.9, (g) 5.7.

3.2. (a) 452.75, (b) 462.5, (c) 8416.2140, (d) 91.7399, (e) 372.5, (f) 532.0, (g) 32.4350.

3.3. 62.

3.4. 39.04.

3.5. (a) 5539.75, (b) 0.9823.

3.6. (a) 0.20007, (b) 0.8398.

3.7.

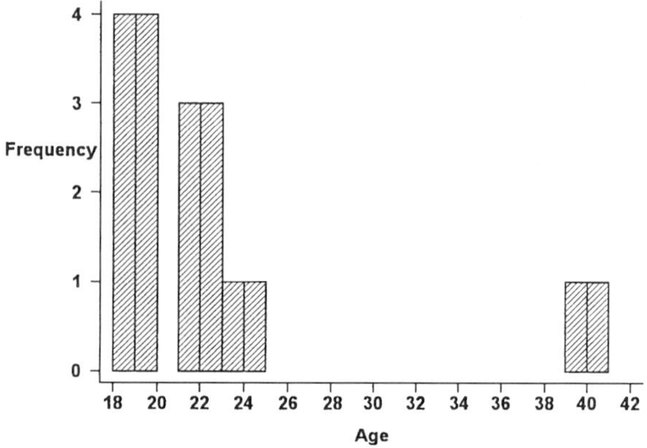

3.8.

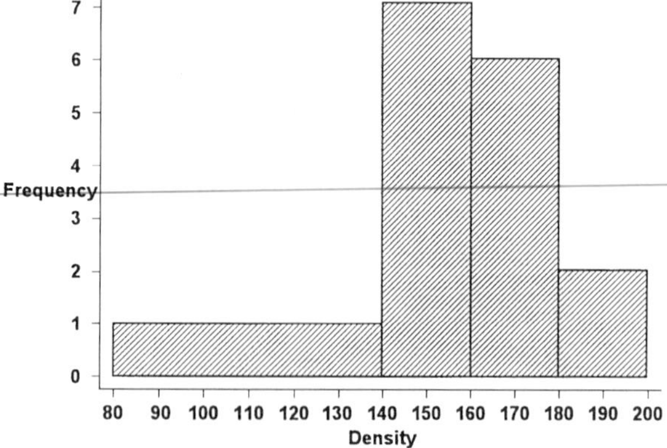

3.9. (a)

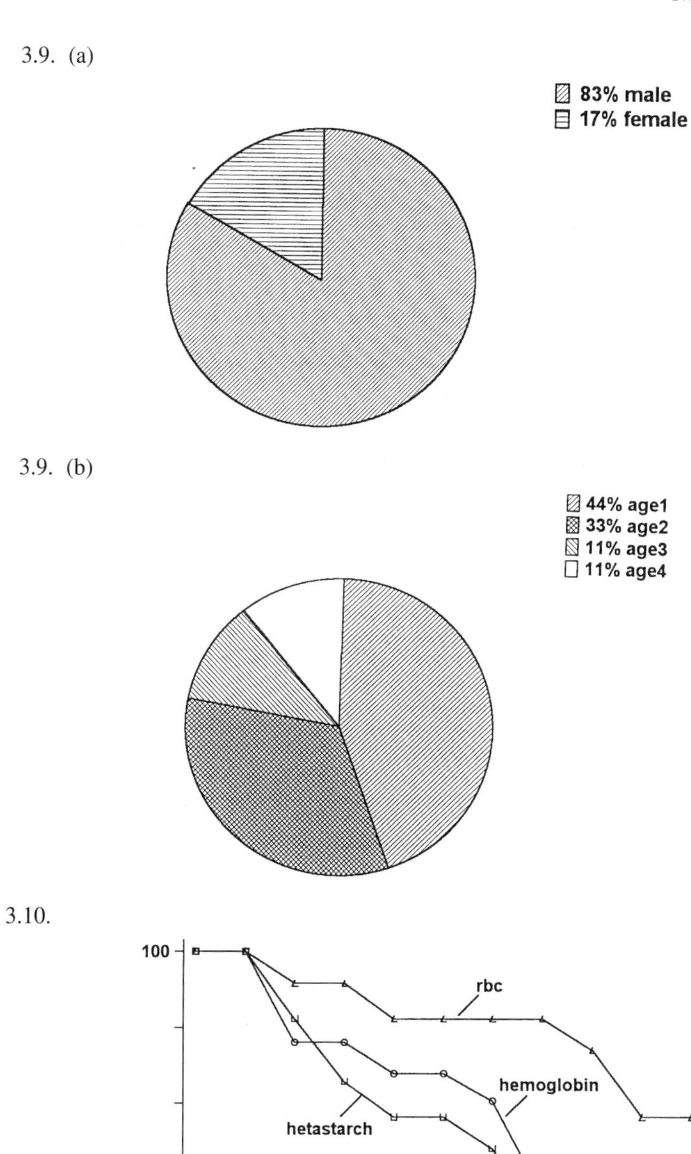
83% male
17% female
44% age1
33% age2
11% age3
11% age4
100
rbc
hemoglobin
hetastarch
23
0
5
10
Day Number

3.9. (b)

3.10.

3.11.

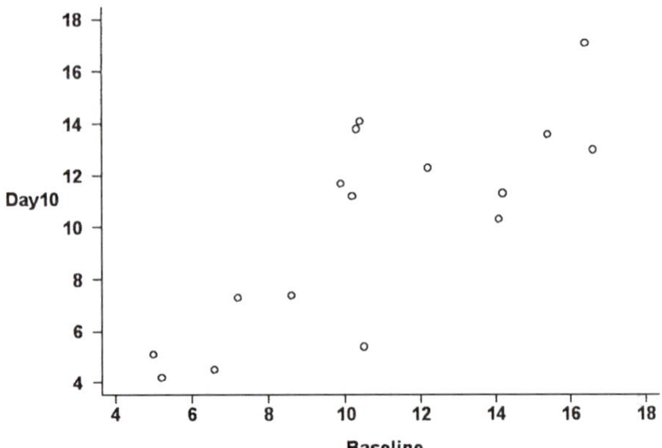

3.12. (a)

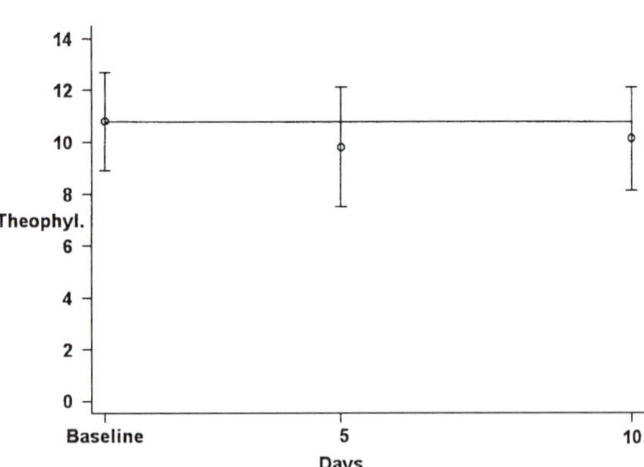

3.12. (b)

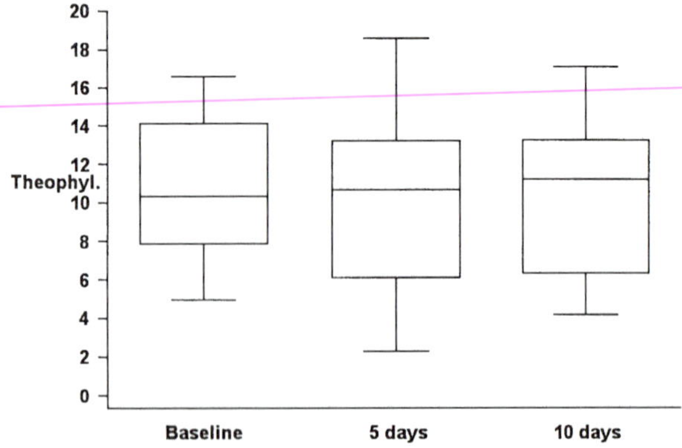

CHAPTER 4

4.1. The 95% confidence limits on individuals are 16.8 and 78.8. Your patient's age lies 2.27 standard deviations below the mean; only 1.2% of patients would be younger (using Table A). Your patient is improbably young.

4.2. Using Table A, (a) (8.59, 9.73); (b) (8.42, 9.90); (c) (8.69, 9.63).

4.3. Using Table B with 19 *df*, (4.42, 8.70).

4.4. Using Table B with 7 *df*, (60.19, 75.31).

4.5. Using Table C in calculating the lower bound and Table D the upper bound, with 19 *df*, (a) (12.08, 44.54); (b) (3.48, 6.67).

4.6. Using Table C in calculating the lower bound and Table D the upper bound, with 7 *df*, (a) (35.73, 338.49); (b) (5.98, 18.40).

CHAPTER 5

5.1. It is a clinical hypothesis, stating what the investigator suspects is happening. A statistical hypothesis would be the following: Protease inhibitors do not change the rate of pulmonary admissions. By stating no difference, the theoretical probability distribution can be used in the test. (If there is a difference, the amount of difference is unknown, so that the associated distribution is unknown.)

5.2. (a) The t distribution is associated with small data sample hypotheses about means. (b) Assumptions include the following: The data are independent from each other. The data samples are drawn from normal populations. The standard deviations at baseline and at 5 days are equal. (c) The Type I error would be concluding that the baseline mean and the 5-day mean are different when in fact they are not. The Type II error would be concluding that the two means are the same when in fact they are different. (d) The risk of a Type I error is designated α. The risk of a Type II error is designated β. The power of the test would be designated $1 - \beta$.

5.3. (a) The χ^2 distribution is associated with a hypothesis about the variance. (b) Assumptions include the following: The data are independent from each other. The data sample is drawn from a normal population. (c) The Type I error would be concluding that the platelet standard deviation is different from 60,000 when in fact it is 60,000. The Type II error would be concluding that the platelet standard deviation is 60,000 when in fact it is not. (d) The risk of a Type I error is designated α. The risk of a Type II error is designated β.

5.4. (a) The F distribution is associated with a hypothesis about the ratio of two variances. (b) Assumptions include the following: The data are independent from each other. The data sample is drawn from normal populations. (c) The Type I error would be concluding that the variance (or standard deviation) of serum silicone before the implant removal is different from the variance (or standard deviation) after when in fact they are the same. The Type II error would be concluding that the before and after variances (or standard deviations) are the same when in fact they are different. (d) The risk of a Type I error is designated α. The risk of a Type II error is designated β.

5.5. (a) A categorical variable. (b) A rating, which might be any type, depending on circumstance. In this case, treatment as a ranked variable is recommended, because it avoids the weaker method of categorical variables and a five-choice is rather small for use as a continuous variable. (c) A continuous variable.

5.6. 1, 6, 4, 7, 5, 8, 2, 3.

5.7. (1) Does the drug reduce nausea score following gall bladder removal? (2 and 3) Drug/no drug against nausea/no nausea. (4) H_0: nausea score is independent of drug use; H_1: nausea score is influenced by drug use. (5) The population of people having laparoscopic gall bladder removals who are treated for nausea with Zofran. The population of people having laparoscopic gall bladder removals who are treated for nausea with a placebo. (6) My samples of treated and untreated patients are selected randomly from patients who present for laparoscopic gall bladder removal. (7) A search of the literature failed to indicate any proclivity to nausea by particular subpopulations. (8) These steps seem to be consistent. (9) A chi-square test of the contingency table is apppropriate; let us use $\alpha = 0.05$. (10) Methodology for step 10 is not given in Part I; the student who wants to pursue this can see Chapter 18.

CHAPTER 6

6.1. Critical value is 3.84. $\chi^2 = 5.44$, which is greater than 3.84. We decide that protease inhibitors are effective. (Actual $p = 0.020$.)

6.2. Critical value is 3.84. $\chi^2 = 10.47$, which is greater than 3.84. We decide that titanium-containing ink is harder to remove. (Actual $p = 0.001$.)

6.3. Critical value is 3.84. $\chi^2 = 10.86$, which is greater than 3.84. We decide that nausea score is reduced by the drug. (Actual $p = 0.001$.)

6.4. (a)

		Diagnosis		
		Appendicitis	Not appendicitis	
Truth	Appendicitis	82	22	104
	Not appendicitis	23	73	96
		105	95	200

(b) 0.24; 24% of cases were diagnosed as appendicitis when in fact they were not.

(c) 0.21; 21% of cases were diagnosed as not appendicitis when in fact they were.

(d) 0.79; 79% of appendicitis cases were diagnosed properly.

(e) 0.76; 76% of nonappendicitis cases were diagnosed properly.

(f) 0.78; 78% of all cases were diagnosed properly.

(g) 11.8; when appendicitis is diagnosed, odds that the diagnosis is correct is nearly 12 to 1.

6.5. $n_1 = 6$, $n_2 = 10\,(>8)$, $T = 72$, $\mu = 51$, $\sigma = 9.22$, $z = 2.278$, $z > 1.96$, the critical value for two-tailed $\alpha = 0.05$. (Actual $p = 0.011$.) Serum theophylline levels drop significantly more in women than in men.

6.6. $n_1 = 3$, $n_2 = 15\,(>8)$, $T = 23$, $\mu = 28.5$, $\sigma = 8.44$, $z = -0.652$, $z < -1.96$, the critical value for two-tailed $\alpha = 0.05$. (Actual $p = 0.257$.) There is inadequate evidence to say that there is a difference in bone density between men and women.

6.7. (a) (Subscript s for survivors, d for died.) $n_s = 117$, $n_d = 17$, $m_s = 48.05$, $m_d = 46.41$, $\sigma = 15.78$, SEM $= 4.10$, $z = 0.4$. $z < 1.96$, the normal's critical value for two-tailed $\alpha = 0.05$. (Actual $p = 0.345$.) The age difference between patients who survived and those who died is not significant in probability.

(b) $n_s = 117$, $n_d = 17$, $m_s = 2.82$, $m_d = 3.96$, $\sigma = 1.54$, SEM $= 0.32$, $z = -3.56$. $z < -1.96$, the normal's critical value for two-tailed $\alpha = 0.05$. (Actual $p < 0.001$.) The extent of resection is significantly greater in patients who died.

6.8. $n_w = 6$, $n_m = 10$, $m_w = 3.335$, $m_m = -0.412$, $s_w = 4.268$, $s_m = 2.067$, $s_d = 1.571$, $t_{14df} = 2.385$, $t > 2.145$, the critical value for two-tailed $\alpha = 0.05$. (Actual $p = 0.032$.) Serum theophylline levels drop significantly more in women than in men; indeed, levels tend to increase in men. The conclusion of the test agrees with the conclusion in Exercise 6.5.

6.9. $n_w = 3$, $n_m = 15$, $m_w = 148.97$, $m_m = 155.27$, $s_w = 15.79$, $s_m = 25.64$, $s_d = 15.57$, $t_{16df} = -0.405$, $t > -2.120$, the critical value for two-tailed $\alpha = 0.05$. (Actual $p = 0.691$.) There is inadequate evidence to say that there is a difference in bone density between men and women. The conclusion of the test agrees with the conclusion in Exercise 6.6.

CHAPTER 7

7.1. (a) One-sided. Ondansetron hydrochloride could decrease nausea score, but does not seem to increase it. Also, the clinical decision not to use the drug is the same whether nausea remains the same or is increased.

(b) Two-sided. There is no reason to believe that the spectrophotometric readings will be higher in one assay than the other.

7.2. (a) A false positive implies that the patient takes the drug when it will not help nausea. A false negative implies that the patient suffers nausea when it could have been reduced. The assessment depends on the side effects and the cost of the drug. If these should be minimal, a false negative is worse than a false positive, so that α should be larger than β. If these are important clinically, the commonly used 5% α and 20% β trade-off should be rethought.

(b) A false positive, i.e., implant appears to raise plasma silicone when it does not, which may lead to unnecessary removal surgery. A false negative, i.e., implant appears to be of no risk when in fact it is, which implies allowing possible side effects. Both errors have undesirable clinical implications, but a β larger than α is reasonable.

7.3. $n_1 = n_2 = 71$.

7.4. $n_1 = n_2 = 53$.

7.5. The minimum sample size estimates provide a sample size that will just barely reach the 5% α *on average*. It is not surprising that repeated sampling yields p values on both sides of $\alpha = 0.05$. A slightly larger sample size than the very minimum requirement would have increased the confidence that a significant p would occur.

CHAPTER 8

8.1. Respiration rate is the dependent variable. Age is the independent variable. The curve goes downward from left to right. No clear pattern is discernible; it would be sensible to start with a simplest straight line model, as in Eq. (8.1).

8.2. Corr(r,a) = −0.195. The form is a downward slope, as conjectured in Exercise 8.1. Some correlation is apparent, but it is not strong.

8.3. $r - 39.0 = -0.34(a - 10.9)$.

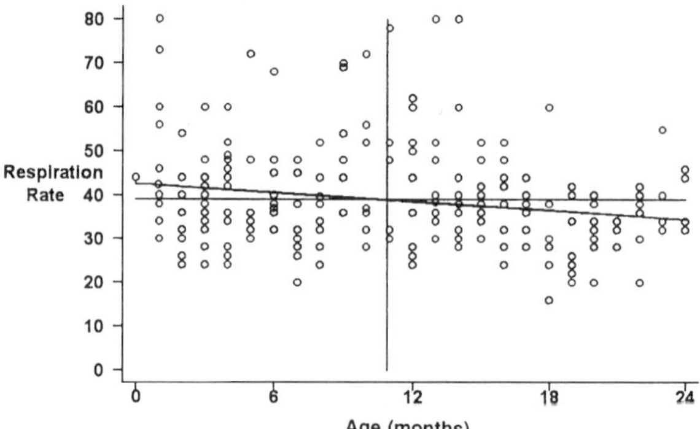

8.4. $R^2 = 0.038$. Age exerts only about 4% of the causal influence on respiration rate. (For the student's information, a t test on the slope of the regression line, which is addressed in Chapter 20, yields a p-value of 0.003, which is strongly significant. We can say that the influence of age on respiration rate is real, but small in comparison to other influences.)

8.5. (a) The MOE is the cost, because no other relevant factors are cited. (b) Using A costs x. Using B costs $y + 0.1x$. Therefore, use y if $y + 0.1x < x$ or if $y < 0.9x$. (c) $15.

CHAPTER 9

9.1. In both, a cause of illness is being sought by trying to isolate a cause from among many potential causes. They are different in that clinical diagnosis seeks to treat an individual, whereas epidemiology seeks to treat a population.

9.2. The steps chosen are somewhat arbitrary. The student's attention to epidemiological history evoked by searching and selecting steps has served the learning purpose.

9.3. Cancer caused by tobacco smoke or occupational exposure. Vitamin or mineral deficiency. Airway obstruction caused by allergic reaction.

9.4. $I_{caff} = 1000 \times$ newly pregnant caffeine consumers/total caffeine consumers $= 1000 \times 236/2355 = 100$ per thousand. $I_{nocaff} = 1000 \times$ newly pregnant not caffeine consumers/ total non-caffeine consumers $= 1000 \times 13/89 = 146$ per thousand. $P_{caff} = 1000 \times$ pregnant women who used caffeine/all pregnant women $= 1000 \times 304/575 = 529$ per thousand. OR = number pregnant who use caffeine/number pregnant who do not use caffeine $= 304/271 = 1.12$.

9.5. Because all of the sailors are exposed to the same air, food, water, and personal habits, and because no outside influences of any type occur, it appears that the cause is not something present, but something absent. You suspect diet. You choose a sample of patients (Lind chose 12), dividing them into experimental groups (Lind chose 2 per group for six treatments). You assign them six different diets, each including a component not regularly eaten aboard ship. It would be sensible to choose foods eaten regularly ashore but not at sea. (Lind did some of this, but some of his treatments were bizarre, such as drinking sea water.) Fortunately, one of your choices is fresh citrus fruits, which quickly cures that group while no other group improves. You have found a cure for scurvy, despite not knowing that vitamins exist or that their deficiency can cause disease.

9.6.

Interval (years)	*begin*	*died*	*lost*	*end*	*S* (survival rate)
0 (outset)	370	0	0	370	1.0000
>0–2	370	33	0	337	0.9108
>2–4	337	20	0	317	0.8567
	317	0	3	314	
>4–6	314	18	0	296	0.8076
>6–8	296	22	0	274	0.7476
	274	0	2	272	
>8–10	272	20	0	252	0.6926

The estimated probability that a diabetic woman survives more than 10 years is 0.69.

9.7.

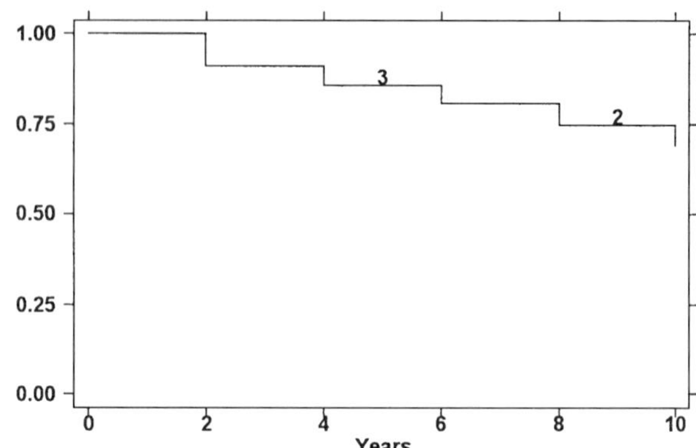

9.8. Many examples are possible. One each is given here for illustration. *Serial correlation*: Cases of yellow fever appearing in a certain tropical nation, suspected to arise from a mutated virus, seem to exhibit longer lasting thrombocytopenia. From records, proportions of patients with below normal platelet counts from before and after the appearance of the new strain are correlated over the course of the disease. The low correlation verifies the mutated behavior. *Cross correlation with lag*: A group of people who traveled recently in a tropical nation contract a new type of viral disease. The dates of visit and symptom onset are correlated with various lags. The lag that provides the largest cross correlation coefficient estimates the average incubation period. *Autocorrelation*: Incidence of aspergillosis is recorded for several years (see Section 19.4 for some data on this). The autocorrelation coefficient is calculated for a lag of 1 year and is seen to be high. It is clear that aspergillosis is a seasonal disease.

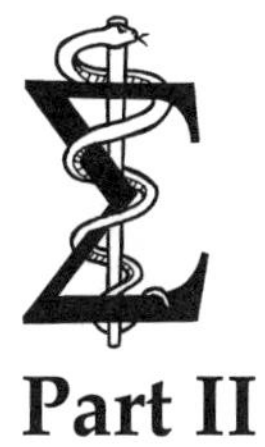

Part II

Reference Handbook

Chapter 10

Reading Articles and Planning Studies

10.1. FINDING AND ORGANIZING MEDICAL INFORMATION FROM AN ARTICLE

The Two Primary Goals in Reading the Medical Literature Are Keeping up with New Developments and Searching for Specific Information to Answer a Clinical Question

The mechanisms to satisfy these goals are not very different. Keeping up is accruing general information on a specialty or subspecialty, whereas searching is accruing information about a particular question; the distinction is just one of focus.

There Are a Number of Ways to Improve Efficiency in Reading Medical Articles

(1) Allow enough time to *think* about the article. A fast scan will not ferret out crucial subtleties. It is what a charlatan author would want the reader to do, but it disappoints the true scientist author.

(2) From the title and beginning lines of the abstract, identify the central question about the subject matter being asked by the author. Read with this in mind, searching for the answer; this will focus and motivate your reading.

(3) Ask yourself, if I were to perform a study to answer the author's question, how would I do it? Comparison of your plan with the author's will improve your

experiment planning if the author's plan is better than yours or show up weaknesses in the article if it is worse.

(4) A multistep process in answering a study question was posed in Section 5.5. Verify that the author has taken these steps.

(5) Read the article repeatedly. Each time, new subtleties will be discovered and new understanding reached. Many times we read an article that appears solid on a first perusal only to discover feet of clay on the third reading.

(6) When seeming flaws are discovered, ask yourself, "Could I do it better?" Many times we read an article that appears to be flawed on a first perusal, only to find upon study and reflection that it is done the best way possible under difficult conditions.

10.2. BIOSTATISTICAL ASPECTS OF ARTICLES FOR WHICH TO WATCH

There Are Several Biostatistical Areas in Which Journal Articles May Fall Short

Some of those giving the most frequent problems will be addressed here.

(1) Statistical versus Clinical Significance

Statistical significance implies that an event is unlikely to have occurred by chance; clinical significance implies that the event is useful in health care. These are very different and must be distinguished. A new type of thermometer may measure body temperature so accurately and precisely that a difference of one-hundredth of a degree is detectable and statistically significant, but it certainly is not clinically important. In contrast, a new treatment that increases recovery rate from 60% to 70% may be very significant clinically, but associated with a level of variability that prevents statistical significance from appearing. When "significance" is used, its meaning should be designated explicitly if it is not totally obvious from the context. Indeed, we might better use the designation clinically important or clinically relevant.

(2) Violating Assumptions upon Which Statistical Methods Are Based

The making of assumptions, more often implicit than explicit, was discussed in Section 2.7. If data are in the proper format, a numerical solution to an equation will always emerge, leading to an apparent statistical answer. The issue is whether the answer can be believed. If the assumptions are violated the answer is spurious, but there is no label on it to say so. It is important for the reader to note whether the author has verified the assumptions.

(3) Generalizing from Poorly Behaved Data

How would we interpret the mean human height, a bimodal distribution? If we made decisions based on the average of such a bimodal distribution, we would judge a typical man to be abnormally tall and a typical woman to be abnormally short. Authors who use descriptors (m, s, ...) from a distribution of sample values of one shape to generalize to a theoretical distribution of another shape mislead the reader. The error seen most frequently is use of the mean and standard deviation of an asymmetric (skewed) distribution to generate confidence intervals assuming a symmetric (normal) distribution. We see a bar chart of means with small standard error whiskers extending above, implying that they would extend below symmetrically, but do they? For example, the pre-op plasma silicone level in DB5 is skewed to the right; it has mean about 0.23 with standard deviation 0.10. Suppose for clinical use, we want to know the level above which lies the upper quarter of the patients. From the data, the 75th percentile is 0.27, but generalization from N(0.23,0.01) claims the 75th percentile to be 0.35. [Recall that N(0.23,0.01) indicates normal distribution with mean 0.23 and variance 0.01 (standard deviation 0.10).] The risk-of-danger level starts much higher using the normal assumption than that shown by the data. The author should verify for the reader the shape of the sample distributions used for generalization.

(4) Failure to Define Data Formats, Symbols, or Statistical Terms

An author labels values in a table as means, but follows the values with a "±", e.g., "5.7 ± 1.2." Are the 1.2 units s, SEM, 1.96σ, $t_{1-\alpha/2} \times s$, etc.? Beware the author who does not define formats and symbols. A further problem is the use of statistical terms. A published paper spoke of data samples "compared for significance using the general linear model procedure." The general linear model is quite general and includes a host of specific tests. Examination of the data and results leads this statistician to conclude that the authors compared pairs of group means using the F test, which is the square of the t test for two means. The authors could have said, "Pairs of means were compared using the t test." However, this may be a wrong conclusion. Are we at fault for failing to understand the jargon used? No. It is incumbent on the author to make the methodology clear to the reader. Beware the author who "snows" rather than informs.

(5) Using Multiple Related Tests That Lead to a Cumulative p-Value

The means of a treatment group are compared to those of a placebo group for systolic blood pressure (BP), diastolic BP, heart rate (HR), and white blood count (WBC) using four t tests, each with a 5% chance of saying that there is a difference when there is not (the p-value). Because the treatment may affect all of these variables, the risk of a false difference accumulates to approximately 20%. (Exactly four such tests yield a risk $= 1 - (1 - p)^4 = 0.185$.) If we performed 20 such tests, we would be almost sure that at least one positive result is spurious. The solution to this problem is to use a multivariate test, which tests the means of several variables simultaneously, such as Hotelling's T^2 or Mahalanobis' D^2 (methods unfortunately outside the realm of this book). Can multiple t or other tests ever be used? Of course. When independent variables do not influence the same dependent variable being tested, they may be tested separately.

10.3. META-ANALYSIS, MULTIVARIABLE ANALYSIS, AND EVOLVING TERMS

Several Terms Not Very Familiar to the Clinician Are Being Seen

A number of terms and methods new to mainstream medicine are beginning to be seen in journal articles, one of the more frequent being meta-analysis. Let us define some of these terms, after which the concept of meta-analysis will be examined in more detail.

Multiple, Multivariate, and Multivariable

"Mult-" connotes several or many, but technical uses vary. "Multiple" implies just that, although sometimes it connotes multivariate, apparently when the adjective multivariate coupled with the noun it modifies generates too many syllables, as "multiple regression." "Multivariate" implies *one dependent* variable depending on *more than one independent* variable. Methods satisfying that definition collectively are called *multivariate analysis* and are mostly beyond what is attempted in this book, but this is a term that is useful to have seen defined prior to encountering it. Consider DB12 on carinal resection, in which we want to identify risk factors for patient death or survival, the dependent variable. To decide whether extent of resection (independent variable) will separate the surviving group from the dying group (dependent variable), we would test mean extent for the two groups using a t test. However, we could test the surviving group's mean extent, age, prior surgery, and intubation against the dying group's means for those variables using a generalization of the t test, the T^2 test of Harold Hotelling. The concept is much the same, except that we are using several independent variables simultaneously. Multiple regression is another form of multivariate analysis. In simple regression, a dependent variable (e.g., heart rate) is predicted from an independent variable (minutes of stair climbing). In multiple regression, a dependent variable (heart rate) is predicted from several independent variables simultaneously (minutes of stair climbing, patient age, number days per week patient exercises). One step further is the case of *more than one dependent variable*, which is termed *multivariable analysis* and is quite far afield from the level of this book. If, in DB3, we want to predict the dependent variables 5-day and 10-day serum theophylline levels simultaneously from the independent variables baseline serum level and age, we would use a form of multivariable analysis. The several terms met in this paragraph are arcane enough to be used without proper care in some articles, and so the reader must be the careful one.

The Concept of Meta-analysis

Meta-analysis is a pooling of data from various journal articles in order to enlarge the sample size and thus reduce the sizes of the Types I and II errors. It treats the different articles as replications of a single study, wherein lies its hazard. The crucial questions are (1) which articles to pool and (2) how to pool them.

Steps to Conduct a Meta-analysis

A meta-analysis should be developed as follows:

(1) Define the inclusion–exclusion criteria for admitting articles.
(2) Search exhaustively and locate all articles addressing the issue.
(3) Assess the articles against the criteria.
(4) Quantify the admitted variables on common scales.
(5) Aggregate the admitted databases. The reader may see one of several aggregation methods referenced, including nonparametric or omnibus combination, vote counting, weighted pooling, ANOVA combining (hopefully following homogeneity tests), linear or regression models, correlation coefficient combining, or clustering. These aggregation methods will not be discussed here. When an author of an article has referred to one of these methods, it may be enough to note that the author is aware of the requirement for methodical aggregation and has attempted it. The meta-analysis that gives no indication of how the databases were combined should be viewed with some reserve.

Biases That May Infiltrate an Integrative Literature Review

(1) Original data. Are original data given? A bias may occur from omitting data that do not support the author's agenda.

(2) Scientific rigor. Various biases can creep in when one article has been done less rigorously than another. Among others are varying enthusiasm in interpreting results, varying quality of randomization, and downplaying or omitting outliers.

(3) Reporting policy. Authors tend to avoid submitting no-result findings and journals tend to reject them when they are submitted, leading to overestimation of the success of an approach.

Criteria for an Acceptable Meta-analysis

As a meta-analysis depends a great deal on the investigator's judgment, clear criteria are crucial. A minimum list of criteria follows, and the reader should verify so far as possible that each criterion has been met.

(1) The study objectives were clearly identified.
(2) Inclusion criteria of articles in general and data to be accepted in specific were established prior to selection.
(3) An active effort was made to find and include all relevant articles.
(4) An assessment of publication bias was made.
(5) Specific data used were identified.
(6) Assessment of article comparability (controls, circumstances, etc.) was made.
(7) The meta-analysis was reported in enough detail to allow replication.

Even after a careful meta-analysis, limitations remain: innate subjectivity, aggregation of data of uneven quality, and forcing results into a mold for which they were not intended.

Sources for Further Information

Perhaps the primary reference in meta-analysis is Hedges and Olkin.[19] Another quite readable reference is Bailar and Mosteller.[1]

10.4. PLANNING A STUDY

A Sequence of Steps Will Aid in Planning a Study

Planning a study is involved, but need not be daunting if well-organized. Total time and effort will be reduced to a minimum by spending organization time at the beginning. An unplanned effort leads to stomach-churning uncertainty, false starts, acquisition of useless data, unrecoverable relevant data, and a sequence of text drafts destined for the wastebasket. Where does one start?

(1) Start with objectives. Do not start with the abstract.

(2) Develop the background and relevance. Become familiar with related efforts made by others. Be clear about why this study will contribute to medical knowledge.

(3) Plan your materials, methods, and data. From where will you obtain your equipment? Will your equipment access mesh with your patient availability? Dry run your procedures to eliminate unforeseen problems. Define the specific data that will satisfy your objectives, and verify that your methods will provide these data.

(4) Define the subject population and verify that your sampling procedures will sample representatively. Assure that your sample size will satisfy your objectives.

(5) Anticipate what statistical analysis will yield results that will satisfy your objectives.

(6) Plan the bridge from results to conclusions. This usually is termed the discussion, which also explains unusual occurrences in the scientific process.

(7) Anticipate the form in which your conclusions will be expressed (but, of course, not what will be concluded).

(8) Now you can write the abstract. It should summarize all the foregoing in approximately half a page.

(9) After drafting this terse summary, review nos.1–8 and revise as required.

10.5. SOME MECHANISMS TO FACILITATE STUDY PLANNING

Devices That Might Be Thought of as "Tricks of the Trade"

In the preceding section, steps to draft a study were given. However, reviewers of study drafts typically see a majority of studies not yet thoroughly planned. Three primary devices to improve study plans, which are used by many investigators but seldom if ever written down, will render most plans "solid."

(1) Work Backward through the Logical Process

After verification that the questions to be asked of the study are written clearly and unequivocally written, go to step 7 of the list in Section 10.4 and work backward. (a) What conclusions are needed to answer these questions? (A conclusion is construed as answering a question such as "Is the treatment efficacious?" rather than providing the specific conclusion the investigator desires.) (b) What data result and how many data will I need to reach these conclusions? (c) What statistical methods will I need to obtain these results? (d) What is the nature and format of the data I need to apply these statistical methods? (e) What is the design and conduct of the study I need to obtain these data? (f) And, finally, what is the ambiance in the literature that leads to the need for this study in general and this design in particular? When the investigator has answered these questions satisfactorily, the study plan will flow neatly and logically from the beginning.

(2) Analyze Dummy Data

If you had your data at this stage, you could analyze them to determine whether you had chosen the appropriate data and the right recording format needed for that analysis. However, although you do not have the data per se, you have a good idea what they will look like. You have seen numbers of that sort in the literature, in pilot studies, or in your clinical experience. Use a little imagination and make up representative numbers of the sort you will encounter in your study. Then subject them to your planned analysis. You do not need more than a few; you can test your planned analysis with 20 patients rather than 200. You do not need to have the data in the relative magnitudes that you want to see; a correlation coefficient of 0.07 rather than the 0.70 that will appear in your later study will tell you whether or not the data form may be used to calculate a legitimate correlation coefficient. This is not lost time, because not only will you learn how to perform any analyses with which you are not intimately familiar, but when you obtain your actual data, your analysis will be much faster and more efficient. This step is worth the time spent to avoid that sinking feeling experienced when you realize that your study will not answer the question because the hematocrits from 200 patients were recorded as low–normal–high rather than as percent.

(3) Play the Role of Devil's Advocate

A device that is useful at the planning stage, but perhaps more so when the finished study is drafted, is to "put on the hat" of a reviewer and criticize your own work. This is not an easy challenge. It requires a complete mental reset followed by self-disciplined focus and rigid adherence to that mind set. Indeed, it requires the investigator to use a bit of acting talent. Many a recognized actor achieves success by momentarily believing he is the character he is playing: in this case a demanding, "I've seen it all," somewhat cynical reviewer. A number of little mechanisms can help. Note everything that can be construed as negative, however trivial. Sneer periodically. Mutter "Good grief! How stupid!" at each new paragraph. When you have finished, and only then, go back and consider which of the criticisms are valid and rewrite to preempt a reviewer's criticism. Remember that you would rather be criticized by a friend than an enemy, and, *if* you carry off this acting job properly, you are being your own best friend. The most difficult problem to recognize and repair in a study draft is lack of clarity. As is often true of computer manual writers, if you know enough to explain, you know too much to explain clearly. The author once had a colleague who advised, "Say it like you would explain it to your mother." Find a patient person who knows nothing about the subject and explain the study, paragraph by paragraph. This technique often uncovers arcane or confusing passages and suggests wordings that can clarify such passages.

The Foregoing Are Simple but Effective Strategies

Their utilization early in the writing game often prevents a great deal of grief.

10.6. TESTS IN DESCRIPTION, EXPLANATION, AND PREDICTION

Stages of Scientific Knowledge

Three stages were described in Section 1.1. We first seek to *describe* events. When we are acquainted with their nature, we seek to *explain* the events, inferring causal factors for these events. When we have identified the primary causes, we seek to *predict* these events from specific values and combinations of the causes. Because biological events tend to include imperfectly controlled variables, we can describe, explain, and predict events only probabilistically. For example, infection with a particular agent will likely, but not certainly, cause a particular symptom. Tests tend to be used in all stages. Much of the mechanics of tests, although pursuing different goals, are used in confidence intervals as part of description. Tests to include or exclude causal factors compose much of explanation. And tests of efficacy of certain levels of causal factors are part of prediction. The largest part of clinical decision making is based on tests. The next section provides a start in the selection of an appropriate test to use in a variety of circumstances.

10.7. A FIRST-STEP GUIDE TO CHOOSING TESTS

Table 10.1 Provides a Guide to Selecting a Statistical Test for a Given Set of Conditions

This table also is given inside the book's back cover. The method of selection is explained in the table's caption. As there are more considerations than can be displayed in a single table, this guide must be taken only as a first suggestion to be

Table 10.1

A First-Step Guide to Choosing Statistical Tests Found in Part II[a]

Type of data:		Counts (nominal)			Ranks	Continuous measurements (including discrete)				
		Proportions								
Questions about:		*p* not near 0 or 1	*p* near 0 or 1	Counted quantities	Position in distribution	Averages		Spread	Distribution normality	Distribution equality
Assumed distributions:		Binomial or multinomial			Not required	Normal curve	Far from normal curve	Chi-square	Any	
Small sample	Single or paired sample	Binomial table *13.6*	Poisson table *13.7*	Matched pairs (McNemar) *13.8*	Signed-rank test *14.2*	Normal test if σ; t if s *15.2*	Go to rank methods	Chi-square *16.2*	Shapiro–Wilk or KS test *17.2*	
	Two samples	Form a 2 × 2 contingency table and use Fisher–Irwin or χ^2 *13.2*			Rank-sum test *14.3*	Normal test if σ's; t if s's *15.3*	Go to rank methods	F test *16.3*		Two-sample KS test *17.3*
	Three or more samples	Form an $r \times c$ contingency table and use Fisher–Irwin or χ^2 *13.3*			Kruskal–Wallis/ Friedman paired *14.4/5*	One-way ANOVA with multiple comparisons *15.4*	Go to rank methods	Bartlett's test *16.4*		
Large sample	Single or paired sample	Normal approximation *13.6*	Poisson approximation *13.7*	Matched pairs (McNemar) *13.8*	Signed-rank normal approx *14.6*	Normal test if σ or if large n; t if s *15.2*		Chi-square *16.2*	KS test or test of fit 17.2	
	Two samples	Form a 2 × 2 contingency table and use Fisher–Irwin or χ^2 *13.2*			Rank-sum normal approximation *4.7*	Normal test if σ_1, σ_2 or if large n; t if s_1, s_2 *15.3*		F test *16.3*		Two-sample KS test *17.3*
	Three or more samples	Form an $r \times c$ contingency table and use Fisher–Irwin or χ^2 *13.3*			Kruskal–Wallis/ Friedman paired *14.4/5*	One-way ANOVA with multiple comparisons *15.4*		Bartlett's test *16.4*		

[a] The column is selected by specifying the type of data you have, the question you are asking of these data, and the distribution you are willing to assume. The row is selected by specifying the sample size and the number of samples. The row–column intersection provides the most apparent test fitting these conditions. This selection does not satisfy all requirements and therefore must be taken as only tentative. Italicized numbers indicate the text section in which the item may be found.

assessed further for appropriateness. The tests themselves are treated in Chapters 6 and 13–17.

Is the PSA Level for 15 Cancer Patients Different after Hormone Therapy?

An example might help the reader use Table 10.1. We want to contrast PSA level before versus after therapy. Type of Data: PSA level is a continuous measurement; go to the Continuous Measurements heading in the right-hand portion of the table. Questions About: averages; go to the Averages heading. Assumed Distributions: we do a quick tally and find that the differences, although a little skewed, are not remarkably different from normal in shape; go to the Normal Curve subheading. Now we know what column to use; we go to the left margin to find the appropriate row. Our sample of 15 is small; go to the Small Sample heading. We have a before-and-after reading on each patient, so that the data arise in pairs; go to the Single or Paired Sample heading, which designates the row. (*Single*: One reading per patient. *Paired*: If the data appear in pairs, e.g., before and after treatment or siblings where one is given a drug and the other a placebo, we are concerned with the difference between pair members, not the actual readings of the individuals. The differences provide one reading per pair and so behave as a single sample.) The intersection of the column and row yields the entry, "Normal if σ; t if s," and directs us to Section 15.2 in the text. We proceed to Section 15.2 and conduct our test as directed.

10.8. SOME ASPECTS OF ETHICS IN STUDY DESIGN

Ethics in the Conduct of Medical Studies Is a Broad Topic

It covers *inter alia* the contrast between research and practice, informed consent issues, the organization, responsibility, and conduct of institutional review boards, adherence to the World Medical Association's Helsinki Declaration and its revisions, issues in the trade-off between care for populations (epidemic containment, immunization, placebo groups in clinical trials) and care for individual patients, and the interaction between the practices of statistics and medicine. The latter issue includes *inter alia* integrity of statistical methods chosen, documentation and availability of statistical methods used, qualifications of a data analyst, patient data privacy, study stopping rules when efficacy is shown prematurely, random patient allocation to treatment groups in the presence of unequal uncertainty about treatment preference, and the issue that poorly done statistics can lead to poorer patient care. The resolution of many of these statistical issues is obvious or has been well-treated. It is the last issue listed that will be addressed here.

Statistical Control Parameters and Sample Sizes Are at Issue

If the statistical design and analysis of a study lead to erroneous conclusions, patients' health care resulting from that study will be degraded. The choice of the appropriate statistical method is a topics of this whole book; the smaller topics addressed in this section are those of the choice of and interaction among error risks (α and β), test sidedness, and sample size.

Ethical Considerations in the Specification of Statistical Test Parameters Will Be Addressed Using Two Examples

(A) A trial investigating the effect of a new muscarinic agent on return of salivary function after head and neck irradiation. How many patients are required for a trial when randomized against pilocarpine? (B) An investigation of a recursive partitioning model in early-stage breast cancer to determine the need for axillary sampling, based on historical control data. How many patients are required for statistical validity?

Relationship among the Statistical Parameters

Required sample size n may be estimated by methods of Chapters 7 and 18. An estimate of the standard deviation of the variable being used is obtained and α and β are chosen. Also chosen is δ, the size of the difference between treatments that will answer the clinical question being posed (often based on the investigator's clinical experience). Medical journal reviewers generally seem to expect choices of $\alpha = 0.05$ and $\beta = 0.20$ (power $= 0.80$). The error risk associated with one tail will be α or $\alpha/2$, depending on whether the test is one- or two-sided. In most cases, a computer operation using these parameters as inputs will provide n.

The Implications of α and β

α is the risk of inferring a difference between cohorts when in fact there is no such difference, and β is the risk of inferring no difference between cohorts when in fact there is such a difference. The choice of $\alpha = 0.05$ and $\beta = 0.20$ (power 80%) implies setting the rate of false negatives at 4 times the rate of false positives.

The Effect on Patients from the Xerostomia Study

A false positive implies inferring the new treatment to be better when it is not; its use subjects patients to the risk of possible serious side effects unnecessarily.

A false negative implies inferring the new treatment to be no better when in fact it is, thereby failing to palliate xerostomia. The false positive is worse for the patient than the false negative. The α/β ratio choice of 0.05/0.20 (or 1/4) is justifiable.

The Effect on Patients from the Breast Cancer Study

In the other trial, however, the false positive implies inferring axillary metastases that are not there and unnecessarily doing an axillary sampling. The false negative implies inferring the absence of cancer when it is present and failing to offer appropriate therapy. In this case, *the false positive represents less loss to the patient than does a false negative.* To set the probability of missing a cancer at 4 times the probability of an unnecessary sampling may not serve patients well. The investigator should take a higher α and lower β. Would this require an untenable increase in the sample size needed? If the error rates were reversed to $\alpha/\beta = 0.20/0.05$ (four unnecessary samplings expected per cancer missed), the sample size would increase by no more than about 10%. [However, if α should be mandated at 0.05 as is usual in medical research (based more on tradition than good reason), the 4/1 ratio would require β to be 0.0125 and the required sample size would increase by about 125%.]

The Choice of α and β Should Be Based on the Clinical Implications to the Patient

The choice, often a hard one, follows as a matter of judgment. Thus, this decision is a clinical one, not a statistical one. Further, whereas the sample size selected will not directly affect patients, the selection of α and β must be carried through into the statistical testing after acquiring the data, and test results *do* affect patients.

The Effect of Test Sidedness on the Patient

After head and neck irradiation, can the muscarinic agent inhibit *or* enhance the return of salivary function, or can it *solely* enhance it? The choice of a one-sided versus two-sided test should be made prior to gathering data. The statistical reason is that an investigator must be a stern self-disciplinarian to choose a two-sided test once the data show on which side of a hypothesized mean the sample mean lies. However, there is an ethical reason as well. When a two-sided test is appropriate, a one-sided test doubles the error rate assigned to the chosen tail, which gives rise to two results. The first is a statistical result of benefit to the investigator: a smaller δ is required to obtain significance in a given sample. The second is a clinical result to the detriment of the patient: too large a number of healthy patients will be treated as ill at the cost of the number of ill patients who will not be treated.

Choice of a two-sided test when a one-sided one is appropriate creates the same classes of mistakes, but with opposite results.

Choosing Sidedness

Often the choice of sidedness is obvious: If we are subjecting the patient to treatments A and B and have no idea which one will be better, two-sidedness is appropriate. If, however, we expect the result associated with one side to be more likely (especially if we *prefer* that result to be chosen), sidedness should be selected thoughtfully. In this case, sidedness should be chosen when the study initially is conceived and should be chosen in answer to the following questions: Can a result on the nonexpected side *possibly* occur physically? If not, select a one-sided test. If so, could a result on the nonexpected (perhaps, nonpreferred) side *affect the patient*? If not, select a one-sided test; if so, select a two-sided test. Note that the choice here, affecting α and β, is made on other grounds, which is why α and β selection and sidedness selection are discussed separately.

The Selection of the Clinical Difference δ

Another potential problem arises when δ is selected. When a study is being developed, a larger δ will require a smaller n. Therefore, for protocols that are expected to accrue slowly or for which a low n is expected, the temptation exists to maximize δ to allow for a small enrollment with subsequent early closure. This clearly is statistical tampering, but it obscures an ethical question: If the proposed new therapy is really *so much* better than the current one, how may the researcher in good faith not offer the patient the superior course? This manipulation of δ poses an ethical dilemma, the answer to which is that we be honest.

The Effect of the Clinical Difference δ on the Patient

Even despite an honest selection of δ, the issue persists of its influence on patients affected by the study results. The smaller the actual δ, the less sensitive the analysis will be in finding a true treatment effect, even with a larger n; the larger the actual δ, the more sensitive the analysis. In the crush for funding and in a forest of competing alternative treatments, it is easier to try many small trials than one enormous one. Are we then reducing our likelihood of improving the lot of all patients in order to reduce the risk to the small group we include in our trial? We must assure ourselves in trial design that such a trade-off is based solely on the potential patient benefit involved, without the influence of personal benefit to the investigator.

Conclusion

A medical study holds the potential, whether explicitly or implicitly, of a deleterious result for all of the patients treated in the future as a result of the information emerging from that study. Ethical soundness in statistical design at present is rarely discussed in the context of study planning. In clinical studies, statistical ethical soundness must be sought side by side with clinical ethical soundness.

Chapter 11

Probability Distributions and Tables

11.1. FINDING PROBABILITIES OF ERRORS IN STATISTICAL INFERENCE

THE RISKS OF ERROR IN A CLINICAL DECISION

In Section 2.7, it was shown that probabilities of occurrences correspond to areas under portions of probability distributions. The probability of inferring an occurrence when it is absent, often the probability of a false positive result on a medical test, usually is denoted α. The probability of inferring the absence of an occurrence when it is present, often the probability of a false negative, usually is denoted β. Rarely must we calculate these probabilities directly, because we may use computers and/or tables to find them.

RELATIONSHIP OF THIS CHAPTER TO CHAPTERS 2 AND 4

The distributions commonly used in statistics were introduced in Section 2.8. Chapter 4 explained how to use tables to find areas under the curves of three of these distributions. This section reviews the use of these three tables and explains how to find areas under the probability curves for the other three common distributions of statistics.

11.2. THE NORMAL DISTRIBUTION

REVIEW OF SECTION 4.2, THE NORMAL DISTRIBUTION

When dealing with variables that follow normal distributions, we want to use the standard normal, symbolized z, which is obtained by subtracting the mean

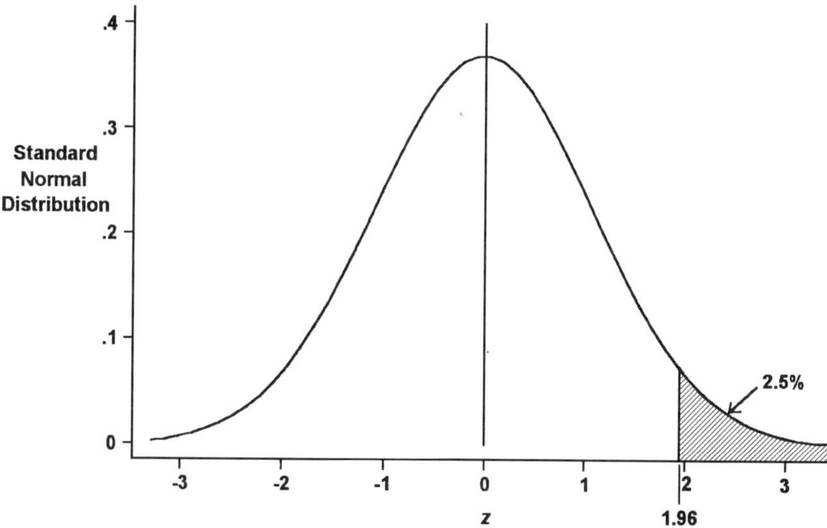

Figure 11.1 A standard normal distribution shown with a 2.5% α and its corresponding z. The α shown is the area under the curve to the right of a given or calculated z. For a two-tailed computation, α is doubled in order to include the symmetric opposite tail. As pictured, 2.5% of the area lies to the right of $z = 1.96$. For a two-tailed use, the frequently used $\alpha = 5\%$ lies outside the ± 1.96 interval, leaving 95% of the area under the curve between the tails.

from each value and dividing by the standard deviation σ. *z represents the number of standard deviations away from the mean.* Figure 4.1, reproduced as Fig. 11.1, shows a standard normal distribution with $z = 1.96$ (frequently seen in practice) and the corresponding area α under the curve to the right of that z. Table A, in the back of the book, contains values of z with four areas: α and $1 - \alpha$ for one tail of the distribution and α and $1 - \alpha$ where α is split between the two tails. The most commonly used areas and their corresponding z-values are italicized in the table.

What Proportion of Carinal Resection Patients Are under 30 Years of Age?

As another illustration of how to find a normal probability, consider the age of patients undergoing resection of the tracheal carina (DB12). Of 134 cases, mean age is about 48 years with standard deviation (taken as σ for this large a sample) of about 16 years. (Values were rounded to make the calculation easier in this illustration.) What percent of patients presenting are less than 30? Age 30 is 18 years below (i.e., to the left of) the mean, or $18/16 = 1.125$ standard deviations below the mean. Our question becomes what proportion of the curve is more than 1.125σ below the mean? Because the distribution is symmetric, the result will

Table 11.1
Segment of Normal Distribution Table A[a]

	One-tailed applications		Two-tailed applications	
z (no. std. deviations to right of mean)	One-tailed α (area in right tail)	$1-\alpha$ (area except right tail)	Two-tailed α (area in both tails)	$1-\alpha$ (area except both tails)
1.10	0.136	0.864	0.272	0.728
1.20	0.115	0.885	0.230	0.770

[a] For selected distances (z) to the right of the mean, given are (a) one-tailed α, the area under the curve in the positive tail; (b) one-tailed $1-\alpha$, the area under all except the tail; (c) two-tailed α, the areas combined for both positive and negative tails; and (d) two-tailed $1-\alpha$, the area under all except the two tails.

be the same as the proportion more than 1.125σ above the mean. By using this property, we need have only one tail of the distribution tabulated. We look up $z = 1.125$ in Table A or Table 11.1, which is a segment of Table A. z lies one-fourth of the way from 1.10 to 1.20, which yields a probability approximately one-fourth of the way from 0.136 to 0.115, or about $0.136 - 0.005 = 0.131$. Thus, the chance of a patient under 30 years presenting is about 13 out of 100.

Exercise 11.1. For a certain population of young healthy adults, diastolic blood pressure (DBP) follows a normal distribution with $\mu = 120$ mmHg and $\sigma =$ 5 mmHg. You have a patient with DBP = 126 mmHg. What percent of the population has DBP higher?

11.3. THE *t* DISTRIBUTION

REVIEW OF SECTION 4.6, THE *t* DISTRIBUTION

The t distribution looks and behaves very much like the normal. It is used where one would choose to use a normal, but where the standard deviation is estimated by s rather than being the known σ. Even the calculations are similar, for example, $(x - m)/s$ provides a standard t-value. The difference is that use of the estimated rather than the known standard deviation yields a less confident and therefore more spread out distribution, with the spread depending on the degrees of freedom (df), a variation of the sample size. Each df yields a member (a curve) of the t family. When using a t arising from one sample, $df = n - 1$; for a t arising from two samples, $df = n - 2$. Figure 11.2 shows a t distribution for 7 df, with 2.5% of the area under the curve's right tail shaded. We note that it is similar in appearance to

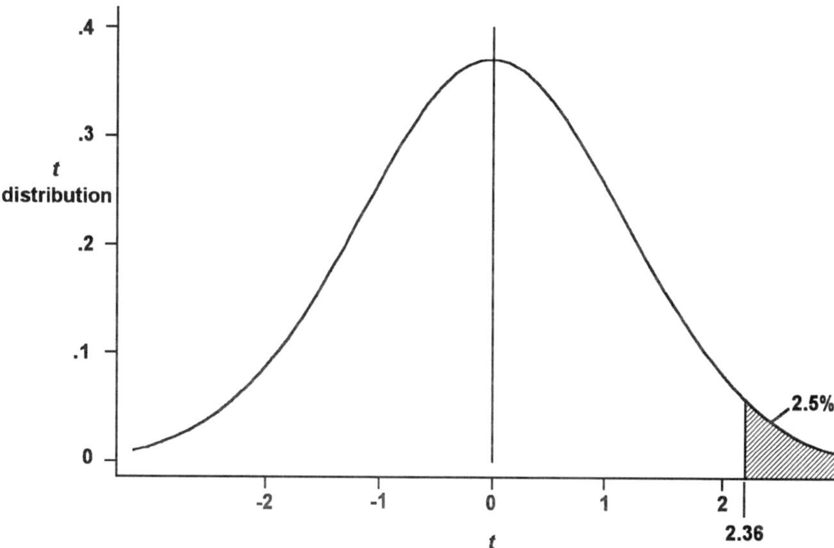

Figure 11.2 A t distribution with 7 *df* shown with $\alpha = 2.5\%$ and its corresponding t. The α shown is the area under the curve to the right of a given or calculated t. For a two-tailed computation, α is doubled in order to include the symmetric opposite tail. As pictured for 7 *df*, 2.5% of the area lies to the right of $t = 2.36$.

the normal distribution depicted in Fig. 11.1, except that the 2.5% critical value lies 2.36s (sample standard deviations) to the right of the mean rather than 1.96σ (population standard deviations).

What Proportion of Hamstring–Quadriceps Surgery Patients (DB10) Can Perform the Triple Hop in Less Than 1.95 Seconds?

By calculating from the database, we find $m = 2.70$ and $s = 0.53$. With $n = 8$ from one sample, $df = 7$. The postulated 1.95 seconds is x, so $t = (1.95 - 2.70)/0.53 = -1.415$. Because the t distribution is symmetric, only the right tail has been tabulated; the area to the left of -1.415 is the same as the area to the right of 1.415. Table 11.2 provides a segment of the t table, Table B. By looking in the row for 7 *df*, we find 1.415 in the first column under the heading for one-tailed $\alpha = 0.10$, implying that 10% of the area under the t curve falls to the right of 1.415. By using the symmetry, we conclude that 10% of the patients will have hop times less than 1.95 seconds.

Exercise 11.2. In DB10, the number of centimeters covered in the hop test using the operated leg has $m = 452.8$ and $s = 91.7$. What interval will include 95% of such patients (i.e., 2.5% in each tail)?

Table 11.2

A Segment of the *t* Distribution[a]

One tailed α	0.10	0.05	0.025	0.01	0.005	0.001
One tailed $1-\alpha$	0.90	0.95	0.975	0.99	0.995	0.999
Two-tailed α	0.20	0.10	0.05	0.02	0.01	0.002
Two-tailed $1-\alpha$	0.80	0.90	0.95	0.98	0.99	0.998
$df = 6$	1.440	1.943	2.447	3.143	3.707	5.208
7	1.415	1.895	2.365	2.998	3.499	4.785
8	1.397	1.860	2.306	2.896	3.355	4.501

[a] Selected distances (t) to the right of the mean are given for various degrees of freedom (df) and for (a) one-tailed α, area under the curve in the positive tail; (b) one-tailed $1-\alpha$, area under all except the tail; (c) two-tailed α, areas combined for both tails; and (d) two-tailed $1-\alpha$, area under all except the two tails.

11.4. THE CHI-SQUARE DISTRIBUTION

Review of Section 4.4, The Chi-Square Distribution

χ^2, the chi-square statistic, is composed of a sum of squares. It occurs in a test of variance, the averaged sum of squares of deviations from a mean, and in a test of contingency, the weighted sum of squares of observed deviations from expected. Statistical applications involving chi-square, being composed of squares, must always have a positive value and can grow to any large size. It is rather like a bell curve with a strong right skew. Figure 11.3 shows the member of the chi-square family of distributions having 19 degrees of freedom.

Is the Variability in Platelet Count among a Sample of Wound Patients Treated with Growth Factor Different from That for Normal Patients?

In DB9, platelet count for $n = 20$ wound patients treated with growth factor has $m = 296{,}000$ and $s = 164{,}900$. If we take the normal platelet count range to include 95% of patients, it will extend about 2σ above and below the mean, implying that $\sigma = 60{,}000$ for normal patients. Is s so much larger than σ that it is improbable to have happened by chance? It turns out that the ratio of s^2 to σ^2, when multiplied by df, is a χ^2 statistic with $n-1$ df, or

$$\chi^2 = \frac{df \times s^2}{\sigma^2}$$

(more in Chapter 16). Thus, $\chi^2 = 19 \times 164{,}900^2/60{,}000^2 = 143.5$. Table 11.3 shows a segment of the right-tailed chi-square table, Table C. For the row $df = 19$,

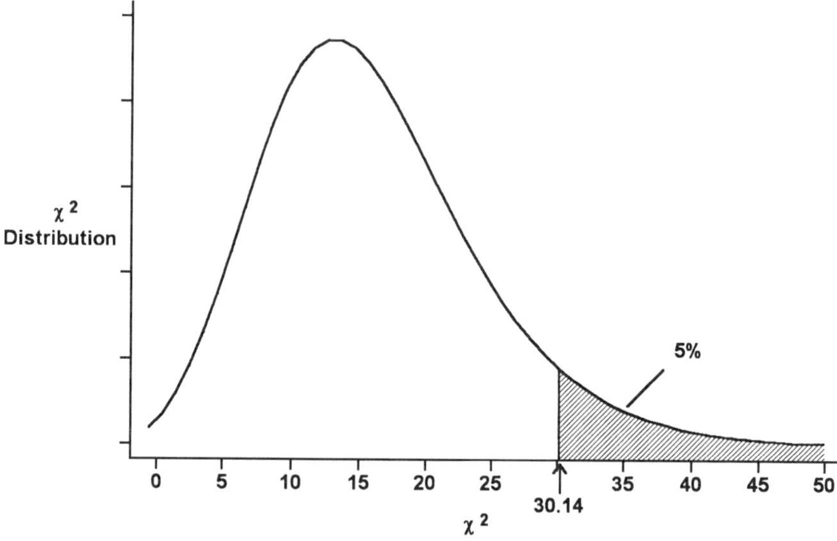

Figure 11.3 The χ^2 (chi-square) distribution for 19 *df* with a 5% α and its corresponding chi-square value of 30.14. The α probability is shown as the shaded area under the curve to the right of a critical chi-square, in this case representing a 5% probability that a value drawn randomly from the distribution will exceed a critical chi-square of 30.14.

we can see that at $\chi^2 = 30.14$, 5% of the area under the curve lies to the right, at $\chi^2 = 36.19$, 1% of the area under the curve lies to the right, and at $\chi^2 = 43.81$, 0.1% of the area under the curve lies to the right. As 143.5 is very much larger than 43.81, the area under the curve to the right is very much smaller than 0.1%. The chance that a standard deviation as large as 164,900 arose from a sample of patients with normal platelet counts is much less than 1 in 1000; we conclude that the variability in the sample of patients who have had growth factor is larger than in normal patients.

Table 11.3

A Segment of the Chi-Square Distribution, Right Tail[a]

α	0.10	0.05	0.025	0.01	0.005	0.001
$1 - \alpha$	0.90	0.95	0.975	0.99	0.995	0.999
$df = 17$	24.77	27.59	30.19	33.41	35.72	40.78
18	25.99	28.87	31.53	34.80	37.16	42.32
19	27.20	30.14	32.85	36.19	38.58	43.81
20	28.41	31.41	34.17	37.57	39.99	45.31

[a] Selected χ^2 values (distances above zero), for various degrees of freedom (*df*), are given for (a) α, the area under the curve in the right tail, and (b) $1 - \alpha$, the area under all except the right tail.

An Effect of Asymmetry in the Chi-Square Distribution

Table C, in the back of the book, provides the chi-square values that yield commonly used values of α, i.e., the probability that a randomly drawn value from the distribution lies in the right tail demarked by the tabulated chi-square value. Because the chi-square distribution is asymmetric, we cannot take an area in one tail and expect that in the other tail to be the same. For areas under the left tail, we need another chi-square table. Table C provides chi-square values for the more commonly used right tail, Table D, those for the left tail. The mechanism of finding areas in a tail from the table is much the same as for the t: the desired area in the tail specifies the column, the *df* specifies the row, and the *critical* chi-square value (the value demarking the tail area) lies at the row–column intersection.

Exercise 11.3. In DB7, the standard deviation of bone density of 18 patients with femoral neck fractures is $s = 24.01$. Take the standard deviation for the normal population as $\sigma = 16.12$. We want to know whether the variability for fracture patients is unusually larger than that for normals and therefore probably different. If we sampled repeatedly from the normal population, how often would we find an s this large or larger? (Hint: by calculating χ^2 as before, what percent of the area under the curve is greater than that value of χ^2?)

11.5. THE F DISTRIBUTION

The Concept of F

Section 2.8 reported that a ratio of two variances drawn from the same population has a distribution named F. Conceptually, F may be thought of as the size of the top variance relative to the bottom variance. An F of 2.5 indicates that the top variance is 2.5 times the bottom variance. If the top is too much larger than the bottom, we believe it is unlikely that the two samples came from populations with the same variance. The probability distribution of F defines "too much."

F and Standard Deviations

Variances, the squares of the respective standard deviations, are used in the computations because they are easier to deal with mathematically. However, the concepts and conclusions are the same for both variances and standard deviations. We may use variances in computations quite legitimately, but make conclusions about the respective standard deviations.

F AND *df*

Each variance (multiplied by a constant) is distributed chi-square, and the resulting F distribution itself looks very much like chi-square. As both top and bottom variances have *df*, any particular F distribution is specified by a *pair* of *df*. The top *df* is always stated first. The member of the family of F distributions specified for the pair 2,6 *df* is shown in Fig. 11.4, with the upper 5% tail area shaded. We note that 5.14 is the critical F for 2,6 *df*, that is, 5% of the F distribution lies to the right of 5.14. Table 11.4, a segment of the F table (Table E) shows from where this critical value comes.

USING THE F TABLE

Table E in the back of the book (also Table 11.4) provides the F-values that yield 5% values of α, i.e., a 5% probability that a randomly drawn value from the distribution exceeds the tabulated F-value. Because the F distribution is asymmetric, we cannot take an area in one tail and expect that in the other tail to be the same. However, for the methods used in this book, the left tail is not used. Finding

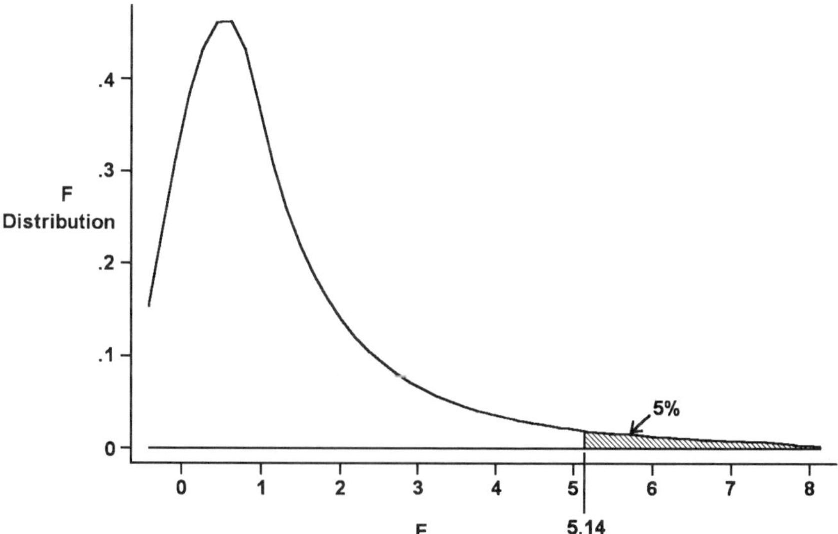

Figure 11.4 F distribution for 2 and 6 *df* with a 5% α and its corresponding F-value of 5.14 is shown. The α probability is shown as the shaded area under the curve to the right of a given or calculated F, in this case representing a 5% probability that a value drawn randomly from the distribution will exceed an F of 5.14.

Table 11.4
A Segment of the F Table[a]

		Numerator *df*				
		1	2	3	4	5
Denominator *df*	3	10.13	9.55	9.28	9.12	9.01
	4	7.71	6.94	6.59	6.39	6.26
	5	6.61	5.79	5.41	5.19	5.05
	6	5.99	5.14	4.76	4.53	4.39

[a] Selected distances (F) are given for various degrees of freedom (*df*) for $\alpha = 5\%$, the area under the curve in the right tail. Numerator *df* appears in column headings, denominator *df* in row headings, and the F-value at the intersection of row and column in the table body.

areas in the right tail is much the same as in chi-square, except for having a pair rather than a single *df*. The *df* of the top variance specifies the column, the *df* of the bottom variance specifies the row, and the distance greater than zero (F) lies at the row–column intersection. Because *df* for both top and bottom must be used in tabulation, an F table can be given for only one α. Several pages of tables could be given, but because $\alpha = 5\%$ is commonly used in almost all medical research, only the 5% table is given here. Calculation of F for other α's may be found in any good statistical computer package or in books of tables.

Is Variability of Prostate Volumes Different for Patients Having Positive and Negative Biopsies?

Let us calculate the variances for the prostate volumes found in Table DB1.1 for the groups of patients having positive and negative biopsies. We want to know whether the variability of volume for the seven negative biopsy patients is significantly larger than that for the three positive biopsy patients. Although variances actually are tested, think of it as a test for standard deviations. The sample sizes 3 and 7 give us the *df* pair 2,6, leading to the 5.14 entry in the table. Because of the 5.14 critical value, the test requires the variance for negative-biopsy volumes to be more than 5 times the size of the variance for positive-biopsy volumes to show evidence that it is larger with no more than a 5% chance of being wrong. Upon calculating the variances, we find $s_-^2 = 326.89$ (standard deviation $= 18.08$) and $s_+^2 = 83.52$ (standard deviation $= 9.14$). The calculated $F = 326.89/83.52 = 3.91$. As this is less than the critical F-value of 5.14, we would be wrong >5% of the time if we concluded that the disparity in variances (or standard deviations) occurred by causes other than chance alone.

F and Sample Size

The effect of sample size can be illustrated dramatically. If we had obtained the same variances from double the sample sizes, i.e., 6 and 14 patients, we would have had 5,13 as the *df* pair, leading to a critical F (from Table E) of 3.03. Our 3.91 F ratio would have well exceeded this value and we would reach the reverse conclusion: we would have enough evidence to say that there is less than a 5% chance that the disparity in variances occurred by chance alone and a causal factor likely is present.

Exercise 11.4. In DB8, means of four GAG levels taken on each of two types of assay were about 0.39 (type 1) and 0.44 (type 2), which are not very different. However, the standard deviations were 0.2421 (type 1) and 0.1094 (type 2). If the type 2 assay averages the same but is less variable, we would choose it as the preferable type of assay. The statistic F is the ratio of the two variances. Is there less than a 5% chance of finding an F this large or larger?

11.6. THE BINOMIAL DISTRIBUTION

Binomial Events Defined

Often we encounter situations in which only two outcomes are possible: ill or well, success or failure of a treatment, a microorganism that does or does not cause a disease. Let us denote by π the probability of occurrence of one of the two outcomes (say the first) on any random trial. (This symbol has nothing to do with the symbol for 3.14... used in the geometry of circles.) If we have n opportunities for the outcome to occur, e.g., n patients, the binomial distribution will tell us how many occurrences of the outcome we would expect by chance alone.

Binomial Table

Table F, in the back of the book, gives the probability of n_0 occurrences of an event under scrutiny out of n trials, given an occurrence rate of π. Table 11.5 shows the segment of Table F needed for the example.

Has the Success of Laser Trabeculoplasty Improved?

As an example, the long-term success of laser trabeculoplasty as therapy for open-angle glaucoma was examined in a Norwegian study.[11] At the end of 2 years, the failure rate was $1/3$. Suppose you perform trabeculoplasty on six patients. At

Table 11.5

A Segment of Table F, Values of the Cumulative Binomial Distribution, Depending on π (Theoretical Proportion of Occurrences in a Random Trial), n (Sample Size), and n_0 (Number of Occurrences Observed)[a]

		π									
n	n_0	0.05	0.10	0.15	0.20	0.25	0.30	0.35	0.40	0.45	0.50
6	1	0.265	0.469	0.629	0.738	0.822	0.882	0.925	0.953	0.972	0.984
	2	0.033	0.114	0.224	0.345	0.466	0.580	0.681	0.676	0.836	0.891
	3	0.002	0.016	0.047	0.099	0.169	0.256	0.353	0.456	0.559	0.656
	4	0.000	0.001	0.006	0.017	0.038	0.071	0.117	0.179	0.255	0.344
	5		0.000	0.000	0.002	0.005	0.011	0.022	0.041	0.069	0.109
	6				0.000	0.000	0.001	0.002	0.004	0.008	0.016

[a] Given π, n, and n_0, the corresponding entry in the table body represents the probability that n_0 or more occurrences (or, alternatively, that n_0/n proportion of observed occurrences) would have been observed by chance alone.

the end of 2 years, you find only one failure. What is the probability that your improved failure rate of 1/6 is due to more than chance, given the Norwegian rate of 1/3? Table 11.5 (or Table F) gives the probability of n_0 or more occurrences of the event under scrutiny out of n trials, given an occurrence rate of π. The table gives only a "$\geq$" value; to find the probability that n_0 is 1 or 0, we must find $1-$ (the probability that $n_0 \geq 2$). The column is indicated by $\pi = 0.333$, lying between 0.30 and 0.35. The row is indicated by $n = 6$ and $n_0 = 2$. The value for our π is bracketed by 0.580 and 0.681, about 0.65. Finally we take 1 $-$ the tabulated value or 0.35 for our result. A more exact value, calculated with the aid of a computer, is 0.351, which is almost the same. With a 35% probability that our result could have occurred by chance alone, our small sample gives us inadequate evidence of an improved success rate.

The Effect of Sample Size

Figure 11.5 shows a binomial distribution for $\pi = 1/3$ and $n = 12$, double the sample size of the example. (The values for 11 and 12 occurrences are not zero, but are too small to appear on the graph.) We can see by combining the first two bars that the probability of $n_0 \leq 1$ is about 8%, much closer to significance. A group of 60 patients with 10 failures rather than 6 patients with 1 failure would have given a probability of 0.003, which is strong evidence of improvement.

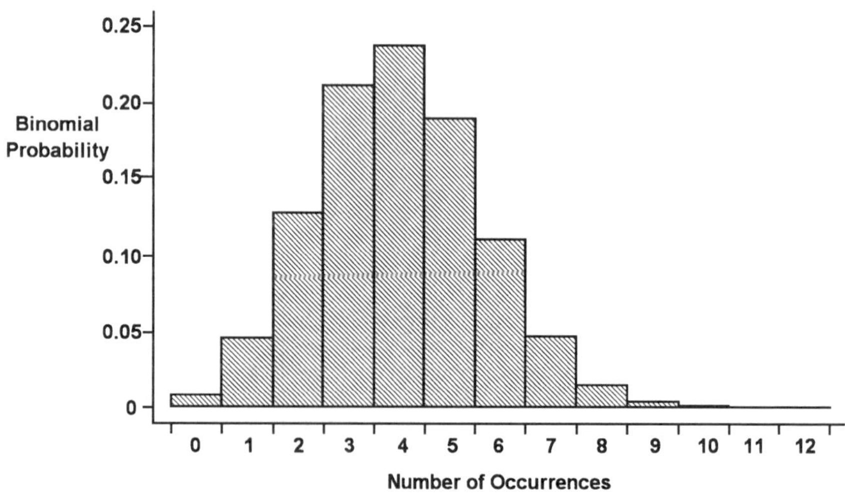

Figure 11.5 The binomial distribution for $n = 12$ and $\pi = 1/3$.

THE BINOMIAL FOR LARGER SAMPLES

The binomial distribution is difficult to calculate when n is more than a few. For medium to large n, we need an easier way to find the required probability. When π, the occurrence rate, is toward the center of the 0–1 interval, the normal distribution adequately approximates the binomial. The mean of the binomial sample is the observed occurrence rate $p = n_0/n$, the number of occurrences observed ÷ sample size, and the variance is $\pi(1 - \pi)/n$. Thus, the mean difference divided by the standard deviation follows approximately the standard normal distribution, as

$$x = \frac{p - \pi}{\sqrt{\frac{\pi(1-\pi)}{n}}}$$

and probability questions may be addressed using Table A. (The approximation can be improved with an adjustment factor; more detail may be seen in Section 13.6.) The similarity to a normal shape can be seen in Fig. 11.5. If π is close to 0 or 1, the binomial becomes too skewed to approximate the normal, but can be approximated adequately by the Poisson distribution.

Exercise 11.5. In a relatively large study on subfascial perforating vein surgery (SEPS),[47] 10% ($=\pi$) of ulcers had not healed by 6 months after surgery. In a particular clinic, $n = 6$ SEPS were performed and $n_0 = 2$ patients had unhealed ulcers after 6 months. What is the probability that, if the clinic shared the theoretical $\pi = 0.10$, 2 out of 6 patients would have had unhealed ulcers?

11.7. THE POISSON DISTRIBUTION

POISSON EVENTS DESCRIBED

The Poisson distribution arises from situations in which there is a large number of opportunities for the event under scrutiny to occur, but a small chance that it will occur on any one trial. The number of cases of bubonic plague would follow Poisson: a large number of patients can be found with chills, fever, tender enlarged lymph nodes, and restless confusion, but the chance of the syndrome being plague is extremely small for any randomly chosen patient. The distribution is named for Siméon Denis Poisson, who published the theory in 1837. The classic use of Poisson was in predicting the number of deaths of Prussian army officers from horse kicks during 1875–1894; there was a large number of kicks, but the chance of death from a randomly chosen kick was very small.

Poisson Table

Table G, in the back of the book, provides the α to test the hypothesis that n_0 or more cases would occur by chance alone, given the occurrence rate λ ($=n\pi$). Table 11.6 shows the segment of Table G needed for the example.

Does Aluminum City Have a Higher Rate of Alzheimer's Disease Than Seattle?

As an example, a survey[63] of medical records of 23,000 people over 60 years of age from a Seattle HMO revealed 200 with indications of Alzheimer's disease, a rate of 0.0087. A clinician in Aluminum City has 100 patients over 60 and finds 4 with Alzheimer's. What would be the probability that his high rate is due to chance alone, if Aluminum City's rate were the same as that of Seattle? Table 11.6 or Table G provides the α to test the hypothesis that n_0 or more cases would occur by chance alone, given the occurrence rate λ. The column in the table must be chosen using the value $\lambda = n\pi = 100 \times 0.0087 = 0.87$, which lies between columns 0.8 and 0.9. The row is indicated by $n_0 = 4$. The Poisson probability is between 0.009 and 0.014, about 0.012. The actual probability from a computer calculation is the same. This result indicates that our chance of being wrong in concluding a difference would be about 1 in 100, which provides adequate evidence to conclude that Aluminum City has a higher rate of Alzheimer's than Seattle.

The Appearance of the Poisson Distribution

Figure 11.6 shows the member of the Poisson family of distributions for $\lambda = 0.87$, the occurrence rate in the example. We might note that theoretically the Poisson distribution has no greatest possible number of occurrences as does the binomial.

The Poisson for Larger Samples

Like the binomial, the Poisson distribution is difficult to calculate when n is more than a few. For medium to large n, when π, the occurrence rate, is close to 0 or 1, the normal distribution adequately approximates the Poisson. Again, like the binomial, the mean of the Poisson sample is the observed occurrence rate $p = n_0/n$, the number of occurrences observed $\div$ sample size, but the variance is π/n. Thus, the mean difference divided by the standard deviation follows approximately the standard normal distribution, as

$$z = \frac{p - \pi}{\sqrt{\pi/n}},$$

Table 11.6

A Segment of Table G, Values of the Cumulative Poisson Distribution, Depending on $\lambda = n\pi$ (Sample Size $\times$ Theoretical Proportion of Occurrences in Random Trials) and n_0 (Number of Occurrences Observed)[a]

	$\lambda\ (=n\pi)$											
n_0	0.1	0.2	0.3	0.4	0.5	0.6	0.7	0.8	0.9	1.0	1.1	1.2
1	0.095	0.181	0.259	0.330	0.394	0.451	0.503	0.551	0.593	0.632	0.667	0.699
2	0.005	0.018	0.037	0.062	0.090	0.122	0.159	0.191	0.228	0.264	0.301	0.337
3	0.000	0.001	0.004	0.008	0.014	0.023	0.034	0.047	0.063	0.080	0.100	0.121
4		0.000	0.000	0.001	0.002	0.003	0.006	0.009	0.014	0.019	0.026	0.034
5				0.000	0.000	0.000	0.001	0.001	0.002	0.004	0.005	0.008
6							0.000	0.000	0.000	0.001	0.001	0.002
7										0.000	0.000	0.000

[a] Given λ and n_0, the corresponding entry in the table body represents the probability that n_0 or more occurrences (or alternatively that n_0/n proportion of observed occurrences) would have been observed by chance alone.

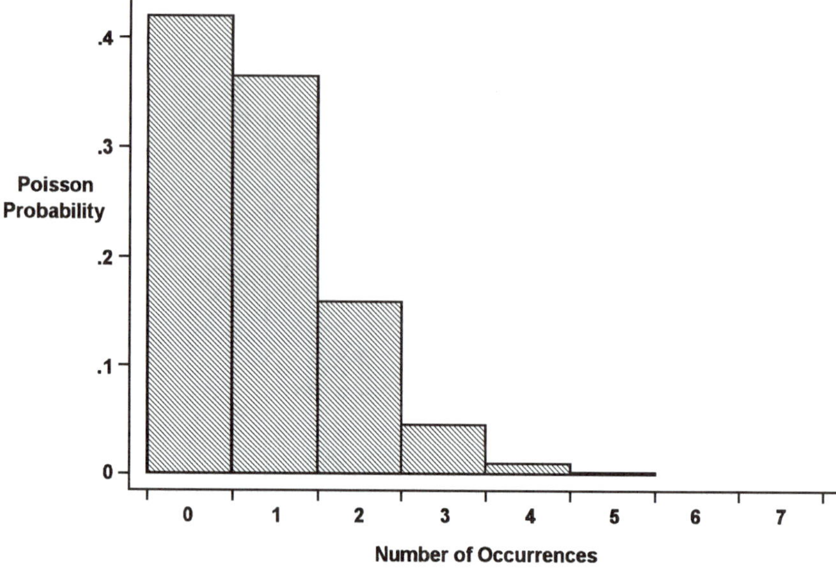

Figure 11.6 The Poisson distribution for an occurrence rate (λ) of 0.87.

and probability questions may again be addressed using Table A. More detail may be found in Section 13.7.

Exercise 11.6. The probability that a person infected with human immunodeficiency virus (HIV) will develop acquired immunodeficiency syndrome (AIDS) during the first year of infection is about 0.01. An investigator reviewed the records of 70 HIV patients. During the year following their reported date of first possible exposure to another HIV-infected person, five developed AIDS. Does the investigator believe their reporting?

ANSWERS TO EXERCISES

11.1. $z = (126 - 120)/5 = 1.20$. Your patient is 1.2σ above the mean. From Table 11.1, the area in the right tail is 0.115. 11.5% of the population have greater DBP.

11.2. For 7 *df*, a two-tailed $\alpha = 0.05$ is obtained by $m \pm 2.365 \times s$, or the interval from 235.9 to 669.7.

11.3. $\chi^2 = 17 \times 576.48/259.85 = 37.71$. From Table 11.3, row for 17 *df*, we see that a χ^2 value of 37.71 lies between 35.72, associated with an area under the curve in the right tail of 0.5%, and 40.78, associated with an area of 0.1%. By interpolation, which is approximate, the area associated with 37.71 will be about 0.4 of the way from 0.5% to 0.1%, or about 0.3%. If we sampled standard deviations repeatedly from a normal–patient population, we would find a standard deviation of 24.01 or larger only about 3 times out of 1000.

11.4. For samples so small, numerator and denominator degrees of freedom are both 3, and the F ratio as shown in Table 11.4 would have to be larger than 9.28. For these types of assay, $F = 0.0586/0.0120 = 4.88$. As $4.88 < 9.28$, we do not have evidence to conclude a difference in variability.

11.5. In Table 11.5, which displays the $n = 6$ block of Table F, the probability 0.114 lies at the intersection of the column $\pi = 0.10$ and the row $n_0 = 2$. The probability that two unhealed-ulcer patients would have occurred is more than 11%.

11.6. $\pi = 0.01$ and $n = 70$, so the expected number of AIDS cases is $\lambda = 0.7$. $n_0 = 5$ cases occurred. In Table 11.6, the intersection of the column $\lambda = 0.7$ and $n_0 = 5$ shows the probability to be 0.001. There is only 1 chance in 1000 that the investigator received true reports.

Chapter 12

Confidence Intervals

12.1. OVERVIEW

Review of Section 4.1

We noted that hematocrit (Hct) values (measured in percent) for healthy patients are not all the same, but range over an interval. What is this interval? Because we see an occasional very high or low value in a healthy patient, we want an interval that we are confident will include most of the healthy population; we name this a *confidence interval*. But what is the width of this interval? We might say that it should include 95% of the population. We denote by α the probability that a healthy patient's Hct will fall outside the healthy interval, usually $\alpha/2$ on each side of the interval. When a patient's Hct does fall outside the healthy interval, we think, "It is likely that the patient has arisen from an unhealthy population, but not certain. We must compare the Hct value with other indicators to derive a total picture."

Statistics and Distributions in Confidence Intervals

The statistic on which a confidence interval is seen most frequently is the population mean, estimated by the sample mean. As the sample mean is distributed normal, the normal most often is associated with the confidence interval. Neither of these choices is required. We can put confidence intervals on any statistic: an individual (Is my patient part of a known healthy population?), a standard deviation (Is the effect of a new drug less variable and therefore more dependable than a prior one?), or others, as well as a mean. The distribution from which the interval values are chosen is specified by the statistic on which the interval is desired: normal for a mean, chi-square for a variance (with the square-root taken of the results to apply to standard deviations), binomial for a proportion, etc.

Level of Confidence in Intervals

The most frequently chosen interval is 95%, which seems to be becoming traditional in medicine. We may be guided, but should not be fettered, by tradition. Note that the greater the variability in the statistic's estimate, the wider the confidence interval. In situations encountering great variability, perhaps in certain psychiatric measures, the clinical need for a tighter interval might dictate a 90% interval. In situations characterized by small variability, perhaps in the control of electronic instruments, a 99% interval might be appropriate.

A Confidence Interval Can Apply to an Individual Patient

We find the extent of resection of the tracheal carina in DB12 to be approximately normal with $m = 2.96$ cm and $s = 1.24$ cm. The sample size is large enough to treat s as σ. In the normal table (Table A), we find that $1 - \alpha = 0.95$ is associated with $z = 1.96$, or the confidence interval on an observation extends $\pm 1.96\sigma$ on either side of m. Thus, the end points of the interval would be $2.96 - 1.96 \times 1.24 = 0.53$ and $2.96 + 1.96 \times 1.24 = 5.39$. This tells us that a new patient presenting is 95% sure to have a resection between about 0.5 and 5.5 cm. In this particular instance, the confidence interval on an individual patient is not very helpful clinically, because the surgically reasonably range is about 1–6 cm anyway. In other cases, such as choosing a healthy range for a laboratory test result, confidence intervals on individuals can be quite useful.

A Confidence Interval on a Statistic

In the preceding paragraph, we used a distribution of patients to obtain a confidence interval in relation to which we interpreted an observation from a single patient. This observation may be thought of as a sample of size 1 from a population with known mean and standard deviation. Although this is useful in clinical practice, in research we often are more interested in the confidence interval on the estimate of a population statistic, such as a mean or a standard deviation. In Chapter 4, Eq. (4.2) expressed a confidence interval separated into its primary and subordinate components as follows:

The probability
that a population statistic
from a distribution of estimates of that statistic
is contained in a specified interval
is given by
the area of the distribution within that interval. (12.1)

By denoting probability as P, the area under the probability curve outside the interval as α, and the interval end points as *critical values*, a somewhat simpler expression is obtained:

$$\text{P[lower critical value} < \text{population statistic} < \text{upper critical value]} = 1 - \alpha. \quad (12.2)$$

Critical values are those values that separate the tails from the main body of the distribution. All we need to implement Eq. (12.2) for any population statistic is the method to find the critical values, which is slightly different for each type of statistic. The methods to calculate the critical values will be the focus for the remainder of this chapter.

One- versus Two-Tailed Confidence Intervals

Whereas most confidence intervals are formed as intervals excluding both tails, an occasional case occurs in which we want to exclude only one tail. An example is given in the next section.

12.2. CONFIDENCE INTERVAL ON A MEAN, KNOWN STANDARD DEVIATION

Example

Let us find a 95% confidence interval on the mean extent of resection of the tracheal carina (DB12), which has been found to be approximately normal with $m = 2.96$ cm and $s = 1.24$ cm. The sample size is large enough to treat s as σ. In Table 12.1 (or Table A), we find that $1 - \sigma = 0.95$ is associated with $z = 1.96$, or the confidence interval on an observation extends $\pm 1.96\sigma_m$ on either side of m. $\sigma_m = \sigma/\sqrt{n} = 1.24/\sqrt{134} = 0.107$. Thus, the end points of the interval would be $2.96 - 1.96 \times 0.107 = 2.75$ and $2.96 + 1.96 \times 0.107 = 3.17$. By using the form

Table 12.1

The Most Used Entries from Table A, the Normal Distribution[a]

	One-tailed applications		Two-tailed applications	
z	One-tailed α	$1-\alpha$	Two-tailed α	$1-\alpha$
1.645	0.050	0.950	0.100	0.900
1.960	0.025	0.975	0.050	0.950
2.326	0.010	0.990	0.020	0.980
2.576	0.005	0.995	0.010	0.990

[a] For distances (z) to the right of the mean, given are (a) one-tailed α, area under the curve in the positive tail; (b) one-tailed $1 - \alpha$, area under all except the tail; (c) two-tailed α, areas combined for both positive and negative tails; and (d) two-tailed $1 - \alpha$, the area under all except the two tails.

in Eq (12.4), the confidence interval would be expressed as

$$P[2.75 < \mu < 3.17] = 0.95$$

and voiced as, "The probability that the interval 2.75 to 3.17 contains μ is 0.95."

One-Tailed Confidence Interval

Suppose we are concerned only with the resections in larger tail, which pose a threat due to their size; the smaller resections do not. Thus, we seek a critical value cutting off α proportion in only the upper tail. Say we still want a 95% confidence interval. This time we look in Table 12.1 (or Table A), under "one-tailed $1-\alpha$ (right tail area)." For $1-\alpha = 0.95$, we find $z_{1-\alpha}$ (no. std. deviations to right of mean) is 1.645, and we substitute these and the values for m and σ_m into Eq. (12.6) to get

$$P[\mu < 2.96 + 1.645 \times 0.107] = P[\mu < 3.136] = 0.95.$$

We are 95% confident that the mean extent of resection will not exceed 3.14 cm.

Method

Equation (12.2) applied to means would be expressed as P[lower critical value $< \mu <$ upper critical value] $= 1 - \alpha$. The critical values on a population mean μ would be given by the sample mean m plus or minus a number of standard errors of the mean (SEMs) as indicated by areas under the normal curve. The SEM is the standard deviations of the individual observations divided by the square root of the number of observations, or SEM $= \sigma/\sqrt{n}$. The number of SEMs is $z_{1-\alpha/2}$, the distance on the normal curve outside of which each tail $\alpha/2$ of the area lies. By substituting these elements in Eq. (12.2), we find

$$P[m - z_{1\alpha/2}\sigma_m < \mu < m + z_{1-\alpha/2}\sigma_m] = 1 - \alpha. \tag{12.3}$$

95% Confidence Interval

Table 12.1 is a segment of Table A, which shows the normal areas most frequently used. If we want 95% confidence, we look in Table 12.1 for 0.950 under "two-tailed $1 - \alpha$ (area except both tails)." To its left in the first column, i.e., under "z (no. std. deviations to right of mean)," we find 1.960. Thus, our critical values are the sample mean m plus and minus $1.96\sigma_m$. In symbols,

$$P[m - 1.96\sigma_m < \mu < m + 1.96\sigma_m] = 0.95. \tag{12.4}$$

One-Tailed Confidence Interval

If we are concerned with the mean falling on one side only, say the larger side, we would seek a critical value cutting off all α proportion in only the upper tail. By rewriting Eq. (12.3), we get

$$P[\mu < m + z_{1-\alpha}\sigma_m] = 1 - \alpha. \tag{12.5}$$

For a 95% confidence interval, we look for 0.95 under the "one-tailed $1 - \alpha$ (right tail area)" column in Table 12.1 and find that $z_{1-\alpha}$ is 1.645. By substitution into Eq. (12.5), we obtain

$$P[\mu < m + 1.645\sigma_m] = 0.95. \tag{12.6}$$

Additional Example

In the initial example of this section, we found a 95% confidence interval on the mean extent of resection of the tracheal carina (DB12). Let us find one on patient age for the same sample of patients: $m = 47.84$ years and we take $\sigma = 15.78$ years, so that $\sigma_m = 15.78/\sqrt{134} = 1.36$. By substituting in Eq. (12.4), we find

$$P[47.84 - 1.96 \times 1.36 < \mu < 47.84 + 1.96 \times 1.36]$$
$$= P[45.17 < \mu < 50.51] = 0.95.$$

We are 95% sure that the interval 45.2–50.5 years will enclose the population mean age.

Exercise 12.1. Find the 90% and 99% confidence intervals on mean age of carinal resection patients.

12.3. CONFIDENCE INTERVAL ON A MEAN, ESTIMATED STANDARD DEVIATION

EXAMPLE

In DB5, plasma silicone level on $n = 30$ patients was measured before and again after silicone implantation. What is the 95% confidence level on the difference pre-op to post-op? The mean difference is $m = 0.0073$ with standard deviation $s = 0.1222$. The SEM $= 0.1222/\sqrt{29} = 0.0227$. A segment of the t table, Table B, appears as Table 12.2. The intersection of the column for two-tailed $1 - \alpha = 0.95$ with the row for 29 *df* gives $t_{1-\alpha/2} = 2.045$, which tells us that the critical values will be the sample mean $\pm$ a bit over 2 SEMs. After substitution in Eq. (12.7), the confidence interval becomes

$$\mathrm{P}[0.0073 - 2.045 \times 0.0227 < \mu < 0.0073 + 2.045 \times 0.0227]$$
$$= \mathrm{P}[0.039 < \mu < 0.054] = 0.95.$$

METHOD

The method was set forth in Section 4.7. Let us review it briefly. The concept of a confidence interval on the mean using s is much the same as that using σ (Section 12.2), the difference being that the t distribution rather than the normal is used to calculate the critical values. The form, seen previously as Eq. (4.6), is quite similar to Eq. (12.3):

$$\mathrm{P}[m - t_{1-\alpha/2}s_m < \mu < m + t_{1-\alpha/2}s_m] = 1 - \alpha. \tag{12.7}$$

Table 12.2

A Segment of the t Table, Table B[a]

Two-tailed α	0.20	0.10	0.05	0.02	0.01	0.002	0.001
Two-tailed $1 - \alpha$	0.80	0.90	0.95	0.98	0.99	0.998	0.999
df = 15	1.341	1.753	2.131	2.602	2.947	3.733	4.073
29	1.311	1.699	2.045	2.462	2.756	3.396	3.659

[a] Selected distances (t) to the right of the mean are given for various degrees of freedom (*df*), for two-tailed α, areas combined for both positive and negative tails, and for two-tailed $1 - \alpha$, area under all except the two tails.

Because the t distribution has a greater spread than the normal, the confidence interval will be slightly wider. If we want 95% confidence, we find the desired t-value in Table B at the intersection the 0.95 column for "two-tailed $1-\alpha$ (except both tails)" and the row for the appropriate *df*.

Additional Example

In DB3, serum theophylline level was measured in emphysema patients before they were given azithromycin, at 5 days, and at 10 days. What are 95% confidence intervals on mean serum theophylline level at these three points in time? $n = 16, m_0 = 10.80, s_0 = 3.77, m_5 = 9.81, s_5 = 4.61, m_{10} = 10.14$, and $s_{10} = 3.989$. SEMs are 0.94, 1.15, and 1.00, respectively. From Table 12.2, the intersection of the column for two-tailed $1-\alpha = 0.95$ with the row for 15 *df* gives $t_{1-\alpha/2} = 2.131$. After substitution in Eq. 12.7, these values yield the following confidence intervals:

$$\begin{aligned}
&P_0[10.80 - 2.131 \times 0.94 < \mu < 10.80 + 2.131 \times 0.94] \\
&\quad = P_0[8.80 < \mu < 12.80] = 0.95, \\
&P_5[9.81 - 2.131 \times 1.15 < \mu < 9.81 + 2.131 \times 1.15] \\
&\quad = P_5[7.36 < \mu < 12.26] = 0.95, \\
&P_{10}[10.14 - 2.131 \times 1.00 < \mu < 10.14 + 2.131 \times 1.00] \\
&\quad = P_{10}[8.01 < \mu < 12.27] = 0.95.
\end{aligned}$$

Exercise 12.2. Among the indicators of patient condition following pyloromyotomy (correction of stenotic pylorus) in neonates is time (hours) to full feeding.[16] A surgeon wants to place a 95% confidence interval on mean time to full feeding. He has readings from $n = 20$ infants. Some of his data are 3.50, 4.52, 3.03, 14.53, ... He calculates $m = 6.56$ and $s = 4.57$. What is his confidence interval?

12.4. CONFIDENCE INTERVAL ON A VARIANCE OR STANDARD DEVIATION

Example

The variability in platelet-derived growth factor (PDGF) has been estimated (DB9) as $s = 19{,}039.7$. What would be a 95% confidence interval on the population σ? We know the probability distribution of s^2 but not that of s, so we shall find the interval on the population variance, σ^2, and take square roots. $s^2 = 19{,}039.7^2 = 362{,}510{,}180$. The distribution of s^2 requires *df* and critical values of

Table 12.3

Segments of the Chi-Square Tables, Tables C (Associated with Right Tail) and D (Associated with Left Tail)[a]

	Right tail			Left tail		
α	0.05	0.025	0.01	0.01	0.025	0.05
$1-\alpha$	0.95	0.975	0.99	0.99	0.975	0.95
18	28.87	31.53	34.80	7.01	8.23	9.39
19	30.14	32.85	36.19	7.63	8.91	10.12
20	31.41	34.17	37.57	8.26	9.59	10.85
28	41.34	44.46	48.28	13.57	15.31	16.93
29	42.56	45.72	49.59	14.25	16.05	17.71
30	43.77	46.98	50.89	14.95	16.79	18.49

[a] Selected χ^2 values (distances above zero) are given for various degrees of freedom (*df*) and for (a) α, the area under the curve in the indicated tail, and (b) $1-\alpha$, the area under all except the indicated tail.

χ^2. $df = n - 1 = 19$. Table 12.3 gives segments of the chi-square tables, Tables C (right tail) and D (left tail). By looking in Table 12.3 under right tail area = 0.025 for 19 *df*, we find 32.85. Similarly, under left tail area = 0.025 for 19 *df*, we find 8.91. By substituting these values in Eq. (12.8), we find

$$\begin{aligned} &P\left[s^2 \times df/\chi^2_R < \sigma^2 < s^2 \times df/\chi^2_L\right] \\ &= P[362{,}510{,}180 \times 19/32.85 < \sigma^2 < 362{,}510{,}180 \times 19/8.91] \\ &= P[209{,}671{,}030 < \sigma^2 < 773{,}029{,}560] = 0.95. \end{aligned}$$

By taking the square root within the brackets, we obtain

$$P[14{,}480.0 < \sigma < 27{,}803.4] = 0.95.$$

Method

We know (from Section 2.8 or 4.9) that s^2 calculated from a random sample from a normal population is distributed as $\chi^2 \times \sigma^2/df$. A confidence-type statement on σ^2 obtained from this relationship, excluding $1-\alpha$ in each tail, is given by

$$P\left[s^2 \times df/\chi^2_R < \sigma^2 < s^2 \times df/\chi^2_L\right] = 1-\alpha, \tag{12.8}$$

where χ^2_R is the critical value for the right tail found from Table C and χ^2_L that for the left found from Table D. The critical values are found separately because the chi-square distribution is asymmetric. To find confidence interval on σ, take the square root of the components within brackets.

Additional Example

Is plasma silicone level (DB5) less variable after implantation? Whereas this question can be tested by a formal hypothesis test as in Section 16.3, we can make an informal comparison by contrasting the confidence intervals on $\sigma_{\text{pre-op}}$ and $\sigma_{\text{post-op}}$. What are these confidence intervals? From Eq. (12.8), we need s^2, *df*, and the critical chi-squares: $s_{\text{pre}} = 0.098565$, $s^2_{\text{pre}} = 0.009715$, $s_{\text{post}} = 0.076748$, $s^2_{\text{post}} = 0.005890$, and $df = 29$. From Table 12.3, the intersections of column $\alpha = 0.025$ and row $df = 29$ yields $\chi^2_{\text{R}} = 45.72$ and $\chi^2_{\text{L}} = 16.05$. Substitution in Eq. (12.8) yields

$$P[0.006162 < \sigma^2_{\text{pre}} < 0.017554] = 0.95$$

and

$$P[0.003736 < \sigma^2_{\text{post}} < 0.010642] = 0.95.$$

By taking the square root within the brackets, we find confidence intervals on the σ's to be

$$P[0.078 < \sigma_{\text{pre}} < 0.132] = 0.95$$

and

$$P[0.061 < \sigma_{\text{post}} < 0.103] = 0.95.$$

The confidence intervals are not very different from a clinical perspective.

Exercise 12.3. An infectious disease specialist samples the WBC of $n = 19$ patients who contracted the same nosocomial infection in an orthopedic ward. She finds that the mean count is not unusual, but suspects that the standard deviation may be larger than normal: $s = 6000$. What is her 95% confidence interval on the standard deviation σ for the population of patients so infected?

12.5. CONFIDENCE INTERVAL ON A PROPORTION

Proportions Fall into Two Types

Proportions fall in the interval 0–1. However, methods must be divided into two types: cases in which the proportion lies away from the extremes 0 and 1 and cases in which the proportion lies very close to 0 or 1. The reason is that they lead to different distributions, as discussed in the following Methods section.

Example, Proportion Not near 0 or 1

Of our 301 urology biopsies from DB1, 95 tested positive, yielding a sample proportion $p = 0.316$. We want a confidence interval on the theoretical proportion π. We know that a large-sample proportion not near 0 or 1 is distributed approximately normal with mean p. The standard deviation σ is given by

$$\sigma = \sqrt{\frac{p(1-p)}{n}} = \sqrt{\frac{0.31 \times 0.684}{301}} = 0.0268.$$

By using Eq. (12.9), we bracket π with 95% confidence as

$$\begin{aligned} &\mathrm{P}[p - 1.96\sigma - 1/2n < \pi < p + 1.96\sigma + 1/2n] \\ &\quad = \mathrm{P}[0.316 - 1.96 \times 0.0268 - 0.00166 < \pi \\ &\qquad < 0.316 + 1.96 \times 0.0268 + 0.00166] \\ &\quad = \mathrm{P}[0.211 < \pi < 0.421] = 0.95. \end{aligned}$$

We are 95% confident that the proportion of positive prostate biopsies in the population of patients presenting with urological problems lies between 21% and 42%.

Example, Proportion near 0 or 1

Children with high lead levels are found in a certain hospital's catchment.[42] Of 2500 children sampled, 30 with high lead levels are found, yielding $p = 0.012$. As π evidently is close to 0, we use the normal approximation to the Poisson distribution: $\sigma = \sqrt{(p/n)} = \sqrt{(0.012/2500)} = 0.00219$. The hospital administration wants to be very sure that it does not have too many high-lead children in its catchment and so chooses a 99% confidence interval. From Table 12.1, the 0.99 two-tailed $1 - \alpha$ yields a corresponding z of 2.576. By replacing the 1.96 in Eq. (12.10) with 2.576, we obtain

$$\begin{aligned} &P[p - 2.576\sigma < \pi < p + 2.576\sigma] \\ &\quad = \mathrm{P}[0.012 - 2.576 \times 0.00219 < \pi < 0.012 + 2.576 \times 0.00219] \\ &\quad = \mathrm{P}[0.0064 < \pi < 0.0176] = 0.99. \end{aligned}$$

By focusing on the right tail, the hospital administration may be 99.5% confident that no more than 1.8% of children in its catchment have high lead levels.

Method

The confidence interval we seek here is on the theoretical but unknown population proportion π, which we estimate by the sample proportion p.

π Is Not near 0 or 1

p is distributed binomial, approximated by the normal with standard deviation estimated as $\sigma = \sqrt{[p(1-p)/n]}$. p and σ are substituted in the 95% confidence interval pattern of Eq. (12.4) to obtain

$$P[p - 1.96\sigma - 1/2n < \pi < p + 1.96\sigma + 1/2n] = 0.95, \qquad (12.9)$$

where the $1/2n$ components are continuity corrections to improve the approximation. If confidence other than 95% is desired, the form of Eq. (12.3) may be used in place of Eq. (12.4). In this case, 1.96 is replaced by the appropriate multiplier chosen from Table A as z (first column) corresponding to the desired two-tailed $1 - \alpha$ (last column).

π Is near 0 or 1

p is distributed Poisson, approximated by the normal with standard deviation estimated as the smaller of $\sigma = \sqrt{(p/n)}$ or $\sqrt{[(1-p)/n]}$. p and σ are substituted in the confidence interval pattern of Eq. (12.4) to obtain

$$P[p - 1.96\sigma < \pi < p + 1.96\sigma] = 0.95. \qquad (12.10)$$

Use Eq. (12.3) in place of Eq. (12.4) for confidence levels other than 95%.

Additional Example

In a study[36] anesthetizing oral surgery patients by a combination of propofol and alfentanil, 89.1% of 110 patients rated the anesthetic as highly satisfactory or excellent. What are 95% confidence limits on π, the proportion of the population satisfied with the anesthetic? As π is not near 0 or 1, the normal approximation to the binomial is appropriate. $p = 0.891$ and $\sigma = \sqrt{(0.891 \times 0.118/110)} = 0.031$ are substituted in Eq. (12.9):

$$\begin{aligned} &P[0.891 - 1.96 \times 0.031 - 1/220 < \pi < 0.891 + 1.96 \times 0.031 + 1/220] \\ &\quad = P[0.826 < \pi < 0.956] = 0.95. \end{aligned}$$

We are 95% confident that at least 83% of patients will be quite satisfied with the combination of propofol and alfentanil, but at least 4% will not.

Exercise 12.4. A 5-year recurrence rate of basal cell carcinoma when lesions measured more than 20 mm was 0.261 based on a sample of 226.[67] Put a 95% confidence interval on the population π for this proportion.

12.6. CONFIDENCE INTERVAL ON A CORRELATION COEFFICIENT

EXAMPLE

An orthopedist is studying hardware removal in broken ankle repair.[23] One of his variables is the maximum angle (degrees) of plantar flexion. He wants to know whether age is related to plantar flexion. He finds the sample correlation coefficient for his 19 patients to be 0.1945 and wants the confidence interval on that coefficient. Equation (12.13) is not so intimidating when he breaks it into pieces: $1 + r = 1.1945$, $1 - r = 0.8055$, $n - 3 = 16$, and $\sqrt{16} = 4$. For 95% confidence, $z_{1-\alpha/2} = 1.96$. The exponent of e will be $\pm 2 \times 1.96/4 = \pm 0.98$. By substituting these components into Eq. (12.13), he finds

$$\mathrm{P}\left[\frac{1+r-(1-r)e^{\frac{2z_{1-\alpha/2}}{\sqrt{n-3}}}}{1+r+(1-r)e^{\frac{2z_{1-\alpha/2}}{\sqrt{n-3}}}} < \rho < \frac{1+r-(1-r)e^{-\frac{2z_{1-\alpha/2}}{\sqrt{n-3}}}}{1+r+(1-r)e^{-\frac{2z_{1-\alpha/2}}{\sqrt{n-3}}}}\right]$$

$$= \mathrm{P}\left[\frac{1.1945 - 0.8055 \times e^{0.98}}{1.1945 + 0.8055 \times e^{0.98}}\right] < \rho < \left[\frac{1.1945 - 0.8055 \times e^{-0.98}}{1.1945 + 0.8055 \times e^{-0.98}}\right]$$

$$= \mathrm{P}[-0.2849 < \rho < 0.5961] = 0.95.$$

Because the population correlation coefficient may be anywhere from about -0.3 to $+0.6$ (the confidence interval crosses 0), he concludes that age has not been shown to be an influence.

METHOD

Confidence intervals on the population correlation coefficient ρ, estimated by r $(=s_{xy}/s_x s_y)$ for small sample sizes usually are too wide to be of much help. If we have a larger sample size, we can transform the correlation coefficient to have approximately the normal distribution. We recall that "ln" denotes "natural logarithm" and "e" denotes the "natural number," 2.71828.... The old base-ten logarithms were used to facilitate certain difficult arithmetic in the days before computers (could we call that BC?) and seldom are used anymore; ln and e are found on every computer and most handheld calculating machines. The normally transformed correlation coefficient has sample mean

$$m = \frac{1}{2}\ln\left(\frac{1+r}{1-r}\right) \tag{12.11}$$

and standard deviation estimated as

$$\sigma = \frac{1}{\sqrt{n-3}}. \tag{12.12}$$

Solution of the transformation Eq. (12.11) for r yields a ratio of exponential expressions, which, along with Eq. (12.12), can be entered into the pattern of Eq. (12.3). This inequality then can be solved mathematically to obtain a $1-\alpha$ confidence interval as

$$\mathrm{P}\left[\frac{1+r-(1-r)e^{\frac{2z_{1-\alpha/2}}{\sqrt{n-3}}}}{1+r+(1-r)e^{\frac{2z_{1-\alpha/2}}{\sqrt{n-3}}}} < \rho < \frac{1+r-(1-r)e^{-\frac{2z_{1-\alpha/2}}{\sqrt{n-3}}}}{1+r+(1-r)e^{-\frac{2z_{1-\alpha/2}}{\sqrt{n-3}}}}\right] = 1-\alpha. \tag{12.13}$$

Equation (12.13) holds for nonnegative correlation coefficients. If r is negative, symmetry properties allow a simple solution. Find the confidence limits as if the r were positive (i.e., use $|r|$), then change the signs on the resulting limits and exchange their positions. This mechanism will be illustrated in the following example.

Additional Example

In a study on increasing red blood cell mass pre-operatively, the correlation between hematocrit (Hct) and serum erythropoietin levels was of interest. An inverse correlation was anticipated for patients with normal renal function. Levels were measured in $n = 126$ patients, and the correlation coefficient was calculated as $r = -0.59$.[14] Let us find a 95% confidence interval on the population correlation coefficient ρ. Because r is negative, we first find the limits as if it were positive; we temporarily use $r = +0.59$. Then, $1+r = 1.59$, $1-r = 0.41$, $n-3 = 123$, and $\sqrt{123} = 11.0905$. The exponent is ± 0.3535. Substitution in Eq. (12.13) yields

$$\mathrm{P}\left[\frac{1+r-(1-r)e^{\frac{2z_{1-\alpha/2}}{\sqrt{n-3}}}}{1+r+(1-r)e^{\frac{2z_{1-\alpha/2}}{\sqrt{n-3}}}} < \rho < \frac{1+r-(1-r)e^{-\frac{2z_{1-\alpha/2}}{\sqrt{n-3}}}}{1+r+(1-r)e^{-\frac{2z_{1-\alpha/2}}{\sqrt{n-3}}}}\right]$$
$$= \mathrm{P}[0.4628 < \rho < 0.6934] = 0.95.$$

To convert the limits to bound $r = -0.59$, we change 0.4628 to -0.4628 and put it in the right (larger limit) position and then change 0.6934 to -0.6934 and put it in the left (smaller limit) position. The resulting confidence interval on ρ when $r = -0.59$ from a sample of 126 becomes

$$\mathrm{P}[-0.6934 < \rho < -0.4628] = 0.95.$$

We are 95% confident that the population correlation coefficient between Hct and serum erythropoietin levels in patients with normal renal function lies between −0.69 and −0.46.

Exercise 12.5. An orthopedist is experimenting with the use of nitronox as an anesthetic in the treatment of children's arm fractures.[21,22] He finds that it provides a shorter duration of surgery and less pain than other procedures he has used. In addition, he expects that the shorter the procedure, the less the perceived pain. Do the data bear out this expectation? More specifically, is the confidence interval on the population correlation coefficient between the two variables entirely within the positive range? He treats $n = 50$ children, recording the treatment time in minutes and the score from a CHEOPS pain scale. He finds $r = 0.267$. Find the 95% confidence interval on this r.

ANSWERS TO EXERCISES

12.1. To substitute in Eq. (12.3), the z-values must be found from Table 12.1 (or Table A). Under the column for two-tailed $1 - \alpha$, 0.900 (90%) yields $z = 1.645$ and 0.990 (99%) yields 2.576. By substituting $m = 47.84$ years and $\sigma_m = 1.36$ years, we find $\text{P}[47.84 - 1.645 \times 1.36 < \mu < 47.84 + 1.645 \times 1.36] = \text{P}[45.60 < \mu < 50.08] = 0.90$ and $\text{P}[47.84 - 2.576 \times 1.36 < \mu < 47.84 + 2.576 \times 1.36] = \text{P}[44.34 < \mu < 51.34] = 0.99$.

12.2. He calculates $s_m = s/\sqrt{n} = 4.57/\sqrt{20} = 1.02$ hr. From Table B, t for 95% "two-tailed $1-\alpha$ (except both tails)" for 19 df is 2.093. He substitutes these values in Eq. (5.7) to obtain $\text{P}[m - t_{1-\alpha/2}s_m < \mu < m + t_{1-\alpha/2}s_m] = \text{P}[6.56 - 2.093 \times 1.02 < \mu < 6.56 + 2.093 \times 1.02] = \text{P}[4.43 < \mu < 8.69] = 0.95$. He is 95% confident that mean time to full feeding will lie between 4.4 and 8.7 hr.

12.3. $s^2 = 36{,}000$ and $df = 18$. From Table 12.3, the intersection of the 0.025 column with 18 df is 31.53 for the right tail and 8.23 for the left. Substitution in Eq. (12.8) yields $\text{P}[20{,}551.855 < \sigma^2 < 78{,}735{,}330] = 0.95$ and taking the square root yields $\text{P}[4533 < \sigma < 8873] = 0.95$. As σ for a healthy population would be around 1200–1300, her variability does indeed appear to be abnormally large.

12.4. p is not near 0 or 1, so $\sigma = \sqrt{[p(1-p)/n]} = \sqrt{[0.261 \times 0.739/226]} = 0.0292$. Substitute in Eq. (5.9) to obtain $\text{P}[p - 1.96\sigma - 1/2n < \pi < p + 1.96\sigma + 1/2n] = \text{P}[0.261 - 1.96 \times 0.029 - 1/452 < \pi < 0.261 + 1.96 \times 0.029 + 1/452] = \text{P}[0.202 < \pi < 0.320] = 0.95$.

12.5. $1 + r = 1.267$, $1 - r = 0.733$, and the exponential term is 0.5718. Substitution in Eq. (12.13) yields $\text{P}[-0.0123 < \rho < 0.5076] = 0.95$. The confidence interval crosses 0, indicating that the population correlation coefficient could be 0 or negative and the 0.267 sample coefficient could have occurred by chance.

Chapter 13

Common Tests on Categorical Data

13.1. CATEGORICAL DATA SUMMARY

Terms and Symbols

A more complete treatment of the basics appeared in Section 6.2. *Categorical* or *nominal* data are data placed into distinct categories rather than being measured as a point on a scale or ranked in order. The basic sample statistics are the *count*, obtained by counting the number of events per category, and the *proportion* of data in a category, the count divided by the total number in the variable. If n denotes the total number of events and n_{a} the number in category a, the proportion in a is $p_{\mathrm{a}} = n_{\mathrm{a}}/n$. Often percent, $100p_{\mathrm{a}}$, is used. π denotes the population proportion, which is known from theory or closely approximated by a very large sample.

Example

A vascular surgeon treated 29 patients endoscopically for thrombosis in the leg,[47] after which 6 recurred. $n = 29$, $n_{\mathrm{a}} = 6$, $p_{\mathrm{a}} = 6/29 = 0.207$. About 21% recurred.

Organizing Data for Categorical Methods

If the relationship between two variables is of interest, such as whether they are independent or associated, the number of observations simultaneously falling into the categories of two variables is counted. For example, the vascular surgeon is interested in the relation between recurrence and ulcer condition. The first variable may be categorized as recurred or not recurred and the second as open ulcers or healed ulcers. This gives rise to the four categories of counts, which are shown along with their counts in Table 13.1. We can see that five is the number of recurrences, contingent upon the ulcers being healed. Tables of this sort are called *contingency tables*, because the count in each cell is the number in that category of that variable contingent upon also lying in a particular category of the other variable.

Contingency Table Symbols

Contingency tables often have more than four categories. For example, if the preulcerous condition of heavy pigmentation were added to the ulcer condition variable, there would be three conditions resulting in a 2×3 table. In general, the number of rows is denoted by r and the number of columns by c to yield an $r \times c$ table. Because the values of r and c are unknown until a particular case is specified, the cell numbers and the marginal (row and column) totals must be symbolized in a way that can apply to tables of any size. The usual symbolism is shown in Table 13.1: n, for "number," with two subscripts, the first indicating the row and the second indicating the column. Thus, the number of cases observed in row 1, column 2 is n_{12}. The row and column totals are denoted by placing a dot in place of the numbers we summed to get the total. Thus, the total of the first row would be $n_{1\cdot}$ and the total of the second column would be $n_{\cdot 2}$. The grand total can be denoted just n (or $n_{\cdot\cdot}$).

Choosing Categorical Methods

Methods exist for counts and proportions. When all cells of the table of counts can be filled in, use the methods for counts. Tests of proportions are appropriate for cases in which some table totals are missing, but for which proportions can still

Table 13.1

Contingency Table of Thrombosis Recurrence and Ulcer Condition

		Ulcers		
		Open	Healed	Totals
Recurred	Yes	$n_{11} = 1$	$n_{12} = 5$	$n_{1\cdot} = 6$
	No	$n_{21} = 7$	$n_{22} = 16$	$n_{2\cdot} = 23$
	Totals	$n_{\cdot 1} = 8$	$n_{\cdot 2} = 21$	$n = 29$

be found. A first-step guide to choosing a test was introduced in Section 10.2. The tests in this chapter address the first three columns in the body of Table 10.1. First decide whether the question of your study asks about proportions (columns 1 and 2) or about counts, i.e., the number of cases falling into the cells of a table (column 3). To select the row of Table 10.1, note whether your sample is small or large and how many subsamples you have. Sections 13.2–13.5 cover methods for count-type data, Sections 13.6 and 13.7 cover proportions, and Section 13.8 covers matched pairs.

Degrees of Freedom for Contingency Tests

Contingency test degrees of freedom (*df*) is given by the minimum number of cells that must be filled to be able to calculate the remainder of cell entries using the totals at the side and bottom. For example, only one cell of a 2×2 table with the sums at the side and bottom needs to be filled, and the others can be found by subtraction; it has 1 *df*. A 2×3 table has 2 *df*. In general, an $r \times c$ table has $df = (r - 1) \times (c - 1)$.

Categories versus Ranks

Cases for which counts or proportions for each sample group can be swapped without affecting the interpretation are constrained to categorical methods. An example would be as follows: group 1, high hematocrit (Hct); group 2, high white blood cell count; group 3, high platelet count. However, if sample groups fall into a natural order in which the logical implication would change by altering this order, such as group 1 low Hct, group 2 normal Hct, and group 3 high Hct, rank methods are appropriate. Although these groups could be considered as categories and categorical methods could be used, rank methods give better results. Whereas rank methods lose power when there is a large number of ties, they still are more powerful than categorical methods, which are not very powerful. *When ranking is a natural option, rank methods of Chapter 14 should be used.*

Methods Addressed in This Chapter

The basic question being tested asks about the relationship between two variables. Different tests exist to answer the question, including the Fisher–Irwin (Fisher's exact) test and the chi-square test of contingency (Sections 13.2 and 13.4) and, less commonly used, a test of logarithm of relative risk (log RR) and a test of logarithm of odds ratio (log OR). RR and OR are measures of association that will be discussed in Section 13.5. Although all of these tests give rather similar results, the choice of test can be aided by noting the question being asked. If we believe that two variables are independent and our goal is to assess the probability that this is true, we would prefer the Fisher–Irwin test or its approximation the chi-square test of contingency, which approximates it in cases of large samples or several categories. If we have a measure of association that we believe is meaningful and our goal is to assess the statistical significance of this association, we would prefer to test the OR (or the RR, although the log OR test is a little more general in that it can be used in more situations than can the log RR test). If we know proportions but do not have the marginal totals required to use the Fisher–Irwin or chi-square tests, we can test the proportions directly (Sections 13.6 and 13.7). Finally, if one of the variables includes matched pairs rather than counts from different samples, the McNemar test would be used (Section 13.8).

13.2. 2 × 2 TABLES: CONTINGENCY TESTS

Are the Row Categories Independent of the Column Categories in 2 × 2 Tables?

A "yes" answer implies that the rows variable has not been shown to be related to the columns variable; knowledge of the outcome of one of the variables gives us no information as to the associated outcome of the other variable. A "no" answer tells us that *some* association exists, but does *not* tell us the strength of this association. (A test of the strength of association may be found in Section 13.5.)

The Chi-Square Contingency Test from Section 6.3

The basic concepts and examples of application of the chi-square contingency test appeared in Section 6.3. A reader new to these ideas should become familiar with that section before continuing. Only a brief summary of that section appears in the methods paragraph herein. The chi-square test of contingency is based on the difference between the observed values and those expected if the variables were independent.

Fisher's Exact Test Is Another Test of Independence between Two Categorical Variables

If the counts within the contingency table cells are small, the probability of independence should be calculated directly by *Fisher's exact test*, which can be found in statistical packages on modern computers. The test should more properly be named the *Fisher–Irwin test*; Irwin and Fisher developed the theory independently, and their work appeared in print almost simultaneously. "Exact" implies that it is calculated by methods from probability theory rather than approximated, as is chi-square; the wide use of the chi-square test arose before there was adequate computing power for the exact test. If there are many cells in the contingency table, the exact method may still be too computation-intensive. In cases where the number of cells is larger than, say, 10 (depending on the speed of the computer), and if there is no cell with a count less than 5 and no expected value less than 1, the Fisher–Irwin result can be well approximated by the chi-square test of contingency.

Example: Dependence of DRE and Biopsy Results

In Chapter 6, we posed the question of whether the digital rectal exam (DRE) is independent of the biopsy result (BIOP). For the 301 urological patients, the 2×2 contingency Table 6.3 reappears here as Table 13.2. The chi-square statistic is calculated as $\chi^2 = 6.62$, which yields a significant p-value of 0.010 that indicates a dependence between DRE and biopsy. The Fisher–Irwin p-value, calculated by a statistical software package, is similar at 0.016, yielding the same interpretation.

Method: 2 × 2 Contingency Table Tests

Two categories of each variable yield a 2×2 contingency table. The two tests of independence are the Fisher–Irwin test or its approximation, the chi-square test of contingency. The basis of the chi-square test was explained in Chapter 6. In summary, the actual chi-square statistic is the sum of these differences squared in ratio to the expected value. The expected value for row i and column j was given by Eq. (6.1) as

$$e_{ij} = \frac{n_{i.} n_{.j}}{n}. \tag{13.1}$$

Table 13.2

Contingency Table of Simultaneous Biopsy and DRE Results from 301 Patients

		DRE		
		1	0	Totals
BIOP	1	$n_{11} = 68$	$n_{12} = 27$	$n_{1.} = 95$
	0	$n_{21} = 117$	$n_{22} = 89$	$n_{2.} = 206$
	Totals	$n_{.1} = 185$	$n_{.2} = 116$	$n = 301$

The chi-square statistic was given by Eq. (6.2) as

$$\chi^2 = \sum_i^2 \sum_j^2 \frac{(|n_{ij} - e_{ij}| - 0.5)^2}{e_{ij}}. \tag{13.2}$$

If this statistic is small, there is little dependence between the variables; a large statistic indicates dependence. If the chi-square statistic is large enough that it is unlikely to have occurred by chance, we say that it is significant and conclude that the rows variable is not totally independent of the columns variable; however, it does *not* follow that one can be well predicted by the other. The reason for this is that the significance is influenced by both sample size and association. The influence of sample size is illustrated in Section 6.3.

Assumptions underlying Chi-Square Contingency

The chi-square method should not be used for extremely small samples. In particular, it is valid *only* if the expected value (row sum $\times$ column sum $\div$ total sum) of every cell is at least 1 and a minimum count of 5 appears in every cell.

The Basis of the Fisher–Irwin Test

The Fisher–Irwin test, or Fisher's exact test, is calculated by a statistical software package. Its p-value gives the probability that the observed deviation from independence would occur by chance alone. A small p-value indicates that causes other than chance are influencing the outcome, and therefore the two variables probably are not independent. The Fisher–Irwin test uses a probability distribution known as the hypergeometric distribution for the observed counts, calculating the probability of all other 2×2 tables with the same marginal totals (n-counts). The p-value is the sum of probabilities of all such outcomes with counts less likely than the observed counts. The interpretation of the Fisher–Irwin p-value is just the same as the chi-square p-value. A significant Fisher–Irwin or chi-square result indicates that the variables are not independent, but does not indicate how closely they are associated.

Additional Example

Improvement with Surgical Experience Tested by Fisher–Irwin

An ophthalmologist investigated his learning curve in performing radial keratotomies.[4] He was able to perform a 1-month post-operative refraction on 78 of his

Table 13.3

Refraction of Post-operative Eyes by Position in Sequence of Surgery

	Eyes in first 50	Eyes in second 50	Totals
20/20 or Better	17	27	44
Worse than 20/20	24	10	34
Totals	41	37	78

first 100 eyes. He classified them as 20/20 or better versus worse than 20/20. His results appear as Table 13.3. He notes that his percent 20/20 or better rose from 41% for earlier surgeries to 73% for later surgeries. His null hypothesis is that resultant visual acuity is independent of when the surgery was done. The Fisher–Irwin test yields $p = 0.005$. He rejects the null hypothesis and concludes that his surgery has gotten significantly better.

Improvement with Surgical Experience Tested by Chi-Square

He could have approximated this result by a chi-square. He calculates his expected value as $e_{ij} = n_i. \times n._j/n. e_{11} = 44 \times 41/78 = 23.13, e_{12} = 20.87$, $e_{21} = 17.87$, and $e_{22} = 16.13$. By substituting in Eq. (13.2), he finds

$$\chi^2 = \sum_i^2 \sum_j^2 \frac{(|n_{ij} - e_{ij}| - 0.5)^2}{e_{ij}}$$

$$= \frac{(|17 - 23.13| - 0.5)^2}{23.13} + \cdots + \frac{(|10 - 16.13| - 0.5)^2}{16.13} = 9.19.$$

From Table C, a fragment of which is reproduced as Table 13.4, the critical value of χ^2 for $\alpha = 0.05$ in one tail with 1 *df* is 3.84, which is much less than 9.19; again the null hypothesis is rejected. Calculation by a software package yields $p = 0.003$, which is similar to the Fisher–Irwin value.

Table 13.4

A Fragment of Table C, the Right Tail of the Chi-Square Distribution[a]

α (area in right tail)	0.10	0.05	0.025	0.01
$df = 1$	2.71	3.84	5.02	6.63

[a] χ^2 values (distances to the right of 0) are tabulated for 1 *df* for four values of α.

Table 13.5
Data on Ankle Ligament Repair

		Treatment		
		MB	CS	Total
Success	Excellent	10	3	13
	Less	10	16	26
	Totals	20	19	39

Exercise 13.1: Comparing Methods of Torn Ankle Ligament Repair. Two methods of torn ankle ligament repair were compared in an orthopedics department in 1994: modified Bostrom (MB) and Chrisman–Snook (CS).[23] The clinical success on 39 patients was rated as excellent or less than excellent. The contingency table is given in Table 13.5. Find the p-values using the Fisher–Irwin test and the chi-square test. Are the two treatments significantly different?

13.3. $r \times c$ TABLES: CONTINGENCY TESTS

Section Topic

This section addresses the following question: *Are the row categories independent of the column categories in tables having r rows and c columns?* A positive answer implies that the rows variable has not been shown to be related to the columns variable.

Example: Is the Use of Smokeless Tobacco Related to Ethnic Origin?

With increased restriction on smoking in ships and shore stations, many Navy and Marine Corps personnel are changing to smokeless tobacco.[42] Navy medicine is concerned about the effect of this pattern on health and seeks causes. Cultural influences may be involved. Is ethnic background related to smokeless tobacco use? A count of the numbers in the various categories yielded Table 13.6. With two rows and three columns, $r = 2$ and $c = 3$. Smokeless tobacco use was ascertained from 2004 sailors and marines of three ethnic backgrounds from a wide variety of unit assignments. A total of 74.8% were of European background but represented 91.2% of users, 15.1% were of African background but represented 2.4% of users, and 10.1% were of Hispanic background but represented 6.0% of users. It was

Table 13.6

Contingency Table (2 × 3) of Smokeless Tobacco Use Associated with Ethnic Origin Categories European, African, and Hispanic from 2004 Patients

		Ethnic background			
		European	African	Hispanic	Totals
Smokeless tobacco	Use	424	13	28	465
	Do not use	1075	290	174	1539
	Totals	1499	303	202	2004

suspected that use is not independent of ethnic background, and the relationship was tested.

Smokeless Tobacco and Ethnic Origin, Fisher–Irwin Test

Here $r + c$ is 5, which is less than 7, so the Fisher–Irwin (FI) test is practical to use when the user has access to a computer statistical package. The (FI) p-value is <0.001. (Statistical software packages may display p-values like 0.000, implying that the first significant digit lies more than three digits to the right of the decimal point. However, values less than 0.001 are not accurate, so $p < 0.001$ should be reported.)

Smokeless Tobacco and Ethnic Origin, Chi-Square Contingency Test

The chi-square approximation formula appears in Eq. (13.3); the critical value may be found in Table C for $(r - 1) \times (c - 1) = 2\,df$. The observed count in row i, column j is n_{ij} ($n_{11} = 424$), and the corresponding expected entry e_{ij} is row i total × column j total/grand total ($e_{11} = 465 \times 1499/2004 = 347.82$). The chi-square component of the first cell is $(|n_{11} - e_{11}| - 0.5)^2/e_{11} = (|424 - 347.82| - 0.5)^2/347.82 = 16.47$. By following this pattern and summing over the six cells, the chi-square statistic becomes

$$\chi^2 = 16.47 + 45.90 + 7.20 + 4.98 + 13.87 + 2.18 = 90.60.$$

In Table 13.7, a fragment of chi-square Table C, the entry for $\alpha = 0.0005$ and $df = 2$ is 15.21, which is much less than the calculated χ^2. Our p-value then is reported as <0.001. Smokeless tobacco use and ethnic background clearly are related.

Method: Fisher–Irwin for $r \times c$ Contingency Tables

When the data are divided into r row and c column categories, an $r \times c$ contingency table is appropriate. The Fisher–Irwin test (also known as Fisher's exact

Table 13.7

A Fragment of Table C, the Right Tail of the Chi-Square Distribution[a]

α (area in right tail)	0.10	0.05	0.025	0.01	0.005	0.001	0.0005
$df = 2$	4.61	5.99	7.38	9.21	10.60	13.80	15.21

[a] χ^2 values (distances to the right of 0 on a χ^2 curve) are tabulated for 2 *df* for seven values of α.

test) uses a distribution named the hypergeometric for calculating the probability of all other $r \times c$ tables with the same marginal totals. The p-value is the sum of probabilities of all such outcomes with counts less likely than the observed counts.

For Larger Tables, Chi-Square Approximates the Result

For large r and c (perhaps $r + c > 7$, depending on computer speed), the Fisher–Irwin test becomes a sizable calculation. This calculation challenge is exacerbated by large cell counts. If $r + c > 7$, the Fisher–Irwin p-value may be too lengthy to be calculated conveniently, and the chi-square contingency calculation of Eq. (13.3), similar to Eq. (13.2), usually is used. By denoting the observed count in row i, column j as n_{ij} and calculating the corresponding expected entry e_{ij} by row i total $\times$ column j total $\div$ grand total, chi-square may be written as

$$\chi^2 = \sum_i^r \sum_j^c \frac{(|n_{ij} - e_{ij}| - 0.5)^2}{e_{ij}}. \tag{13.3}$$

The difference from Eq. (13.2) is that, instead of summing over 2 rows and 2 columns, we sum over r rows and c columns. Table C gives the chi-square p-value (looking it up as if it were α) using degrees of freedom equal to 1 less than r multiplied by 1 less than c, or $df = (r-1)(c-1)$. For example, a 3×4 contingency table has $(3-1)(4-1) = (2)(3) = 6$ *df*. Choose the largest α having a table entry less than the calculated χ^2; the p-value of the test, that is, the chance of being wrong when a "dependent" decision is made, is less than that α. Alternatively, use a statistical package on a computer and calculate the p-value directly. (The distinction between using a tabulated critical value and a calculated p-value is discussed in Section 5.3.)

Assumptions Underlying a Valid Chi-Square

In order for the chi-square approximation to be valid, all cell entries should be at least 5 and the expected value for all cells should be at least 1. If this assumption is violated and the Fisher–Irwin test cannot be used, cells with small entries or expectations may have to be amalgamated, which, of course, reduces the *df* and the information contained.

Additional Example: Who Chooses Type of Therapist for Psychiatry Residents?

In a study on the desirability of psychotherapy for psychiatry residents,[9] a question asked was whether the choice of therapist was independent of who paid for the therapy. Responses gave rise to Table 13.8. A Fisher–Irwin test using a computer yielded a p-value of <0.001. The choice of type of analyst clearly is related to who pays for the analyst. To perform the chi-square test, the expected values $e_{ij} = n_{i}.. \times n._{j}/n$, which are $e_{11} = 45 \times 38/155 = 11.032$, $e_{12} = 102 \times 38/155 = 25.006, \ldots, e_{43} = 0.413$, are calculated first. (Note that the last expected value is less than 1, which violates the assumptions required for the chi-square approximation. However, the term involving that value contributes very little to the total sum, which is huge, so we may continue. We must remember, however, that the resulting chi-square will be a little off.) We note that $df = (4 - 1) \times (3 - 1) = 6$. Substitution of the values in Eq. (13.3) yields $\chi^2 = (|15 - 11.032| - 0.5)^2/11.032 + \cdots = 24.45$. The α associated with 24.45 in the row for 6 *df* in Table C is a little less than 0.0005. We record $p < 0.001$, which is similar to the Fisher–Irwin p. Psychiatrists and psychoanalysts were chosen by the overwhelming majority of residents and residency programs, but not by insurance companies. Psychologists were chosen by 63% of insurance companies, although the costs, interestingly, were not very different.

Exercise 13.2: Change in Blood Pressure Resulting from Change in Position. The influence of patient position during the measurement of blood pressure

Table 13.8

Type of Therapist Chosen as Contingent upon the Chooser for Psychotherapy Given to Psychiatry Residents as Part of Their Training

Type of therapist chosen	Who paid for therapy: Resident	Residency program	Insurance company	Totals
Psychoanalyst	15	22	1	38
Psychiatrist	18	64	1	83
Psychologist	7	14	5	26
Social worker	5	2	1	8
Totals	45	102	8	155

Table 13.9
Data on Change in Blood Pressure in Response to Change in Position

	Rise in BP	No change in BP	Fall in BP	
Systolic BP	8	20	72	100
Diastolic BP	11	30	54	95
Totals	19	50	126	195

(BP) has long been questioned. A 1962 paper[76] examined alterations in BP of 195 pregnant women resulting from a change from upright to supine position. We ask the following: Is the pattern of change the same or different for systolic and diastolic BPs? The data are given as Table 13.9.

13.4. RISKS AND ODDS IN MEDICAL DECISIONS

Example and Method Combined: Accuracy and Errors in the Diagnosis of Appendicitis

Pain and tenderness in the lower right quadrant of the abdomen may or may not be appendicitis. Clinical diagnoses often are wrong. Of 250,000 cases treated yearly in the United States, 20% of appendicitis cases are missed, leading to ruptures and complications, and the appendix is removed unnecessarily in 15–40% of cases. In a study at Massachusetts General Hospital,[53] 100 cases of abdominal pain were diagnosed by computed tomography (CT) scans and followed for eventual verification of diagnosis. Fifty-two of 53 cases diagnosed as appendicitis were correct and 46 of 47 cases diagnosed as other causes were correct. We can ask several questions about the risks of being wrong and the odds of being right. The possible errors and their risks were discussed in Section 5.2. A case may be diagnosed as appendicitis when it is not (false positive) or it may not be diagnosed when it is (false negative).

True and False Positive and Negative Events

A special case of the contingency table is the case in which one variable represents a prediction that a condition will occur and the other represents the outcome, i.e., "truth." For example, the occurrence of appendicitis among a sample of patients was predicted by a CT scan, and outcomes were known from followup. (The appendicitis example will be followed as an exercise at the end of this section.) Such a table and some of its implications were discussed in Section 6.4. The

Table 13.10

Truth Table Showing Relationships and Counts of the Prediction of Presence or Absence of a Malady as Related to the Truth of That Presence or Absence

		PREDICTION (Exposure or test result)		
		Have disease	Do not have	Totals
TRUTH	Have disease	True positive correct decision (probability $1 - \beta$) frequency n_{11}	False negative Type II error (probability β) frequency n_{12}	$n_{1\cdot}$ (Yes)
	Do not have	False positive Type I error (probability α) frequency n_{21}	True negative correct decision (probability $1 - \alpha$) frequency n_{22}	$n_{2\cdot}$ (No)
	Totals	$n_{\cdot 1}$ (predict yes)	$n_{\cdot 2}$ (predict no)	n (or $n_{\cdot\cdot}$)

frequencies of possible prediction and outcome combinations can be counted and arrayed as n_{11}–n_{22} in a 2×2 *truth table*, as illustrated in Table 13.10. The true and false positives and negatives are shown along with names for the associated risks (probabilities of error).

Example Data

In Table 13.11, reproducing the data of Table 6.7, the format of Table 13.10 is used to show DRE and PSAD values of the 301 prostate patients in predicting biopsy results. The DREs are symbolized + for predicted positive biopsy and − for predicted negative biopsy. By using a PSAD value of 0.14 ng/ml/ml as a critical value (decision criterion), PSAD > 0.14 predicts a positive biopsy and PSAD ≤ 0.14 predicts a negative biopsy.

Table 13.11

Tables of Biopsy Results Predicted by DRE and by PSAD > 0.14 as Related to the True Outcomes of the Biopsies for 301 Patients

		Predicted by DRE			Predicted by PSAD > 0.14		
		+	−		+	−	
Truth	+	68:n_{11}	27:n_{12}	95	75: n_{11}	20:n_{12}	95
(biopsy)	−	117:n_{21}	89: n_{22}	206	88:n_{21}	118:n_{22}	206
		185	116	301	163	138	301

Truth Table Statistics Are Explained in Table 13.12

A number of truth table statistics introduced in Section 6.4 plus some additional concepts are given in Table 13.12, an expansion of Table 6.8. Column 1 gives the names of the concepts, and column 2 gives the formulas for computing them from the sample truth table. Columns 3 and 4 give population definitions and the relationships these concepts are estimating, respectively, i.e., what they would be if all data in the population were available. These are the values that relate to error probabilities in statistical inference, as discussed in Sections 2.1 and 2.2. As before, a vertical line, |, is read as "given." Columns 5 and 6 show numerical estimates of the probabilities and odds, respectively, in predicting biopsy results from DRE and PSAD values calculated from the counts displayed in Table 13.11. Next, interpretations of the statistics introduced in Chapter 6 are summarized and new concepts are discussed in more detail.

Sensitivity, Specificity, Accuracy, and Odds Ratio

Definitions of a number of concepts related to estimates of correct and erroneous predictions from the sample truth table were introduced in Section 6.4. These included sensitivity, the chance of detecting a disease when present, specificity, the chance of ruling out a disease when absent, accuracy, the chance of making a correct prediction, and the odds ratio (OR), the odds of being correct when disease is predicted. It is important to note that the OR can be tested for statistical significance, which is addressed in the next section.

Positive and Negative Predictive Values

Predictive values indicate the relative frequency of a predictor being correct. The PPVs of $68/185 = 37\%$ for DRE and $75/163 = 46\%$ for PSAD indicate that PSAD better predicts the chance of a patient having cancer when the test predicts he does. Similarly, the NPVs of $89/116 = 77\%$ for DRE and $118/138 = 86\%$ for PSAD indicate that PSAD better predicts the chance of a patient being free of cancer when the test predicts he is.

Relative Risk

The RR gives the rate of disease given exposure in ratio to the rate of disease given no exposure. It also could represent the ratio of incidence rates of disease under two different conditions or strategies (including treatment as one strategy and nontreatment as the other). It should be noted that RR cannot be measured directly

Table 13.12

Concepts of False Positive and Negative, Sensitivity, Specificity, Accuracy, Positive and Negative Predictive Values, Relative Risk, Odds Ratio, and Likelihood Ratio Based on Sample Error Rates[a]

Values found from a sample truth table		Population definitions of probabilities and odds of values being estimated		Examples of prediction	
Names of estimates	Sample computing formulas	Definitions	Relationships	by DRE	by PSAD
False positive sample rate (p-value)	$n_{21}/n_{2\cdot}$	Probability of a false positive (α)	P(predict yes|no)	0.568	0.427
False negative sample rate	$n_{12}/n_{1\cdot}$	Probability of a false negative (β)	P(predict no|yes)	0.284	0.210
Sensitivity	$n_{11}/n_{1\cdot}$	Probability of a true positive: *power* $(1-\beta)$	P(predict yes|yes)	0.716	0.790
Specificity	$n_{22}/n_{2\cdot}$	Probability of a true negative $(1-\alpha)$	P(predict no|no)	0.433	0.573
Accuracy	$(n_{11}+n_{22})/n$	Overall probability of a correct decision	P(predict no|no or yes|yes)	0.522	0.641
Positive predictive value (PPV)	$n_{11}/n_{\cdot 1}$	Probability that a positive prediction is correct	P(yes|predicted yes)	0.368	0.460
Negative predictive value (NPV)	$n_{22}/n_{\cdot 2}$	Probability that a negative prediction is correct	P(no|predicted no)	0.767	0.855
Relative risk (RR)	$n_{11}n_{\cdot 2}/n_{12}n_{\cdot 1}$	Probability of a disease when predicted in ratio to probability of the disease when not predicted	$\frac{\text{P(yes\|predicted yes)}}{\text{P(yes\|predicted no)}}$ or $\frac{PPV}{1-NPV}$	1.579	3.175
Odds ratio (OR)	$n_{11}n_{22}/n_{12}n_{21}$	Odds of a disease when predicted in ratio to odds of the disease when not predicted	$\frac{\text{Ratio(yes/no\|predicted yes)}}{\text{Ratio(yes/no\|predicted no)}}$	1.916	5.028
Likelihood ratio (LR)	$n_{11}n_{2\cdot}/n_{21}n_{1\cdot}$	Probability of correctly predicting a disease in ratio to probability of incorrectly predicting the disease	$\frac{\text{P(predict yes\|yes)}}{\text{P(predict yes\|no)}}$ or $\frac{1-\beta}{\alpha}$	1.260	1.848

[a] Third and fourth columns show the population entities these values are estimating. The rightmost two columns show biopsy outcome predictions of these values from the data of Table 13.11.

in retrospective case–control studies. In this application, the RR gives the rate of cancer among *yes* predictions in ratio to the rate of cancer among *no* predictions. The PSAD RR of $(75 \times 138) \div (20 \times 163) = 3.17$ indicates that PSAD's chance of cancer when predicted is more than 3 times its chance when not predicted. The PSAD RR is double the DRE RR of $(68 \times 116) \div (27 \times 185) = 1.58$.

The Relationship between RR and OR

The relative risk and the odds ratio seem rather similar in their definitions. The relationship between them is worth noting. If the disease or malfunction is rare, a and b are small so that their product ab is almost 0 and drops out of the RR $= a(b + d)/b(a + c) = (ab + ad)/(ab + bc) \approx ad/bc$. In this case, the OR approximates the RR.

Likelihood Ratio

The likelihood ratio (LR) gives the probability of correctly predicting cancer in ratio to the probability of incorrectly predicting cancer. The LR indicates by how much a diagnostic test result will raise or lower the pretest probability of the suspected disease. A LR of 1 indicates that no diagnostic information is added by the test. A LR greater than 1 indicates that the test increased the assessment of the disease probability; if less than 1, it decreased. The DRE PSAD of 1.848 indicates that the chance of correctly predicting a positive biopsy is nearly twice that of incorrectly predicting a positive biopsy, but the DRE LR of 1.260 is only about one-quarter again. Both tests increase the chance of correctly predicting prostate cancer, although the DRE only very slightly.

Be Wary of the Term Likelihood Ratio

Likelihood ratio as used here is a useful concept in describing and assessing diagnosis and treatment options, but the name is somewhat unfortunate. The term likelihood ratio has long been used in statistical theory for concepts other than that adopted in the medical community described here. The user should be careful to differentiate interpreting results and presenting results to others so that the meaning will not be misunderstood.

Receiver Operating Characteristic (ROC) Curve

A receiver operating characteristic curve is a graph displaying the relationship between the true positive rate (on the vertical axis) and the false positive rate (on the horizontal axis). Brought into the medical field from engineering usage, the receiver

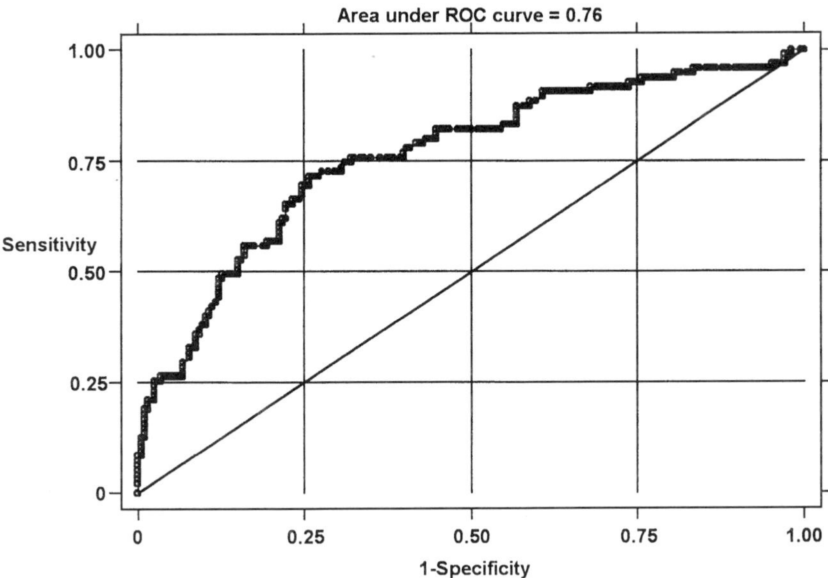

Figure 13.1 ROC curve for biopsy result as predicted by PSAD.

operating characteristic curve usually is abbreviated ROC curve. Figure 13.1 shows the ROC curve for PSAD. A ROC curve helps to choose the critical value at which a predictor best discriminates between choices, such as choosing the value of PSA or PSAD that best predicts the presence or absence of a positive biopsy. The critical value is found as the value at which the curve's deviation from the diagonal line from (0,0) (lower left) to (1,1) (upper right) is the greatest. However, there is an additional advantage in being able not just to maximize the correct response, but to weight it for relative loss associated with the two types of error. For example, a missed cancer (false negative) is more costly to the patient than an unnecessary biopsy (false positive). If a false negative error is assessed as 4 times as serious as a false positive error, the corresponding position on the ROC curve can be located and the associated critical value determined.

Calculating a ROC Curve

In our urological data, a DRE is either positive or negative. There is no ROC curve for it. (More exactly, its ROC curve would consist of a single point.) However, for PSAD, we could choose any critical value. As one error grows smaller, the other grows larger. The issue is choosing the trade-off of the two error values.

In Fig. 13.1, calculation started with the critical value of PSAD at 0, where all patients are classed as cancerous, and the error rates were counted. The critical value was taken as 0.1, then 0.2, etc.; the error rates for each critical value were calculated, and the points were plotted on the evolving ROC curve. Such a procedure is time-consuming and best done with computer software.

Choosing the Best Critical Value

The strongest predictor of biopsy result will be indicated by where the perpendicular distance from (and above) the (45°) line of equality is a maximum, which can be seen by inspection to be about at the point (0.26,0.73). We use these coordinates to select the number of negative biopsies predicted that led to that point, and from that number we find the critical value of PSAD. If we calculated the ROC values ourselves, we just select it from the list of calculations. If the ROC curve was done on a computer, we have to "back-calculate" it. We know that 95 patients have a positive biopsy, i.e., $n_{1\cdot} = 95$, and that 206 have a negative biopsy, i.e., $n_{2\cdot} = 206$. We use this information to find the $n_{11} \ldots n_{22}$ elements of a new 2×2 table. Sensitivity $\times n_{1\cdot} = n_{11}$ or $0.73 \times 95 = 69.35$, which rounds to 69. Because $n_{1\cdot} = n_{11} + n_{12}$, $n_{12} = 95 - 69 = 26$. Similarly, $n_{21} = (1 - \text{specificity}) \times n_{2\cdot} = 0.26 \times 206 = 53.56$, which rounds to 54. $n_{22} = n_{2\cdot} - n_{21} = 206 - 54 = 152$. Finally, $n_{12} + n_{22} = 26 + 152 = 178$. Prediction of the smallest 178 values of PSAD to have a negative biopsy would lead to $1 -$ specificity $= 0.26$ and sensitivity $= 0.73$. We rank the PSAD values in order smallest to largest and note that the PSAD value lying between the 178th and 179th PSAD values is 0.184, the required PSAD critical value.

Choosing a Best Weighted Critical Value

Suppose we were to require that the rate of false positive errors (the number of unnecessary biopsies) be 4 times the rate of false negative errors (the number of missed cancers), or $1 -$ specificity $= 4 \times$ sensitivity. What critical value of PSAD would provide this result? By inspection, $1 -$ specificity would be about 0.56 and sensitivity about 0.14. By following a procedure similar to that in the preceding paragraph, we find $n_{21} = 115$, $n_{12} = 13$, $n_{22} = 91$, and negative predictions number -104, which lead to critical PSAD $- 0.106$.

Using the ROC to Choose the Better of Two Indicators (Risk Factors)

Another use of ROC curves is to compare two indicators, for example, PSA and PSAD, the ROC curves for which are shown superposed in Fig. 13.2. A ROC curve that contains a larger area below it is a better predictor than one with a lesser area. However, if the curves cross, an indicator with a lesser area can be better in some regions of the indicator. The area under the PSAD curve is greater than that under the PSA curve, and the PSAD curve is uniformly higher than or equal to the PSA curve.

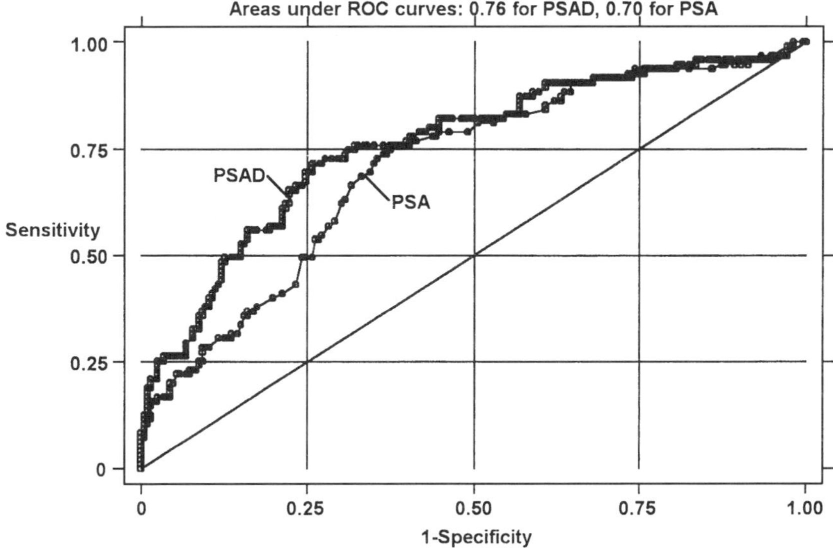

Figure 13.2 Superposed ROC curves for biopsy result predicted by PSAD and PSA.

Additional Example: Truth Tables as Related to Survival Rates

The risks and odds related to various medical occurrences follow the same numerical patterns, but must be interpreted according to their own definitions. Survival as related to treatment represents an interpretation rather different from the results of a lab test.

Pancreatic Cancer Data

Oncologists examined the effect of re-operation for pancreatic cancer on patient survival 1 year after surgery.[30] Of 28 patients, 16 were resectable and 12 were not. All were followed for 1 year or until death, whichever came first. We know which patients survived for 1 year and which did not; we are interested in what resection portends about that survival. Results are given in Table 13.13.

False Positive and False Negative Rates

The false positive rate is the chance of having been resected given no survival for 1 year, or $n_{21}/n_{2\cdot} = 8/18 = 44\%$. The false negative rate is the chance of not

Table 13.13

Data on Survival as Related to Treatment for Pancreatic Cancer

	Resection	No Resection	
Survive for 1 year	8 (n_{11})	2 (n_{12})	10 ($n_{1}.$)
Not survive for 1 year	8 (n_{21})	10 (n_{22})	18 ($n_{2}.$)
	16 ($n._{1}$)	12 ($n._{2}$)	28 (n)

having been resected given survival, or $n_{12}/n_{1}. = 2/10 = 20\%$. In the prostate example, the values for false positive and negative rates, sensitivity, and specificity dealt with the rates at which our predictions came true and had considerable meaning. In this example, they have less meaning, but the PPV and NPV relate more to what interests us.

Sensitivity, Specificity, and Accuracy

The sensitivity is the chance of having had a resection, given survival for 1 year, or $n_{11}/n_{1}. = 8/10 = 80\%$. The *specificity* is the chance of having had no resection given no survival, or $n_{22}/n_{2}. = 10/18 = 56\%$. The accuracy, i.e., the overall chance of an appropriate resection, is $(n_{11} + n_{22})/n = (8 + 10)/28 = 64\%$.

Positive and Negative Predictive Values

The PPV is the chance of survival given a resection, or $n_{11}/n._{1} = 8/16 = 50\%$. This useful information is the relative frequency with which resected patients survive. Similarly, NPV, the chance of nonsurvival given no resection, or $n_{22}/n._{2} = 10/12 = 83\%$, is the relative frequency with which nonresected patients die.

Relative Risk

The RR provides the rate of survival given resection in ratio to the rate of survival given no resection, which is essentially the improvement in survival rate due to resection. RR $= n_{11}n._{2}/n_{12}/n._{1} = 8 \times 12/2 \times 16 = 3$ indicates that the resected patient's chance of survival to 1 year is 3 times that of the nonresected patient.

Odds Ratio

The OR gives the odds of resected patients' survival in ratio to the odds of nonresected patients' survival. OR $= n_{11}n_{22}/n_{12}n_{21} = 8 \times 10/2 \times 8 = 5$. The improvement in survival odds due to resection is 5 times that for no resection.

Likelihood Ratio

The LR gives the ratio of appropriate resections to inappropriate resections, or $n_{11}n_{2\cdot}/n_{21}n_{1\cdot} = 1.8$. The rate of appropriate resections is nearly double the rate of inappropriate ones.

Exercise 13.3. Table 13.14 displays the Massachusetts General Hospital appendicitis data[53] as a truth table. Calculate and interpret sensitivity, specificity, accuracy, PPV, NPV, RR, OR, and LR.

13.5. 2 × 2 TABLES: TESTS OF ASSOCIATION

The Reason for This Section and What Is in It

The chi-square and Fisher–Irwin tests of contingency are so influenced by sample size that they are poor indicators of association. A small sample is unlikely to indicate a significant relationship between variables, however strong the association may be. However, take a large enough sample and you will find evidence, however weak the influence of association. A better test of the level of association is needed. Two such tests exist: the log OR test and the log RR test. The log OR test is more general and has a better mathematical foundation, so that it is the only one treated here. In addition, there is a clinical indicator, termed attributable risk, of the relationship between two variables. This indicator has inadequate mathematical foundation to relate it to probabilistic tests, but it adds another dimension to the understanding of interrelationships just on a clinical basis.

Is the Odds Ratio (OR) Large Enough to Indicate That the Association between the Two Types of Category Is Significant in Probability?

This is the first question addressed in this section. If we have estimated the level of association by the OR, we can go directly to a test using that value. The

Table 13.14
Truth Table for Appendicitis Data

		Appendicitis Predicted		
		Yes	No	
Appendicitis verified	Yes	52 (n_{11})	1 (n_{12})	53 ($n_{1\cdot}$)
	No	1 (n_{21})	46 (n_{22})	47 ($n_{2\cdot}$)
		53 ($n_{\cdot 1}$)	47 ($n_{\cdot 2}$)	100 (n)

OR has a difficult, asymmetric distribution (as does the RR). To put it into a form with a known and usable probability distribution, the natural logarithm of the OR, the *log odds ratio*, which we will denote by L, is used. L is symmetric about 0, unlike the OR. The square of L divided by its standard deviation is distributed as chi-square with 1 *df*. (The chi-square test of log OR is not the same test as the chi-square test of contingency; they just both use the chi-square probability distribution.)

EXAMPLE: IS OR FOR POSITIVE TO NEGATIVE DRE PREDICTING A POSITIVE BIOPSY RESULT SIGNIFICANT?

From Table 13.2 giving DRE and biopsy counts, the OR is $(68 \times 89)/(117 \times 27) = 1.92$. This OR is greater than the value of 1, which would indicate no association, but is 1.9 significant in probability? (Because the Fisher–Irwin test showed dependence in the example of Section 13.2, we expect the log odds ratio to be significant.)

$$L = \ln\left[\frac{(n_{11} + 0.5) \times (n_{22} + 0.5)}{(n_{12} + 0.5) \times (n_{21} + 0.5)}\right] = \ln\left[\frac{68.5 \times 89.5}{27.5 \times 117.5}\right] = 0.6404.$$

Its standard error is

$$\text{SEL} = \sqrt{\left(\frac{1}{n_{11} + 0.5}\right) + \left(\frac{1}{n_{12} + 0.5}\right) + \left(\frac{1}{n_{21} + 0.5}\right) + \left(\frac{1}{n_{22} + 0.5}\right)}$$

$$= \sqrt{\left(\frac{1}{68.5}\right) + \left(\frac{1}{27.5}\right) + \left(\frac{1}{117.5}\right) + \left(\frac{1}{89.5}\right)} = 0.2658.$$

The chi-square statistic to test against $\lambda = 0$ is

$$\chi^2 = \left(\frac{L - \lambda}{\text{SEL}}\right)^2 = \left(\frac{0.6404 - 0}{0.2658}\right)^2 = 5.8049,$$

with 1 degree of freedom. This chi-square value falls between 0.025 and 0.01, as seen in Table 13.4 (or Table C), so we may say that the p-value is significant, as we had thought. The actual p-value for chi-square with 1 *df* calculated from a software package is 0.016, which is the same as the Fisher–Irwin result. We have adequate evidence from the sample to conclude that DRE result is associated with biopsy result.

Method: 2 × 2 Table Test of Association

A test of the significance of 2 × 2 association requires the probability distribution of the measure. The *log odds ratio, L* (see Section 6.4 for odds ratio), is one that can be put into a form having a chi-square distribution. (The log relative risk also might be used, but it is slightly less general than L. Others exist, for example, the Mantel–Haenszel chi-square test, but are more complicated and no better for the simpler cases treated in this book.) By using the n notation introduced in Section 6.2, L is given by

$$L = \ln\left[\frac{(n_{11}+0.5)\times(n_{22}+0.5)}{(n_{12}+0.5)\times(n_{21}+0.5)}\right], \tag{13.4}$$

where "ln" denotes the natural logarithm. The 0.5 values are a continuity correction added to improve the approximation. The standard error of L is

$$\mathrm{SEL} = \sqrt{\left(\frac{1}{n_{11}+0.5}\right)+\left(\frac{1}{n_{12}+0.5}\right)+\left(\frac{1}{n_{21}+0.5}\right)+\left(\frac{1}{n_{22}+0.5}\right)}. \tag{13.5}$$

To test L against a hypothesized log odds ratio λ (for example, $H_0: \lambda = 0$ if the category types are independent), the quantity

$$\chi^2 = \left(\frac{L-\lambda}{\mathrm{SEL}}\right)^2 \tag{13.6}$$

may be looked up in the chi-square table, Table C, for 1 degree of freedom. The resulting p-value is the probability that such an association would occur by chance alone.

Additional Example: Does a Surgeon's RK Experience Affect the Visual Acuity of the Patients?

In the additional example on RK surgery from Section 13.2, the ophthalmologist found that post-operative visual acuity and position in his surgical sequence were dependent. The OR, calculated from the formula in Table 13.12, is 0.26, which is much less than 1, suggesting a negative relationship: the greater the number of surgeries, the fewer the eyes with poor refraction. Is the association as indicated by the OR significant? He substitutes data from Table 13.3 in Eqs. (13.4), (13.5), and finally (13.6) to calculate

$$L = \ln\left[\frac{(n_{11}+0.5)\times(n_{22}+0.5)}{(n_{12}+0.5)\times(n_{21}+0.5)}\right] = \ln\left[\frac{17.5\times 10.5}{27.5\times 24.5}\right] = -1.2993,$$

$$\text{SEL} = \sqrt{\frac{1}{n_{11}+0.5} + \frac{1}{n_{12}+0.5} + \frac{1}{n_{21}+0.5} + \frac{1}{n_{22}+0.5}}$$

$$= \sqrt{\frac{1}{17.5} + \frac{1}{27.5} + \frac{1}{24.5} + \frac{1}{10.5}} = 0.4791,$$

$$\chi^2 = \left(\frac{L-\lambda}{\text{SEL}}\right)^2 = \left(\frac{-1.2993-0}{0.4791}\right)^2 = 7.35.$$

From Table 13.4 (or Table C), the critical value of χ^2 for $\alpha = 0.05$ for 1 *df* is 3.84. Because 7.35 still is much larger than 3.84, he concludes that there is a significant association between the two factors. (The actual $p = 0.007$.)

Exercise 13.4: Is the Quality of Ligament Repair Significantly Associated with the Method? Use the data in Exercise 13.2 (on ligament repair) to calculate L and SEL and test the hypothesis that $\lambda = 0$, i.e., that there is no difference between the modified Bostrom and Chrisman–Snook methods of repair.

What Is the Clinical Relevance of the Dependence between the Two Types of Category?

This is the second question addressed in this section. The relative risk and the odds ratio do not answer this question, because the actual rates of occurrence have been factored out. The clinical relevance may be indicated by the *difference* in odds, termed the *attributable risk*. The importance and interpretation of this statistic lie in direct clinical judgment and not in a probability statement.

Example: Is the Prediction of Prostate Biopsy Result from DRE Clinically Relevant?

From Table 13.2, attributable risk $= (n_{11}/n_{21}) - (n_{12}/n_{22}) = 68/117 - 27/89 = 0.2778$. We get a 28% greater chance of predicting an existing positive biopsy correctly from a positive DRE than from a negative DRE.

Method: 2 × 2 Table Clinical Relevance

The clinical relevance is well indicated, not by the ratio of odds, but by the *difference* in odds, termed the attributable risk. By using the n notation introduced in Section 6.2, the odds of a positive prediction being positive is n_{11}/n_{21} and the odds of a negative prediction being positive is n_{12}/n_{22}. The attributable risk is the difference, given by

$$\frac{n_{11}}{n_{21}} - \frac{n_{12}}{n_{22}}. \tag{13.7}$$

Attributable risk estimates the increased probability in predicting the outcome characteristic from a positive risk factor compared to a negative risk factor.

Additional Example: What Is the Attributable Risk for the Learning Advantage of Repeated Surgery?

Let us use the data of Table 13.3 to find the advantage of eye surgery done later in the learning curve over that done earlier. The odds of a good result in the earlier surgery is $17/24 = 0.71$, whereas the odds of a good result later is $27/10 = 2.70$. From Eq. (13.7), the attributable risk is $0.71 - 2.70 = -1.99$. The odds of a good result for later surgery is much greater.

13.6. Tests of a Proportion (Proportion Not Close to 0)

What a Test of a Proportion Will Do and Why It Is Needed

Suppose we are concerned with the efficacy of an antibiotic in treating pediatric otitis media accompanied by fever. We know that, say, 85% of patients get well within 7 days without treatment. We learn that, of 100 such patients, 95% of those treated with the antibiotic got well within 7 days. Is this improvement statistically significant? Note that we cannot fill in a contingency table because we do not have the number of untreated patients nor the total number of patients. However, we do have the theoretical proportion and so can answer the question using a test of proportions. Testing a *proportion* will answer the following question: *Is a sample proportion the same as or different from a theoretical or population proportion?*

Basis of the Binomial Distribution and Test

Proportions for binary data (yes–no, plus–minus, heads–tails, etc.) follow the *binomial distribution*, because outcomes from a sampling must fall into one category or the other. Probabilities for the binomial distribution appear in Table F in the back of the book. Suppose we wanted to compare our 30% positive biopsy rate from Table DB1.1 with a theoretical result of long standing in which 25% of patients over 50 years of age presenting to urology clinics had positive biopsies. We would use the binomial distribution with theoretical proportion $\pi = 0.25$. (The Greek π is used for the binomial population proportion and the Roman p for the sample proportion. This p is completely unrelated to the p of p-value; the use of the same letter is coincidental. We must keep track of the usage by context.) We ask, "Could a rate as large as or larger than our $p = 0.30$ rate have occurred by chance alone?" (The "larger than" portion arises because we really are considering 1 minus the probability that the rate is less than 0.30.) The probability of obtaining a proportion $p \geq 0.30$ by chance alone, given $\pi = 0.25$, can be calculated or looked up in a table. The resulting probability is the p-value of the binomial test of proportion. In Table F, the binomial probabilities are given for π values no larger than 0.50; for larger values of π, just reverse the tails of the distribution. For example, for a particular disease occurring in an undeveloped country, the mortality rate is 80%. Instead of examining the chance of death, examine the chance of survival having $\pi = 20\%$.

A Different Method Is Used if n Is Large

For a large sample n, exact probabilities do not appear in the tables and would be very time-consuming to calculate. Fortunately, good approximations have been found for large samples. For the binomial distribution, the sample proportion is distributed approximately *normal* with mean equal to the theoretical proportion, that is, normal $\mu = \pi$, and standard deviation $\sigma = \sqrt{[\pi(1 - \pi)/n]}$. By knowing μ and σ, we may calculate a z score and use normal tables to find p-values, as detailed in the examples and method paragraphs to follow.

A Different Distribution Is Used if the Proportion Being Examined Is Very close to Zero

Suppose we are concerned with a rare disease having prevalence 0.002. Slightly different methods should be used, as addressed in Section 13.7.

Tests of Two Proportions

A method exists to test for a significant difference between two sample proportions. This is a generalization of the large-sample test of a single proportion.

However, in order to use the method, the proportions and the sample sizes must be known. From these values, the actual counts can be found, which will permit the data to be posed in the form of a contingency table. Use the methods of Section 13.2.

The Case of Three or More Proportions

When three or more proportions are to be compared, the associated distribution is the multinomial distribution, a generalization of the binomial. However, we can get by without the multinomial in many cases in which a proportion can be examined by combining the probabilities of occurrence in the two or more other categories together.

Examples

Small *n*: Comparison of a Sample Biopsy Result Rate with a Theoretical Rate

We want to compare the positive biopsy rate $p_s = 0.30$ (30%) from Table DB1.1's sample of size 10 with a theoretical positive biopsy rate defined as 0.25 (25%) of patients over 50 years of age presenting to a urology clinic. We use the binomial distribution with theoretical proportion $\pi = 0.25$. To find the probability of drawing $n_s \geq 3$ out of $n = 10$ by chance alone, given $\pi = 0.25$, we go to Table F. A portion of Table F appears as Table 13.15. The table entry is 0.474; the chance is nearly one-half that we would find such a result by chance alone (the p-value). Thus, we conclude that there is insufficient evidence to say that our proportion of positive biopsies is larger than that found in the clinic.

Table 13.15

A Portion of Table F[a]

		π									
n	n_0	0.05	0.10	0.15	0.20	0.25	0.30	0.35	0.40	0.45	0.50
9	4	0.001	0.008	0.034	0.086	0.166	0.270	0.391	0.517	0.639	0.746
10	3	0.012	0.070	0.180	0.322	0.474	0.617	0.738	0.833	0.900	0.945

[a] Values of cumulative binomial distribution, depending on π, n, and n_0 (number of occurrences observed). The corresponding entry in the table body represents the probability that n_0 or more occurrences (or n_0/n proportion) would have been observed by chance alone.

Large *n*: 150 Years Ago, This Method Would Have Shown the Advantage of Physician Cleanliness

In 1847, Ignaz Semmelweis in Vienna experimented with the effect on patient mortality of physician hand cleansing between patients.[57] Whereas original data are not available (if they ever were), a reconstruction from medical history accounts yields results something like this: The long-term mortality rate for patients treated without the cleansing had been about 18%. Subsequently, for 500 patients treated with the cleansing, the mortality was 1.2%. The requirement $n > 5/\pi (500 > 28)$ is satisfied. Because hand cleansing could not increase the mortality, a one-tailed test is appropriate. We substitute in the formula for a normal z-value, obtaining

$$z = \frac{|p_s - \pi| - \frac{1}{2n}}{\sqrt{\pi(1-\pi)/n}} = \frac{|0.012 - 0.18| - 0.001}{\sqrt{0.18 \times 0.82/500}} = 9.720.$$

The area in the tails is far less than the smallest tabulated in Table A for one-tailed α, which yields $p < 0.002$ for $z = 3.5$. The cleansing significantly reduced the mortality. Nonetheless, as a matter of historical interest, the local medical society attacked Semmelweis' findings viciously. He was reduced in rank and his practicing privileges were curtailed. He was broken and died in an asylum.

Method: Test of Proportion (for Proportions Not Close to 0)

This method tests a sample proportion against a theoretical (or previously known) population proportion, π. We sample n observations randomly from a population with probability π_s of a "success." (A "success" is the occurrence of the event for which we are testing, not necessarily what we would want clinically.) We want to know whether π_s, the proportion for the population from which we sampled, is the same as π, the proportion for the theoretical population. Thus, H_0 is $\pi_s = \pi$. We obtain n_s successes, estimating π_s by the sample proportion $p_s = n_s/n$.

Case of Small *n*

If n is less than 17, Table F gives the p-value, the probability that, for expected chance of a success π, we would find n_s successes or p_s proportion successes by chance alone.

Case of Large n

For larger n, a normal approximation to the binomial distribution is adequate, so binomial tables are not required. Specifically, if $n > 16$, and also if $n \geq 5/\pi$, the difference between the sample and theoretical proportions is transformed to a normal variate z by

$$z = \frac{|p_s - \pi| - \frac{1}{2n}}{\sqrt{\pi(1-\pi)/n}}. \tag{13.8}$$

(The $1/2n$ is a correction to bring the normal approximation closer to the exact binomial result.) The two-tailed p-value corresponding to the calculated z then is found from the normal table (Table A).

Additional Examples

Small n: Does Radiation Therapy Improve the Proportion of Survival?

The 2-year survival rate of an unusual form of malignant cancer has been $\pi = 0.20$. A radiation oncology department treated nine patients.[29] Two years later, four patients survived. Does the treatment improve survival? From Table 13.15, a portion of Table F, the column for $\pi = 0.20$ and row for $n = 9$, and $n_0 = 4$ yield a probability of 0.086 that four or more patients with the 20% untreated survival rate would survive by chance alone. There is not enough evidence to infer treatment effectiveness on the basis of this small a sample.

Large n: Does Absorbable Mesh in Closure of Large Abdominal Wall Openings Reduce the Proportion of Dense Adhesion Formation?

The use of permanent prosthetic mesh has led to the formation of dense adhesions with later obstructions and fistula formations. We ask whether the population proportion π_a of these problems is less using absorbable mesh. Then H_0: $\pi_a = \pi$ and H_1: $\pi_a < \pi$. A number of studies in the literature report the proportion of dense adhesion formation from permanent mesh to be in the vicinity of 0.63, which is taken as π. An experiment[42] on 40 rats found the proportion of dense adhesions from absorbable mesh to be $p_a = 0.125$ (five rats), which estimates π_a. The clinical difference is obvious, but we need to state the risk of error. $\sigma = \sqrt{[\pi(1-\pi)/n]} = \sqrt{[0.63 \times 0.37/40]} = 0.0763$. By using Eq. (13.8), $z = (|p_a - \pi| - 1/2n)/\sigma = (|0.125 - 0.63| - 1/80)/0.0763 = 6.45$. The area under the tail of a normal distribution more than 6.45 standard deviations away from the mean is smaller than any tabulated, certainly <0.001, which is as small as should be quoted. (The normal assumption breaks down in the far tails, so

p-values smaller than 0.001 should not be listed, even though they can be calculated.)

Exercise 13.5: Small n. Are More Boys Than Girls Born in This Town? A small-town obstetrician has been delivering babies from a particular family for three generations. He notes a high proportion of male babies and suspects he may be seeing a genetic phenomenon. Of 16 babies born during his experience, 11 are boys. Does he have evidence of a nonrandom causative factor, or could it have occurred by chance?

Exercise 13.6: Large n. Do Boys and Girls Present with Fractures of the Limbs in Equal Numbers? Theoretically, the population proportion would be $\pi = 0.5$ if the proportion were sex-independent. We recorded the sex of the next 50 children presenting to the orthopedic clinic with limb fractures and found 34 boys. What do we conclude?

13.7. TESTS OF A PROPORTION (PROPORTION CLOSE TO 0)

What a Test of a Proportion Will Do and Why It Is Needed

Suppose we suspect a sudden increase in the prevalence of a rare disease, having prevalence known to be 0.002 under ordinary conditions. Testing of our sample proportion will answer the question: *Is a sample proportion the same as or different from a theoretical or population proportion?* The proportion 0.002 is too small to use the binomial methods discussed in Section 13.6. If π is near 0, and if the relationship $n \gg n\pi \gg \pi$ may be assumed, the result can be well approximated using the *Poisson distribution*, for which probabilities appear in Table G. Suppose our sample shows a prevalence of 0.006, which is 3-fold greater than the expected prevalence. The probability of obtaining a proportion $p \geq 0.006$ by chance alone, given $\pi = 0.002$, can be calculated or looked up in a table, as detailed in the examples and method paragraphs to follow. The resulting probability is the p-value of the binomial test of proportion. (p denoting proportion and p denoting p-value use the same letter only coincidentally and must be differentiated by context.)

What Is Done if π Is Very Close to 1 Rather Than 0

If π is near 1, we can use the complementary proportion, $1 - \pi$. If the prevalence of freedom from a rare disease is 0.098, we examine the prevalence of the disease itself as 0.002.

A Different Method Is Used for Large Samples

If n is large enough that the input value $\lambda = n\pi$ does not appear in Table G (i.e., $\lambda > 9$), a large-sample approximation is used. It has been shown that, for the Poisson distribution, the sample proportion is distributed approximately *normal* with mean equal to the theoretical proportion, that is, normal $\mu = \pi$ and standard deviation $\sigma = \sqrt{[\pi/n]}$. By knowing μ and σ, we may calculate a z score and use normal tables to find p-values, as detailed in the examples and method paragraphs to follow.

Examples

Small λ: Are There Too Many Large Prostates in a Distribution?

The sample of $n = 301$ urological patients contains 3 men with prostate volumes in excess of 90 ml. We might hypothesize that the distribution of volumes in the general population is normal. If so, would we be likely to find $x = 3$ volumes greater than 90 ml by chance alone, or should we suspect that our sample is not normal in form? In a normal curve with $\mu = 36.473$ ml and $\sigma = 18.039$ ml, 90 ml would lie 2.967σ above the mean. From Table A, the area in the right tail would be about $0.002 = \pi$. We have a large number of opportunities for a volume to be >90, but a small chance that any one randomly chosen volume would be, suggesting the Poisson process. The Poisson constant is $\lambda = n\pi = 301 \times 0.002 = 0.602$. The Poisson assumption $n \gg n\pi \gg \pi$ is satisfied: $301 \gg 0.6 \gg 0.002$. From Table 13.16, a portion of Table G, the Poisson probability of observing three or more volumes greater than 90 ml given a Poisson constant of 0.6 is 0.023. With this small a p-value, we reject the hypothesis and conclude that our sample is not normal in form.

Large λ: Does a New Drug Cause Birth Defects?

It has been established that 1.75% ($\pi = 0.0175$) of babies born to women exposed during pregnancy to a certain drug have birth defects. It is believed that an

Table 13.16

A Portion of Table G[a]

	$\lambda\ (= n\pi)$												
n_0	0.1	0.2	0.3	0.4	0.5	0.6	0.7	0.8	0.9	1.0	1.1	1.2	1.3
3	0.000	0.001	0.004	0.008	0.014	0.023	0.034	0.047	0.063	0.080	0.100	0.121	0.143

[a] Values of the cumulative Poisson distribution, depending on $\lambda = n\pi$ and n_0 (no. of occurrences observed). Given λ and n_0, the table entry represents the probability that n_0 or more occurrences would have been observed by chance alone.

Table 13.17

A Fragment of Normal Distribution Table A[a]

z (no. std. deviations to right of mean)	One-tailed α (area in right tail)	Two-tailed α (area in both tails)
1.20	0.115	0.230
1.30	0.097	0.194
1.40	0.081	0.162
1.50	0.067	0.134

[a] For selected distances (z) to the right of the mean, given are one-tailed α, the area under the curve in the positive tail, and two-tailed α, the areas combined for both tails.

adjuvant drug will reduce the risk of a birth defect. The two drugs are used together on 638 pregnant women, and 7 of their babies have birth defects.[42] Did the adjuvant drug reduce the rate of defects? A large number of opportunities to occur but a small chance of occurring on any one indicates Poisson. Because the adjuvant drug would be used clinically if defects decrease but not if they stay the same or increase, a one-tailed test is appropriate. $\lambda = n\pi = 638 \times 0.0175 = 11.165$, which is larger than appears in Table G, so the normal approximation is used. $p_s = 7/638 = 0.0110$. Substitution in Eq. (13.9) yields $z = (0.0110 - 0.0175)\sqrt{(638/0.0175)} = -1.2411$. By normal curve symmetry, we can look up 1.2411 in Table 13.17. By interpolation, we can see that the p-value, i.e., the α that would have given this result, is about 0.108. A reduction in the defect rate has not been shown.

Method: Test of Proportion (for Proportion near 0)

This method tests a sample proportion against a theoretical (or previously known) population proportion, π, where π is close to 0 or to 1 and where the Poisson assumption $n \gg n\pi \gg \pi$ is satisfied. We sample n observations randomly from a population with probability π_s of a "success." We want to know whether π_s, the proportion for the population sampled, is the same as π. Thus, H_0 is $\pi_s = \pi$. We obtain n_s successes, estimating π_s by the sample proportion $p_s = n_s/n$. The Poisson assumes that the relationship $n \gg n\pi \gg \pi$ is fulfilled. (Recall that $\gg$ denotes "much greater than.") The Poisson constant is $\lambda = n\pi$, which is also the number of occurrences expected on average. Calculate $\lambda = n\pi$ and verify the assumption.

Case of Small λ

Table G gives the probability of n_s or more successes by chance alone, which is also the p-value for the test that the sample observations have π proportion success.

Case of Large λ

If $\lambda > 9$ (for example, $n = 500$ and $\pi = 0.02$), a normal approximation to the Poisson distribution is adequate. Calculate

$$z = \frac{p_s - \pi}{\sqrt{\pi/n}} = (p_s - \pi)\sqrt{n/\pi} \tag{13.9}$$

and test it using the normal Table A. (Either the expression in the middle or that on the right may be used, as convenient.)

Additional Examples

Small λ: Does the Site of IM Injection Affect the Incidence of Sarcoma?

A veterinarian[42] finds that cats contract vaccine-associated feline sarcoma when vaccinated in the back at a rate of 2 in 10,000 ($\pi = 0.0002$). She initiates a study in which 5000 cats are given their rabies and feline leukemia vaccinations in the rear leg. She finds $n_0 = 3$ cases of the sarcoma. Is the incidence of sarcoma for leg vaccination different from that for the back? There are many opportunities for the sarcoma to occur, but the probability of it occurring in any randomly chosen case is near 0, indicating Poisson methods. If the incidences at the two sites are different, either one could be greater, so a two-tailed test is appropriate. In Table G, the table entry is the probability that n_0 or more sarcomas would have occurred by chance alone, so the critical values for $\alpha = 5\%$ will be 0.975 (i.e., $1 - 0.025$) for the case of fewer sarcomas in the new site and 0.025 for the case of more sarcomas in the new site. $\lambda = n\pi = 5000 \times 0.0002 = 1$. In Table G, the probability is 0.080 between the two critical values. She concludes that the data did not provide evidence that leg vaccination gives a sarcoma rate different from back vaccination.

Large λ: Is Anorexia in the Military Different from That in the General Public?

Anorexia among the general U.S. population of women is known to be $\pi = 0.020$ (2%). We want to know whether this rate also is true for female military officers.[40] Let us use π_m to represent the true but unknown female military officer population proportion, which we will estimate by p_m. $H_0\colon \pi_m = \pi; H_1\colon \pi_m \neq \pi$. We take a sample of 539 female Navy officers and find $p_m = 0.011$. Do we reject H_0 or H_1? As $\lambda = 0.02 \times 539 = 10.79$ is larger than the tabulated values, we use the normal approximation to the Poisson distribution. By using Eq. (13.9), we find

$$z = \frac{p_m - \pi}{\sqrt{\pi/n}} = \frac{0.011 - 0.020}{\sqrt{0.020/539}} = -1.48.$$

By the symmetry of the normal curve, the result is the same as for $z = 1.48$, which lies between $z = 1.40$ and $z = 1.50$ in Table 13.13 (or Table A). The two-tailed p-values (found in the table as if they were α's) for these z's are 0.162 and 0.135. Interpolation to $z = 1.48$ yields $p = 0.157$, a result not statistically significant. We do not reject H_0 and conclude that we have no evidence that military officers have a rate of anorexia different from that of the general population.

Exercise 13.7: Does Blood-Bank Screening Reduce Hepatitis-Infected Blood? Studies through 1992 found the rate of viral hepatitis infection due to red blood cell transfusions in the United States to be 1 per 3000 units transfused, or $\pi = 0.000333$. Introduction of second- and third-generation hepatitis C screening tests is expected to reduce this rate.[32] Test the significance of results from 15,000 transfused units reducing the rate to 1:5000, or $p = 0.000200$.

13.8. MATCHED PAIR SAMPLE (McNEMAR'S TEST)

McNEMAR'S TEST ASSESSES THE DEPENDENCE OF CATEGORICAL DATA THAT ARE MATCHED OR PAIRED

EXAMPLE

We want to know whether smoking is associated with lung cancer. We randomly choose the records of 10 patients with lung cancer and find 10 control patients without lung cancer for a one-for-one match for age, sex, health history, socioeconomic level, and air quality of living region.[42] Then we record whether each patient smokes (yes) or not (no) in the format of Table 13.18. For McNemar's test, we tally the number of pairs falling into the yes–yes, yes–no, etc., categories in the two-way table Table 13.19. The difference in proportion of smokers is $(b - c)/n = (5 - 0)/10 = 0.5$ and its standard error is $[\sqrt{(b + c)}]/n = \sqrt{5}/10 = 0.224$. Chi-square, which has 1 degree of freedom, the same as in contingency tables for unpaired data, is

$$\chi^2_{1\,df} = \frac{(|b - c| - 1)^2}{b + c} = \frac{(5 - 1)^2}{5} = 3.2.$$

Table 13.18

Smoking Records of Patients Paired for Lung Cancer and Control

Pair no.	Cancer	Control
1	yes	no
6	no	no
2	no	no
7	no	no
3	yes	yes
8	yes	yes
4	yes	no
9	yes	no
5	yes	no
10	yes	no

From Table C or Table 13.4, a chi-square of 3.2 with 1 *df* lies between 5% and 10%; for an α of 5%, we do not have quite enough evidence to say that smoking is related to lung cancer. The actual p-value, calculated using a statistical software package, is 0.074.

Method: McNemar's Test

McNemar's test assesses the dependence of categorical data that are matched, or paired. We want to determine whether a certain characteristic is associated with a disease (or other malady). We identify n patients having the disease and pair them one-for-one with control patients without that disease, but with other possibly relevant characteristics being the same. Then we record the presence or absence of the characteristic in each patient and summarize the result in a two-way table. The data are listed in the format of Table 13.20, where "yes" and "no" indicate the presence or absence of the characteristic.

Table 13.19

Tally of Counts from Table 13.18

		Control	
		Yes	No
Lung cancer	Yes	$a = 2$	$b = 5$
	No	$c = 0$	$d = 3$

Table 13.20

Recording Format for Patients Paired for Disease and Nondisease

	Factor present for	
Pair no.	Diseased member of pair	Nondiseased member of pair
1	yes	no
2	yes	yes
3	no	no
etc.	etc.	etc.

A tally of the results can be recorded in a two-way table, as Table 13.21, where a is the number of pairs with a yes–yes sequence (as in patient no. 2), b is the number of pairs with a yes–no sequence (as in patient no. 1), etc. The difference in proportion of cases having and not having the characteristic under study is given by $(b - c)/n$ and its standard error by $[\sqrt{(b + c)}]/n$. Chi-square with 1 degree of freedom is calculated by Eq. (13.10) and the p-value is obtained from Table C.

$$\chi^2_{1\,df} = \frac{(|b - c| - 1)^2}{b + c}. \tag{13.10}$$

The p-value is the probability of being wrong if we conclude that the characteristic is associated with the disease.

Additional Example: Is There a Genetic Predisposition to Stomach Cancer?

A company physician suspects a genetic predisposition to stomach ulcers and targets a specific gene.[42] He chooses workers in the company who have ulcers. He matches each with a nonulcerous co-worker in the same job (same work environment) with similar personal characteristics (sex, marital state, etc.). He then checks all subjects for the presence of the suspect gene, obtaining the data

Table 13.21

Recording Format for Tallying the Data of Table 13.20

		Control members of pair	
		Yes	No
Diseased members of pair	Yes	a	b
	No	c	d

Table 13.22

Presence of a Suspect Gene in Patients Paired for Ulcerous and Healthy

	Gene present?	
Pair no.	Ulcers	Healthy
1	Yes	No
2	Yes	Yes
3	No	No
4	No	No
5	No	Yes
6	Yes	Yes
7	Yes	No
8	Yes	No
9	Yes	No
10	Yes	No
11	No	No
12	Yes	Yes
13	Yes	No
14	Yes	No
15	Yes	No

in Table 13.22. From those data, he completes two-way Table 13.23. $\chi^2_{1df} = (|b-c|-1)^2/(b+c) = (7-1)^2/9 = 4.0$. From Table C or Table 13.4, the critical value of χ^2 for $\alpha = 0.05$ with 1 *df* is 3.84. Because $4.0 > 3.84$, he concludes that evidence is present for a genetic predisposition. The actual $p = 0.046$.

Exercise 13.8: Are Boys More Accident Prone Than Girls? You suspect that male children between the ages of 3 and 5 are more accident prone than girls. You identify families with a boy and a girl and check their medical records for accidents during those ages.[42] Your data are given in Table 13.24. Use McNemar's test to decide whether boys have significantly more accidents.

Table 13.23

Tally of Counts from Table 13.22

		Gene in healthy member of pair	
		Yes	No
Gene in ulcerous member of pair	Yes	$a = 3$	$b = 8$
	No	$c = 1$	$d = 3$

Table 13.24

Accident Occurrence in Patients Paired for Male and Female

	Had accident(s)	
Pair no.	Boy	Girl
1	Yes	No
2	Yes	Yes
3	No	No
4	Yes	No
5	No	Yes
6	Yes	No
7	Yes	Yes
8	No	No
9	Yes	No
10	Yes	No
11	Yes	No
12	No	Yes

ANSWERS TO EXERCISES

13.1. FI p-value = 0.026, indicating a significant difference between the success of the two treatments with a risk of error less than 5%; MB is better than CS. $\chi^2 = 6.775$, yielding p just less than 0.01, also showing a significant difference. A cell entry of less than 5 indicates that the chi-square approximation may not be adequate. FI is the appropriate test.

13.2. $e_{11} = 19 \times 100/195 = 9.7436$, etc. $\chi^2 = (8 - 9.7436)^2/9.7436 + \cdots = 0.085$. $df = 2$. From Table C, 0.085 for 2 df is far less than any tabulated figure. There is no evidence of a systolic and diastolic difference.

13.3. Sensitivity = 0.981, the chance of detecting appendicitis using MRI. Specificity = 0.979, the chance of correctly diagnosing non-appendicitis. Accuracy = 0.980, the overall chance of making a correct diagnosis. PPV = 0.981, the chance that a diagnosis of appendicitis is correct. NPV = 0.979, the chance that a diagnosis of non-appendicitis is correct. That these values are the same as sensitivity and specificity is an unusual coincidence due to the equality of the marginal totals. RR = 46.11, the chance of appendicitis when predicted in ratio to the chance of appendicitis when not predicted. OR = 2392, the odds of correctly diagnosing appendicitis in ratio to the odds of incorrectly diagnosing appendicitis. LR = 46.11, the chance of correctly diagnosing appendicitis in ratio to the chance of incorrectly diagnosing appendicitis, which coincidentally is the same as RR due to identical marginal totals.

13.4. $L = 1.5506$; SEL $= 0.7327$; $\chi^2 = (1.5506/0.7327)^2 = 4.4787$. From Table C, the p-value for this result is between 0.025 and 0.05, which is a significant result. The actual p is 0.034, which compares to the 0.026 Fisher–Irwin result in Exercise 13.2. We have shown that quality of result is associated significantly with method of ligament repair.

13.5. $n = 16$ and $n_0 = 11$. From Table F, the probability of $11/16$ occurring by chance alone is 0.105, which is too large to infer evidence of a nonrandom phenomenon.

13.6. If π_b is the true population proportion of boys presenting, $H_0: \pi_b = \pi$ and $H_1: \pi_b \neq \pi$. Then $p_b = 0.68$. By using the normal approximation, $\sigma = \sqrt{[\pi(1-\pi)/n]} = \sqrt{[0.5 \times 0.5/50]} = 0.0707$. From Eq. (13.8), $z = (|p_b - \pi| - /2n)/\sigma = 0.17/0.0707 = 2.40$. From Table A, $z = 2.40$ yields two-tailed $p = 0.016$. We reject H_0 and conclude that more boys than girls present with limb fractures.

13.7. We judge that the introduction of better testing can only reduce the rate, so the test is one-sided. From Table A, a critical value of z at $\alpha = 0.05$ will be -1.645. We note that $\lambda = n\pi = 5$, so we may use Table G. We want the probability of 3 or fewer [P(3 or fewer)], which is 1 – P(4 or more), occurring by chance alone. By using $n_0 = 4$, P(3 or fewer) $= 1 - 0.735 = 0.265$. There is inadequate evidence to infer an improvement due to the additional screening tests. For illustration, let us calculate the normal approximation, although we know the result will be erroneously different from the Table G result due to the small λ. From Eq. (7.8), $z = (p_s - \pi)\sqrt{(n/\pi)} = (0.000200 - 0.000333) \times \sqrt{(15000/0.000333)} = -0.893$, which is less distant from 0 than the critical value, so again there is inadequate evidence to infer an improvement. From a statistical software package, $p = 0.186$.

13.8. The data tally appears in Table 13.25. $\chi^2_{1df} = (|b - c| - 1)^2/(b + c) = (4 - 1)^2/8 = 1.125$. From Table C, the critical value of χ^2 for $\alpha = 0.05$ with 1 *df* is 3.84. Because $1.125 < 3.84$, you conclude that boys are not shown to have a higher accident rate. The actual $p = 0.289$.

Table 13.25

Tally of Counts from Table 13.24

		Female member of pair had accident(s)	
		Yes	No
Male member of pair had accident(s)	Yes	$a = 2$	$b = 6$
	No	$c = 2$	$d = 2$

Chapter 14

Common Tests on Ranked Data

14.1. BASICS OF RANKS

WHAT RANKS ARE

This section summarizes the basics of ranked data as seen in Section 6.5. Ranked data are values put in order according to some criterion, e.g., smallest to largest, etc. Rank-order data may arise from ranking events directly or from putting already recorded continuous-type quantities in order. If categories fall into a natural ordering (most to least severe skin lesions would, cultural groups would not), they may be treated as rank-order data.

WHEN AND WHY DO WE USE RANKS?

Continuous measurements contain more information than ranks, and ranks more information than counts. When the user can rank events but cannot measure them on a scale, rank-order statistical methods will give the best results. When the sampling distribution of continuous data is skewed or otherwise poorly behaved, the assumptions underlying continuous-based methods may be violated, giving rise to spurious results. Ranks do not violate these assumptions. When sample sizes are too small to verify the satisfaction of these assumptions, rank-order methods are safer. In summary, rank-order methods should be used (1) when the primary data consist of ranks, (2) when samples are too small to form conclusions about the underlying probability distributions, or (3) when data indicate that necessary assumptions about the distributions are violated.

Ties in Ranked Data

If ranks should be tied, the usual procedure is to average the tied ranks. The heart rates 64, 67, 67, 71 would have ranks 1, 2.5, 2.5, 4. Ties reduce the quality of rank methods somewhat, but they are still stronger than categorical methods.

14.2. SINGLE OR PAIRED SMALL SAMPLES: THE SIGNED-RANK TEST

Examples

Single Sample: Are Our First 10 PSAs from the Same Population as the Remainder of Our Sample?

Table DB1.1 gives PSA for the first 10 of the 301 urology patients. The median PSA of the next 291 is 5.8. We ask whether the first 10 have an average (more exactly, a median) like the remaining 291. (We removed the initial 10 from the second group to avoid contamination of the dependent data, i.e., using the same data in two groups being compared.) As the second median could be either more or less than the first, we use a two-tailed test. If the averages are alike, the ranks of the deviations of the first 10 from the median of the remainder should vary approximately equally about 0. We rank these deviations without regard to the sign (+ or −), then reattach these signs to the ranks and add the positive and the negative ranks. If the first 10 observations are like the remainder, the positive rank sum will be similar to the negative rank sum. These deviations and their ranks are as follows:

Deviations	1.8	−1.7	0.1	3.2	1.0	2.2	1.9	−1.4	0.3	2.1
Signless ranks	6	1	3	10	5	9	7	2	4	8
Signed ranks	6	−1	3	10	5	9	7	−2	4	8

The sum of positive ranks is 52 and that of negative ranks is −3, which are quite different. Denote by T the unsigned value of the smaller sum; in this case, $T = 3$. Table 14.1 shows a portion of Table H, signed-rank probabilities, from the back of the book. In Tables 14.1 and H, the intersection of the row for $T = 3$ and the column for $n = 10$ yields $p = 0.010$. For this low a risk of error, we conclude that the median of the first 10 PSA readings is different from that of the next 291.

Paired Observations: Does a Drug Change the Heart Rate?

Anecdotal information suggests that heart rate (HR) changes in response to a certain ophthalmologic drug designed to reduce intraocular pressure. For a sample

Table 14.1
A Portion of Table H, Signed-Rank Probabilities, Two-Tailed Probabilities of T^a

	Sample size n								
T	4	5	6	7	8	9	10	11	12
3	0.625	0.313	0.156	0.078	0.039	0.020	0.010	0.005	0.003
4	0.875	0.438	0.219	0.109	0.055	0.027	0.014	0.007	0.004
6		0.801	0.438	0.219	0.109	0.055	0.027	0.014	0.007

[a] For a sample of size n and value of T, the entry gives the p-value.

of eight patients,[42] the heart rates prior to beginning treatment and 24 hr following the first dosage are as follows:

Before	After	Difference	Magnitude rank	Signed rank
64	66	−2	2	−2
67	58	8	5	5
67	68	−1	1	−1
71	65	6	4	4
72	75	−3	3	−3
76	67	9	6	6
78	59	19	8	8
89	74	15	7	7

The two unsigned-rank sums are 6 for negative and 30 for positive; $T = 6$. In Table 14.1, the intersection of the $n = 8$ column and the $T = 6$ row yields $p = 0.109$, which is too large a p-value to conclude that the drug changed the intraocular pressure.

Method: The Signed-Rank Test

Often referred to as the Wilcoxon signed-rank test, this method tests the hypothesis that the distribution of differences has a median equal to 0. It may test

(1) a set of observations deviating from a hypothesized common value or
(2) pairs of observations on the same individuals, such as before-and-after data.

Steps to perform the test are as follows:

1. Calculate the differences of the observations as in (1) or (2) (0 differences are omitted from the calculation, and the sample size is reduced accordingly).

2. Rank the magnitudes, i.e., the differences without signs, the smallest being rank 1. (For ties, use the average of the ranks that would have occurred without ties in the same positions.)
3. Reattach the signs to the ranks.
4. Add up the positive and negative ranks.
5. Denote by T the unsigned value of the smaller sum.
6. Look up the p-value for the test in Table H. If $n > 12$, go to Section 14.6.

One Tail or Two?

If we have some sound nonstatistical reason why the result of the test must lie in only one tail, such as a physiological impossibility to occur in the other tail, we can halve the tabulated value to obtain a one-tail error probability.

Additional Example: Does Certain Hardware Restore Adequate Functionality in Ankle Repair?

An orthopedist installs hardware in the broken ankles of nine patients.[23] He scores the percent functionality of the joint. He asks, "Is the average functionality 90% of normal?" His data in % are 75, 65, 100, 90, 35, 63, 78, 70, 80. A quick frequency plot of the data show that they are far from normal, so he uses a rank-based test. He subtracts 90% from each (to provide a base of 0) and ranks them, ignoring signs. Then he attaches the signs to the ranks to obtain the signed ranks. These results are as follows:

Deviation from 90%	−15	−25	10	0	−55	−27	−12	−20	−10
Unsigned ranks	5	7	2.5	1	9	8	4	6	2.5
Signed ranks	−5	−7	2.5	1	−9	−8	−4	−6	−2.5

The sum of positive signs obviously will be the smaller sum, namely, $3.5 = T$. From Table 14.1 (or Table H), the p-value for $n = 9$ with $T = 3.5$ lies between 0.020 and 0.027, which clearly is significant. He concludes that the patients' average functionality is significantly different from 90%.

Exercise 14.1: Are a Certain Thermometer's Readings on a Healthy Patient Normal? We are investigating the reliability of a certain brand of tympanic thermometer (temperature measured by a sensor inserted into the patient's ear).[55] Eight readings (degree Fahrenheit) were taken in the right ear of a healthy patient at 2-min intervals. Data were 98.1, 95.8, 97.5, 97.2, 97.7, 99.3, 99.2, 98.1. "Is the median different from the population average of 98.6°F?"

14.3. TWO SMALL SAMPLES: THE RANK-SUM TEST

THIS METHOD WAS INTRODUCED IN SECTION 6.6

The rank-sum test uses sample ranks to compare two samples in which the observations are not paired; n_1 observations are drawn from one sample and n_2 from the other. (n_1 is always assigned to the smaller of the two n's.)

EXAMPLE: REVIEW OF THE EXAMPLE FROM SECTION 6.6

We compared PSA levels for the $n_1 = 3$ patients from Table DB1.1 with positive biopsy results with the $n_2 = 7$ patients with negative biopsy results. We ranked the PSA levels and then added up the ranks for the smaller sample, naming this rank sum T. We converted T to the Mann–Whitney U statistic by the formula $U = n_1 n_2 + n_1(n_1 + 1)/2 - T$ and looked up the probability that a U-value this small would have arisen by chance alone. n_2 was 7, n_1 was 3, T was 18, U was 9, and the p-value associated with $U = 9$ was 0.834. We concluded that we had no evidence from the Table DB1.1 data that the PSA distributions are different for positive and negative biopsy results.

METHOD: THE RANK-SUM TEST

Given two samples, the hypothesis being tested is whether the value for a randomly chosen member of the first sample is probably smaller than one of the second sample, a slightly technical concept. For practical purposes, the user may think of it informally as testing whether the two distributions have the same median. Sampling and choosing hypotheses and α were discussed in Section 6.6. The steps to conduct the test may be summarized as follows:

1. Name the sizes of the samples n_1 and n_2; n_1 is the smaller. If $n_2 > 8$, go to Section 14.7.
2. Combine the data, keeping track of the sample from which each datum arose.
3. Rank the data.
4. Add up the ranks of the data from the smaller sample and name it T.
5. Calculate $U = n_1 n_2 + n_1(n_1 + 1)/2 - T$.
6. Look up p-value from Table I and use it to accept or reject the null hypothesis.

One-Tailed Test

Table I gives a two-tailed p-value. If we have a sound nonstatistical reason why the result of the test must lie in only one tail, we can halve the tabulated value to obtain a one-tailed p-value.

Other Names of This Test

The rank-sum test may be seen named as the Mann–Whitney test, Wilcoxon rank-sum test, or Wilcoxon–Mann–Whitney test.

Additional Example: Hct Compared for Laparoscopic versus Open Pyloromyotomies

Among the indicators of patient condition following pyloromyotomy (correction of stenotic pylorus) in neonates is hematocrit percent (Hct). A surgeon[16] wants to compare average Hct on 16 randomly allocated laparoscopic versus open pyloromyotomies ($n_1 = n_2 = 8$.) A quick frequency plot shows the distributions to be far from normal; a rank method is appropriate. Data were as follows: Open: 46.7, 38.8, 32.7, 32, 42, 39, 33.9, 43.3. Laporoscopy: 29.7, 38.3, 32, 52, 43.9, 32.1, 34, 25.6. He puts the data in order and assigns ranks, obtaining the following data.

Hct	Rank	Open (0) versus laparoscopy (1)
25.6	1	1
29.7	2	1
32.0	3.5	0
32.0	3.5	1
32.1	5	1
32.7	6	0
33.9	7	0
34.0	8	1
38.3	9	1
38.8	10	0
39.0	11	0
42.0	12	0
43.3	13	0
43.9	14	1
46.7	15	0
52.0	16	1

He finds the rank sums to be 77.5 for open pyloromyotomy and 58.5 for laparoscopy. Because of symmetry, either may be chosen; $T = 77.5$. He calculates

Table 14.2

A Segment of Table I, Rank-Sum U Probabilities[a]

	n_2:	8							
	n_1:	1	2	3	4	5	6	7	8
U	22						0.852	0.536	0.328
	23						0.950	0.612	0.382

[a] Two-tailed probabilities for the distribution of U, the rank-sum statistic. For two samples of size n_1 and n_2 ($n_2 > n_1$) and the value of U, the entry gives the p-value.

$U = n_1n_2 + n_1(n_1 + 1)/2 - T = 8 \times 8 + 8(9)/2 - 77.5 = 22.5$. Table 14.2 is a segment of Table I. From Table 14.2 or I, the p-value for $n_1 = n_2 = 8$ and $U = 22.5$ falls between 0.33 and 0.38, or about 0.335. He concludes that post-operative Hct has not been shown to be different for open versus laparoscopic pyloromyotomy.

Exercise 14.2: Does a Certain Tympanic Thermometer Measure the Same in Both Ears? We are investigating[55] the reliability of a certain brand of tympanic thermometer (temperature measured by a sensor inserted into the patient's ear). Sixteen readings (degrees Fahrenheit), eight per ear, were taken on a healthy patient at intervals of 1 min, alternating ears. Data were as follows:

Left ear	95.8	95.4	95.3	96.0	96.9	97.4	97.4	97.1
Right ear	98.1	95.8	97.5	97.2	97.7	99.3	99.2	98.1

Are the medians for the two ears different?

14.4. THREE OR MORE INDEPENDENT SAMPLES: THE KRUSKAL–WALLIS TEST

EXAMPLE: IS PSA THE SAME AMONG BPH, CAP, AND NED PATIENTS?

A urologist asks whether PSA level is different among the three patient groups: six with benign prostatic hypertrophy (BPH), eight with positive biopsy for prostate cancer, and eight with negative biopsy and no evidence of disease.[27] Thus, $k = 3$, $n_1 = 6$, $n_2 = 8$, $n_3 = 8$, and $n = 22$. The PSA levels are as follows:

BPH	5.3	7.9	8.7	4.3	6.6	6.4		
Positive biopsy	7.1	6.6	6.5	14.8	17.3	3.4	13.4	7.6
Negative biopsy	11.4	0.5	1.6	2.3	3.1	1.4	4.4	5.1

We rank all 22 data in order, keeping track of the sample each came from, as shown at the bottom of this page. We calculate the Kruskal–Wallis H statistic as

$$H = \frac{12}{n(n+1)}\left(\frac{T_1^2}{n_1} + \frac{T_2^2}{n_2} + \frac{T_3^2}{n_3}\right) - 3(n+1)$$

$$= \frac{12}{22(23)}\left(\frac{2916}{6} + \frac{13689}{8} + \frac{2916}{8}\right) - 3(23) = 6.80.$$

Table 14.3 is a portion of Table C. In Table 14.3 or Table C, the critical chi-square for $k-1=2$ degrees of freedom (df) for $\alpha=0.05$ is 5.99. The p-value for $H=6.801$ is calculated as 0.033. As H is greater than the critical χ^2, our urologist has sufficient evidence to conclude that the PSA levels are different among BPH patients, patients with positive biopsies for prostate cancer, and non-BPH patients with negative biopsies.

PSA	Rank for BPH patients	Rank for positive biopsy patients	Rank for negative biopsy patients
0.5			1
1.4			2
1.6			3
2.3			4
3.1			5
3.4		6	
4.3		7.5	
4.3	7.5		
4.4			9
5.1			10
5.3	11		
6.4	12		
6.5		13	
6.6		14.5	
6.6	14.5		
7.1		16	
7.6		17	
7.9	18		
8.7	19		
11.4			20
13.4		21	
17.3		22	
$T=$	82	117	54

Table 14.3

A Portion of Table C, Chi-Square Distribution, Right Tail[a]

α (area in right tail)	0.10	0.05	0.025	0.01	0.005	0.001
$df = 2$	4.61	5.99	7.38	9.21	10.60	13.80
3	6.25	7.81	9.35	11.34	12.84	16.26
4	7.78	9.49	11.14	13.28	14.86	18.46

[a] Selected χ^2 values (distances above zero) for various *df* and for α, the area under the curve in the right tail.

Method: The Kruskal–Wallis Test

Methodologically, the Kruskal–Wallis test is just the rank-sum test extended to three or more samples. It is used when rank-order data arise naturally in three or more groups or if the assumptions underlying the one-way analysis of variance test are not satisfied. The hypothesis being tested is whether the value for a randomly chosen member of one sample is probably smaller than one of another sample. For practical purposes, the user may think of it informally as testing whether the several distributions have the same median. The chi-square approximation is valid only if there are five or more members in each sample.

1. Name the number of samples k (3 or 4 or ...).
2. Name the sizes of the several samples $n_1, n_2, \ldots, n_k$; n is the grand total.
3. Combine the data, keeping track of the sample from which each datum arose.
4. Rank the data.
5. Add the ranks from each sample separately, naming the sums $T_1, T_2, \ldots, T_k$.
6. Calculate the Kruskal–Wallis H statistic, which is distributed as chi-square, by

$$H = \frac{12}{n(n+1)}\left(\frac{T_1^2}{n_1} + \frac{T_2^2}{n_2} + \cdots + \frac{T_k^2}{n_k}\right) - 3(n+1). \qquad (14.1)$$

7. Obtain the p-value (looked up as if it were α) from Table C (χ^2 right tail) for $k - 1$ degrees of freedom.

ADDITIONAL EXAMPLE: DO SURGICAL INSTRUMENTS FROM FIVE DIFFERENT MANUFACTURERS PERFORM DIFFERENTLY?

As part of an instrument calibration, we want to compare $k = 5$ disposable current-generating instruments used in surgery to stimulate (and thereby help locate) facial nerves.[48] Among the variables recorded is current (milliamperes). $n_1 = n_2 = n_3 = n_4 = n_5 = 10$ readings are taken from each machine for a total of $n = 50$. A quick plot shows that the data clearly are not normal, and Bartlett's test of equal variances yields $p < 0.001$, so that a rank method must used. The ordered current readings, separated by instrument from which each datum arose, and their corresponding ranks are as follows:

Instrument 1	Ranks 1	Instrument 2	Ranks 2	Instrument 3	Ranks 3	Instrument 4	Ranks 4	Instrument 5	Ranks 5
		1.90	1						
		1.95	2.5	1.95	2.5				
		1.96	6	1.96, 1.96	6 × 2	1.96	6	1.96	6
		1.97	9						
				1.98	12	1.98, 1.98	12 × 2	1.98, 1.98	12 × 2
2.00, 2.00	16.5 × 2			2.00	16.5			2.00	16.5
2.01	20.5	2.01	20.5	2.01	20.5	2.01	20.5		
2.03, 2.03	25 × 2	2.03	25					2.03, 2.03	25 × 2
2.04	29.5	2.04	29.5	2.04	29.5	2.04	29.5		
		2.06	33.5	2.06	33.5	2.06	33.5	2.06	33.5
2.07, 2.07	38 × 2	2.07	38	2.07	38			2.07	38
						2.08	41		
20.9	42								
						2.10	43		
						2.11	44.5	2.11	44.5
2.12	46								
		2.31	47						
				2.76	48				
						3.02	49		
								3.03	50
$T =$	297		212		212.5		291		262.5

We calculate the H statistic to obtain

$$H = \frac{12}{n(n+1)}\left(\frac{T_1^2}{n_1} + \frac{T_2^2}{n_2} + \cdots + \frac{T_5^2}{n_5}\right) - 3(n+1)$$

$$= \frac{12}{50(51)}\left(\frac{88209}{10} + \frac{44944}{10} + \frac{45156.25}{10} + \frac{84681}{10} + \frac{68906.25}{10}\right) - 3(51)$$

$$= 3.187.$$

From Table 14.3 or Table C, the critical value of χ^2 for $\alpha = 0.05$ with 4 *df* is 9.49, which is much larger than 3.187, so H_o is accepted; the current is not different from instrument to instrument. By using a statistical software package, we find $p = 0.527$.

Exercise 14.3: Are Three Methods of Removing Excess Fluid in Infected Bursitis Different? An orthopedist compares an inflow–outflow catheter (treatment 1), needle aspiration (treatment 2), and incision-and-drain surgery (treatment 3).[77] Among his measures of effectiveness is posttreatment sedimentation rate (Sed). He uses each method on $n_1 = n_2 = n_3 = 10$ patients for a total of $n = 30$. Data are as follows:

Treatment 1	28	10	94	29	2	27	1	58	25	26
Treatment 2	64	30	30	11	30	9	9	30	9	25
Treatment 3	16	22	108	18	45	10	15	40	15	24

Draw rough frequency plots of Sed for groups of 10 to show that they are not normal and that a rank method is appropriate. Use the Kruskal–Wallis method to test the null hypothesis that Sed is the same for all treatments.

14.5. THREE OR MORE "PAIRED" SAMPLES: THE FRIEDMAN TEST

EXAMPLE: ARE TWO SKIN TESTS FOR SENSITIVITY TO AN ALLERGEN DIFFERENT?

An allergist applies three skin prick tests (two stimuli and a control) to the inside forearms, randomizing the order proximal to distal, to each of eight patients.[31] Thus, $k = 3$ and $n = 8$. After 15 min, he ranks the wheal-and-erythema reactions by severity (most severe being 1). The results (ranks and rank sums) were as follows:

Patient no.	Test 1	Test 2	Control
1	1	2	3
2	2	1	3
3	1	3	2
4	3	2	1
5	1	2	3
6	1	2	3
7	2	1	3
8	1	2	3
$T =$	12	15	21

We calculate the Friedman statistic:

$$F_r = \frac{12}{nk(k+1)}\left(T_1^2 + T_2^2 + \cdots + T_k^2\right) - 3n(k+1)$$

$$= \frac{12}{8(3)(4)}(144 + 225 + 441) - 3(8)(4) = 5.25.$$

In Table 14.3 or Table C, the critical chi-square for $k - 1 = 2$ degrees of freedom for $\alpha = 0.05$ is 5.99. As F_r is less than critical χ^2, our allergist has insufficient evidence to infer any difference in efficacy between the two tests or that the tests are more efficacious than the control. The p-value is calculated as 0.072.

Method: The Friedman Test

If three or more treatments are given to each patient of a sample, we have an extension of the paired-data concept. More exactly, it is called a randomized block design. In the example, a dermatologist applied three skin patches to each of eight patients to test for an allergy. The three skin test results for each patient are called a "block." (In contrast, three groups of patients with a different skin test being used in each would call for the Kruskal–Wallis test.) The hypothesis being tested is that the several treatments have the same distributions. The chi-square approximation is valid only if there are five or more blocks, e.g., patients, in the sample.

1. Name the number of treatments (3 or 4 or ...) k and blocks (e.g., patients) n.
2. Rank the data within each block (e.g., rank the treatments for each patient).
3. Add the ranks for each treatment separately; name the sums $T_1, T_2, \ldots, T_k$.
4. Calculate the Friedman statistic, F_r, which is distributed as chi-square, by

$$F_r = \frac{12}{nk(k+1)}\left(T_1^2 + T_2^2 + \cdots + T_k^2\right) - 3n(k+1). \qquad (14.2)$$

5. Obtain the p-value (as if it were α) from Table C (χ^2 right tail) for $k - 1$ *df*.

Additional Example: Does the Systemic Level of Gentamicin Treatment Decline over Time?

In treating an infected ear, gentamicin, suspended in a fibrin glue, can be inserted in the middle ear, and some makes its way into the system. The time after application that it resides in the system is unknown. $n = 8$ chinchillas, which have large ears anatomically similar to those of humans, were used.[24] The serum gentamicin level (microgram/milliliter) was measured at 8 hr, 24 hr, 72 hr, and 7 days after the administration. If the declining levels at these times test significantly different, an approximate "fade-out" time can be inferred. A quick plot showed that the data per time grouping were far from normal, and Bartlett's test of equal variances yielded $p < 0.001$; a rank method must be used. As the data arose through time from the same animal, Friedman's test was appropriate. The data, listed and then ranked for each animal, were as follows:

	8 hr		24 hr		72 hr		7 days	
Animal no.	Level	Rank	Level	Rank	Level	Rank	Level	Rank
1	482	3	877	4	0	1.5	0	1.5
2	124	3	363	4	66	2	0	1
3	280	3	1730	4	50	2	13	1
4	426	4	102	3	0	1.5	0	1.5
5	608	4	2	3	0	1.5	0	1.5
6	161	4	0	1.5	0	1.5	23	3
7	456	3	1285	4	48	2	0	1
8	989	4	189	2	378	3	0	1
$T =$		28		25.5		15		11.5
$T^2 =$		784		650.25		225		132.25

The results were substituted in Eq. (14.2) to obtain

$$F_r = \frac{12}{nk(k+1)}\left(T_1^2 + T_2^2 + \cdots + T_k^2\right) - 3n(k+1)$$

$$= \frac{12}{8 \times 4 \times 5}(1791.5) - 3 \times 8 \times 5 = 14.36.$$

From Table 14.3 or Table C, the critical value of χ^2 for $\alpha = 0.05$ with $k - 1 = 3$ *df* is 7.81. F_r is much greater than 7.81, so the null hypothesis of equal levels over time was rejected. The *p*-value calculated from a statistical software package is 0.002.

Exercise 14.4: Do Posttherapy CaP Patients' PSAs Remain Stable? $n = 9$ cancer-of-the-prostate (CaP) patients clinically had been without evidence of disease 10 years after a negative staging pelvic lymphadenectomy and definitive radiation therapy.[29] Prostate specific antigen (PSA) levels then were measured in three successive intervals about a year apart. Data were as follows:

	Patient number								
	1	2	3	4	5	6	7	8	9
First PSA	3.90	3.70	1.80	0.80	3.80	1.80	1.80	3.60	0.62
Second PSA	3.95	3.80	1.86	0.30	7.68	2.10	1.67	4.51	0.65
Third PSA	4.95	0.10	3.03	0.30	13.5	2.54	0.80	6.80	0.42

The data are not distributed normal, and Bartlett's test shows that the variances are significantly different; a rank test is appropriate. Test the hypothesis that PSA level is not changing through time.

14.6. SINGLE LARGE SAMPLES: NORMAL APPROXIMATION TO SIGNED-RANK TEST

EXAMPLE: IS THE EARLY SAMPLING OF OUR 301 PROSTATE BIOPSY PATIENTS BIASED RELATIVE TO THE LATER SAMPLING?

We ask whether the PSA levels of the first 20 significantly differ from 8.96 (the average of the remaining 281). We compute the differences of the first 20 from 8.96 and rank them by magnitude (i.e., regardless of sign).

PSA difference	Rank	Negative ranks	Positive ranks
−0.04	1	1	
0.06	2		2
0.96	3		3
1.06	4		4
1.26	5		5
1.26	6		6
1.36	7		7
1.36	8		8
2.16	9		9
2.63	10		10
2.86	11		11
3.06	12		12
3.26	13		13
3.36	14		14
3.66	15		15
4.16	16		16
4.36	17		17
4.56	18		18
4.86	19		19
7.66	20		20
Sums of ranks =		1	209

$T = 1$, the unsigned value of the smaller sum of ranks; $\mu = n(n+1)/4 = 20(21)/4 = 105$; $\sigma^2 = (2n+1)\mu/6 = 41(105)/6 = 717.5$; $\sigma = \sqrt{717.5} = 26.7862$; $z = (T - \mu)/\sigma = (1 - 105)/26.7862 = -3.8826$. This large a z is off the scale in Table A, telling us that $p < 0.001$; the early values are different. (Calculated exactly, two-tailed $p = 0.0001$.) We have strong evidence that PSA levels from early sampling were different from those from later sampling. The claim of bias is credible.

Method: The Signed-Rank Test for Large Samples

This method, the normal approximation to the Wilcoxon signed-rank test for samples larger than 12, tests the hypothesis that the distribution of differences has a median of 0. It may test (1) a set of observations deviating from a hypothesized common value or (2) pairs of observations on the same individuals, such as before-and-after data.

1. Calculate the differences of the observations as in (1) or (2).
2. Rank the magnitudes (i.e., the differences without signs).
3. Reattach the signs to the ranks.
4. Add up the positive and negative ranks.
5. Denote by T the unsigned value of the smaller; n is sample size (number of ranks).
6. Calculate $\mu = n(n+1)/4$, $\sigma^2 = (2n+1)\mu/6$, and then $z = (T - \mu)/\sigma$.
7. Obtain the p-value (as if it were α) from Table A for a two- or one-tailed test as appropriate.

Additional Example: Does a Certain Type of Hardware Installed in Broken Ankles Restore Functionality?

An orthopedist installs the hardware in ankle repair in $n = 19$ patients.[23] (This example is similar to the Additional Example of Section 14.2 but with a larger sample size.) He scores the percent functionality of the joint. He asks, "Is the average functionality 90% of normal?" Because it could be more or less, his test is two-sided. His data in percent are 75, 65, 100, 90, 35, 63, 78, 70, 80, 98, 95, 45, 90, 93, 85, 100, 72, 99, 95. A quick frequency plot of the data show that they are far from normal, so he uses a rank test. As he has more than 12 data, the normal approximation is adequate. He subtracts 90% from each (in order to test against a basis of 0), obtaining -15, -25, 10, 0, -55, -27, -12, -20, -10, 8, 5, -45, 0, 3, -5, 10, -18, 9, 5. He puts them in order and assigns ranks to them, ignoring signs. Then he attaches signs to the ranks to obtain the signed ranks. These rankings are as follows:

Deviations ranked	Unsigned ranks	Signed ranks
−55	1	−1
−45	2	−2
−27	3	−3
−25	4	−4
−20	5	−5
−18	6	−6
−15	7	−7
−12	8	−8
−10	9	−9
−5	10	−10
0	11.5	11.5
0	11.5	11.5
3	13	13
5	14.5	14.5
5	14.5	14.5
8	16	16
9	17	17
10	18.5	18.5
10	18.5	18.5

Calculations and Outcome

The sum of negative signed ranks (−55) is smaller, so $T = 55$. $\mu = n(n-1)/4 = 19 \times 20/4 = 95$, $\sigma^2 = (2n+1)\mu/6 = 39 \times 95/6 = 617.5$, and $\sigma = 24.85$. Then $z = (T - \mu)/\sigma = (55 - 95)/24.85 = -1.61$. The critical value of a 5% two-tailed α is the usual ± 1.96. Because the calculated z is inside these bounds, the orthopedist concludes that the post-operative patients' average ankle functionality is not different from 90%. Table 14.4 shows the relevant portion of Table A, the normal distribution. From Table 14.4 or Table A, interpolation gives the p-value as 0.108.

Table 14.4

A Portion of Table A, Normal Distribution[a]

z (no. std. deviations to right of mean)	Two-tailed α (area in both tails)
0.60	0.548
0.70	0.484
1.60	0.110
1.70	0.090
1.80	0.072
1.90	0.054

[a] For selected distances (z) to the right of the mean, given are two-tailed α, the areas combined for both positive and negative tails.

Exercise 14.5. In Exercise 8.2, $n = 8$ temperature readings were taken on a patient. The question was, "Is the median different (implying a two-tailed test) from the population average of 98.6°F?" As an exercise, answer the question using the normal approximation to the signed-rank test, even though the sample is smaller than appropriate. Data were 98.1 95.8 97.5 97.2 97.7 99.3 99.2 98.1.

14.7. TWO LARGE SAMPLES: NORMAL APPROXIMATION TO RANK-SUM TEST

EXAMPLE: IS PSA FOR THE 10 TABLE DB1.1 PATIENTS THE SAME AS THAT FOR BPH PATIENTS?

We obtain a sample of 12 patients with BPH. We want to compare the PSA for these patients with that for the 10 patients in Table DB1.1. $n_1 = 10$ and $n_2 = 12$. The data are as follows:

PSA from Table DB1.1	7.6	4.1	5.9	9.0	6.8	8.0	7.7	4.4	6.1	7.9		
PSA for BPH patients	5.3	7.9	8.7	4.3	6.6	6.4	20.2	8.5	6.5	6.5	12.5	7.1

We then rank all 22 data in order, keeping track of the sample each came from:

PSA	Rank for BPH patients	Rank for Table DB1.1 patients
4.1		1
4.3	2	
4.4		3
5.3	4	
5.9		5
6.1		6
6.4	7	
6.5	8.5	
6.5	8.5	
6.6	10	
6.8		11
7.1	12	
7.6		13
7.7		14
7.9	15.5	
7.9		15.5
8.0		17
8.5	18	
8.7	19	
9.0		20
12.5	2	
20.2	22	
Sum of ranks =	147.5	105.5

$T = 105.5$, the smaller rank sum; $\mu = n_1(n_1+n_2+1)/2 = 10(10+12+1)/2 = 115$; $\sigma^2 = n_1n_2(n_1+n_2+1)/12 = 10(12)(10+12+1)/12 = 230$; $\sigma = \sqrt{230} = 15.1658$; $z = (T - \mu)/\sigma = (105.5 - 115)/15.1658 = -0.626$. From Table 14.4 or Table A, $z = 0.60$ yields an area in both tails of 0.548, which is slightly larger than the p-value that would arise from a z of 0.626. (An exact calculation gives an area of 0.532.) There is no evidence that the two samples have differing PSA levels.

Method

The Rank-Sum Test for Large Samples

This method is a normal approximation to the rank-sum test for cases in which $n_2 > 8$. Given two samples, the hypothesis being tested is whether the value for a randomly chosen member of the first sample is probably smaller than one of the second sample. For practical purposes, the user may think of it informally as testing whether the two distributions have the same median.

1. Name the sizes of the two samples n_1 and n_2; n_1 is the smaller.
2. Combine the data, keeping track of the sample from which each datum arose.
3. Rank the data.
4. Add up the ranks of the data from each sample separately.
5. Denote as T the sum associated with n_1.
6. Calculate $\mu = n_1(n_1 + n_2 + 1)/2$, $\sigma^2 = n_1n_2(n_1 + n_2 + 1)/12$, and $z = (T - \mu)/\sigma$.
7. Obtain the p-value (as if it were σ) from Table A for a two- or one-tailed test as appropriate.

Other Names for the Rank-Sum Test

This test may be referred to in the literature as the rank-sum test, Mann–Whitney U test, Wilcoxon rank-sum test, or Wilcoxon–Mann–Whitney test. Mann and Whitney published what was thought to be one test and Wilcoxon another. Eventually they were seen to be only different forms of the same test.

Additional Example: Does Removal of Hardware in Broken Ankle Repair Alter Joint Functionality?

An orthopedist installs hardware in $n = 19$ broken ankles.[23] He removes the hardware in $n_1 = 9$ of the patients, randomly selected, and leaves it permanently in place in the remaining $n_2 = 10$. He judges the post-operative percent functionality of the ankle joint and asks, "Is the average functionality different for the two treatments?" Because either one might be better, his test is two-sided. His data are as follows. Remove: 75, 65, 100, 90, 35, 63, 78, 70, 80. Retain: 98, 95, 45, 90, 93, 85, 100, 72, 99, 95. A quick frequency plot of the data show that they are far from normal, so he uses a rank test. As $n_2 > 8$, the normal approximation is adequate. His data, put in order with ranks assigned, become

Percent Functionality	Rank	Removed
35	1	yes
45	2	no
63	3	yes
65	4	yes
70	5	yes
72	6	no
75	7	yes
78	8	yes
80	9	yes
85	10	no
90	11.5	yes
90	11.5	no
93	13	no
95	14.5	no
95	14.5	no
98	16	no
99	17	no
100	18.5	yes
100	18.5	no

By summing the smaller group ("yes"), he finds $T = 67$. $\mu = n_1(n_1+n_2+1)/2 = 9(9+10+1)/2 = 90$, $\sigma^2 = n_1 n_2(n_1+n_2+1)/12 = 150$, and $\sigma = 12.25$. Then $z = (67-90)/12.25 = -1.88$. From Table 14.4 or Table A, the critical value of a 5% two-tailed test is ± 1.96. Because the calculated z is just inside these bounds, the orthopedist must conclude that he has inadequate evidence to show that leaving or removing the hardware provides a different percent functionality. From a computer package, the p-value is 0.060.

Exercise 14.6. In Exercise 14.3, $n_1 = n_2 = 8$ temperature readings were taken from a patient's left and right ears, respectively.[55] The question was, "Are the medians for the two ears different (implying a two-tailed test)?" As an exercise, answer the question using the normal approximation to the rank-sum test, even though the sample size is just barely smaller than appropriate. Data were as follows:

Left ear	95.8	95.4	95.3	96.0	96.9	97.4	97.4	97.1
Right ear	98.1	95.8	97.5	97.2	97.7	99.3	99.2	98.1

ANSWERS TO EXERCISES

14.1. The data differences (98.6 minus each datum) are 0.5, 0.8, 1.1, 1.4, 0.9, −0.7, −0.6, 0.5. The unsigned ranks are 1.5, 5, 7, 8, 6, 4, 3, 1.5, and the signed ranks are 1.5, 5, 7, 8, 6, −4, −3, 1.5. The smaller rank sum is 7. From Table H, the probability that a signed rank sum is 7, given $n = 8$, is 0.149. This p-value is too large to infer a difference; the patient's median temperature is shown not to be different from 98.6°F.

14.2. Rank the combined data, keeping track of which ear gave rise to each datum. The ranks are 3.5, 2, 1, 5, 6, 9.5, 9.5, 7, 13.5, 3.5, 11, 8, 12, 16, 15, 13.5. The first eight ranks for the left ear sum to 43.5; the remainder for the right sum to 92.5. Because the n's are the same, either n could be designated n_1. The associated U-values are $U = n_1n_2 + n_1(n_1 + 1)/2 - 43.5 = 56.5$ and $U = n_1n_2 + n_1(n_1 + 1)/2 - 92.5 = 7.5$. Because 56.5 is off the table, we choose $U = 7.5$. (The test is symmetric.) In Table I, for $n_1 = n_2 = 8$, $U = 7.5$ designates a p-value lying halfway between 0.006 and 0.010, or 0.008. The data provide strong evidence that the median temperature readings for the two ears are different.

14.3. Frequency plots per group are as follows:

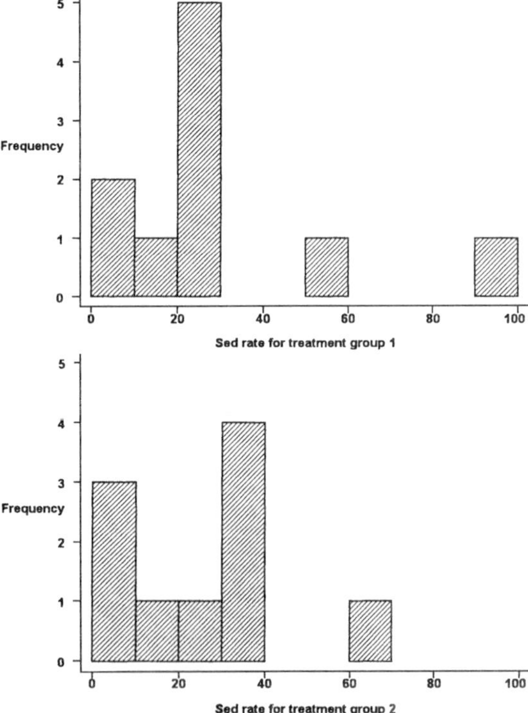

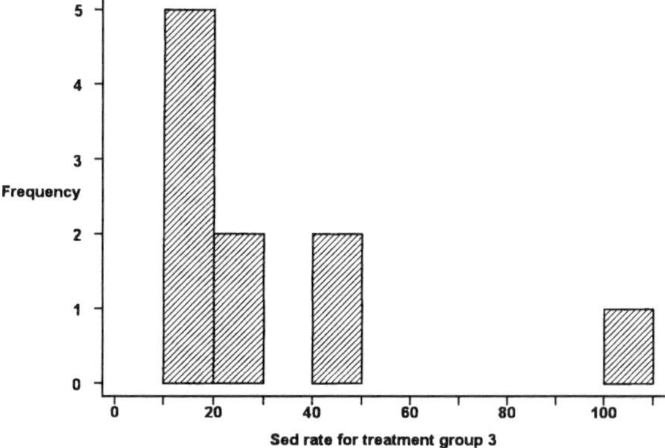

Sed rates, separated by treatment from which each datum arose, and their corresponding ranks are as follows:

Sed 1	Ranks 1	Sed 2	Ranks 2	Sed 3	Ranks 3
1	1				
2	2				
		9, 9, 9	4 × 3		
10	6.5			10	6.5
		11	8		
				15, 15	9.5 × 2
				16	11
				18	12
				22	13
				24	14
25	15.5	25	15.5		
26	17				
27	18				
28	19				
29	20				
		30, 30, 30, 30	22.5 × 4		
				40	25
				45	26
58	27				
		64	28		
94	29				
				108	30
$T =$	155		153.5		156.5
$T^2 =$	24,025		23,562.25		24,492.25

$$H = \frac{12}{n(n+1)}\left(\frac{T_1^2}{n_1} + \frac{T_2^2}{n_2} + \frac{T_3^2}{n_3}\right) - 3(n+1)$$

$$= \frac{12}{30 \times 31}\left(\frac{24025}{10} + \frac{23562.25}{10} + \frac{24492.25}{10}\right) - 3 \times 31 = 0.0058.$$

From Table C, the 5% critical value for 2 *df* is 5.99, which is much larger than H; Sed is not different for the three treatments. From a statistical software package, $p = 0.997$.

14.4. The ranks for each patient of his PSA levels, with rank sums at the bottom, are as follows:

Patient	Rank of first PSA	Rank of second PSA	Rank of third PSA
1	1	2	3
2	2	3	1
3	1	2	3
4	3	1.5	1.5
5	1	2	3
6	1	2	3
7	3	2	1
8	1	2	3
9	2	3	1
$T =$	15	19.5	19.5
$T^2 =$	225	380.25	380.25

$$F_r = \frac{12}{nk(k+1)}\left(T_1^2 + T_2^2 + \cdots + T_k^2\right) - 3n(k+1)$$

$$= \frac{12}{9(3)(4)}(225 + 380.25 + 380.25) - 3(9)(4) = 1.50.$$

From Table C, the critical chi-square for $k - 1 = 2$ degrees of freedom for $\alpha = 0.05$ is 5.99. On average, PSA level is not increasing over time in this population. The p-value is 0.472.

14.5. Follow the answer to Exercise 14.2 until the smaller rank sum $T = 7$ is found. Calculate $\mu = n(n+1)/4 = 8 \times 9/4 = 18$, $\sigma^2 = (2n+1)\mu/6 = 17 \times 18/6 = 51$, and then $z = (T - \mu)/\sigma = (7 - 18)/\sqrt{51} = -1.54$. From Table A, the two-tailed α lies between 0.134 and 0.110, or 0.124 by interpolation. We accept the null hypothesis of no difference. Note that use of Table H yielded $p = 0.149$. The discrepancy is due to too small a sample for a good approximation.

14.6. Follow the answer to Exercise 14.3 until the rank sums $T = 43.5$ and 92.5 are found. Calculate $\mu = n_1(n_1 + n_2 + 1)/2 = 8 \times 17/2 = 68$, $\sigma^2 = n_1 n_2(n_1 + n_2 + 1)/12 = 8 \times 8 \times 17/12 = 90.67$, $\sigma = 9.57$, and then $z = (T - \mu)/\sigma = (43.5 - 68)/9.52 = -2.57$. (The other $T = 92.5$ yields $+2.57$; note symmetry.) From Table A, $p = 0.010$. Because it is a borderline sample size for adequate approximation, the result differs little from Table I's 0.008.

Chapter 15

Common Tests on Continuous Data Means

15.1. SUMMARY OF MEANS TESTING

THE BASIC QUESTION BEING ASKED

Is a sample mean the same as a population mean, or, alternatively, do two or more samples have the same population mean? The question is answered by testing the null hypothesis that the means are equal and then accepting or rejecting this hypothesis. The concept of a hypothesis test was discussed in Sections 5.1 and 5.2.

ASSUMPTIONS UNDERLYING A HYPOTHESIS TEST

Tests of means using continuous data were developed under the assumptions that (1) the sample observations are independent from each other and (2) they were drawn from a normal distribution. Additionally, when two sample means are being tested, the hypothesis that they arose from the same distribution implies (3) equal standard deviations. These assumptions were discussed in Section 6.7. Also discussed was the property of *robustness*, i.e., how impervious the test is to violations of the assumptions. Whereas these assumptions usually are not satisfied exactly, the robustness of the test allows it to be valid if the assumptions are roughly approximated. Assumption (1) is essential for all types of test; if it is violated badly, the results of any test will be spurious. If assumption (2) is violated badly, a valid test may still be made using the rank methods of Chapter 14. If assumption (3) is violated in a test of two means, the user should use either an unequal-variance form of the test or a rank test. Further guidance will be given in Section 15.3.

We Must Specify the Null and Alternate Hypotheses

The null hypothesis states that the mean of the population from which the sample is drawn is not different from a theorized mean or from the population mean of another sample. The alternate hypothesis may say that the two means are not equal or that one is greater than the other. The form of the alternate hypothesis was discussed in Section 6.7. We should specify the hypotheses before seeing the data so that our choice will not be influenced by the outcome.

15.2. SINGLE OR PAIRED NEAR-NORMAL SAMPLES: NORMAL (z) AND t TESTS

Equivalence of Single Samples and Paired Samples

Single and paired samples are treated by the same method, because we may create a single observation from a pair by subtraction, e.g., the after measurement minus the before or the patient's response to drug 1 minus the response to drug 2.

Examples

Normal: Do the Beginning Members of our PSA Sample Average the Same as Later Ones?

We ask whether the mean PSA ($m = 6.75$) of the 10 patients of Table DB1.1 is different from that of the remaining 291, a sample large enough for its sample mean and standard deviation to be treated as if they were population mean and standard deviation. Thus, $\mu = 8.86$ and $\sigma_m = \sigma/\sqrt{n} = 17.19/\sqrt{291} = 1.01$. The distribution is about like that shown for all 301 patients in Fig. 2.3, close enough to normal in shape for the test to be valid. The null hypothesis is that m is drawn from the population having mean μ, so that m and μ should be different only by random influence. We have no reason to anticipate whether m should be larger or smaller than μ, so we use a two-tailed test. The null hypothesis is tested by the normal statistic $z = (m - \mu)/\sigma_m = (6.75 - 8.86)/1.01 = -2.09$. Because the normal curve is symmetric, we are concerned with how far z is from 0 regardless of the direction, so we can look up $+2.09$ in the table. Table 15.1 is a portion of Table A. In either table, the two-tailed p-value (looked up as if it were α) for this z is a bit more than 0.036 (actually 0.037 from exact calculation). The chance that the difference between m and μ occurred by a random influence is less than 4%; we conclude that they are different.

Table 15.1
A Portion of Table A, Normal Distribution[a]

z (no. std deviations to right of mean)	Two-tailed α (area in both tails)
0.50	0.619
0.60	0.548
1.90	0.54
1.960	*0.050*
2.00	0.046
2.10	0.036
2.30	0.022
2.326	*0.020*
2.40	0.016

[a] For selected distances (z) to the right of the mean, given are two-tailed α values, the areas combined for both tails. Entries for the most commonly used areas are italicized.

t: Does Asthma Training of Pediatric Patients Reduce Acute Care Visits?

We include all asthma patients satisfying inclusion criteria presenting over a period of time, in this case 32, and record the number of acute care visits during 1 year.[15] We then provide them a standardized course of asthma training and record the number of acute care visits for the following year. These "before-and-after" data allow us to analyze the change per patient: d (named for "difference" or "delta") = number of visits before training minus number after. A plot of the data shows an approximately normal shape, satisfying that assumption. H_0: $\mu_d = 0$.

What Is the Alternate Hypothesis?

We would *expect* the training to reduce the number of visits, but we are not *certain*. Perhaps the training will increase the child's awareness and fear, causing an increase in visits; this is unlikely, but we cannot rule it out. Therefore, we cannot in good faith say that the error can lie in only one direction, so we must use a two-tailed test. H_1: $\mu_d \neq 0$.

Data and Results

The d values were 1, 1, 2, 4, 0, 5, −3, 0, 4, 2, 8, 1, 1, 0, −1, 3, 6, 3, 1, 2, 0, −1, 0, 3, 2, 1, 3, −1, −1, 1, 1, 5. $m_d = 1.66$ and $s_d = 2.32$. $t = (m - \mu)/s_m = (1.66 - 0)/(2.32/\sqrt{32}) = 1.66/0.41 = 4.05$. Table 15.2 is a portion of Table B.

Table 15.2

A Portion of Table B, t Distribution[a]

Two-tailed α	0.10	0.05	0.02	0.01	0.002	0.001
$df = 11$	1.796	2.201	2.718	3.106	4.025	4.437
14	1.761	2.145	2.624	2.977	3.787	4.140
26	1.706	2.056	2.479	2.779	3.435	3.707
30	1.697	2.042	2.457	2.750	3.385	3.646
40	1.684	2.021	2.423	2.704	3.307	3.551
100	1.660	1.984	2.364	2.626	3.174	3.390
∞	1.645	1.960	2.326	2.576	3.090	3.291

[a] Selected distances (t) to the right of the mean are given for various degrees of freedom (df) and for two-tailed α, areas combined for both positive and negative tails.

In either table, look under the two-tailed α column for $df = 30$ (df, degrees of freedom) to find the critical value of t; our $df = 31$ will be just less than the tabulated value or about 2.04. Because 4.05 is greater than that, and in fact greater than the critical 3.64 for $\alpha = 0.001$, we can say there is less than a 1 in 1000 chance of being wrong if we conclude that the asthma training was efficacious.

METHOD: THE ONE-SAMPLE–PAIRED-SAMPLE z AND t TESTS

We want to test the hypothesis that the mean of the distribution from which we draw our sample, denoted μ_0, is the same as the known (theoretical) mean μ, or H_0: $\mu_0 = \mu$. The alternative hypothesis may be that μ_0 is greater than or less than μ, giving a one-tailed test, or either, giving a two-tailed test (H_1: $\mu_0 > \mu$, H_1: $\mu_0 < \mu$, or H_1: $\mu_0 \neq \mu$). Choose an appropriate α. We must assume that the basic data are distributed roughly normal. The test is a normal z test or a t test in the form of a standardized mean. When the standard error of the mean σ_m is known theoretically or the sample is large enough that s_m is close to σ_m (say >30, although extreme accuracy may require >50 or >100), use z, calculated as in Eq. (15.1), and Table A:

$$z = \frac{m - \mu}{\sigma_m} = \frac{m - \mu}{\sigma/\sqrt{n}}. \tag{15.1}$$

When σ_m is unknown and therefore estimated by s_m, and n is smaller than the preceding guide, use t, calculated as in Eq. (15.2), and Table B with $n - 1$ df:

$$t = \frac{m - \mu}{s_m} = \frac{m - \mu}{s/\sqrt{n}}. \tag{15.2}$$

Follow these steps for either test:

1. Specify null and alternate hypotheses and choose α.
2. Make a quick, informal frequency plot of the basic data to check for normal shape.
3. Look up the critical value in the appropriate table for the chosen α.
4. Calculate the appropriate statistic from Eq. (15.1) or (15.2).
5. Make the decision to accept or reject the null hypothesis.

Additional Example: Is a New Dyspepsia Treatment Effective in the ED?

An emergency medicine physician wants to test the effectiveness of a "GI cocktail" (antacid plus viscous lidocaine) to treat emergency dyspeptic symptoms as measured on a 1–10 pain scale.[42] H_0: $\mu = 0$. He suspects that the treatment will not worsen the symptoms, but he is not totally sure, so he uses H_1: $\mu \neq 0$, implying a two-sided test; he chooses $\alpha = 0.05$. He decides to accept as the population standard deviation that for scoring of a large number of patients without treatment, $\sigma = 1.73$. He samples $n = 15$ patients, measuring the difference in pain before treatment minus that after treatment. Data are 6, 7, 2, 5, 3, 0, 3, 4, 5, 6, 1, 1, 1, 8, 6. $m = 3.87$. He substitutes in Eq. (15.1) to find $z = (m - \mu)/\sigma_m = (3.87 - 0)/(1.73/\sqrt{15}) = 8.66$. Because the critical value from Table 15.1 or Table A is 1.96, which is much less than 8.66, he rejects H_0 and concludes that the treatment is effective. The actual p-value is 0 to more than three decimal places and so is stated as $p < 0.001$.

Suppose the Standard Deviation Came from a Small Sample Instead of a Large Sample

If he had decided not to use $\sigma = 1.73$ because it arose from untreated patients, he would have estimated the standard deviation from the data as $s = 2.23$ and used the t test. From Table 15.2 or Table B, the critical value for a two-tailed t with 14 *df* is 2.145. By substituting in Eq. (15.2), he finds $t = (m - \mu)/s_m = (3.87 - 0)/(2.23/\sqrt{15}) = 6.72$. The conclusion is identical to that for the case of large sample statistics.

Exercise 15.1: The Original Example That "Student" Used for His *t*. In W. S. Gossett's classic 1908 paper[69] introducing the t test, he used the following data. Two soporific drugs were used in turn on 10 insomniac patients and the number of hours of additional sleep each provided were recorded. Data were as follows:

Patient	Dextro	Laevo	Difference (d)
1	0.7	1.9	1.2
2	−1.6	0.8	2.4
3	−0.2	1.1	1.3
⋮	⋮	⋮	⋮
10	2.0	4.3	1.4
mean =	0.75	2.33	1.58
standard deviation =			1.23

We denote the unknown population's mean of differences as δ, estimated from the sample by the mean of d. At the $\alpha = 0.05$ level of significance, test H_0: $\delta = 0$ against H_1: $\delta \neq 0$.

15.3. TWO NEAR-NORMAL SAMPLES: NORMAL (z) AND t TESTS

A Test of Means of Two Samples

The particular form of the test to contrast two means depends on the relationship of the variances, which are pooled to obtain an overall estimate of variability. Unequal variances are pooled differently from equal variances. Fortunately, the tests are rather robust against differing variances, provided the sizes of the two samples are about the same. If sample sizes are quite different or if one variance is more than double the other, the variances should be tested for equality before making the means test. Methods for testing the equality of variances appear in Section 16.3. The logic for selecting which form to use appears in Table 15.3.

Table 15.3

Guide for Selecting Appropriate Two-Sample Means Test

Total sample size	Subgroup sample size	Variances about equal	Variances somewhat different	Variances extremely different
Large size *or* σ's known	About equal	(1) Normal (z) test, equal variances	(1) Normal (z) test, equal variances	Rank-sum test
	Very different		(3) Normal (z) test, unequal variances	Rank-sum test
Small size	About equal	(2) t test, equal variances	(2) t test, equal variances	Rank-sum test
	Very different		(4) t test, unequal variances	Rank-sum test

Format of This Section

This section presents tests in four of the five cases of Table 15.3, in numbered order: (1) normal (z) test, equal variances; (2) t test, equal variances; (3) normal (z) test, unequal variances; and (4) t test, unequal variances. The rank-sum test was discussed in Sections 6.6 and 14.3.

Not Everyone Agrees with the Logic of Table 15.3

There is some controversy in the field of statistics about using unequal-variance normal and t methods. Although they are approximately correct and acceptably usable, some statisticians prefer to use the rank-sum test whenever variances are unequal.

Assumptions Required

As discussed at the beginning of this chapter, the two-sample means test requires the assumptions that data sampled are independent one from another and that their frequency distributions are approximately normal, i.e., roughly bell-shaped.

Examples

Normal (z) Test, Equal Variances: Is Age a Risk Factor for Prostate Cancer?

This question was addressed in Section 6.8, exemplifying this method. The user is encouraged to review this example.

t Test, Equal Variances: Continuation of This Example

Also addressed in Section 6.8 is the effect had the t test been used rather than the z test of means. The user should continue the review through this example.

Normal, Unequal Variances: Is Prostate Volume a Risk Factor for Prostate Cancer?

Because the population to which we want to generalize is composed of patients with possible prostate cancer, we omit the five patients with known benign prostate hypertrophy (BPH), as they arose from a different population. We ask whether the mean volume for $n_1 = 201$ patients with negative biopsies is different from that for $n_2 = 95$ patients with positive biopsies. The sample sizes are large enough to use methods for normal instead of t, H_0: $\mu_1 = \mu_2$. As it is theoretically possible for either mean to be the larger, H_1: $\mu_1 \neq \mu_2$.

Examining the Normality Assumption

We make a quick plot of the frequency distribution of volumes using a statistical package with normal fits superposed, as shown in Fig 15.1. We see that the plots are roughly normal in shape, but skewed a little to the right. The normality assumption is not unequivocal, but probably is adequate. If we were insecure in making this assumption, we could find additional evidence by testing it using the methods of Section 17.2.

The descriptive data are as follows:

	Sample size	Mean volume (ml)	Standard deviation (ml)
Negative biopsy	201	36.85	17.33
Positive biopsy	95	32.51	13.68

The standard deviations are somewhat, but not extremely, different and the sample sizes are quite different, so that the method for unequal variances is appropriate. Indeed, by using the methods of Section 16.3, the variances test significantly different with $p = 0.01$.

$$\sigma_d = \sqrt{\frac{\sigma_1^2}{n_1} + \frac{\sigma_2^2}{n_2}} = \sqrt{\frac{17.33^2}{201} + \frac{13.68^2}{95}} = 1.86,$$

so that

$$z = (m_1 - m_2)/\sigma_d = (36.85 - 32.51)/1.86 = 2.33.$$

From Table 15.1 or Table A, $z = 2.33$ corresponds to $p = 0.020$, which is statistically significant. We have evidence that the mean prostate volume for patients with negative biopsies is larger than that for those with positive biopsies.

t, Unequal Variances: Using the *t* Test on the Question of Prostate Volume as a Risk Factor in CaP

Would the t test of means have been appropriate in the preceding example? Yes, for large samples, the normal and t tests are a little different. (See the discussion

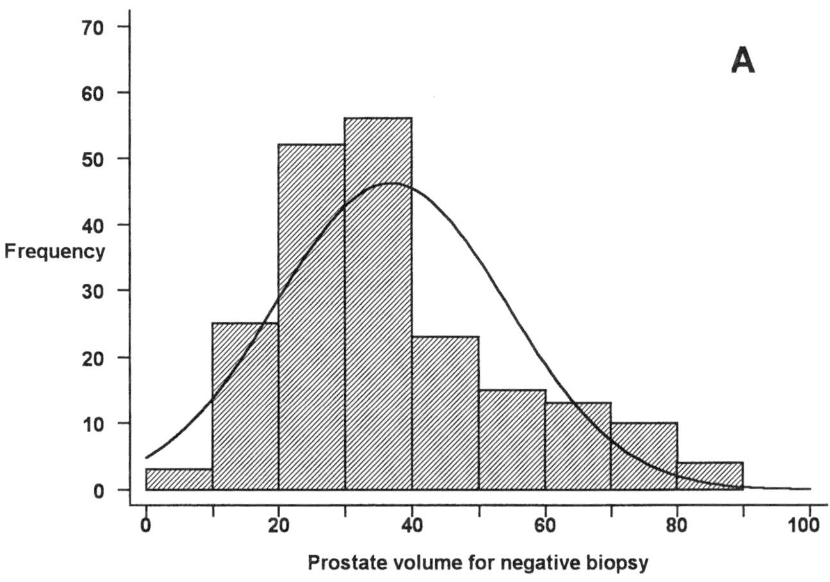

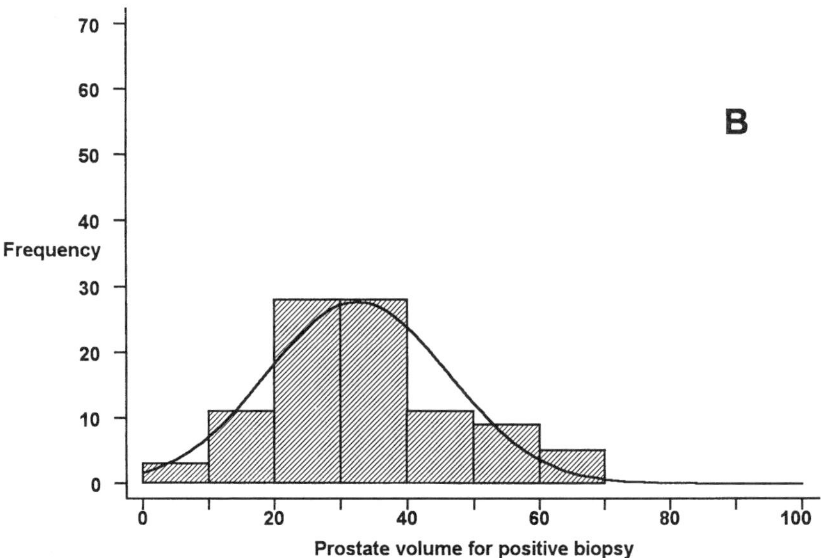

Figure 15.1 A plot of prostate volume distribution by biopsy result for 296 non-BPH patients

in Section 6.8.) We have the same hypotheses and normality assumptions.

$$s_d = \sqrt{\frac{s_1^2}{n_1} + \frac{s_2^2}{n_2}} = \sqrt{\frac{17.33^2}{206} + \frac{13.68^2}{95}} = 1.85$$

$$t = (m_1 - m_2)/s_d = (36.85 - 32.51)/1.85 = 2.35.$$

From Table 15.2 or Table B, $t = 2.35$ for 299 *df* approximately corresponds to $p = 0.02$, which is statistically significant. Because *df* is so large, the normal table gives the same result. An exact calculation on a computer yields $p = 0.019$.

Suppose We Had Used the Rank-Sum Test

Because the equal-variance assumption was violated, we could have used the rank-sum test from Section 6.3 or 14.3, which does not require such an assumption. What we sacrifice to do so is to use a slightly different null hypothesis and lose some of the accuracy of information contained in continuous data. Upon doing so, the p-value turns out to be 0.097. We lost enough accuracy to no longer have probabilistic evidence of a difference. See Section 14.3 for further details.

Method: Tests between Means from Two Samples

We have two samples of size n_1 and n_2. H_0: $\mu_1 = \mu_2$. Select the alternate as H_1: $\mu_1 \neq \mu_2$ (two-tailed α) or as H_1: $\mu_1 < \mu_2$ or H_1: $\mu_1 > \mu_2$ (one-tailed α). We must assume that the basic data are independent from each other and distributed roughly normal in shape. Choose an appropriate α. The test is a normal (z) test or a t test in the form of a standardized difference between means.

Normal (z) Test

m_1 and m_2 are the sample means, respectively. When the σ's that compose σ_d are known theoretically or the samples are large enough that s_d will be close to σ_d, calculate z using Eq. (15.3) and find the p-value from Table A:

$$z = \frac{m_1 - m_2}{\sigma_d}. \tag{15.3}$$

t Test

When the σ's are unknown and the n's are small (say <30, although extreme accuracy may require <50 or <100), calculate t using Eq. (15.4) and find the p-value from Table B:

$$t = \frac{m_1 - m_2}{s_d}. \tag{15.4}$$

What Are the σ_d and s_d in These Formulas?

The standard error of the difference, σ_d or s_d, is calculated according to whether the variances of the two samples are equal or unequal. In addition, the calculation of *df* for s_d also is different. These four cases follow.

Standard Error, z Test, Equal Variances

Variances taken as equal, theoretical σ^2 known *or n* large:

$$\sigma_d = \sigma\sqrt{\frac{1}{n_1} + \frac{1}{n_2}}. \tag{15.5}$$

For large n, an unknown σ_d is approximated by Eq. (15.6), but the normal form of Eq. (15.3) is still used.

Standard Error, t Test, Equal Variances

Variances taken as equal, σ^2 estimated by s^2, small samples:

$$s_d = \sqrt{\left(\frac{1}{n_1} + \frac{1}{n_2}\right)\left[\frac{(n_1 - 1)s_1^2 + (n_2 - 1)s_2^2}{n_1 + n_2 - 2}\right]}, \tag{15.6}$$

with $df = n_1 + n_2 - 2$.

Standard Error, z Test, Unequal Variances

Unequal variances, known σ_1^2 and σ_2^2:

$$\sigma_d = \sqrt{\frac{\sigma_1^2}{n_1} + \frac{\sigma_2^2}{n_2}}. \tag{15.7}$$

For large n_1 and n_2, an unknown σ_d is approximated by Eq. (15.8), but the normal form of Eq. (15.3) is still used.

Standard Error, t Test, Unequal Variances

Unequal variances σ_1^2 and σ_2^2 estimated by s_1^2 and s_2^2 , sample size small:

$$s_d = \sqrt{\frac{s_1^2}{n_1} + \frac{s_2^2}{n_2}}, \tag{15.8}$$

with *df* rounded to the next smallest integer below the rather peculiar expression of Eq. (15.9):

$$\text{approx}\ (df) = \frac{\left(s_1^2/n_1 + s_2^2/n_2\right)^2}{\dfrac{\left(s_1^2/n_1\right)^2}{n_1 - 1} + \dfrac{\left(s_2^2/n_2\right)^2}{n_2 - 1}}. \tag{15.9}$$

Steps to Follow in Testing

Follow these steps for either the z or the t test:

1. Specify null and alternate hypotheses and choose α.
2. Make quick frequency plots of the two samples' basic data to check for normality.
3. In light of the assumption about variances, choose the appropriate form from Table 15.3.
4. Look up the critical value in the appropriate table for the chosen α.
5. Calculate as appropriate the statistic from Eq. (15.3) or (15.4), which will include the standard error calculation from among Eqs. (15.5)–(15.9).
6. Make the decision to accept or reject the null hypothesis.

Additional Examples, z and t Tests, Equal Variances

Comparing the Effectiveness of Two Treatments: z Test

An emergency medicine physician wants to compare the relative effectiveness of a "GI cocktail" (antacid plus viscous lidocaine) (treatment 1) versus IV ranitidine hydrochloride (treatment 2) to treat emergency dyspeptic symptoms as measured on a 1–10 pain scale.[42] He records data as pain before treatment minus pain 45 min after treatment for $n = 28$ patients, randomly assigned to the two treatments; 15 fall into the first group and 13 into the second. Not having data on the pain ratings of the treatments, he uses a known standard deviation of pain difference in the absence of treatment, $\sigma = 1.73$, as an estimate of both s_1 and s_2, H_0: $\mu_1 = \mu_2$. He takes $\alpha = 0.05$, which is two-tailed, because either treatment could be the more effective one, H_1: $\mu_1 \neq \mu_2$. The critical values of z from Table 15.1 or Table A are ± 1.96. Data are as follows:

Treatment 1	6	7	2	5	3	0	3	4	5	6	1	1	1	8	6
Treatment 2	0	1	8	4	7	4	7	7	6	1	0	4	4		

$m_1 = 3.87$ and $m_2 = 4.08$. He substitutes in Eqs. (15.5) and (15.3) to find

$$\sigma_d = \sigma\sqrt{\frac{1}{n_1} + \frac{1}{n_2}} = 1.73\sqrt{\frac{1}{15} + \frac{1}{13}} = 0.6556$$

and

$$z = \frac{m_1 - m_2}{\sigma_d} = \frac{3.87 - 4.08}{0.6556} = -0.32.$$

z is within ± 1.96, so he accepts H_0; his data demonstrated no difference between the treatments. He interpolates from Table A to find $p = 0.75$.

Comparing the Effectiveness of Two Treatments: *t* Test

To continue the example, suppose he decides that the population σ of untreated patients is not an appropriate estimate for treated patients and chooses to estimate it by s_d. He finds $s_1 = 2.50$ and $s_2 = 2.84$. He substitutes in Eq. (15.6) and then Eq. (15.4) to find

$$s_d = \sqrt{\left(\frac{1}{n_1} + \frac{1}{n_2}\right)\left[\frac{(n_1 - 1)s_1^2 + (n_2 - 1)s_2^2}{n_1 + n_2 - 2}\right]}$$

$$= \sqrt{\left(\frac{1}{15} + \frac{1}{13}\right)\left[\frac{14 \times 2.5^2 + 12 \times 2.84^2}{15 + 13 - 2}\right]} = 1.0475$$

and

$$t = \frac{3.87 - 4.08}{-1.0475} = -0.20.$$

From Table 15.2 or Table B, the critical t-value for 26 *df* is 2.056. t is within ± 2.056, so he accepts H_0; no difference between treatments has been shown. From a computer package, the p-value is 0.84.

Exercise 15.2: Equal Variances. Are tympanic temperatures the same for left and right ears? We are investigating the reliability of a certain brand of tympanic thermometer (temperature measured by a sensor inserted into the patient's ear). Sixteen readings (degrees Fahrenheit), eight per ear, were taken on a healthy patient at intervals of 1 min, alternating ears.[55] Data are given in Exercise 8.3. As either ear may be higher, the alternative hypothesis is two-sided. "L" denotes left, "R," right. $m_L = 96.41°F$, $s_L = 0.88°F$, $m_R = 97.86°F$, and $s_R = 1.12°F$. At the $\alpha = 0.05$ level of significance, are the means of the two ears different?

Additional Example, Means Test, Unequal Variances: Comparing Pain Relief from Two Drugs

In 1958, a study[42] compared a new post-operative pain relief drug (treatment 1) to the established Demerol (treatment 2). Data, consisting of reduction in pain measured on a 1–12 rating scale, for patients who completed the protocol were as follows:

Treatment 1	2	0	3	3	0	0	7	1	4	2	2	1	3
Treatment 2	2	6	4	12	5	8	4	0	10	0			

$m_1 = 2.15, s_1 = 1.9513, s_1^2 = 3.8077, m_2 = 5.10, s_2 = 4.0125, s_2^2 = 16.1000.$ The variances seem quite different. (For a test of these variances, see Additional Example in Section 16.3.) We substitute in Eq. (15.8) and then Eq. (15.4) to find

$$s_d = \sqrt{\frac{s_1^2}{n_1} + \frac{s_2^2}{n_2}} = \sqrt{\frac{3.8077}{13} + \frac{16.1000}{10}} = 1.3795$$

and

$$t = \frac{m_1 - m_2}{s_d} = \frac{2.15 - 5.10}{1.3795} = -2.14.$$

The degrees of freedom calculation is a bother in this case. From Eq. (15.9),

$$\text{approx } (df) = \frac{\left(\frac{s_1^2}{n_1} + \frac{s_2^2}{n_2}\right)^2}{\frac{(s_1^2/n_1)^2}{n_1-1} + \frac{(s_2^2/n_2)^2}{n_2-1}} = \frac{\left(\frac{3.0877}{13} + \frac{16.1000}{10}\right)^2}{\frac{\left(\frac{3.0877}{13}\right)^2}{12} + \frac{\left(\frac{16.1000}{10}\right)}{9}} = 11.66.$$

The next smallest integer gives $df = 11$. From Table 15.2 or Table B, the critical value for two-tailed $\alpha = 0.05$ for 11 df is 2.201. Our calculated t is just shy of the critical value, so we do not have quite enough evidence to conclude that the new drug is better than Demerol. A computer package gives the p-value as 0.054.

Exercise 15.3: Unequal Variances. Testing the effectiveness of a vaccine to inhibit HIV. The vaccine was tested by randomizing HIV patients into unvaccinated (treatment 1) and vaccinated (treatment 2) groups and comparing number of HIV per milliliter of blood.[72] Data format was as follows:

Patient no.	1	2	3	⋯	24	25	⋯	44	45	46
No. of virus	134	19,825	38,068	⋯	4,315	8,677	⋯	292	67,638	4,811
Treatmt	1	1	1	⋯	1	2	⋯	2	2	2

$n_1 = 24$, $m_1 = 21{,}457.3$, $s_1 = 29{,}451.98$, $n_2 = 22$, $m_2 = 32{,}174.5$, $s_2 = 50{,}116.50$. The standard deviations appear quite different, so an unequal-variance t test was chosen. (An F test of the variances as in Section 16.3 yielded $p < 0.001$.) At the $\alpha = 0.05$ level, test H_0: $\mu_1 = \mu_2$ against H_1: $\mu_1 \neq \mu_2$.

15.4. THREE OR MORE NEAR-NORMAL SAMPLES: ONE-WAY ANOVA

Example: Do Prostate Cancer's Risks of Low, Uncertain, and High Relate to Age?

PSA often is used to screen patients for risk of cancer. PSA < 4 represents low risk, PSA between 4 and 10 is uncertain, and PSA > 10 is high risk. Could age be associated with these PSA levels? We want to know whether average ages (m_1, m_2, and m_3) are different for these groups. We will label the groups $i = 1, 2, 3$, respectively. H_0: There are no differences among the m_i. The alternate hypothesis is H_1: A difference exists somewhere among the groups.

Satisfaction of Assumptions

Are the assumptions of normality and equal variance (or standard deviation) in the original data satisfied? We make a quick plot of the distributions, shown in Fig. 15.2, and see that they are approximately normal. We also examine the three standard deviations and decide that 9.1, 7.8, and 6.4 are not strikingly different. (If we wanted to be more formal, for example, in preparing for journal publication, we could add evidence to our procedure by testing normality group by group using the methods of Section 17.2 and testing equal variances using the methods of Section 16.4.)

Calculations

We choose $\alpha = 0.05$. Degrees of freedom are $k - 1 = 3 - 1 = 2$ and $n - k = 301 - 3 = 298$. For 2,298 *df*, Table E gives a critical value of F falling between 3.06 and 3.00, approximately 3.03. We calculate (carrying six significant digits)

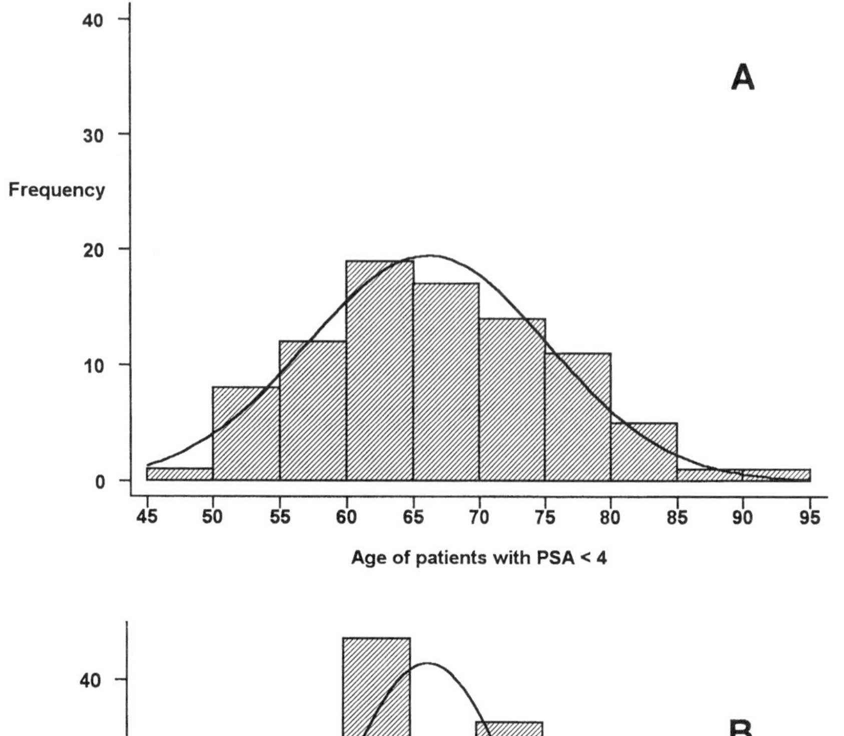

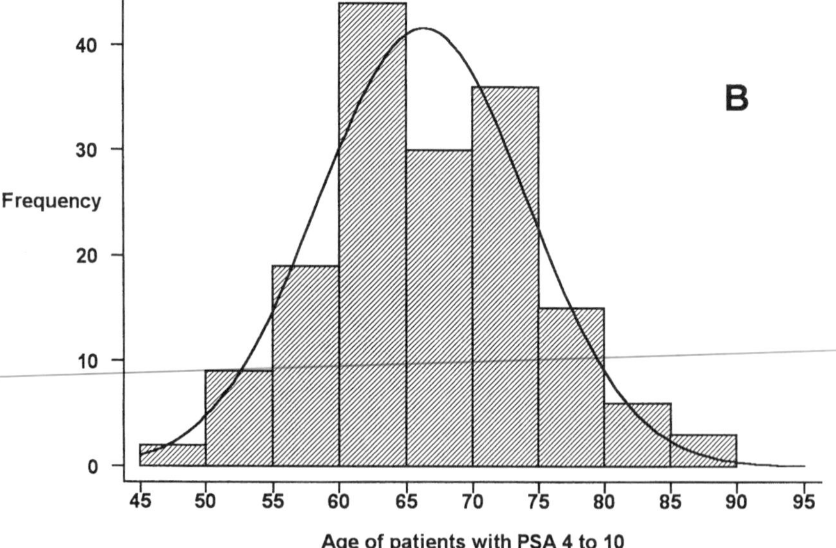

Figure 15.2 A plot of age distributions of 301 patients for groups: PSA $<$ 4, PSA $=$ 4 $-$ 10, and PSA $>$ 10.

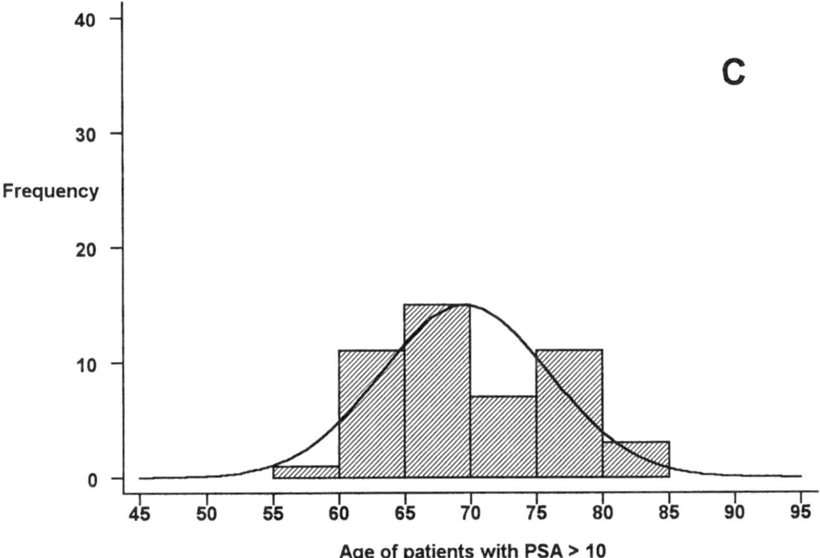

Figure 15.2 *(Continued)*

the following:

$m = 66.7641$	$n_1 = 89$	$m_1 = 66.1124$
$\text{SST} = 19{,}670.3$	$n_2 = 164$	$m_2 = 66.2988$
$s^2 = 65.5675$	$n_3 = 48$	$m_3 = 69.5625$

$$\text{SSM} = \Sigma n_i(m_i - m)^2 = 89(66.1124 - 66.7641)^2 + \cdots = 449.2230$$
$$\text{SSE} = \text{SST} - \text{SSM} = 19{,}221.046$$
$$s_m^2 = \text{SSM}/(k-1) = 449.223/2 = 224.612$$
$$s_e^2 = \text{SSE}/(n-k) = 19{,}221.046/298 = 64.5002$$
$$F = s_m^2/s_e^2 = 224.612/64.5002 = 3.48$$

As 3.48 is greater than critical 3.03, we have evidence that a difference exists among means. From a computer calculation, the p-value is 0.032.

Which among the Possible Mean Differences Account(s) for the Significance?

We still must answer that question. Is it m_1 versus m_2, m_1 versus m_3, and/or m_2 versus m_3? Different software packages will provide a variety of multiple comparison tests. The differences mostly are too subtle to concern the user at this level. In this case, a good method available was the test developed by Henry Scheffé (University of California, Berkeley). We find the p-values for the three pairs, adjusted so that we can interpret them according to our original 5% criterion, to be

	Group 1	Group 2
Group 2	0.985	
Group 3	0.058	0.048

Thus, we find no difference between the averages of groups 1 and 2, a marginal but not quite significant difference between the averages of groups 1 and 3, and a just significant difference between the averages of groups 2 and 3. We conclude that the ages of patients with PSA < 4 and PSA $= 4$–10 are not different, but patients in the PSA > 10 group are on the borderline of being older than the others. The result is not strong and we decide that age probably is not very helpful in anticipating PSA groups.

What Do We Do if We Do Not Have a Statistical Software Package?

If we have no access to statistics software, we can use Bonferroni's method to contrast the pairs. We make two-sample t tests on each pair, but choose the critical t from an adjusted α rather than $\alpha = 5\%$. As the number of possible pairings is $q = 3$, the Bonferroni adjusted $\alpha/q = 0.05/3 = 0.016$. For all pairs, *df* well exceeds 100. In Table 15.2 or Table B, we see that the t-value for *df* a little over 100 lies one-third of the way from two-tailed $\alpha = 0.02$ to two-tailed $\alpha = 0.01$, in the vicinity of 2.4. (A computer tells us that it is exactly 2.393.) Thus, the calculated t's in the tests of mean pairs must exceed 2.4 to drop below the overall 5% level. The t-values obtained from the three t tests, using a format similar to the preceding p-value display, is

	Group 1	Group 2
Group 2	0.17	
Group 3	2.33	2.64

We see that the t for m_1 versus m_2 is far from significant, whereas the other two are a little below and a little above the critical value, respectively. The conclusion is just the same as that made from the Scheffé method.

Method: One-Way Analysis of Variance (ANOVA)

We want to know whether the means from k groups are the same. (For first-time reading, just replace k by three until the material is familiar.) Should we make t tests for each possible pair? No. Each t test would increase the size of the error.

(For two 5% tests, we would have the chance of error on the first *or* the second *or* both, which is 1− the chance of no error on any or $1 - [0.95]^2 = 0.0975$, which is nearly double.) For three groups, our 5% risk of error would become nearly 15% ($1 - [1 - \alpha]^3 = 14.3\%$); the risk of error would exceed 26% for four groups and exceed 40% for five. We need to use a single test to detect any overall difference and, if one difference or more is embedded, find a way to detect which one(s) is significant without increasing the risk of error. This single overall test is called a *one-way analysis of variance (ANOVA)*.

One-Way ANOVA Is Like the *t* Test Generalized to Three or More Means

Our total sample has n observations, mean m, and variance s^2. This sample is divided into k groups having $n_1, n_2, \ldots, n_k$ observations with group means $m_1, m_2, \ldots, m_k$. The method of one-way ANOVA may be thought of as a three-or-more-mean extension of the two-mean t test. It looks very different, but underneath the mechanics is similar. If we took k to be 2, using ANOVA to test two means, we would find that ANOVA's F statistic is just the square of t and the α's come out the same. (The one-way ANOVA bears a relationship to the t test much as the Kruskal–Wallis bears a relationship to the rank-sum test, as seen in Chapter 14.)

Assumptions Required for ANOVA

A legitimate ANOVA, as would be expected from a generalization of the two-sample t test, requires the same three assumptions: (1) the data are independent from each other; (2) the distribution of each group in the original data is normal; and (3) the variances (or standard deviations) are the same for all groups. ANOVA is fairly robust against these assumptions so we need not be stringent about them, but the data should not be extremely far off.

ANOVA Uses a Couple of New Terms: Mean Square (MS) and Sum of Squares (SS)

These are only new names for familiar concepts. The mean square is just the sample variance, and the sum of squares is the numerator in the sample variance calculation. To analyze the variance (in the classic sense of separating it into components), the total sum of squares is separated into its components due to variability among the means and the remaining (*residual* or *error*) component. These component sums of squares are divided by their *df* to obtain variances (or mean squares). The differences-among-means variance (MSM or mean square of means) divided by the error variance (MSE or mean square of error) yields the F statistic. This is because conceptually the differences-among-means component is a variance due to an identified cause and the error variance is a variance

Table 15.4
Relationship of Components of One-Way Analysis of Variance

Source of variability	Sum of squares			Variances or Mean squares	
	Designation	Formula	*df*	Designation	Formula
Mean	SSM	$\Sigma n_i(m_i - m)^2$	$k - 1$	s_m^2 (or MSM)	$\text{SSM}/(k-1)$
Error	SSE	SST − SSM	$n - k$	s_e^2 (or MSE)	$\text{SSE}/(n-k)$
Total	SST	$\Sigma(x_i - m)^2$	$n - 1$	s^2 (or MST)	$\text{SST}/(n-1)$

assumed to be due to random influences alone. If the differences-among-means variance is sufficiently larger than the error variance that it is unlikely to have happened by chance, we say a significant difference exists among the means. The relationships among the various components in the ANOVA are shown in Table 15.4.

Interpretation of ANOVA

In actuality, the error variance is due to random influences *plus* unidentified causal influences. Part of a good study design is to control the variability so that the influence of unidentified causes is small. The test is conservative in that a significant outcome implies that the numerator variance (MSM) is larger than random *plus* other causal variability, so that it certainly is larger than random variability alone. If the design is not controlled carefully, large unidentified causes may enter and an outcome that would have been significant when tested against random variability alone will not show its significance. Thus, a significant result allows the investigator to conclude a difference, but a nonsignificant result does not allow the investigator to conclude no difference; it may only be said that significance *has not been shown*.

Most statistical software packages will perform a one-way ANOVA upon command. The logic of a one-way ANOVA follows these steps:

1. Pose H_0: There are no differences among the means, and H_1: There are one or more differences somewhere among the means.
2. Verify approximate satisfaction of the assumptions: (a) normal distributions and (b) equal variances in the original data of the k groups.
3. Choose the error probability α, such as 5%, you are willing to accept and look up the associated critical value of F, named F_0, in Table E for $k - 1$ (numerator) and $n - k$ (denominator) *df*.
4. Calculate m and s^2 for the total sample as usual, noting the sum of squares for the total (SST) before dividing by $n - 1$.
5. Calculate the means m_i for the k groups.

6. Calculate the sum of squares for means (SSM) by squaring each difference $m_i - m$ and adding them.
7. Calculate the sum of squares for error (SSE) by SST − SSM.
8. Calculate s_m^2 (or MSM) = SSM/($k - 1$) and s_e^2 (or MSE) = SSE/($n - k$).
9. Calculate F = MSM/MSE = s_m^2/s_e^2.
10. Compare the calculated F with F_0. If $F < F_0$, do not reject H_0; if $F > F_0$, reject H_0.

Finding the Mean Difference(s) That Caused the Significance: Multiple Comparisons Tests

Suppose we reject H_0 and conclude that differences exist among the group means. Which are different and which are not? Recall that we cannot just make t tests of all possible pairings. Methods testing the several subgroups without increasing α are called *multiple comparisons* tests (sometimes termed *post hoc* comparisons). Several, named after their developers, have been published, including Duncan, Scheffé, Tukey, Newman-Keuls, Šidák, Bonferroni, and perhaps others. They have different theoretical justifications, but do not give very different results; in the Bonferroni and Šidák, slightly greater differences are required for significance to appear because they are more conservative tests. The Bonferroni is the simplest to use and so will be demonstrated here when the procedure is carried out by hand. This choice does not indicate preference.

Multiple Comparisons Using Statistical Software

When statistical software is used to make a multiple comparisons test, the outcome is given as p-values adjusted so that each may be compared with our chosen overall α. Different software packages display the results using various schemes. One common display type is presented here; the user who understands it can follow other schemes with little difficulty. The display forms a table in which the group names are shown as both columns and rows, providing a position for every possible pair. (Of course, positions in which row and column show the same group are omitted.) If we denote the p-value for the pair i and j as p_{ij}, it appears as follows:

	Mean 1	Mean 2	...	Mean $k-1$
Mean 2	p_{12}			
Mean 3	p_{13}	p_{23}		
⋮	⋮	⋮		
Mean k	p_{1k}	p_{2k}	...	$p_{k,k-1}$

We then identify the pairs for which the displayed p-value exceeds the overall α.

Multiple Comparisons Carried Out by Hand

Sometimes a requirement for multiple comparisons arises when no statistical software is available or when using methods that the software does not include. Without much effort, we can use the Bonferroni method to contrast the pairs. We make two-sample t tests on each pair, but choose the critical t from an adjusted α rather than from $\alpha = 5\%$. The number of pairs is $q = k(k-1)/2$ and the Bonferroni adjusted α is α/q. We find the *df* for each pair's t test. In Table B, we obtain a critical t-value for that *df*, using α/q instead of α and interpolating as required. The calculated t's in the test of the pair's mean must exceed that critical t-value. The t-values obtained from the q t tests may be displayed in a format similar to the preceding p-value display, each compared with its critical t one by one.

Additional Example: Does Steroid Decrease Edema Following Rhinoplasty?[7] If So, What Level Should Be Used?

Following rhinoplasty, swelling may cause deformity during healing. Steroids may decrease the swelling, but the required level of steroid has not been known. $n = 50$ rhinoplasty patients were randomized into $k = 5$ groups of increasing steroid level having $n_1 = \cdots = n_5 = 10$. Swelling reduction was measured by MRIs before and after administration of the steroid.[7] H_0: $\mu_1 = \mu_2 = \mu_3 = \mu_4 = \mu_5$ was to be tested using $\alpha = 0.05$. The first few data are given in Table 15.5. The total mean (all data pooled) was $m = 5.52$ and total variance $s^2 = 4.2074$. The following calculations are needed:

$$\text{SST} = (n-1)s^2 = 49 \times 4.2074 = 206.16,$$

$$\text{SSM} = 10[(3.77-5.52)^2 + (5-5.52)^2 + \cdots + (6.35-5.52)^2] = 56.57,$$

$$\text{SSE} = \text{SST} - \text{SSM} = 206.16 - 56.57 = 149.59.$$

Table 15.5

Data on Edema Following Rhinoplasty

Swelling reduction (ml):	Level 1	Level 2	Level 3	Level 4	Level 5
Patients 1–5	1.6	4.4	5.5	4.0	8.0
Patients 6–10	2.3	5.8	6.4	8.3	6.2
Patients 11–15	2.3	6.4	6.9	5.8	3.1
⋮	⋮	⋮	⋮	⋮	⋮
Means m_i	3.77	5.00	5.67	6.79	6.35

Table 15.6
ANOVA Table for Rhinoplasty Data

Source	SS (sum of squares)	*df*	MS (mean square)	Calculated F
Mean	SSM = 56.57	4	MSM = 56.57/4 = 14.14	MSM/MSE = 4.26
Error	SSE = 149.57	45	MSE = 149.57/45 = 3.32	
Total	SST = 206.16	49	($s^2 = 4.2074$)	

Table 15.6 gives the ANOVA table. From Table E, the critical $F_{4,45\,df} = 2.58$. The calculated $F = 4.26$ is much larger, so H_0 is rejected; steroid level does affect swelling. From a statistical software package, the calculated $p = 0.005$.

Identifying the Steroid Dosage

Steroid level affects swelling, but which level should be selected for clinical use? A Bonferroni multiple comparisons procedure using a statistical software package yields the following significance levels (p-values), adjusted to be interpreted according to the usual 5% α, although the computer calculations were made so that the true α's used accumulated to 5% in total.

	Level 1	Level 2	Level 3	Level 4
Level 2	1.000			
Level 3	0.243	1.000		
Level 4	0.006	0.333	1.000	
Level 5	0.028	1.000	1.000	1.000

(The p-values showing 1.000 really are slightly less, but round to 1.000.) We see that level 1 is significantly worse than levels 4 or 5; we reject level 1 as an acceptable steroid level. The other levels are not significantly different. Any one of levels 2–5 may be chosen for clinical use. By examining the means, we see that level 4 gives the greatest reduction in swelling, so one would tend to choose level 4 pending additional information.

Exercise 15.4: Are Animals Supplied for Experimentation Equally Resistant to Parasites? In a study on the control of parasites,[41] rats were injected with 500 larvae each of the parasitic worm *Nippostrongylus muris*. Ten days later, they were sacrificed and the number of adult worms counted. The question arose, "Is there a batch-to-batch difference in resistance to parasite infestation by groups of rats received from the supplier?" $k = 4$ batches of $n_i = 5$ rats each were tested.

Data were as follows:

	Group 1	Group 2	Group 3	Group 4
	279	378	172	381
	338	275	335	346
	334	412	335	340
	198	265	282	471
	303	286	250	318
Mean m_i =	290.4	323.2	274.8	371.2

Total mean $m = 314.9$ and total variance $s^2 = 4799.358$. At the $\alpha = 0.05$ level of significance, test H_0: $\mu_1 = \mu_2 = \mu_3 = \mu_4$.

15.5. EQUIVALENCE TESTING

CONCEPT

In hypothesis testing, we establish a null hypothesis of no difference and use a test to evaluate if there is sufficient evidence to reject it. A very common question asked is if a new treatment is superior on average to a placebo (addressed in Chapter 5 and previously in this chapter), in which case the null hypothesis is one of no difference between means. Suppose, in contrast, we ask if a new treatment is as good on average as an established one, perhaps because it is less invasive or less costly. In this case the null hypothesis states: The difference in means equals or exceeds a magnitude judged to represent clinical inferiority. The alternative hypothesis states: The mean difference is less than the clinically important amount and thus the treatments are deemed equivalent. This recent development in statistical methodology has been termed *equivalence testing* or *bioequivalence testing*. Only one case will be treated here.

EXAMPLE

A method of measuring cardiac index (CI; cardiac output normalized for body surface area) is thermodilution (TD), in which a catheter is placed in the heart. A proposed noninvasive method is bioimpedance (BI), in which an instrument attached to the patient's skin by electric leads indicates CI. We judge BI to be equivalent if, on average, it falls within 20% of the TD mean, known to be 2.75 ($1/\text{min/m}^2$). Twenty percent of 2.75 is $0.55 = \delta$, so that H_0: $|\mu_T - \mu_B| = |\Delta| = 0.55$ and H_1: $|\mu_T - \mu_B| = |\Delta| < 0.55$. We sample $n = 96$ patients[61] and find BI has mean $m_B = 2.68$ (1/min/m^2). $D = 2.75 - 2.68 = 0.07$ with standard deviation $s = 0.26$, so that $s_D = s\sqrt{n} = 0.0265$. From Table B, $t_{0.975}$ for 95 $df = 1.984$. Substituting, we find $|D| + t_{1-\alpha}s_D = 0.07 + 1.984 \times 0.0265 = 0.1226$. Because $0.1226 < 0.55$, the null hypothesis is contradicted and we conclude that mean BI is equivalent to mean TD.

METHOD

Let δ represent the clinically important difference; μ_E and μ_N, the population means of the established (E) and the new (N) treatments; and Δ, the difference between the means. H_0: $\Delta = \delta$ and H_1: $\Delta < \delta$ are hypotheses for a one-sided test asking if $\mu_N < \mu_E$. Similarly, H_0: $|\Delta| = \delta$ and H_1: $|\Delta| < \delta$ are hypotheses for a two-sided test asking if $\mu_N \neq \mu_E$. Let n denote sample size and m_N the sample estimate of μ_N. Then $D = \mu_E - m_N$ estimates Δ, s_D is its standard error, and our test statistic with $n-1$ *df* becomes $t = D/s_D$ or $t = |D|/s_D$, depending on one- or two-sidedness. For a one-sided test, if $D + t_{1-\alpha}s_D \geq \delta$ the null hypothesis is not rejected and the new treatment is not demonstrated to be equivalent to the established one. If $D + t_{1-\alpha}s_D < \delta$, the null hypothesis is rejected and the new treatment is considered equivalent. For a two-sided test, replace D by $|D|$ and $1-\alpha$ by $1-\alpha/2$.

ANSWERS TO EXERCISES

15.1. Substitution in Eq. (15.2) (with renamed elements) yields $t = (d-0)/s_d = 1.58/(1.23/\sqrt{10}) = 4.06$. From Table B, the critical value for a 5% two-tailed t with 9 *df* is 2.26. As 4.06 is much larger, we reject H_0; Laevo is more effective. A statistical software package gives the p-value as 0.001.

15.2. Equal Variances. From Table 15.3, the sample sizes are small, σ's are only estimated, and the standard deviations are not significantly different (refer to Exercise 16.3), so we choose a two-sample t test with equal standard deviations. From Eq. (15.6),

$$s_d = \sqrt{\left(\frac{1}{n_1} + \frac{1}{n_2}\right)\left[\frac{(n_1-1)s_1^2 + (n_2-1)s_2^2}{n_1+n_2-2}\right]}$$

$$= \sqrt{\left(\frac{1}{8} + \frac{1}{8}\right)\left[\frac{7 \times 0.88^2 + 7 \times 1.12^2}{8+8-2}\right]} = 0.5036.$$

From Eq. (15.4),

$$t = \frac{m_1 - m_2}{s_d} = \frac{96.41 - 97.86}{0.5036} = -2.88.$$

From Table A, the p-value for a z-value of 2.88 standard deviations from the mean is 0.002. We have strong evidence to infer a difference in mean readings between ears.

15.3. Unequal Variances. By substituting in Eq. (15.8) and then Eq. (15.4), we find

$$s_d = \sqrt{\frac{s_1^2}{n_1} + \frac{s_2^2}{n_2}} = \sqrt{\frac{29{,}451.98^2}{24} + \frac{50{,}116.50^2}{22}} = 12{,}260.06$$

and

$$t = \frac{21{,}457.3 - 32{,}174.5}{12{,}260.06} = -0.874.$$

To find the critical value of t, we need df. By substituting in Eq. (15.9), we find

$$\text{approx}\ (df) = \frac{\left(\frac{s_1^2}{n_1} + \frac{s_2^2}{n_2}\right)^2}{\frac{\left(s_1^2/n_1\right)^2}{n_1-1} + \frac{\left(s_2^2/n_2\right)^2}{n_2-1}} = \frac{\left(\frac{29{,}451.98^2}{24} + \frac{50{,}116.50^2}{22}\right)}{\frac{\left(\frac{29{,}451.98^2}{24}\right)^2}{23} + \frac{\left(\frac{50{,}116.50^2}{22}\right)^2}{21}} = 33.35.$$

From Table B, the critical value of t for a two-tailed 5% α for 34 df is ± 2.03; -0.874 is not outside the ± 2.03 critical values, so H_0 is accepted. From a statistical software package, $p = 0.195$.

15.4. From the formulae in Table 15.4, calculate SST $= (n-1)s^2 = 19 \times 4799.358 = 91{,}187.805$, SSM $= 5[(291.4 - 314.9)^2 + (323.2 - 314.9)^2 + (274.8 - 314.9)^2 + (371.2 - 314.9)^2 = 27,234.20$, and SSE $=$ SST $-$ SSM $= 91{,}187.80 - 27{,}234.20 = 63{,}953.60$. Table 15.7 gives the ANOVA table. From Table E, the critical $F_{3,16df} = 3.24$. The calculated $F = 2.27$ is smaller, so H_0 is accepted; mean parasite infestation does not differ from batch to batch. (When F is not significant, no subordinate pair will be significant, so a multiple comparisons procedure is unnecessary.) From a statistical software package, the calculated $p = 0.120$.

Table 15.7

ANOVA Table

Source	SS (sum of squares)	df	MS (mean square)	Calculated F
Mean	SSM = 27234.20	$k - 1 = 3$	MSM = 27234.20/3 = 9078.07	MSM/MSE = 2.27
Error	SSE = 63953.60	$n - k = 16$	MSE = 63953.60/16 = 3997.10	
Total	SST = 91187.80	$n - 1 = 19$	($s^2 = 4799.36$)	

Chapter 16

Common Tests on Continuous Data Variances

16.1. BASICS OF TESTS ON VARIABILITY

Why Should We Be Interested in Testing Variability?

The average does not tell the whole story. As a metaphor, consider two bowmen shooting at a target. Bowman A always hits the bullseye. Half of bowman B's arrows fall to the left of the bullseye and half to the right. Both bowmen have the same average, but bowman A is the better shot. As an example in medicine, small amounts of two orally administered drugs reach a remote organ. The mean level is the same for both, but drug B is more variable (has a larger standard deviation) than drug A. In some cases, too little of drug B gets through to be effective and in other cases a dangerously high level gets through. Thus, the less variable drug is the better.

A Test of Variability Serves Two Main Purposes

(1) The need to detect differences in variability per se was just illustrated, and (2) it tests the assumption of equal variances used in means testing.

How Are Two Variances Compared?

In dealing with variability, we usually use the *variance*, which is the square of the standard deviation. The decisions made using it are the same, and the difficult mathematics associated with square roots are avoided in the derivation of probability functions. To compare the relative size of two variances, we take their ratio, adjusted for degrees of freedom (*df*). The tabulated critical value of the ratio for statistical significance also depends on the *df*.

A Sample Variance May Be Compared with a Population Variance or Another Sample Variance

If we compare a sample variance s^2 against a population variance σ^2 (the topic of Section 16.2), we find the significance level of $\chi^2 = df \times s^2/\sigma^2$ in chi-square Tables C or D for $df = n - 1$. If we compare two sample variances s_1^2 and s_2^2 (the topic of Section 16.3), assigning subscript 1 to the larger, we find the significance level of $F = s_1^2/s_2^2$ in Table E. This table involves *df* for both variances, $df_1 = n_1 - 1$ and $df_2 = n_2 - 1$.

A Negative Test Result Must Be Interpreted Carefully

Tests of variance often are useful in assessing the validity of the equal-variance assumption required for normal (z) and t tests and the analysis of variance, but we must understand the limitation of this use. A significant difference between variances implies the conclusion that they are different, whereas, like all tests of hypotheses, a negative result implies only that no difference has been demonstrated, not that one does not exist. However, a negative result provides some evidence of no difference and represents all the evidence we have, which leads us to carry out the analysis as if the variances had in fact been shown to be the same.

16.2. SINGLE SAMPLES

Example: Is the PSA Variance of the First 10 Urology Patients (Table DB1.1) Different from That of the Remaining 291?

Let us follow the steps given in the following Methods paragraph. We assume normality: we have seen that PSA data are roughly bell-shaped, although right-skewed. We believe the deviations are not so great as to invalidate this rather robust test. H_0: $\sigma_0^2 = \sigma^2$. We have no reason to anticipate whether s^2 should be larger or smaller than σ^2, so we use H_1: $\sigma_0^2 \neq \sigma^2$ and, if α is chosen as 5%, must allow a 2.5% α for each tail. The remaining 291 PSAs form a sample large

Table 16.1
A Fragment of Table D, Chi-Square Distribution, Left Tail[a]

α (area in left tail)	0.0005	0.001	0.005	0.01	0.025	0.05	0.10
$df = 9$	0.97	1.15	1.73	2.09	2.70	3.33	4.17

[a] Selected χ^2 values (distances above zero) are given for 9 *df* for various α, the area under the curve in the left tail.

enough that its variance has closely converged to the population variance, so we may use the calculated variance as σ^2. This implies that we will test s^2/σ^2, which, when multiplied by *df*, is distributed χ^2. The left-tail critical value must be found from Table D and the right from Table C, because the chi-square distribution is not symmetric like z or t. $df = 10 - 1 = 9$. Table 16.1 gives a fragment of Table D. From Table 16.1 or Table D, $\alpha = 0.025$ and $df = 9$ yields $\chi^2 = 2.70$. If $df \times s^2/\sigma^2 < 2.70$, we reject H_0. Similarly, the same inputs into Table C or Table 16.2 yield $\chi^2 = 19.02$; if $df \times s^2/\sigma^2 > 19.02$, we reject H_0. Now we can calculate our statistic. For the first 10 data, $s^2 = 1.61^2 = 2.59$. For the remaining 291 data, $\sigma^2 = 17.19^2 = 295.50$. $\chi^2 = df \times s^2/\sigma^2 = 9 \times 2.59/295.50 = 0.0789$, which is far less than 2.70, the left critical value. We reject H_0 and conclude that the first 10 patients have smaller variability than the remaining 291. Indeed, from Table D, the χ^2 for an 0.0005 α with 9 *df* is 0.97. As $0.0789 < 0.97$, we have a less than 0.001 chance of error by rejecting H_0.

Method: Test of One Sample Variance

We ask whether the variance σ_0^2 of a population from which we draw a sample is the same as a theoretical variance σ^2. σ_0^2 is estimated by the sample variance s^2. We assume that the sample data are distributed normal. σ^2 may be known from some theory or may be estimated by a very large sample, because the sample variance converges on the population variance as the sample size grows large. The null hypothesis is that s^2 is drawn from the population having variance σ^2, or H_0: $\sigma_0^2 = \sigma^2$, and the ratio s^2/σ^2 should be different from 1 only by a random influence. The statistic calculated is

$$\chi^2 = \frac{df \times s^2}{\sigma^2}. \tag{16.1}$$

This is a relatively simple test except for one aspect: the test statistic is distributed chi-square, which is not symmetric, so that a different table must be used for each tail. The alternate hypothesis H_1 specifies the probability table(s) to be used. For a chosen α, the cases are as follows:

(a) $\sigma_0^2 > \sigma^2$: the χ^2 critical value for α is found from Table C.
(b) $\sigma_0^2 < \sigma^2$: the χ^2 critical value for α is found from Table D.
(c) $\sigma_0^2 \neq \sigma^2$: split α; the left χ^2 critical value for $\alpha/2$ is found from Table D and the right χ^2 critical value for $\alpha/2$ is found from Table C.

The steps to be are as follows:

1. Verify that the sample frequency distribution is roughly normal.
2. Specify null and alternate hypotheses and choose α.
3. Identify the theoretical σ.
4. Look up the critical value(s) for the chosen α in the appropriate χ^2 table(s).
5. Calculate the statistic from Eq. (16.1): $\chi^2 = df \times s^2/\sigma^2$.
6. Make the decision to accept or reject the null hypothesis.

Additional Example: A Treatment for Dyspepsia in the ED Is Effective on Average, But Is It Too Variable?

In the Additional Example of Section 15.2, an emergency medicine physician tested the effectiveness of a "GI cocktail" (antacid plus viscous lidocaine) to treat emergency dyspeptic symptoms as measured on a 1–10 pain scale.[42] He concluded that the treatment was effective on average, but was it more variable? This question implies a one-tailed test. He will sample the treatment for 15 patients, so $df = 14$. Table 16.2 provides a portion of Table C. From Table 16.2 or Table C with 14 *df*, the critical value of χ^2 for $\alpha = 0.05$ is 23.69. The population standard deviation for the scoring difference upon being seen minus that after a specified number of minutes for a large number of patients without treatment was $\sigma = 1.73$. He treated $n = 15$ patients, measuring the difference in pain before minus after treatment. Data were 6, 7, 2, 5, 3, 0, 3, 4, 5, 6, 1, 1, 1, 8, 6. He calculated $m = 3.87$ and $s = 2.23$. He tested the variance of his sample ($s^2 = 4.9729$) against the

Table 16.2

A Portion of Table C, Chi-Square Distribution, Right Tail[a]

α (area in right tail)	0.10	0.05	0.025	0.01	0.005	0.001	0.0005
$df = 2$	4.61	5.99	7.38	9.21	10.60	13.80	15.21
4	7.78	9.49	11.14	13.28	14.86	18.46	20.04
9	14.68	16.92	19.02	21.67	23.59	27.86	29.71
14	21.06	23.69	26.12	29.14	31.32	36.12	38.14

[a] Selected χ^2 values (distances above zero) are given for various *df* and for selected α, the area under the curve in the right tail.

variance of untreated patients ($\sigma^2 = 2.9929$) at the $\alpha = 0.05$ level of significance. By substituting in Eq. (16.1), he found

$$\chi^2 = \frac{df \times s^2}{\sigma^2} = \frac{14 \times 4.9729}{2.9929} = 23.26.$$

The calculated χ^2 is just less than the critical value, although it is near the borderline. We have to conclude that the treated patients' pain has not been shown to be more variable than that of untreated patients, although we would be better satisfied if we took a larger sample to gain more confidence. From a statistical software package, $p = 0.056$.

Exercise 16.1: Is the Variability of Readings from a Tympanic Thermometer Too Large? We are investigating the reliability of a certain brand of tympanic thermometer (temperature measured by a sensor inserted into the patient's ear). Sixteen readings (degrees Fahrenheit) were taken on a healthy patient at intervals of 1 min.[55] (Data are given in Exercise 14.2.) In our clinical judgment, a reliable thermometer will be no more than 1°F off 95% of the time. This implies that 1°F is about 2σ, so that $\sigma = 0.5$°F. $s = 1.238$. At the $\alpha = 0.05$ level of significance, is the variability of the tympanic thermometer reading on a patient unacceptably large?

16.3. TWO SAMPLES

Example: Is the Nonrepresentativeness in the PSAs Only from the First 10 or Also from Other Sections of the Sample?

In the Example of Section 16.2, we concluded that the PSA variances (and therefore standard deviation) for the first 10 and the remaining 291 patients were quite different. We want to know whether the first 10 per se are nonrepresentative or whether the variability increased gradually or at a later point. Let us test the variance of the first 10 against each successive 10 and list the result. The normal data assumption remains. By using "first" to denote the first sample of 10 and "later" to denote each later sample, H_0: $\sigma^2_{\text{first}} = \sigma^2_{\text{later}}$ and H_1: $\sigma^2_{\text{first}} < \sigma^2_{\text{later}}$. We choose $\alpha = 5\%$. Table 16.3 is a portion of Table E. From Table 16.3 or Table E, we find that the critical value of F for 9,9 df is 3.18. The F ratio must exceed 3.18 to become significant.

Calculations

The second 10 (numbers 11–20) yielded a standard deviation of 2.11. $F = (2.11)^2/(1.61)^2 = 4.45/2.59 = 1.72$. As $1.72 < 3.18$, we conclude that the variances (and, of course, the standard deviations) are not different for the first and

Table 16.3

A Portion of Table E, F Distribution[a]

		Numerator *df*		
		8	9	10
Denominator *df*	9	3.23	3.18	3.14
	10	3.07	3.02	2.98
	11	2.95	2.90	2.85
	12	2.85	2.80	2.75

[a] Selected distances (F) are given for $\alpha = 5\%$, the area under the curve in the positive tail. Numerator *df* appears in column headings, denominator *df* in row headings, and F in the table body.

second sets of 10. A list of comparisons of the first 10 with successive samples of 10, compiled using the same numerical procedures, is as follows:

Sample numbers	*F* ratio
11–20	1.72
21–30	1.20
31–40	0.92
41–50	1794.06
51–60	11.14
61–70	27.28
71–80	511.72
81–90	61.11
⋮	⋮

Interpretation

We note that the 41–50 set yielded a huge F. By examining the data, we find that PSA = 221 for patient 47! This turned out to be a useful way to discover *outliers*, those data so far different from the bulk of data that we suspect they arose from a unique population. However, even if we dropped the 221 reading, F would equal 8.88 for the remaining data, which is still significant. It appears that there are patterns of nonhomogeneity scattered throughout the data.

Method: Test of Two Sample Variances

Are two population variances, or standard deviations, the same? We assume that the data of both samples are distributed normal. H_0: $\sigma_1^2 = \sigma_2^2$. Because we test the larger variance over the smaller, Table E may be used for any H_1. Choose α.

Sample 1 has sample variance s_1^2 calculated from n_1 observations and sample 2, s_2^2 from n_2, where the number 1 is assigned to the larger variance. The statistic is

$$F = s_1^2/s_2^2, \tag{16.2}$$

with $n_1 - 1$ and $n_2 - 1$ *df*. Look up the critical value of F in Table E or calculate the p-value with a statistical software package. The steps are as follows:

1. Verify that the data of each sample are roughly normal.
2. State the null and alternate hypotheses (H_0: $\sigma_1^2 = \sigma_2^2$ and H_1: $\sigma_1^2 > \sigma_2^2$); choose α.
3. Look up the critical value for the chosen α in Table E.
4. Calculate the statistic in Eq. (16.2), $F = s_1^2/s_2^2$ (where s_1^2 designates the larger variance).
5. Make the decision to accept or reject the null hypothesis.

Additional Example: Compare the Variability of Two Pain Relief Drugs

In 1958, a study[42] compared a new post-operative pain relief drug (treatment 1) to the established Demerol (treatment 2). Data consisted of reduction in pain measured on a 1–12 rating scale. For patients who completed the protocol, data were as follows:

Treatment 1	2	6	4	12	5	8	4	0	10	0			
Treatment 2	2	0	3	3	0	0	7	1	4	2	2	1	3

In order to test the means, we need to know whether we can assume equal variances. We want to test H_0: $\sigma_1^2 = \sigma_2^2$ against H_1: $\sigma_1^2 \neq \sigma_2^2$ at $\alpha = 0.05$. $m_1 = 5.10$, $s_1 = 4.0125$, $s_1^2 = 16.1000$, $m_2 = 2.15$, $s_2 = 1.9513$, $s_2^2 = 3.8077$. We substitute in Eq. (16.2) to find

$$F = s_1^2/s_2^2 = 16.10/3.81 = 4.23.$$

From Table 16.3 or Table E, the critical value of F for 9,12 *df* is 2.80. As 4.23 is much larger, the variances (and, of course, the standard deviations) are significantly different. From a statistical software package, $p = 0.012$. A test of means must use either the unequal-variances form of the t test or the rank-sum test from Sections 6.6 or 14.3.

Exercise 16.2: Is the Variability of the Tympanic Thermometer Readings the Same in Both Ears? We are investigating the reliability of a certain brand of tympanic thermometer (temperature measured by a sensor inserted into the patient's ear). Sixteen readings (degrees Fahrenheit), eight per ear, were taken on a healthy patient at intervals of 1 min, alternating ears.[55] (Data are given in Exercise 14.2.) We want to test the hypothesis that the mean temperatures are the same in the left ("L") and right ("R") ears (Exercise 15.3), but we want evidence that the equal-variance t test is appropriate. $m_{\mathrm{L}} = 96.41°\mathrm{F}$, $s_{\mathrm{L}} = 0.88°\mathrm{F}$, $m_{\mathrm{R}} = 97.86°\mathrm{F}$, and $s_{\mathrm{R}} = 1.12°\mathrm{F}$. At the $\alpha = 0.05$ level of significance, are the variances (standard deviations) of the two ears different?

16.4. THREE OR MORE SAMPLES

Example: Can We Assume Equal Variances in the Test of Classifying Patients by Risk of CaP?

Of our sample of 301 patients, 19 are known to have cancer already and therefore are not in the risk population, so we must delete them to obtain an unbiased population, leaving 282. Three groups remain, identified by a clinical decision algorithm: those whose risk of prostate cancer is (1) low, (2) moderate, and (3) high. We note that mean prostate specific antigen density (PSAD) seems quite different for the three groups: 0.07, 0.21, and 0.35. We want to test this difference using a one-way ANOVA, but require the assumption of equal variances, which can be examined by Bartlett's test.

Is the Normal Assumption Satisfied?

We make quick plots of the PSAD frequency distributions for the three groups, as shown in Fig. 16.1. We are not very happy with the one or two extremely high PSAD values in each group. It would be advisable to go to rank methods and perform a Kruskal–Wallis test from Section 14.4. However, we will continue with Bartlett's test for the sake of illustration.

Calculations

H_0: $\sigma_1^2 = \sigma_2^2 = \sigma_3^2$. H_1: not H_0. We choose $\alpha = 0.05$. The 0.05 critical value from Table 16.2 or Table C for 2 *df* is 5.99; if $M > 5.99$, we reject H_0. We obtain the following values, carrying six significant digits in the calculations (so that we can take precise square roots). The s_i^2 are just the ordinary variances (standard deviations before taking the square root). Those variances and the associated n's are as follows:

$n_1 = 89$	$s_1^2 = 0.00557546$
$n_2 = 164$	$s_2^2 = 0.0139188$
$n_3 = 29$	$s_3^2 = 0.0227769$

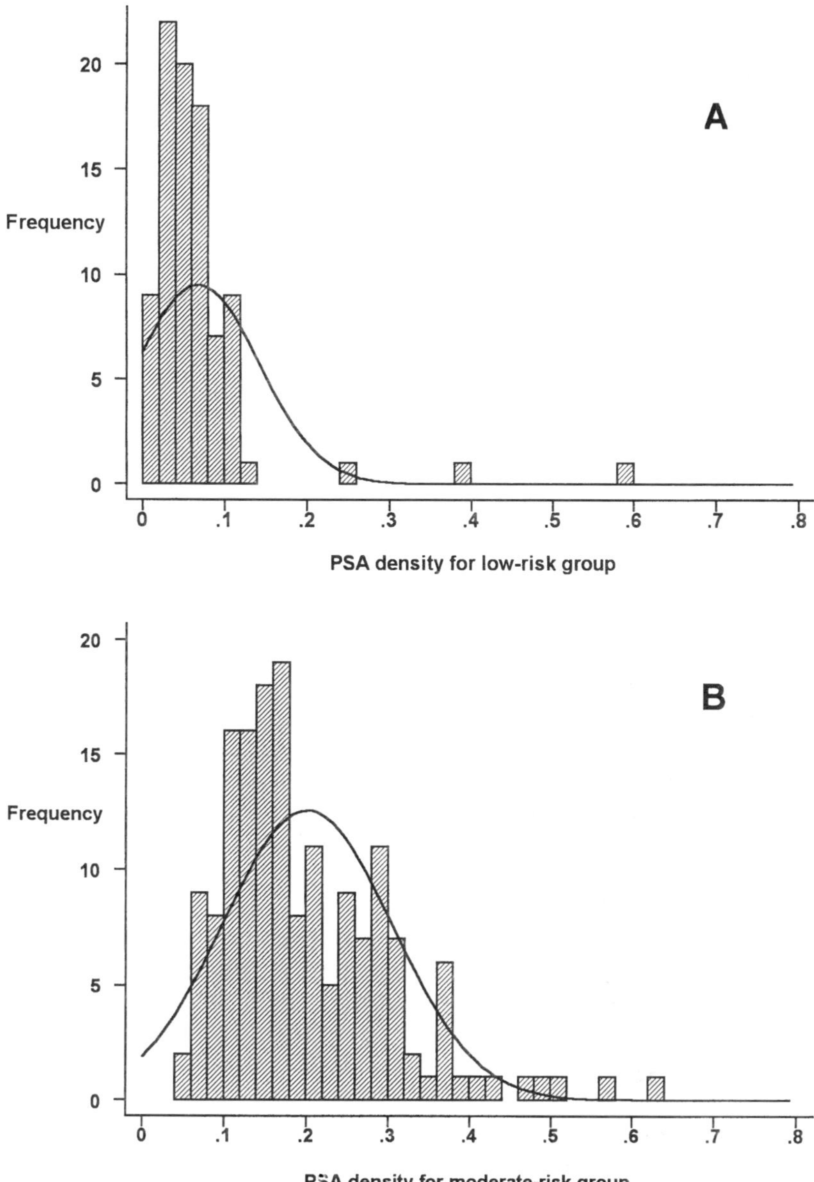

Figure 16.1 A plot of PSAD distributions of 282 patients for groups of low, moderate, and high risk of prostate cancer.

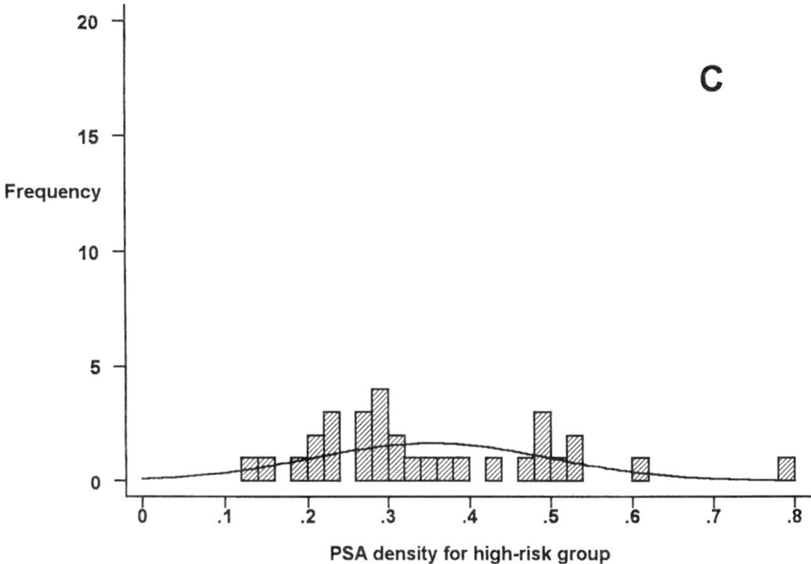

Figure 16.1 *(Continued)*

Substitution in Eq. (16.4) from yields (summing over the index i)

$$s^2 = \frac{\sum(n_i - 1)s_i^2}{n - k}$$

$$= \frac{88 \times 0.00557546 + 163 \times 0.0139188 + 29 \times 0.0227769}{282 - 3} = 0.0122578.$$

Finally, substitution in Eq. (16.5) yields

$$M = \frac{(n-k)\ln(s^2) - \sum(n_i - 1)\ln\left(s_i^2\right)}{1 + \frac{1}{3(k-1)}\left(\sum \frac{1}{n_i - 1} - \frac{k}{n-k}\right)}$$

$$= \frac{279\ln(0.0122578) - 88\ln(0.00557546) - \cdots - 28\ln(0.0227769)}{1 + \frac{1}{6}\left(\frac{1}{88} + \frac{1}{163} + \frac{1}{28} - \frac{3}{279}\right)}$$

$$= 31.0436.$$

The M of 31.04 is greater than the critical 5.99, so H_0 is rejected. In fact, M exceeds the critical value for the smallest chi-square in the table, 15.21 for $\alpha = 0.0005$. We may state that $p < 0.001$. We have strong evidence that the variances are quite different and an ANOVA would not be appropriate.

Suppose We Had Used the Kruskal–Wallis Test, as It Seemed Most Appropriate

The result is so dramatic that, had we not had the skew from normal symmetry in the plots, the decision clearly would be the same. Out of interest, a Kruskal–Wallis test yields a chi-square of 158, even larger than the M, which agrees with our conclusion.

METHOD: BARTLETT'S TEST OF HOMOGENEITY OF VARIANCES

We want to know whether three or more variances are the same. Bartlett's test compares the variances of k independent random samples, assumed to be distributed normal. It tests H_0: $\sigma_1^2 = \sigma_2^2 = \cdots = \sigma_k^2$ against the alternative H_1: not H_0. Choose α. Let i denote sample number, $i = 1, 2, \ldots, k$. There are n observations in total in the k samples with n_i observations x_{ij} in the ith sample. First find the variance s_i^2 for each sample, just the way the usual sample variance is found (where j is the index to sum over):

$$s_i^2 = \frac{\sum x_{ij}^2 - n_i m_i^2}{n_i - 1}. \tag{16.3}$$

Then pool the k sample variances to find the overall variance s^2 (now summing over i):

$$s^2 = \frac{\sum (n_i - 1) s_i^2}{n - k}. \tag{16.4}$$

Note that Eq. (16.4) is not the same as the overall variance of the n observations, as each is the variance about its own sample mean. The test statistic, Bartlett's M, is given by

$$M = \frac{(n-k)\ln(s^2) - \sum (n_i - 1)\ln\left(s_i^2\right)}{1 + \frac{1}{3(k-1)}\left(\sum \frac{1}{n_i - 1} - \frac{k}{n-k}\right)}. \tag{16.5}$$

The α for M arises from the right tail of a chi-square distribution with $k-1$ *df*. A critical value for M may be found in Table C. If M is less than this critical value, there is inadequate evidence to reject H_0; otherwise, reject H_0. The steps are as follows:

1. Note the null and alternate hypotheses (H_0: $\sigma_1^2 = \sigma_2^2 = \cdots = \sigma_k^2$ and H_1: not H_0).
2. Choose α.
3. Look up the critical value for the chosen α in Table C for $k - 1$ *df*.
4. Calculate the variances s_i^2 for each sample and the overall variance s^2 [note that s^2 is not exactly the same as the variance for the entire n observations combined; calculate it from Eq. (16.4) using the s_i^2].

5. Calculate Bartlett's M as in Eq. (16.5).
6. Make the decision whether or not to reject the null hypothesis.

Additional Example: Is the Equal-Variance Assumption Satisfied for the One-Way ANOVA of Medication Levels to Reduce Edema following Rhinoplasty?

Following rhinoplasty, swelling may cause deformity during healing. Steroids may decrease the swelling, but the required level of steroid was not known. A total of $n = 50$ rhinoplasty patients were randomized into $k = 5$ groups of increasing steroid level having $n_1 = \cdots = n_5 = 10$. Swelling reduction was measured by MRIs before and after administration of the steroid.[7] The means, variances, and first few data are given in Table 16.4. The requirement was to carry out a one-way analysis of variance (ANOVA) to learn whether the means were all the same or whether there were differences among them (Additional Example from Section 15.4). The ANOVA requires the assumption that the variances of the various groups are equal, which may be examined by Bartlett's M. We choose $\alpha = 0.05$. From Table 16.2 or Table C, the critical value of M (which follows the χ^2 distribution) with $k - 1 = 4$ *df* is 9.49. By substituting in Eq. (16.4) and then Eq. (16.5), we find

$$s^2 = \frac{\sum(n_i - 1)s_i^2}{n - k} = \frac{9 \times 6.30 + 9 \times 3.80 + \cdots + 9 \times 2.25}{50 - 5} = 3.326$$

and

$$M = \frac{(n - k)\ln(s^2) - \sum(n_i - 1)\ln\left(s_i^2\right)}{1 + \frac{1}{3(k-1)}\left(\sum \frac{1}{n_i - 1} - \frac{k}{n-k}\right)}$$

$$= \frac{45 \times \ln(3.326) - 9 \times \ln(6.30) - \cdots - 9 \times \ln(2.25)}{1 + \frac{1}{3 \times 4}\left(\frac{1}{9} + \cdots + \frac{1}{9} - \frac{5}{45}\right)} = 4.51.$$

Table 16.4

Data on Edema following Rhinoplasty

Swelling reduction (ml):	Level 1	Level 2	Level 3	Level 4	Level 5
Patients 1–5	1.6	4.4	5.5	4.0	8.0
Patients 6–10	2.3	5.8	6.4	8.3	6.2
Patients 11–15	2.3	6.4	6.9	5.8	3.1
⋮	⋮	⋮	⋮	⋮	⋮
Means m_i	3.77	5.00	5.67	6.79	6.35
Variances s_i^2	6.30	3.80	1.85	2.43	2.25

As 4.51 < 9.49, we do not have evidence to reject H_0; the variances are not shown to be different. As we have some evidence that the variances are not different, we will carry on with the one-way ANOVA. From a statistical software package, the calculated $p = 0.341$.

Exercise 16.3: Is There a Batch-to-Batch Variability of Laboratory Animals' Resistance to Parasitic Infestation? In a study[41] on the control of parasites, rats were injected with 500 larvae each of the parasitic worm *Nippostrongylus muris*. Ten days later, they were sacrificed and the number of adult worms counted. In Exercise 15.3, we concluded that there was no batch-to-batch difference in *average* resistance to parasite infestation by groups of rats received from the supplier. However, is there a batch-to-batch difference in the *variability* of resistance? We answer this question with Bartlett's test on the homogeneity of variances. $k = 4$ batches of $n_i = 5$ rats each were tested. Data were given in Exercise 15.3. The four variances are 3248.30, 4495.70, 4620.70, 3623.70. At the $\alpha = 0.05$ level of significance, test H_0: $\sigma_1^2 = \sigma_2^2 = \sigma_3^2 = \sigma_4^2$.

ANSWERS TO EXERCISES

16.1. H_0: $\sigma_0^2 = \sigma^2$ and H_1: $\sigma_0^2 > \sigma^2$. From Table C, the critical χ^2 value for $\alpha = 0.05$ with 15 *df* is 25.00. By substituting in Eq. (16.1), we find

$$\chi^2 = \frac{df \times s^2}{\sigma^2} = \frac{15 \times 1.238^2}{0.5^2} = 91.96.$$

As the calculated χ^2 is much larger than the critical value, we reject H_0; the tympanic thermometer is too variable for clinical use. From a computer package, the p-value is 0 to a dozen decimal places; we would say $p < 0.001$.

16.2. H_0: $\sigma_L^2 = \sigma_R^2$ and H_1: $\sigma_L^2 \neq \sigma_R^2$. From Table E, the critical F-value for $\alpha = 0.05$ with 7,7 *df* is 3.79. By substituting in Eq. (16.2), we find $F = s_R^2/s_L^2 = 1.12^2/0.88^2 = 1.620$. As $1.62 < 3.79$, we accept the null hypothesis; we may use the equal-variance t test. From a statistical software package, the actual $p = 0.270$.

16.3. From Eq. (16.4) and then Eq. (16.5), calculate

$$s^2 = \frac{\sum(n_i - 1)s_i^2}{n - k} = \frac{4 \times 3248.30 + \cdots + 4 \times 3623.70}{16} = 3997.10$$

and

$$M = \frac{(n-k)\ln(s^2) - \sum(n_i - 1)\ln\left(s_i^2\right)}{1 + \frac{1}{3(k-1)}\left(\sum \frac{1}{n_i-1} - \frac{k}{n-k}\right)}$$

$$= \frac{16 \times \ln(3.997.10) - 4 \times \ln(3248.30) - \cdots - 4 \times \ln(3623.70)}{1 + \frac{1}{3\times 3}\left(\frac{1}{4} + \cdots + \frac{1}{4} - \frac{4}{16}\right)}$$

$$= 0.1587.$$

From Table C, the critical χ_3^2 $df = 7.81$. The calculated $M = 0.1587$ is very much smaller, so we do not have evidence to reject H_0; variability of parasite infestation does not differ from batch to batch. From a statistical software package, the actual $p = 0.984$.

Chapter 17

Common Tests on the Distribution Shape of Continuous Data

17.1. OBJECTIVES OF TESTS ON DISTRIBUTIONS

What Do We Usually Ask about Distributions?

Of the many questions that could be asked about distribution shape, two are most common: "Is the distribution normal?" and "Do two distributions have the same shape?"

The First Type of Test Addressed in This Chapter Is a Test of Normality of a Distribution

Normality of underlying data is assumed in many statistical tests, including the normal test for means, the *t* test, and the analysis of variance. A user who is not sure that the assumption of normality is justified is on firmer ground by testing the sampling distribution(s) for normality before deciding on the appropriate test, although we must understand a limitation of this use. A significant outcome implies the conclusion that the distribution is not normal, whereas, like all tests of hypotheses, a nonsignificant outcome implies only that no deviation from normality has been demonstrated, not that it does not exist. However, a negative result is some evidence of normality and all the evidence we have, which leads us to carry out the analysis as if normality had been demonstrated.

The Second Type of Test Is a Test of Equality of Two Distributions

The user encountering two distributions may want to know whether they have the same or a different form, in some cases to satisfy assumptions required for tests and in other cases to learn whether the natural forces giving rise to these distributions are similar.

17.2. TEST OF NORMALITY OF A DISTRIBUTION

Tests of Normality and Their Comparison

Keep in mind that the robustness of most tests, some more than others, allows the test to be used if the underlying data are *approximately* normal. Thus, barring quite unusual circumstances, any good test of normality will be adequate. The better tests are more complicated, as one might expect. Also as one might expect, the better tests are more recent. (The chi-square goodness-of-fit test was first published in 1900, the Kolgorov–Smirnov, usually abbreviated KS, test in 1933, and the Shapiro–Wilk test in 1965.) The choice of the test to use depends on both the sample size and whether the user would rather err on the side of being too conservative or the opposite. The Shapiro–Wilk tends to reject the null hypothesis more readily than one would wish, whereas the KS and chi-square tests are too conservative, retaining the null hypothesis too often. The selection can be made with the help of Table 17.1.

The Shapiro–Wilk Can Test Only Sample Data, Not Population or Theoretical Data

One limitation of the Shapiro–Wilk test is that some software packages allow only the sample parameters (mean and standard deviation) to be used for the

Table 17.1

Guide to Selecting a Test of Normality of a Distribution

	Prefer less conservative test	Prefer more conservative test
Small sample (5–50)	Shapiro–Wilk test	Kolmogorov–Smirnov test (one-sample)
Medium to large sample (>50)	Shapiro–Wilk test	Chi-square goodness-of-fit test

theoretical normal against which the data are being tested, whereas we would prefer to allow specification of the normal being tested by either theoretical or sample parameters.

Computer Packages Usually Are Used, but Not Required

Attention here will be focused on what the tests do and how they do it, not on commands required to conduct computer-based tests. Enough detail on the KS and chi-square goodness-of-fit methods is given to allow the user to apply the method even in the absence of a comprehensive statistical software package. Such a package should be accessed for the Shapiro–Wilk test.

Small-Sample Test of Normality of a Distribution: Kolmogorov–Smirnov (KS) Test (One-Sample Form)

The two-sample form of the KS test is used in Section 17.3 to test the equality of two distributions.

Example: Are the Ages of the Patients in Table DB1.1 Distributed Normal?

H_0: The distribution from which the sample was drawn is normal. H_1: The distribution is different. $n = 10$. From Eq. (17.1b), and choosing $\alpha = 0.05$, the critical value is found as

$$\frac{1.36}{\sqrt{n}} - \frac{1}{4.5n} = \frac{1.36}{\sqrt{10}} - \frac{1}{4.5 \times 10} = 0.408.$$

We set up Table 17.2 with headings representing the values that will be required in the calculation.

1. The first column consists of the ages in increasing order.
2. The second column (x) consists of the sample values at each change. The first change occurs as age goes from 54 to 61 years.
3. The third column (k) consists of the number of sample members less than x. For the first x, there is only one age less than 61 years, so $k = 1$.
4. The fourth column consists of the values k/n. For the first $x, k/n = 1/10 = 0.1$.
5. Column five consists of z, the standardized values of x. We note the mean $m = 65.1$ years and the standard deviation $s = 7.0$ years from Table DB1.1 and, for each x, calculated $(x - m)/s$.
6. The sixth column consists of normal distribution probabilities, the area under

Table 17.2

Example Data (Ages of 10 Patients from Table DB1.1) with the Corresponding Calculations Required for the Kolmogorov–Smirnov (KS) Test of Normality

Ages	x	k	$F_n(x)$	z	$F_e(x)$	$\|F_n(x) - F_e(x)\|$
54						
61	61	1	0.1	$(61 - 65.1)/7 = -0.586$	0.279	0.179
61						
61						
62	62	4	0.4	$(62 - 65.1)/7 = -0.443$	0.329	0.071
62						
68	68	6	0.6	$(68 - 65.1)/7 = 0.414$	0.661	0.061
73	73	7	0.7	$(73 - 65.1)/7 = 1.129$	0.870	0.170
74	74	8	0.8	$(74 - 65.1)/7 = 1.271$	0.898	0.098
75	75	9	0.9	$(75 - 65.1)/7 = 1.414$	0.921	0.021

the normal curve to the left of z. For the first x, we want to find the area under a normal curve from the left tail up to the -0.586 standard deviation position (just over half a standard deviation to the left of the mean). A statistical package gives it as 0.278938, which rounds to 0.279. If we do not have such access, we can interpolate from Table A. Because Table A gives only the right half of the curve, we use the knowledge of symmetry; the area to the left of -0.586 will be the same as the area to the right of $+0.586$, lies 86% of the way from 0.50 to 0.60. We need the one-tailed area given by α for 0.50 plus 0.86 of the difference between the α's for 0.50 and 0.60, or $0.308 + 0.86 \times (0.274 - 0.308) = 0.27876$, which rounds to 0.279 as did the result from the statistical package.

7. The last column consists of the absolute difference (difference without regard to sign) between the entries in columns 4 and 6. For the first x, $|0.1 - 0.279| = |-0.179| = 0.179$.

8. The largest value in the rightmost column is $L = 0.179$.

9. Finally, we compare L with the critical value. Because $(L=)\,0.179 \leq 0.408$ (= critical value), we do not reject H_0: the distribution from which the sample was drawn has not been shown to be different from normal. The p-value was computed to be 0.4719 using a statistical software package.

Method: One-Sample Kolmogorov–Smirnov (KS) Test

There are two questions we might ask: (1) Did the sample arise from a particular normal distribution with a postulated mean and standard deviation? (2) Is the sample normal in shape without any *a priori* mean and standard deviation specified? The latter is the question we ask to satisfy the normality assumption in tests of hypothesis. In the first case, we use the postulated normal distribution's mean μ and standard deviation σ in the method that follows. In the second case, we use the sample's m and s in the method that follows. The hypotheses are H_0: The distribution from which the sample was drawn is not different from (a specified) normal; two-tailed H_1: The distribution is different. Calculate the critical value for a 1%, 5%, or 10% test, whichever is desired, from Eqs. (17.1a), (17.1b), or (17.1c), respectively. (These critical values are approximations, but are accurate to within 0.001.)

$$\frac{1.63}{\sqrt{n}} - \frac{1}{3.5n} \quad \text{for } \alpha = 0.01 \tag{17.1a}$$

$$\frac{1.36}{\sqrt{n}} - \frac{1}{4.5n} \quad \text{for } \alpha = 0.05 \tag{17.1b}$$

$$\frac{1.22}{\sqrt{n}} - \frac{1}{5.5n} \quad \text{for } \alpha = 0.10 \tag{17.1c}$$

1. Arrange the n sample values in ascending order.
2. Let x denote the sample value each time it changes. (If sample values are 1, 1, 2, 2, 2, 3, the first x is 2, the second 3.) Write these x's in a column in order.
3. Let k denote the number of sample members less than x. (When the preceding sample values changed from 1 to 2 and x became 2, there were $k = 2$ values less than x. At the next change, x takes on the value 3 and there are $k = 5$ values less than that x.) Write these k's next to their corresponding x's.
4. Let $F_n(x)$ denote k/n for each x. This is the sample cumulative frequency distribution (CDF). Write down each $F_n(x)$ in the next column corresponding to the associated x.
5. Now we need the expected CDF against which to test the sample. Calculate $z = (x - \mu)/\sigma$ for each x for case (1) or $z = (x - m)/s$ for each x for case (2).
6. For each z, find an expected $F_e(x)$ as the area under the normal distribution to the left of z. This area can be found using a statistical software package or from a very complete table of normal probabilities. If neither of these sources is available, interpolate from Table A. Write down these $F_e(x)$ next to the corresponding $F_n(x)$.
7. Write down next to these the absolute value (value without any minus signs) of the difference between the F's, namely, $|F_n(x) - F_e(x)|$.
8. The test statistic is the largest of these differences, say L.
9. If L is greater than the critical value, reject H_0. Otherwise, do not reject H_0.

Additional Example: A Test of Normality on a Potential HIV Vaccine

In a study on a potential vaccine for human immunovirus (HIV), the number of HIV per milliliter of blood (denoted h) was measured on a baseline sample of $n = 45$ patients.[72] It was required that the data be approximately normal in order to conduct other statistical procedures. A quick frequency plot shows clearly that it is far from a normal distribution, which is superposed (Fig. 17.1A). Natural

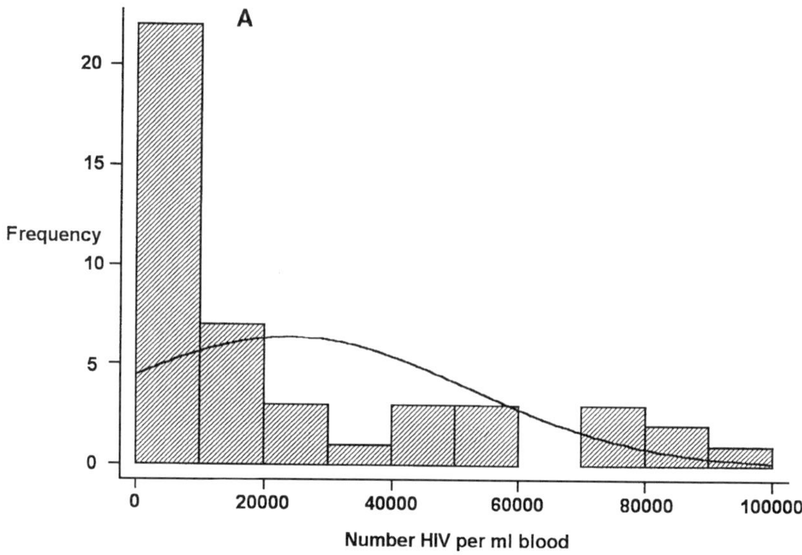

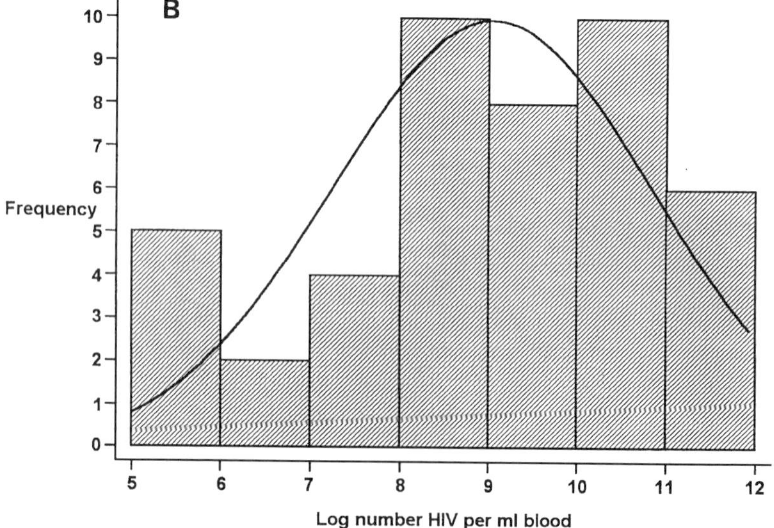

Figure 17.1 Plots of number of HIV per milliliter of blood (h) (A) and ln h (B) with superposed normal distributions based on m and s from the data.

logarithms (ln) were taken in the hope of transforming the data to normal. A quick plot of ln h with a superposed normal (based on the mean and standard deviation of the data) appears somewhat better (Fig. 17.1B), but is deviant enough from bell-shaped to require a test of normality.

Stepping through the Test Procedure

α is chosen as 5%. The critical value of the test for $\alpha = 0.05$ is found from Eq. (17.1b): $(1.36)/\sqrt{n}) - (1/4.5n) = 0.1978$. Data arranged in ascending order appear in Table 17.3 in the format of Table 17.2. $m = 9.04$ and $s = 1.80$. As there are no ties in ln h, x will be the same as the sample values. k is one less than the count number of each datum. As before, $F_n(x) = k/n$, $z = (x - m)/s$, and $F_e(x)$ is the area under the normal curve to the left of the z associated with that x. The last column is the absolute value of the difference between the two F's. The largest value in the last column is the last, $L = 0.1030$. As $L < 0.1978$, we accept the hypothesis of normality; nonnormality has not been shown.

Exercise 17.1: KS. Hct's need to be distributed normally to find a confidence interval. In the Additional Example of Section 14.3, we examined post-operative hematocrit (Hct) on pyloromyotomized neonates[16] and concluded that Hct was not different for laparoscopic versus open surgeries; thus, we pool the data. To put a confidence interval on mean Hct, we need to assume that the distribution is normal. The $n = 16$ Hct readings in ascending order are 25.6, 29.7, 32.0, 32.0, 32.1, 32.7, 33.9, 34.0, 38.3, 38.8, 39.0, 42.0, 43.3, 43.9, 46.7, 52.0. Test for normality using Kolmogorov–Smirnov.

Large-Sample Test of Normality of a Distribution: Chi-Square Goodness-of-Fit Test

Characteristics of the Chi-Square Goodness-of-Fit Test

The time-honored Pearson's goodness-of-fit test is a relatively easy concept but has limitations, which include the fact that it is an approximate test and the fact that the calculated value of χ^2 depends on the user's choice of interval widths and starting points. The test is similar to a chi-square contingency table test, but uses areas under the normal curve for expected values.

Example: Is the Distribution of Ages of the 301 Prostate Patients Normal?

We ask whether the data are drawn from just a normal, not a specific normal, so we use $m = 66.76$ years and $s = 8.10$ years from DB1. We choose $\alpha = 0.05$. The

Table 17.3

HIV per Milliliter of Blood Data in the Format of Table 17.2

ln *h* and *x*	*k*	$F_n(x)$	*z*	$F_e(x)$	$\lvert F_n - F_e \rvert$
5.2575					
5.3613	1	0.0222	−2.0437	0.0205	0.0017
5.6095	2	0.0444	−1.9058	0.0283	0.0161
5.8111	3	0.0667	−1.7938	0.0364	0.0302
5.8377	4	0.0889	−1.7790	0.0376	0.0513
6.2206	5	0.1111	−1.5663	0.0586	0.0525
6.4599	6	0.1333	−1.4334	0.0759	0.0575
7.4719	7	0.1556	−0.8711	0.1918	0.0363
7.7841	8	0.1778	−0.6977	0.2427	0.0649
7.8466	9	0.2000	−0.6301	0.2537	0.0537
7.9124	10	0.2222	−0.6264	0.2655	0.0433
8.0830	11	0.2444	−0.5316	0.2975	0.0530
8.1026	12	0.2667	−0.5208	0.3013	0.0346
8.1158	13	0.2889	−0.5134	0.3038	0.0149
8.4036	14	0.3111	−0.3536	0.3618	0.0507
8.4602	15	0.3333	−0.3221	0.3736	0.0404
8.5834	16	0.3556	−0.2537	0.3999	0.0443
8.6778	17	0.3778	−0.2012	0.4203	0.0425
8.8796	18	0.4000	−0.0891	0.4645	0.0645
8.9383	19	0.4222	−0.0565	0.4775	0.0552
8.9408	20	0.4444	−0.0551	0.4780	0.0336
9.1607	21	0.4667	0.6701	0.5267	0.0601
9.4340	22	0.4889	0.2189	0.5866	0.0977
9.5623	23	0.5111	0.2902	0.6141	0.1030
9.5645	24	0.5333	0.2914	0.6146	0.0813
9.5988	25	0.5556	0.3104	0.6219	0.0663
9.7200	26	0.5778	0.3778	0.6472	0.0694
9.7600	27	0.6000	0.4000	0.6554	0.0554
9.7712	28	0.6222	0.4062	0.6577	0.0355
10.1036	29	0.6444	0.5909	0.7227	0.0783
10.1956	30	0.6667	0.6420	0.7396	0.0729
10.1963	31	0.6889	0.6424	0.7397	0.0508
10.4942	32	0.7111	0.8079	0.7904	0.0793
10.6105	33	0.7333	0.8725	0.8085	0.0752
10.6144	34	0.7556	0.8747	0.8091	0.0536
10.6794	35	0.7889	0.9108	0.8188	0.0410
10.8751	36	0.8000	1.0195	0.8460	0.0460
10.9183	37	0.8222	1.0435	0.8516	0.0294
10.9501	38	0.8444	1.0612	0.8557	0.0113
11.2159	39	0.8667	1.2089	0.8866	0.0200
11.2270	40	0.8889	1.2150	0.8878	0.0011
11.2511	41	0.9111	1.2284	0.8904	0.0208
11.3553	42	0.9333	1.2863	0.9008	0.0325
11.3634	43	0.9556	1.2907	0.9016	0.0540
11.4586	44	0.9778	1.3437	0.9105	0.0673

Table 17.4

Excerpt of Table C, Chi-Square Distribution, Right Tail[a]

α (area in right tail)	0.10	0.05	0.025	0.01	0.005	0.001
df = 6	10.64	12.59	14.45	16.81	18.54	22.46
df = 8	13.36	15.51	17.53	20.09	21.95	26.10
df = 9	14.68	16.92	19.02	21.67	23.59	27.86

[a] χ^2 values (distances above zero) are given for 6, 8, and 9 *df* for various α, the area under the curve in the right tail.

critical value of chi-square uses 9 *df* (number of intervals −1). From Table 17.4 (or Table C), chi-square (9 *df*) for $\alpha = 0.05$ is 16.92.

1. We define 10 intervals as <50, 50 up to but not including 55, ..., 85 up to but not including 90, and ≥90. We form a blank table in the format of Table 17.5.
2. To use a normal probability table, we need to standardize the ends of the intervals by subtracting the mean and dividing by the standard deviation. We standardize the end of the first interval by $(50-66.76)/8.1 = -2.0691$. The second is $(55 - 66.76)/8.1 = -1.4519$.
3. We need to relate areas under the normal curve to the intervals, which we do by finding the area to the end of an interval and subtracting the area to the end of the preceding interval. Table A includes only positive z-values, so we use the normal symmetry: we change the sign of z and use α instead of $1 - \alpha$. For the first interval, $z = -2.0691$ interpolates as $0.023 + 0.691 \times (0.018 - 0.023) = 0.0195$. There is no prior interval yielding a probability to subtract, so 0.0195 is the

Table 17.5

Table of Values Required to Compute the Chi-Square Goodness-of-Fit Statistic[a]

Interval	Standard normal z to end of interval	Probability	Expected frequencies (e_i)	Observed frequencies (n_i)
<50	−2.0691	0.0195	5.87	3
50–<55	−1.4519	0.0542	16.31	17
55–<60	−0.8346	0.1286	38.71	32
60–<65	−0.2173	0.2120	63.81	74
65–<70	0.3999	0.2407	72.45	62
70–<75	1.0173	0.1900	57.19	57
75–<80	1.6346	0.1035	31.15	37
80–<85	2.2519	0.0359	10.81	14
85–<90	2.8691	0.0145	4.36	4
≥90	∞	0.0019	0.57	1

[a] The entries arise from the example, but the format may be used in general.

probability for the first interval. For the second, $z = -1.4519$ gives $0.081 + 0.519 \times (0.067 - 0.081) = 0.0737$. Subtraction of 0.0195 for the prior area results in a second-interval probability of 0.0542.

4. To obtain the expected frequencies (e_i), we multiply the probability associated with an interval by n. $e_1 = 0.0195 \times 301 = 5.87$, etc.

5. To obtain the observed frequencies (n_i), we tally the data for each data interval and enter the frequencies (3, 17, 32, ...) in the table.

6. The chi-square statistic is obtained as

$$\chi^2 = \sum \frac{n_i^2}{e_i} - n = \frac{3^2}{5.87} + \frac{17^2}{16.31} + \cdots - 301 = 7.895.$$

7. The calculated chi-square of 7.895 is less than the critical chi-square of 16.92, so the result is taken to be not significant and we do not reject H_0; the distribution from which the data arise is normal. The p-value was computed on a statistical software package to be 0.555.

Method: Chi-Square Goodness-of-Fit Test of Normality

The hypotheses are H_0: The distribution from which the sample was drawn is not different from (a specified) normal; two-tailed H_1: The distribution is different. Choose α. Look up the critical χ^2 in Table C.

1. We define the data intervals, say k in number, as we would were we to form a histogram of the data. We form a blank table in the format of Table 17.5.

2. To use a normal probability table, we standardize the ends of the intervals by subtracting the mean and dividing by the standard deviation. The "expected" normal usually is specified by the sample m and s, although it could be specified by a theoretical μ and σ.

3. To relate areas under the normal curve to the intervals, we find the area to the end of an interval from a table of normal probabilities, such as Table A, and subtract the area to the end of the preceding interval.

4. To find the frequencies expected from a normal fit (name them e_i), we multiply the normal probabilities for each interval by the total number of data n.

5. We tally the number of data falling into each interval and enter the tally numbers in the table. Name these numbers n_i.

6. Calculate a χ^2 value [reminiscent of Eq. (6.2) in pattern] using Eq. (17.2):

$$\chi^2 = \sum \frac{(n_i - e_i)^2}{e_i} = \sum \frac{n_i^2}{e_i} - n, \qquad (17.2)$$

where the first form is easier to understand conceptually and the second is easier to compute.

Table 17.6
HIV per Milliliter of Blood Data in the Format of Table 17.5

Interval	Standard normal z to end of interval	Probability	Expected frequencies (e_i)	Observed frequencies (n_i)
5–<6	−1.6864	0.0459	2.0635	5
6–<7	−1.1318	0.0830	3.7349	2
7–<8	−0.5722	0.1530	6.8867	4
8–<9	−0.0226	0.2091	9.4086	10
9–<10	0.5320	0.2117	9.5244	8
10–<11	1.0866	0.1588	7.1442	10
11–<12	1.6412	0.0882	3.9704	6

7. If calculated χ^2 is greater than critical χ^2, reject H_0; otherwise, do not reject H_0.

Additional Example

Let us test the normality of the HIV data[72] introduced earlier by the chi-square goodness-of-fit test, even though the sample size is just borderline smaller than we would choose. We use $\alpha = 0.05$. From Table 17.4 (or Table C), the critical value of $\chi^2_{6\ df} = 12.59$. Recall that $m = 9.0408$ and $s = 1.8031$. To form a table, we can use the intervals and frequencies chosen for Fig. 17.1B. Results in the format of Table 17.5 appear in Table 17.6. By substituting in Eq. (17.2), we find

$$\chi^2 = \sum \frac{n_i^2}{e_i} - n = \frac{5^2}{2.0635} + \frac{2^2}{3.7349} + \cdots + \frac{6^2}{3.9704} - 45 = 10.92.$$

Because $10.92 < 12.59$, we conclude that deviation from normality is not demonstrated. (The actual $p = 0.091$.)

Exercise 17.2: χ^2. Was our prior judgment of normality of PSA = 4–10 data correct? In the Example of Section 15.4, we looked at a plot of age for $n = 164$ patients with PSA in the uncertain region of 4–10 and judged that it was distributed approximately normal. Test this judgment using the χ^2 goodness-of-fit test at the $\alpha = 5\%$ level. Use the intervals chosen for the 4–10 plot of Fig. 15.2. Intervals and observed frequencies follow (where "45–<50" represents the interval 45 up to but not including 50, etc.). $m = 66.2988$ and $s = 7.8429$.

45–<50	50–<55	55–<60	60–<65	65–<70	70–<75	75–<80	80–<85	85–<90
2	9	19	44	30	36	15	6	3

17.3. TEST OF EQUALITY OF TWO DISTRIBUTIONS

THE TWO-SAMPLE KS IS USED FOR THIS TEST

The two-sample Kolmogorov–Smirnov (KS) test will compare two data sets to decide whether they were sampled from population distributions of the same shape. (The one-sample form can be seen in Section 17.2.)

EXAMPLE: IS PSA FROM THE FIRST MEMBERS OF THE DB1 SAMPLE DISTRIBUTED THE SAME AS THE LATER ONES?

We want to know whether the distribution from which the first 10 PSA values were drawn is the same as that for the next 16 PSA values. We choose $\alpha = 0.05$. The larger sample is designated number 1. Then $n_1 = 16$ PSA readings, which are 5.3, 6.6, 7.6, 4.8, 5.7, 7.7, 4.6, 5.6, 8.9, 1.3, 8.5, 4.0, 5.8, 9.9, 7.0, and 6.9, and $n_2 = 10$, with the PSA values from Table DB1.1. We use Eq. (17.3b) to find the critical value:

$$1.36\sqrt{\frac{n_1 + n_2}{n_1 n_2}} = 1.36\sqrt{\frac{26}{160}} = 0.5482.$$

1. Combine the two data sets, keeping track of which datum belongs to which sample, and record in ascending order, using the format (headings) as in Table 17.7.
2. Going down the data list, each time a datum belonging to sample 1 is different from the datum above it, record an entry for k_1, the number of data in sample 1 preceding it. 1.3 has no datum preceding it, so we enter $k_1 = 0$. 4.0 has one datum preceding it. 4.1 is not from sample 1; we skip to 4.6, which has two sample 1 data preceding it. And so forth until PSA value 9.9, for which $k_1 = 15$. Repeat the process for sample 2 data, recording entries for k_2.
3. For every k_1, calculate $F_1 = k_1/n_1$ and enter it under the F_1 column. Wherever a blank appears (corresponding to sample 2 data), write down the F_1 from the line above. $F_1 = 0/16 = 0$ for the first PSA value. $F_1 = 1/16 = 0.0625$ for the second. The third PSA value is from sample 2 and no k_1 was recorded, so we repeat 0.0625. We follow the same process for sample 2 data, recording entries for F_2 and writing down the F_2 value from the preceding line to fill in blanks. The F's are the cumulative sums, i.e., cumulative data frequencies (CDFs), for the two samples.
4. Calculate and record $|F_1 - F_2|$, the absolute difference (difference without any minus signs) between the two cumulative sums (CDFs), for every datum. For example, for the fourth PSA value, 4.4, $|F_1 - F_2| = |0.0625 - 0.1| = |-0.0375| = 0.0375$.

Table 17.7

Example Data (PSA for 10 Patients from Table DB1.1 and the Next 16 Patients Presenting) along with the Corresponding Calculations Required for the Two-Sample Kolmogorov–Smirnov (KS) Test of Equality of Distribution

Ordered data	k_1	k_2	F_1	F_2	$\|F_1 - F_2\|$
1.3	0		0	0	0
4.0	1		0.0625	0	0.0625
4.1		0	0.0625	0	0.0625
4.4		1	0.0625	0.1	0.0375
4.6	2		0.1250	0.1	0.0250
4.8	3		0.1875	0.1	0.0875
5.3	4		0.2500	0.1	0.1500
5.6	5		0.3125	0.1	0.2125
5.7	6		0.3725	0.1	0.2725
5.8	7		0.4375	0.1	$0.3375 = L$
5.9		2	0.4375	0.2	0.2375
6.1		3	0.4375	0.3	0.1375
6.6	8		0.5000	0.3	0.2000
6.8		4	0.5000	0.4	0.1000
6.9	9		0.5625	0.4	0.1625
7.0	10		0.6250	0.4	0.2250
7.6	11	5	0.6875	0.5	0.1875
7.7	12	6	0.7500	0.6	0.1500
7.9		7	0.7500	0.7	0.0500
8.0		8	0.7500	0.8	0.0500
8.5	13		0.8125	0.8	0.0125
8.9	14		0.8750	0.8	0.0750
9.0		9	0.8750	0.9	0.0250
9.9	15		0.9395	0.9	0.0395

5. The test statistic L is the largest of these differences. We can see that it is 0.3375.

6. L (=0.3375) is less than 0.5482, the critical value, so we do not reject H_0. (The actual p-value calculated by a statistical software package is 0.3995.)

Method: The Hypotheses and the Nature of the Two-Sample KS Test

The hypotheses are H_0: The population distributions from which the samples arose are not different from one another; two-tailed H_1: The samples arose from different population distributions. Choose α. The sample sizes are n_1 and n_2, where n_1 is the larger. Calculate the critical value for the chosen 1%, 5%, or

10% α from Eqs. (17.3a), (17.3b), or (17.3c), respectively. (These critical values are approximations. They are adequate for $n_2 > 10$. For smaller n's, they may be used if the calculated statistic is much greater or lesser than the critical value; if borderline, the user should arrange for calculation using a statistical software package.)

$$1.63\sqrt{\frac{n_1+n_2}{n_1 n_2}} \quad \text{for } \alpha = 0.01 \tag{17.3a}$$

$$1.36\sqrt{\frac{n_1+n_2}{n_1 n_2}} \quad \text{for } \alpha = 0.05 \tag{17.3b}$$

$$1.22\sqrt{\frac{n_1+n_2}{n_1 n_2}} \quad \text{for } \alpha = 0.10 \tag{17.3c}$$

The test consists of calculating the cumulative data frequencies (CDFs) for the two samples and finding the probability of the greatest difference between these CDFs.

1. Combine the two data sets, keeping track of which datum belongs to which sample, and arrange in ascending order, using the format (headings) as in Table 17.7.
2. Going down the data list, each time a datum belonging to sample 1 is different from the datum above it, record an entry for k_1, the number of data in sample 1 preceding it. Repeat the process for sample 2 data, recording entries for k_2.
3. For every k_1, calculate $F_1 = k_1/n_1$ and enter it under the F_1 column. Wherever a blank appears (corresponding to sample 2 data), write down the F_1 from the line above. Repeat the process for sample 2 data, recording entries for F_2 and writing down the F_2 value from the preceding line to fill in blanks. The F's are the CDFs (cumulative sums) for the two samples.
4. Calculate and record $|F_1 - F_2|$, the absolute difference (difference without any minus signs) between the two CDFs, for every datum.
5. The test statistic is the largest of these differences; call it L.
6. If L is greater than the critical value, reject H_0. Otherwise, do not reject H_0.

The Two-Sample KS on Large Samples

If the sample sizes are large, the number of differences to be computed may be reduced to a manageable number by collapsing the data into class intervals as one would do in making a histogram. The method, however, then acquires the faults of the goodness-of-fit test: it becomes an approximation and becomes dependent on the choice of interval position and spacing.

Additional Example: A Study on a Potential Vaccine for Human Immunovirus (HIV)

The study included a control sample of $n_1 = 24$ patients and an experimental vaccine sample of $n_2 = 20$ patients, randomly allocated into the two groups.[72] The treatment was a placebo saline injection for the control group and a vaccine injection for the experimental group. The knowledge of whether the experimental and control groups follow the same distribution aided in the development of the physiological theory. The number of HIV per milliliter of blood (denoted h) was measured before treatment and a fixed period of time after treatment. Its natural logarithm ($\ln h$) was calculated in order to reduce the extreme skewness of the frequency distribution. Then the difference $d \ln h = \ln h$ before $- \ln h$ after was taken. A quick frequency plot of the two samples appears in Fig. 17.2. The distributions are not obviously different, but enough so to warrant a test. We use the KS test of equality of distributions with a two-sided $\alpha = 0.05$.

The data and analysis operations appear in Table 17.8 in the format of Table 17.7. The values of $d \ln h$, the difference in log number HIV per milliliter of blood before minus after treatment, are put in order. The number of data in the respective sample preceding the current observation are listed for control (k_1) and vaccine (k_2). $F_1 = k_1/24$, $F_2 = k_2/20$, and $|F_1 - F_2|$ are entered. Inspection of the last column shows that the largest value is $L = 0.3583$, indicated by an asterisk. The critical value for the test is found from Eq. (17.3b):

$$1.36\sqrt{\frac{n_1 + n_2}{n_1 n_2}} = 1.36\sqrt{\frac{24 + 20}{24 \times 20}} = 0.4118.$$

Because $0.3583 < 0.4118$, we do not reject H_0 and we proceed on the premise that the distributions are not different.

Exercise 17.3: Is the Distribution of Functionality the Same for Two Types of Ankle Repair? An orthopedist installs hardware in the repair of broken ankles in $n = 19$ patients.[23] He randomly selects two groups: (1) remove the hardware after adequate healing ($n_1 = 9$) and (2) leave it in place ($n_2 = 10$). He judges the posthealing percent functionality of the ankle joint. In assessing the relative success of the two groups, he observes that their distributions are far from normal in shape. However, are the distributions both the same, whatever they may be? His data are as follows:

Remove hardware		75	65	100	90	35	63	78	70	80
Leave hardware	95	98	95	45	90	93	85	100	72	99

Perform a KS test of equality of distribution using $\alpha = 0.05$.

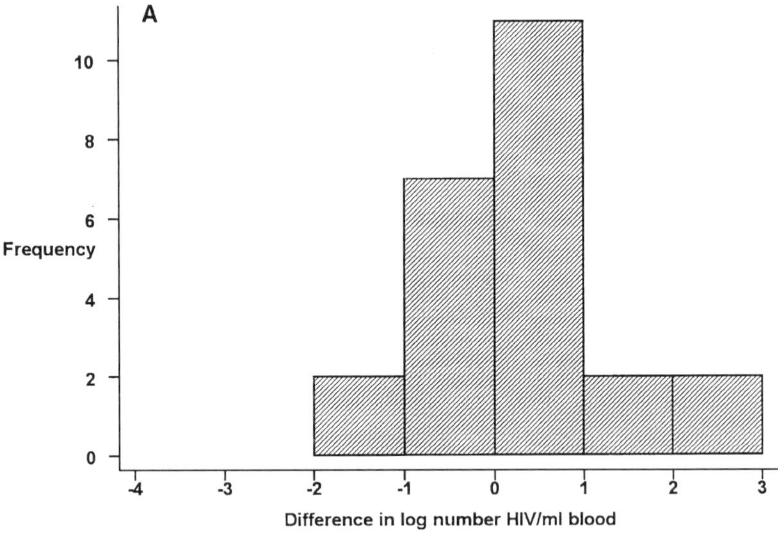

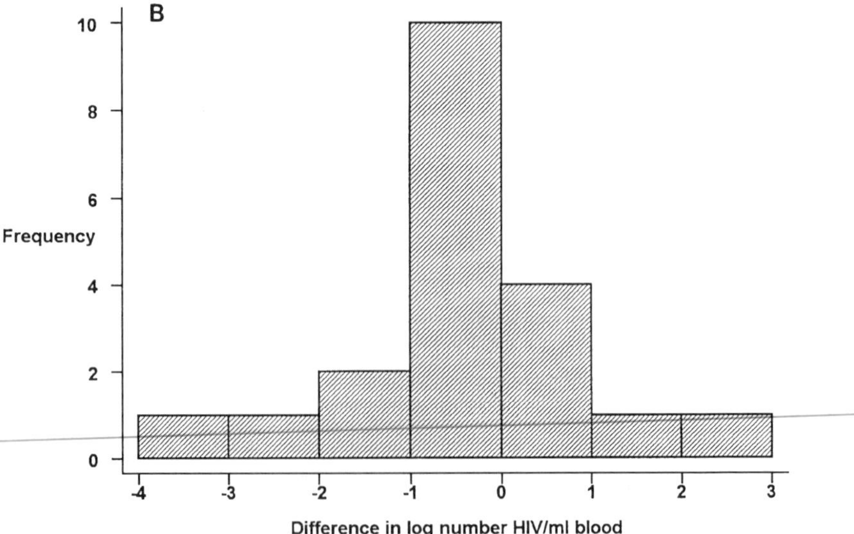

Figure 17.2 Plots of distributions of control (A) and vaccine-treated (B) differences in log number HIV per milliliter of blood before minus after treatment.

Table 17.8

HIV per Milliliter of Blood Data in the Format of Table 17.7

$d \ln h$	k_1	k_2	F_1	F_2	$\|F_1 - F_2\|$
−3.4009		0	0	0	0
−2.4125		1	0	0.05	0.0500
−1.2169	0		0	0.05	0.0500
−1.1564	1		0.0417	0.05	0.0083
−1.1453		2	0.0417	0.10	0.0583
−1.0750		3	0.0417	0.15	0.1083
−0.7466		4	0.0417	0.20	0.1583
−0.6159	2		0.0833	0.20	0.1167
−0.5456	3		0.1250	0.20	0.0750
−0.5114		5	0.1250	0.25	0.1250
−0.4494		6	0.1250	0.30	0.1750
−0.4158		7	0.1250	0.35	0.2250
−0.4153		8	0.1250	0.40	0.2750
−0.4152	4		0.1667	0.40	0.2333
−0.3644	5		0.2083	0.40	0.1917
−0.3628		9	0.2083	0.45	0.2417
−0.2673	6		0.2500	0.45	0.2000
−0.2372		10	0.2500	0.50	0.2500
−0.2148		11	0.2500	0.55	0.3000
−0.1302		12	0.2500	0.60	0.3500
−0.1298		13	0.2500	0.65	0.4000
−0.0851	7		0.2917	0.65	0.3583*
−0.0030	8		0.3333	0.65	0.3167
0.6257	9		0.3750	0.65	0.2750
0.0989	10		0.4167	0.65	0.2333
0.1054	11		0.4583	0.65	0.1917
0.1756	12		0.5000	0.65	0.1500
0.2982	13		0.5417	0.65	0.1083
0.3122	14		0.5833	0.65	0.0667
0.4635	15		0.6250	0.65	0.0250
0.7133		14	0.6250	0.70	0.0750
0.7277	16		0.6667	0.70	0.0333
0.7371		15	0.6667	0.75	0.0833
0.7550	17		0.7083	0.75	0.0417
0.7907		16	0.7083	0.80	0.0917
0.8137	18		0.7500	0.80	0.0500
0.9115	19		0.7917	0.80	0.0083
0.9980		17	0.7917	0.85	0.0583
1.1957	20		0.8333	0.85	0.0167
1.4076	21		0.8750	0.85	0.0250
1.6083		18	0.8750	0.90	0.0250
2.1146	22		0.9167	0.90	0.0167
2.3530	23		0.9583	0.90	0.0583
2.7834		19	0.9583	0.95	0.0083

ANSWERS TO EXERCISES

17.1. KS. For $n = 16$, our 5% critical value is $1.36/4 - 1/(5.5 \times 16) = 0.329$. The data were given in ascending order. We prepare Table 17.9 in the format of Table 17.2. x is Hct each time the value is different from the preceding value. k is the number of values preceding x. From the Hct readings, we calculate $m = 37.25$ and $s = 6.9937$. We calculate $z = (x - m)/s$. F_e is the area under the normal curve to the left of z. And finally, the last column is the absolute value of the difference between the F's. From inspection of the last column, the largest is $L = 0.1164$. As $0.1164 < 0.329$, we accept the hypothesis of normality.

17.2. χ^2. With nine intervals, $df = 8$. From Table 17.5 (or Table C), the critical value of χ^2 is 15.51. The data and calculations are set up in Table 17.10 in the format of Table 17.5. By using Eq. (17.2), we find

$$\chi^2 = \sum \frac{n_i^2}{e_i} - n = \frac{2^2}{3.0832} + \frac{9^2}{9.1840} + \cdots - 164 = 9.2448,$$

which is less than the critical value. We accept the H_0 of normality and conclude that our initial judgment was correct.

17.3. The 5% critical value from Eq. (17.3b) is

$$1.36\sqrt{\frac{n_1 + n_2}{n_1 n_2}} = 1.36\sqrt{\frac{9 + 10}{9 \times 10}} = 0.6249.$$

He rank-orders the values of percent functionality (% func.) in Table 17.11

Table 17.9

Hct Data in the Format of Table 17.2

x	k	$F_n(x)$	z	$F_e(x)$	$\|F_n - F_e\|$
29.7	1	0.0625	−0.0795	0.1402	0.0777
32.0	2	0.1250	−0.7507	0.2264	0.1014
32.1	4	0.2500	−0.7364	0.2308	0.0192
32.7	5	0.3125	−0.6506	0.2577	0.0548
33.9	6	0.3750	−0.4790	0.3160	0.0590
34.0	7	0.4375	−0.4647	0.3211	0.1164
38.3	8	0.5000	0.1501	0.5597	0.0597
38.8	9	0.5625	0.2216	0.5877	0.0252
39.0	10	0.6250	0.2502	0.5988	0.0262
42.0	11	0.6875	0.6792	0.7515	0.0640
43.3	12	0.7500	0.8651	0.8065	0.0565
43.9	13	0.8125	0.9501	0.8292	0.0167
46.7	14	0.8750	1.3512	0.9117	0.0367
52.0	15	0.9375	2.1090	0.9825	0.0450

Table 17.10

PSA = 4–10 Data in the Format of Table 17.4

Interval	Standard normal z to end of interval	Probability	Expected frequencies (e_i)	Observed frequencies (n_i)
45–<50	−2.0782	0.0188	3.0832	2
50–<55	−1.4406	0.0560	9.1840	9
55–<60	−0.8031	0.1362	22.3368	19
60–<65	−0.1656	0.2232	36.6048	44
65–<70	0.4719	0.2473	40.5572	30
70–<75	1.1094	0.1849	30.3236	36
75–<80	1.7470	0.0933	15.3012	15
80–<85	2.3845	0.0317	5.1988	6
85–<90	3.0220	0.0073	1.1972	3

in the format of Table 17.7. The number in the respective sample preceding each current observation is listed for remove (k_1) and leave in place (k_2). $F_1 = k_1/9$ and $F_2 = k_2/10$ and finally $|F_1 - F_2|$ are entered. Inspection of $|F_1 - F_2|$ shows the largest value as $L = 0.5778$, denoted by an asterisk. L is barely smaller than critical; there is not enough evidence to conclude that the distributions are different.

Table 17.11

Functionality of Repaired Ankles Data in the Format of Table 17.7

% func.	k_1	k_2	F_1	F_2	$\|F_1 - F_2\|$
35	0		0	0	0
45		0	0	0	0
63	1		0.1111	0	0.1111
65	2		0.2222	0	0.2222
70	3		0.3333	0	0.3333
72		1	0.3333	0.1	0.2333
75	4		0.4444	0.1	0.3444
78	5		0.5556	0.1	0.4556
80	6		0.6667	0.1	0.5667
85		2	0.6667	0.2	0.4667
90	7		0.7778	0.2	0.5778*
90		3	0.7778	0.3	0.4778
93		4	0.7778	0.4	0.3778
95		5	0.7778	0.5	0.2778
95		6	0.7778	0.6	0.1778
98		7	0.7778	0.7	0.0778
99		8	0.7778	0.8	0.0222
100	8		0.8889	0.8	0.0889
100		9	0.8889	0.9	0.0111

Chapter 18

Sample Size Required in a Study

18.1. OVERVIEW

Chapter 7 examined the basic ideas of estimating the minimum sample size required in a study. More exactly, it is the size required in a test or confidence interval, as sample size may be estimated for multiple tests in a study. The conservative strategy is to choose for the study the largest of those sample sizes. It was pointed out that statistical needs may compete with limitations of time, money, support facilities, and ethics of patient use, but speaking solely from a statistical viewpoint, *the larger the sample, the better*, because the character of the sample approaches that of the population as the sample grows larger. Larger samples provide better estimates, more confidence, and smaller test errors. Ideally, we would obtain all the data our time, money, support facilities, and ethics will permit. The purely statistical purpose of minimum sample size estimation is to *verify that we will have enough* data to make the study worthwhile.

Number Needed to Treat

A related concept is the number needed to treat, as in the number of mammograms required to detect one breast cancer that otherwise would have been missed. The methods for this question are rather different and so are examined in Chapter 19 on modeling.

Summary of Minimum Sample Size Concept

In Chapter 7, the concept was introduced as estimating that sample size n that has $1 - \beta$ probability of detecting a clinically chosen difference δ when it is present and $1 - \alpha$ probability of rejecting such a difference when it is absent. The calculation of the probabilities depends on the standard error of the mean (SEM), σ_m. Figure 7.1 illustrated the effect of increasing the sample size from n to $4n$, which halved σ_m and reduced the error rates α and β. The difference δ was termed *clinical relevance*. The method of estimating minimum required sample size often is called *power analysis*, because $1 - \beta$, the power of the test, is a component in the estimation process.

Test Sidedness

Sample size estimation may be based on a one- or two-sided alternate hypothesis. For one-sided cases, the more commonly used two-sided form of the normal tail area ($z_{1-\alpha/2}$) is replaced by $z_{1-\alpha}$ wherever it appears. For example, replace the two-tailed 5% α's $z = 1.96$ by the one-tailed 5% α's $z = 1.645$.

Test Parameters

Although $\alpha = 5\%$ and power $= 80\%$ ($\beta = 20\%$) have been the most commonly selected error sizes in the medical literature, a 20% β is larger than appropriate in many cases. Furthermore, the false negative rate to false positive rate (β/α) ratio of 4/1 may affect the care of patients in treatments based on the outcome of the study, because the false positive sometimes is worse for the patient than the false negative. The β/α ratio should be chosen with thought and care for each study.

Clinical Relevance

The size of the difference between treatment outcomes (often denoted d or δ) that will answer the clinical question being posed usually is the statistical parameter that most influences the sample size and also may affect patient care. Too often it is chosen rather casually. Because a larger difference will require a smaller n, the temptation exists to maximize the difference to allow for a small enrollment in the study. The choice should be made on clinical rather than statistical grounds.

Sequential Analysis in Relation to Sample Size Estimation

The concept of sequential analysis is to test the hypothesis successively with each new datum. The result of the test falls into the following classes: accept hypothesis, reject hypothesis, or continue sampling. At first, due to a very small sample size, the test result falls into the continue sampling class. Sampling is continued until it falls into one of the other classes, at which point sampling is stopped. The purpose is to minimize the sample size required in a study. Whereas it does serve this purpose, it does not give the investigator any advance idea of required sample size. On the contrary, it prevents a planned sample size. Thus, sequential analysis will be categorized as a time-dependent analysis and addressed in Chapter 21.

18.2. RELATION OF SAMPLE SIZE CALCULATED TO SAMPLE SIZE NEEDED

The Calculated Sample Size Is Just a Rather Poor Estimate

Remember that the calculation of the minimum required sample size estimate is based on judgmental inputs and data different from those that will be used in the ensuing study. This estimate, therefore, is one of low confidence. Inasmuch as the SEM used in the sample size calculation arose from a sample other than that of the study, there is a *wrong data* source of possible error in the calculation. Also, sample size is estimated on data that are subject to randomness, so that there also is a *randomness* source of possible error in the estimate. Due to these errors, the calculated sample size is likely to be different from that actually needed. In case the calculated size is smaller than truly needed, the calculated size should be increased by a "safety factor" to allow for these two sources of possible error. The size of this safety factor is an educated guess.

18.3. SAMPLE SIZE FOR A CONFIDENCE INTERVAL ON A MEAN

Example

In DB12, the extent of carinal resection (centimeters) is distributed approximately normal and the sample size is large enough to use the estimated standard deviation 1.24 as σ. Suppose that in a new study we will require the sample mean m of the extent of resection to be no more than 0.5 cm from the population mean μ, i.e., $d = |m - \mu| = 0.5$. How large of a sample will we need to obtain 95% confidence on this interval? Confidence at 95% implies that $z_{1-\alpha/2} = 1.96$ (the frequently seen entry from Table A). From Eq. (18.1), we find that

$$n = \frac{(z_{1-\alpha/2})^2\sigma^2}{d^2} = \frac{1.96^2 \times 1.24^2}{0.5^2} = 24.$$

We need a sample of at least 24 patients and should take a few more, as per Section 18.2.

Method

From the confidence intervals of Chapter 4, the end values of a $1-\alpha$ confidence interval on the mean μ of a normal distribution with known σ was given by Eq. (4.5) as $\mu = m \pm z_{1-\alpha/2}\sigma_m$. We subtract m from μ to generate $d = |\mu - m|$, the difference between the observed and theoretical means. We square throughout and substitute $\sigma_m^2 = \sigma^2/n$ to obtain $d^2 = (z_{1-\alpha/2}\sigma)^2/n$, or

$$n = \frac{(z_{1-\alpha/2})^2\sigma^2}{d^2}. \quad (18.1)$$

The n calculated in Eq. (18.1) is a very minimum; it would be wise to take a slightly larger sample for the reasons discussed in Section 18.2. Note that σ is estimated from a sample of pilot data or a sample from an earlier study found in the literature. The form using σ rather than s is employed regardless of sample size. A confidence form using s would involve the t distribution, and t cannot be found without the degrees of freedom (*df*), which is unknown. Furthermore, the nicety of difference between σ and s is lost in the distinction between the past data and those to be obtained for the ensuing study. For 95% confidence, we have seen repeatedly from Table A and elsewhere that $z_{1-\alpha/2} = 1.96$ for $1-\alpha = 95\%$; we need only replace $z_{1-\alpha/2}$ by 1.96.

Additional Example

In the example from DB12 at the beginning of this section, the minimum sample size required in a new study was estimated for 95% confidence on a 0.5-cm mean difference of the extent of carinal resection. Suppose we required greater confidence, say 99%, and greater accuracy, say 0.25 cm. σ was taken as 1.24, derived from the data already at hand. $d = |m - \mu| = 0.25$. In Table A, the 0.990 entry in the column under two-tailed $1-\alpha$ lies in the row for $z_{1-\alpha/2} = 2.576$. By substituting in Eq. (18.1), we find that

$$n = \frac{(z_{1-\alpha/2})^2\sigma^2}{d^2} = \frac{2.576^2 \times 1.24^2}{0.25^2} = 163.25.$$

We require a minimum of 164 patients and would be advised to have a few more for the reasons of Section 18.2.

Exercise 18.1. In DB7, the distribution of bone density is not far from normal. $m = 154$ and $s = 24$. Estimate n for a 95% confidence interval on a deviation of the sample mean from the theoretical mean of no more than $d = 10$.

18.4. SAMPLE SIZE FOR A CONFIDENCE INTERVAL ON A PROPORTION

EXAMPLE

In the additional example of Section 12.5, oral surgery patients were anesthetized by a combination of propofol and alfentanil, and 89.1% of patients rated the anesthetic as highly satisfactory.[36] We placed a 95% confidence interval on π as 83–96%. The width of the half-interval $w = |p_s - \pi|$ is 6.5%. How many patients would we need to reach $w = 5\%$? π is not near 0 or 1, so we use Eq. (18.2) from the following Methods section:

$$n = \frac{1.96^2 p_s(1 - p_s)}{w^2} = \frac{1.96^2 \times 0.811 \times 0.112}{0.05^2} = 153.3.$$

We would need a very minimum of 154 and would be advised to take a few more. Suppose we wanted to be 98% confident, that is, to risk 1% chance of error on each tail. From Table A, the 0.98 two-tailed $1 - \alpha$ yields a corresponding z of 2.326. By replacing the 1.96 in the preceding calculation by 2.326, we obtain

$$n = \frac{2.326^2 p_s(1 - p_s)}{w^2} = 216.0.$$

METHOD

Conceptually, we may think of estimating the sample size needed for a confidence interval as specifying the interval we require and back-solving the equation for n. However, there are other considerations. The width of the interval is $w = |p - \pi|$, where we do not yet have p and usually we never know π exactly, so this interval is rather arbitrary. Because we need p to estimate σ, but will not have it until data have been gathered, we must use some rough indicator of p, the proportion found in a pilot study or a similar study found in the literature. As a result of these uncertainties, the n obtained is not an accurate sample size, but just some idea of the size as discussed in Section 18.2. We would be better assured of reaching our target confidence if we take a slightly larger n, although there is no way to know just how much larger. By solving one side of the confidence interval equations of Section 12.5 for n for 95% confidence, we find

$$n = \frac{1.96^2 p(1 - p)}{w^2} \tag{18.2}$$

for the case of π not near 0 or 1 and

$$n = \frac{1.96^2 p}{w^2} \tag{18.3}$$

when π is near 0 or 1. Confidence levels other than for 95% can be found by replacing 1.96 with the appropriate probability from Table A. [Note that because the maximum value of $p(1-p) = 0.25$, the numerator of Eq. (18.2) cannot exceed 0.49. The numerator of Eq. (18.3) cannot exceed 3.842.]

Additional Example

A dermatologist is studying the efficacy of tretinoin in treating $n = 15$ women's post-partum abdominal stretch marks.[68] Tretinoin was used on a randomly chosen side of the abdomen and a placebo on the other. Neither patient nor investigator knew which side was medicated. The dermatologist rated one side or the other as better where he could make a distinction, and afterward the code was broken and the treated side identified. The treated side was chosen in 9 of 13 abdomens for an observed proportion of 0.69. If the treatment were of no value, the theoretical proportion π would be 0.5. How many patients would be needed to have 95% confidence on the $w = |p-\pi| = 0.19$? π is not near 0 or 1, so he uses Eq. (18.2). By substituting, he finds

$$n = \frac{1.96^2 p(1-p)}{w^2} = \frac{3.8416 \times 0.69(1-0.69)}{(0.69-0.5)^2} = 22.8.$$

He requires a minimum of 23 patients.

Exercise 18.2. A pediatric surgeon is studying indicators of patient condition following pyloromyotomy (correction of stenotic pylorus) in neonates.[16] He finds that 14 out of 20 infants, i.e., a proportion of 0.7, suffered from emesis after surgery. How large of a sample will he require to be 95% sure that he is within 0.1 of the true proportion?

18.5. SAMPLE SIZE FOR A CONFIDENCE INTERVAL ON A CORRELATION COEFFICIENT

Example

In a study on broken ankle repair,[23] an orthopedist found the correlation coefficient between age and plantar flexion of a repaired ankle to be 0.1945. How large of a sample would he have required to be able to show evidence of flexion

Table 18.1

Samples Sizes Required to Infer a ρ Larger Than Would Occur Due to Chance at 95% Confidence for Various Values of the Sample Correlation Coefficient r

r	n	r	n
0.01		0.31	41
0.02		0.32	39
0.03	4269	0.33	37
0.04	2401	0.34	34
0.05	1538	0.35	32
0.06	1068	0.36	30
0.07	785	0.37	29
0.08	601	0.38	27
0.09	475	0.39	26
0.10	385	0.40	25
0.11	319	0.41	24
0.12	268	0.42	26
0.13	228	0.43	22
0.14	197	0.44	21
0.15	172	0.45	20
0.16	149	0.46	19
0.17	134	0.47	18
0.18	120	0.48	17
0.19	107	0.49	17
0.20	97	0.50	16
0.21	88	0.55	13
0.22	80	0.60	11
0.23	74	0.65	9
0.24	68	0.70	8
0.25	63	0.75	7
0.26	58	0.80	6
0.27	54	0.85	5
0.28	50	0.90	4
0.29	47		
0.30	44		

depending on age? From Table 18.1, $r = 0.1945$ corresponds to an n between 97 and 107; he would have needed a minimum of about 100 patients.

METHOD

When a correlation coefficient between two variables is small enough to have occurred by chance alone, we cannot infer evidence of a relationship between these variables. What sample size will make the correlation coefficient r larger than would occur by chance? More precisely, how large of a sample is required for the 95% confidence interval to exclude $\rho = 0$? When $\rho = 0$ is true and the two variables are approximately normal, a transformation to the t distribution can be made, namely,

$$t = \frac{r\sqrt{n-2}}{\sqrt{1-r^2}}. \tag{18.4}$$

A little algebra will solve this equation for n and provide Table 18.1. The last line of Table 18.1 carries the sample size smaller (<12 or so) than would be wise to use in practice. It is given to show the pattern of reduction in n. What is done if r is negative? A symmetry property of the distribution from which Table 18.1 arose allows the same n to emerge as if the r were positive, so just drop the minus sign for sample size purposes.

Statistical Significance and Clinical Meaning

A look at the first row or two of Table 18.1 will show the reader that an investigator can find a correlation coefficient to be "larger than chance" just by taking a large enough sample. The fact of being larger than chance statistically may have no relationship to clinical meaning. Increased sample size is useful up to the value of the coefficient that is clinically meaningful; beyond that, further increases are just a statistical exercise that should be avoided as the result could be misleading.

Additional Example

An anesthesiologist wanting to predict the requirement for deep sedation during surgery found a correlation coefficient between surgical difficulty and surgical duration of 0.17 on a small sample of patients.[42] If this sort of coefficient holds, how many patients would she need to conclude that surgical difficulty is a factor in predicting surgical duration? From Table 18.1, $r = 0.17$ corresponds to $n = 134$.

Exercise 18.3. An ophthalmologist suspects that the effect of a beta-blocker (timolol) on intraocular pressure (IOP) diminishes with age.[5] He takes a pilot sample of $n = 30$ patients, recording their ages and their reduction in IOP 4 weeks after initiation of treatment. He calculates the sample correlation coefficient as $r = -0.23$. How large of a sample will he need to conclude that the population ρ is truly less than 0, based on his pilot result?

18.6. SAMPLE SIZE FOR TESTS ON CATEGORICAL DATA

Methods for testing categorical data are treated in Chapters 6 and 13. From categorical data, proportions can always be obtained; minimum sample size is calculated from such proportions. Values used in such calculations are the error risks α and β, the proportions involved, and the difference between the proportions. This difference, often denoted δ, is the value to be tested. It should be chosen as the difference clinically important to detect. The minimum sample size depends more on this difference than on the other inputs. The sample size grows large quickly as this difference grows small.

Contingency Tables

Methods for the estimation of minimum required sample size are not well developed for contingency tests, but we can use the method for two proportions. The cell entries over their marginal totals (the totals for each category) provide two proportions. If the contingency table is bigger than 2×2, an *ad hoc* approach is to calculate the required sample size for the various pairs by using the method for two proportions repeatedly and then accept as the estimate the largest sample size that emerges.

Test of a Sample Proportion against a Theoretical Proportion

A proportion follows the binomial or Poisson distributions, depending on whether the proportion is *not* near 0 (or 1) or *is* near 0 (or 1), respectively. A proportion from an at least moderately sized sample is distributed approximately normal for either the binomial or the Poisson. The proportion behaves like a mean for either, leaving the only difference in the method as the mode of estimating the standard deviation: the binomial form

$$\sigma = \sqrt{\frac{\pi(1-\pi)}{n}}, \qquad s = \sqrt{\frac{p(1-p)}{n}}$$

(depending on the proportion known or estimated by p, respectively) versus the Poisson form

$$\sigma = \sqrt{\pi/n}, \qquad s = \sqrt{p/n}.$$

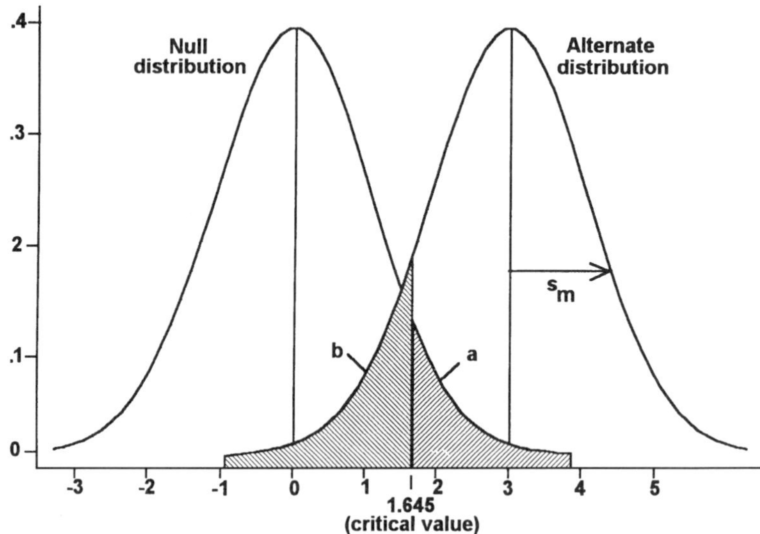

Figure 18.1 Distributions of null and alternate hypotheses showing Types I and II errors separated by the critical value, chosen at 1.645 (standard errors) to provide $\alpha = 5\%$. We specify the difference in standard errors between the means (here about three) that we want the test to detect. The error probabilities are dictated by the overlap of distributions, which in turn is dictated by the standard error $\sigma_m = \sigma/\sqrt{n}$. As we increase n, σ_m shrinks, and therefore the areas under the overlap giving the error sizes shrink until the specified error probabilities are reached. The resulting n is the minimum sample size required to detect the specified difference in means.

Thanks to the normal approximation, the required sample size estimation follows the concept and logic depicted first in Fig. 7.1 and again in Fig. 18.1.

Example

In Section 6.1, we proposed testing an observed 30% rate of positive prostate cancer biopsies (DB1) against a smaller theoretical proportion $\pi = 0.25$. How many patients do we need for a $p = 0.30$ proportion testing positive to be significant with a one-tailed $\alpha = 0.05$ and power $= 0.80$? (Note that we have a one-sided alternate hypothesis.) From Table A, the z-values are 1.645 and 0.84, respectively. Because π is not near 0 or 1, we use the binomial form, Eq. (18.5). By substituting the z-values, π, and p, we obtain $n = [1.645 \times \sqrt{(0.25 \times 0.75)} + 0.84 \times \sqrt{(0.31 \times 0.69)}]^2/(0.31 - 0.25)^2 = (0.7123 + 0.3885)^2/(0.06)^2 = 1.2118/0.0036 = 337$. To be safe from unforeseen sampling fluctuations (see Section 18.2), we should take a slightly larger sample.

Method

We assume normal theory, with mean difference $p-\pi$ divided by the appropriate standard deviation given earlier, which gives rise to the sample size Eqs. (18.5) and (18.6). We know the theoretical proportion π and we calculate the sample proportion p from our data. If π is not near 0 or 1, we use a binomial form, Eq. (18.5). If π is near 0 or 1, we use a Poisson form, Eq. (18.6). We choose the risk required of a false positive (α) and a false negative (β or $1-$ power). We look up the z-values in Table A associated with these two risks (areas in the tails of the normal curve), $z_{1-\alpha/2}$ and $z_{1-\beta}$. We then substitute the z-values, π, and p in Eq. (18.5) or (18.6) to find n, the minimum sample size required.

$$n = \left[\frac{z_{1-\alpha/2}\sqrt{\pi(1-\pi)} + z_{1-\beta}\sqrt{p(1-p)}}{p-\pi}\right]^2 \tag{18.5}$$

$$n = \left[\frac{z_{1-\alpha/2}\sqrt{\pi} + z_{1-\beta}\sqrt{p}}{p-\pi}\right]^2. \tag{18.6}$$

We should note that $p-\pi$ is a major determinant in the sample size estimation, and therefore p should be chosen carefully in line with its clinical implications.

Additional Example

A Navy specialist in internal medicine, sent to an African nation, must decide whether female residents of a particular rural region lying along an often stagnant river have a prevalence of schistosomiasis greater than the national average, which dictates hypotheses H_0: $\pi_s = \pi$ (subscript s for "sample") and H_1: $\pi_s > \pi$ (a one-sided alternative).[58] He plans an informal study to compare the local mean to the national mean and must estimate how many patients he needs to sample. Clinical judgment leads him to believe that he needs to detect a difference of 2%. He finds an article in the literature that quotes a prevalence of 24% over 1600 patients examined. He chooses one-tailed $\alpha = 5\%$ and power $= 80\%$. His z-values from Table A are 1.645 and 0.84. By substituting these values in Eq. (18.5), he finds

$$n = \left[\frac{z_{1-\alpha}\sqrt{\pi(1-\pi)} + z_{1-\beta}\sqrt{p(1-p)}}{p-\pi}\right]^2$$
$$= \left[\frac{1.645\sqrt{(0.24)(0.76)} + 0.84\sqrt{(0.26)(0.74)}}{0.02}\right]^2 = 2867.63.$$

He will require nearly 2900 patients to be able to detect a 2% difference.

Exercise 18.4: One Proportion. Radial keratotomy (RK) is performed by residents in ophthalmology in a certain hospital. A review of records shows that 18%

of residents performed enhancements in more than one-fifth of their cases.[4] This frequency of enhancements is thought to arise from the surgery learning curve. Training in the surgery by a computer simulation may shorten the learning curve. How many residents will need to be monitored to detect a decrease of 6% (i.e., a drop from 18% to 12%) in the number of residents performing enhancements in more than one-fifth of their cases? Use $\alpha = 5\%$ and power $= 80\%$.

Test of Two Proportions

A test of two proportions can be used in place of a contingency test, such as appeared in Section 6.3, but usually is less convenient as it does not appear in many software packages. For sample size estimation, we use it, reformatted for this purpose.

Example

A psychiatrist wants to know whether the proportion of people having a personality disorder is the same for those committing violent crimes (p_1) and those committing nonviolent crimes (p_2).[42] Theoretically, either p could be the larger, so he chooses a two-sided alternative hypothesis. He examines a few of his past records to serve as a pilot survey and estimates p_1 as 0.06 and p_2 as 0.02. How many patients does he need to detect a difference $p_1 - p_2 = 0.04$ significant at two-tailed $\alpha = 0.05$ and power $= 0.80$? From Table A, the z-values are 1.96 and 0.84, respectively. From Eq. (18.7), p_m, the mean p, is $(p_1 + p_2)/2 = 0.04$. Because p_m is near 0, he uses the Poisson form Eq. (18.9):

$$n_1 = n_2 = \left[\frac{(z_{1-\alpha/2} + z_{1-\beta})\sqrt{p_1 + p_2}}{p_1 - p_2}\right]^2 = \left[\frac{(1.96 + 0.84)\sqrt{0.08}}{0.04}\right]^2$$

$$= 19.80^2 = 392.04.$$

He will need a very minimum of 393 patients in each group. To include a safety factor (see Section 18.2), a slightly larger number would be wiser.

Method

We assume normal theory. We calculate the sample proportions p_1 and p_2 from our data and then p_m (m for mean) as the average of p_1 and p_2:

$$p_m = \frac{p_1 + p_2}{2}. \qquad (18.7)$$

If p_m is not near 0 or 1, we use Eq. (18.8), derived from the binomial form. If p_m

is near 0 or 1, we use Eq. (18.9), derived from the Poisson form:

$$n_1 = n_2 = \left[\frac{z_{1-\alpha/2}\sqrt{2p_m(1-p_m)} + z_{1-\beta}\sqrt{p_1(1-p_1)+p_2(1-p_2)}}{p_1 - p_2} \right]^2 \tag{18.8}$$

$$n_1 = n_2 = \left[\frac{(z_{1-\alpha/2} + z_{1-\beta})\sqrt{p_1 + p_2}}{p_1 - p_2} \right]^2. \tag{18.9}$$

We choose α, the risk of a wrong rejection of H_0, and $\beta(1-\text{power})$, the risk of a wrong acceptance of H_0. We look up the z-values in Table A associated with these two risks (areas in the tails of the normal curve), $z_{1-\alpha/2}$ and $z_{1-\beta}$. We substitute the z-values and the p's in Eq. (18.8) or (18.9) to find n, the minimum sample size required in each group.

Estimates on the Borderline between Binomial and Poisson

If π is close to the borderline for using the Poisson approximation, a correction of the normal approximation is appropriate, especially if n_1 is small. The corrected n for each group will be n_{corr}:

$$n_{corr} = \frac{n_1}{4}\left[1 + \sqrt{1 + \frac{4}{n_1|p_1 - p_2|}}\right]^2. \tag{18.10}$$

Additional Example

An emergency medicine specialist finds that 15% of patients report having a fever.[42] She wants to know whether there is a difference between reporting rates of men and women. She does not know which would be the greater, which implies a two-tailed test. How many patients would she have to monitor to find a difference of 6% (e.g., 12% for one group and 18% for the other) with $\alpha = 0.05$ and power $=$ 0.80? $z_{1-\alpha/2} = 1.96$ and $z_{1-\beta} = 0.84$. $p_m = 0.15$, not near 0 or 1, so the binomial form Eq. (18.8) is used:

$$\begin{aligned} n_1 = n_2 &= \left[\frac{z_{1-\alpha/2}\sqrt{2p_m(1-p_m)} + z_{1-\beta}\sqrt{p_1(1-p_1)+p_2(1-p_2)}}{p_1 - p_2} \right]^2 \\ &= \left[\frac{1.96\sqrt{2 \times 0.015 \times 0.085} + .084\sqrt{0.12 \times 0.88 + 0.18 \times 0.82}}{0.12 - 0.18} \right]^2 \\ &= 554.16. \end{aligned}$$

The minimum sample size per group is 555. In line with Section 18.2, she should take a few more.

Exercise 18.5: Two Proportions. An eye surgeon is performing radial keratotomies using hand surgery and is considering a laser device.[3] His hand surgery record shows that 23% of eyes require surgical enhancement. He plans a prospective study in which patients are randomized into the hand and laser groups. On how many eyes per method would he need to operate to detect an improvement of 10% (i.e., a reduction in enhancement rate from 23% to 13%)? Use $\alpha = 5\%$ and power = 80%.

18.7. SAMPLE SIZE FOR TESTS ON RANKED DATA

Methods for testing ranked data are treated in Chapters 6 and 14. Not much attention has been paid to estimating minimum required sample sizes for ranked (nonparametric) data, as the largest application is for cases in which standard deviations are markedly different or in which the distributions are "poorly behaved." For these cases, the method of Section 18.8, Case 3, may be used, although this method is very conservative and tends to overestimate the minimum required sample size.

18.8. SAMPLE SIZE FOR TESTS ON MEANS

What Goes into the Calculation

Methods for testing means of continuous data are treated in Chapters 6 and 15. Values used in minimum sample size calculations are the error risks, the standard deviation of the population data, and the difference between the two means being tested. This difference, often denoted d or δ, should be chosen as the difference clinically important to detect. The minimum sample size depends more on this difference than on the other inputs. The sample size grows large quickly as this difference grows small.

Explanation Instead of Derivation

The following cases for calculating minimum sample size provide only formulas, which are not derived here. In lieu of derivation, a comment on where they come from may help the user understand them. The comment will treat a test of a sample mean against an established mean using the normal distribution; concepts for other tests are similar.

Where the Formulas Come From

A population exists with mean μ. We are sampling from some population that may or may not be the same. Our sample distribution has a population mean μ_s (subscript s for "sample"). We want to learn whether μ_s is the same as μ or, let us say, larger, implying hypotheses H_0: $\mu_s = \mu$ and H_1: $\mu_s > \mu$. However, we do not know the value of μ_s, so we estimate it with the sample mean m. Thus, to decide whether $\mu_s = \mu$, we test m against μ. Figure 18.1 shows the two distributions involved: the null distribution, with its mean $\mu = 0$ (standard normal) indicated by a vertical line, and a possible alternate distribution, with its mean μ_s, estimated by m, indicated by a vertical line at about 3. σ is the standard deviation of the population data, so σ_m, the standard error of the mean (the standard deviation of distribution shown in the figure) is $\sigma/\sqrt{n}$, where n is the sample size we seek. We use the form of a test for a significant difference between means, $m - \mu$, with $\alpha = 5\%$ and $\beta = 20\%$ (power $= 1-\beta = 80\%$). The critical value (here $\mu + 1.645\sigma_m$) is the position separating the two types of error, shown in Fig. 18.1 as the number of standard errors to the right of μ that yields a 5% α (area under a tail of the null distribution; 1.645 is the critical value from the normal table for $\alpha = 5\%$). Similarly, β is the area under a tail of the alternate distribution specified by the number of standard errors to the left of m that the critical value lies, or $m - 0.84\sigma_m$ (where 0.84 is the value from the normal table for 20% in the tail area). Because these two expressions both equal the critical value, we set them equal to each other, or $\mu + 1.645\sigma/\sqrt{n} = m - 0.84\sigma/\sqrt{n}$. Solution of the equation for n yields $n = (1.645 + 0.84)\sigma^2/(m - \mu)^2$. Other formulas for minimum required sample size follow equivalent logic.

Suppose We Do Not Know σ

Note that the methods given here use mostly normal distribution theory and the population or large-sample σ rather than a small-sample s. If s is all we have, we just use it in place of σ. The reason for this is two-fold. First, by not knowing n, we have no *df* to use in finding the appropriate t-values to use in the calculation. Second, the nicety of using t would be lost in the grossness of the approximation, because the process depends on pilot data or results from other studies and not the data to be used in the actual analysis.

Case 1: One Mean, Normal Distribution

Example

We want to determine whether BPH patients treated with an experimental hormonal therapy have larger prostates than those of non-BPH patients. The prostate volume (milliliters) of our 296 patients without BPH (see DB1) has mean

μ =35.46 ml and standard deviation $\sigma = 18.04$ ml. What is the smallest sample size that can detect a sample mean m (of the experimental group) at least 10 ml larger than μ (implying a one-sided alternative hypothesis)? We choose $\alpha = 0.05$ and $\beta = 0.20$, as is common in medicine, giving us $z_{1-\alpha} = 1.645$ and $z_{1-\beta} = 0.84$. Substitution in Eq. (18.11) yields $n = (1.645 + 0.84)^2 18.04^2/10^2 = 6.175 \times 325.44 \div 100 = 20.1$; we must round up to 21. In line with Section 18.2, we should take a larger n to allow for deviations due to sampling fluctuations.

Method

What size of sample do we need to decide whether m is different from μ? (More exactly, if the mean of the sample's population as estimated by m is different from μ) Choose the smallest distance d between m and μ, i.e., $d = m - \mu$, that you want to detect with statistical significance. Choose the risk you will accept of concluding that there is a difference when there is not (α) and of concluding that there is no difference when there is (β or $1-$power). Look up the z-values in Table A associated with these two risks, $z_{1-\alpha/2}$ and $z_{1-\beta}$. If the test is to be one-sided, use $z_{1-\alpha}$ instead of $z_{1-\alpha/2}$. Substitute the z-values and d along with the standard deviation σ in Eq. (18.11) to find n, the minimum sample size required:

$$n = \frac{(z_{1-\alpha/2} + z_{1-\beta})^2 \sigma^2}{d^2}. \tag{18.11}$$

Additional Example

An emergency medicine physician wants to test the effectiveness of a "GI cocktail" (antacid plus viscous lidocaine) to treat emergency dyspeptic symptoms as measured on a 1–10 pain scale.[42] The standard deviation without treatment has been scored for a large number of patients as $\sigma = 1.73$. He considers a reduction in pain rating of $d = 1.5$ points as clinically meaningful. He believes that the treatment cannot increase pain, so the test will be one-sided. By taking $\alpha = 0.05$ and $\beta = 0.20$ (power = 80%), $z_{1-\alpha} = 1.645$ and $z_{1-\beta} = 0.84$. By substituting in Eq. (18.11), he finds

$$n = \frac{(z_{1-\alpha} + z_{1-\beta})^2 \sigma^2}{d^2} = \frac{(1.645 + 0.84)^2 \times (1.73)^2}{1.5^2} = 8.21.$$

He sees that he needs only nine patients to be able to just detect significance. However, he anticipates that the posttreatment standard deviation might be larger and he wants a safety factor in line with Section 18.2, so he decides to sample 14 patients.

Exercise 18.6: One Mean. An emergency medicine physician wants to know whether mean heart rate following a particular type of trauma differs from the healthy population rate of 72 beats per minute (bpm).[55] He considers a mean difference of 6 bpm clinically meaningful. He takes σ to be the 9.1 bpm reported in a large study. How many patients will he need? Use $\sigma = 0.05$ and power $= 0.80$.

Estimation of Required *n* without Using Power $(1 - \beta)$

Some (mostly older) statistics books give methods for finding n without using power. If μ, m, and σ are known, it is possible to solve for n without factoring in power, that is, by letting the power fall where it may. If a known population heart rate has $\mu = 68$ bpm and $\sigma = 3$ bpm and we want to detect a difference in an experimental population having $m = 69$ bpm with $\alpha = 5\%$, solution of the equation $(m - \mu)/(\sigma/\sqrt{n}) = 1.96$ yields $n = 35$. However, μ, m, σ, and the assumption of normality specify the alternate distribution, so that the better method including the power could and should be used. The power in the preceding estimate can be calculated to be 0.50. If we specify a power of 0.80, which is common in medical research, we would require $n = 71$. Methods that do not use power are best avoided.

Case 2: Two Means, Normal Distributions

This case was detailed in Section 7.4. The example given was a comparison of range of motion between two types of artificial knee. Another example might be helpful.

Example

As another example, let us use the carinal resection surgery (DB12) data to estimate standard deviations. We want to find the minimum required sample size to detect a 2-year mean difference in age at surgery between patients who survive and those who die. We might propose older patients to be more at risk, but unanticipated factors that might create a risk in the younger cannot be ruled out, so a two-tailed test is appropriate. For the 117 surviving patients, $s_1 = 16.01$, and for the 17 dying patients, $s_2 = 15.78$, which we take as σ-values for the calculation. $\sigma_1^2 = 256.32$ and $\sigma_2^2 = 209.09$. α is chosen as 5% and $1 - \beta$ (the power) as 80%. From Table A, $z_{1-\alpha/2} = 1.96$ and $z_{1-\beta} = 0.84$. Substitution in Eq. (18.12) yields

$$n_1 = n_2 = \frac{(z_{1-\alpha/2} + z_{1-\beta})^2(\sigma_1^2 + \sigma_2^2)}{d^2} = \frac{2.80^2 \times 465.41}{2^2} = 912.20.$$

The required minimum sample size is 913. For the reasons discussed in Section 18.2, a few more would be advisable.

Method

We ask whether μ_1 (estimated by m_1) is different from μ_2 (estimated by m_2). Choose the smallest distance d between m_1 and m_2, i.e., $d = m_1 - m_2$, that you want to detect with statistical significance. This usually is a clinical choice: the size of the difference that is clinically important. Also find σ_1^2 and σ_2^2, as estimated by s_1^2 and s_2^2. Choose the risk you will accept of concluding that there is a difference when there is not (α) and of concluding that there is no difference when there is (β or $1-$ power). Look up the z-values in Table A for these two risks, $z_{1-\alpha/2}$ and $z_{1-\beta}$. Substitute the z-values and d along with the standard deviations in Eq. (18.12) to find $n_1(=n_2)$, the minimum sample size required in *each* sample. Replace $z_{1-\alpha/2}$ with $z_{1-\alpha}$ for a one-sided test.

$$n_1 = n_2 = \frac{(z_{1-\alpha/2} + z_{1-\beta})^2 \left(\sigma_1^2 + \sigma_2^2\right)}{d^2}. \tag{18.12}$$

Additional Example

An emergency medicine physician wants to compare the relative effectiveness of two treatments, the "GI cocktail" (antacid plus viscous lidocaine) (treatment 1) versus IV ranitidine hydrochloride (treatment 2) to treat emergency dyspeptic symptoms as measured on a 1–10 pain scale.[42] Not having data on the pain ratings of the treatments, he estimates s_1 and s_2 as the standard deviation without treatment $\sigma = 1.73$. He considers a reduction in pain rating of $d = 1.5$ points as clinically meaningful. Either treatment can either be more effective, so the test will be two-tailed. Taking $\alpha = 0.05$ and $\beta = 0.20$ (power = 80%), $z_{1-\alpha/2} = 1.96$ and $z_{1-\beta} = 0.84$. By substituting in Eq. (18.12), he finds

$$n_1 = n_2 = \frac{(z_{1-\alpha/2} + z_{1-\beta})^2 \left(\sigma_1^2 + \sigma_2^2\right)}{d^2} = \frac{(1.96 + 0.84)^2 (2 \times 1.73^2)}{1.5^2} = 20.86.$$

He requires a minimum of 21 per sample just to show significance. However, he suspects that sample standard deviations will be larger than the untreated σ and plans a larger sample size.

Exercise 18.7: Two Means. An emergency medicine physician wants to know whether mean heart rate following two particular types of trauma are different.[55] He considers a mean difference of 6 bpm clinically meaningful. From pilot data, he finds $s_1 = 6.13$ bpm and $s_2 = 6.34$ bpm, which he uses to estimate σ_1 and σ_2. How many patients will he need in each group? Use $\alpha = 0.05$ and power $= 0.80$.

Case 3: Nonnormal (Poorly Behaved or Unknown) Distributions

One relationship that sometimes is helpful in sizing samples needed to detect a difference between m and μ arises in an inequality named for the Russian mathematician P. L. Chebychev (and other spellings, e.g., Tchebysheff). The relationship actually is due to I. J. Bienaymé (1835); Chebychev discovered it independently a bit later. The inequality is known as the Law of Large Numbers. Of interest to us is a form of the inequality relating sample size n to the deviation of the sample mean from the population mean. *This relationship is useful when an underlying data distribution is very poorly behaved or when nothing is known about the distribution. It also is useful when there are no data at all to estimate the variability.* As this inequality is solved without any information as to the distribution of the statistic involved, it is a rather gross overestimate of the sample size that would be required were the distribution known and wellbehaved. The sample size given by Chebychev's inequality certainly will be enough in any case and therefore is a conservative sample size, but *it is more than required for most applications.*

Example

Suppose we want to know the required minimum sample size to find a difference between mean intraocular pressure (IOP in mmHg) between patients who have been treated with a new drug and those who have not.[5] The units of this difference must be standard deviations, i.e., the unit is 1 standard deviation. For example, the detectable difference $m - \mu$ might be expressed as 0.5, 1, or 2 standard deviations. In this case, the standard deviation is 4 mmHg; we decide as a clinical judgment that we want to detect a 2 mmHg decrease in IOP, which yields a difference $k = 0.5\sigma$. We choose $\alpha = 0.05$, i.e., we are willing to take a 5% risk of being wrong in our choice. By using these quantities, Eq. (18.14) becomes

$$n = \frac{\sigma^2}{\alpha k^2} = \frac{\sigma^2}{0.05 \times 0.25\sigma^2} = 80.$$

Method

Choose k, the difference you want to detect between the sample mean and population mean (a clinical choice), expressed as the number of standard deviations apart they are. The form of the Chebycheff Inequality useful in this case is

$$\mathrm{P}[-k \leq m - \mu \leq k] \geq 1 - \frac{\sigma^2}{k^2 n}, \qquad (18.13)$$

where m denotes the sample mean, μ the hypothesized population mean, and σ the population standard deviation. Choose α, the risk of error you are willing to accept, which will be equivalent to the rightmost portion of Eq. (18.13). Then $1 - \alpha = 1 - \sigma^2/k^2 n$, which reduces to

$$n = \frac{\sigma^2}{\alpha k^2}. \qquad (18.14)$$

Substitution for k in terms of σ allows the σ^2s to cancel and provides a number for n.

Case 4: No Objective Prior Data

If we have neither data nor experience with a phenomenon being studied, we have no way to guess a required sample size. However, if we have some experience with the quantitative outcome of the variable to be measured, but no objective data at all, we have recourse to a very rough idea of needed sample size as a starting point.

Example

The wife of an internist has been treating her common colds with an herbal remedy for 3 years and claims it reduces the number of days to disappearance of all symptoms. Her best time was 8 days and the worst 15 days. The internist decides to conduct a prospective randomized double-masked study to evaluate the remedy's efficacy.[55] How many data should he take? He decides that a reduction of $d = 1$ day would be clinically meaningful. He chooses $\alpha = 5\%$ and power $= 80\%$, which yields one-tailed z-values of 1.645 and 0.84, respectively. In the absence of objectively recorded data, he guesses σ from her range: $\sigma \approx 0.25$ (largest $-$ smallest) $= 0.25(15 - 8) = 1.75$. (The symbol "$\approx$" often is used to indicate "approximately equal to".) By substituting these values in Eq. (18.11), with the one-sided $z_{1-\alpha}$ replacing $z_{1-\alpha/2}$, he finds

$$n = \frac{(z_{1-\alpha} + z_{1-\beta})^2\sigma^2}{d^2} = \frac{(1.645 + 0.84)^2 \times 1.75^2}{1^2} = 18.91.$$

Nineteen in each group (the experimental group and the placebo-treated group) is indicated as a minimum. He chooses a large safety factor (see Section 18.2) in light of the poor estimation of σ and plans 25 in each group.

Method

From experience, guess the smallest and largest values of the variable you have noticed. Take the difference between them as a guess of the interval: mean $\pm$ 2 standard deviations. This is equivalent to assuming that the data are roughly normal and your experience covers about 95% of the possible range. Then σ is estimated as 0.25 (largest – smallest). Use this value of σ in the method of Case 1. Clearly, this "desperation" estimate is of extremely low confidence, but may be better than picking a number out of the air.

18.9. SAMPLE SIZE FOR TESTS ON VARIANCES AND DISTRIBUTIONS

Estimation of Sample Size *n* for Tests on Variances and Distributions Are Not Easy

The χ^2 and F probabilities used to estimate n depend on n. Such estimates exist as tables, but they are based only upon the Type I error and therefore are not dependable. It is possible to develop estimates based on both types of error, but this entails using the difficult mathematical distributions noncentral χ^2 and noncentral F, which is far beyond the level of this text. The best advice for an investigator who requires such sample sizes is to seek the assistance of an accomplished statistician.

ANSWERS TO EXERCISES

18.1. By substituting in Eq. (18.1), we find

$$n = \frac{(z_{1-\alpha/2})^2\sigma^2}{d^2} = \frac{1.96^2 \times 24^2}{10^2} = 22.1.$$

We will need a sample of at least 23 patients and should take a few more, as per Section 18.2.

18.2. π is not near 0 or 1, so he uses Eq. (18.2). $p = 0.7$, $w = 0.1$, and, for 95% confidence, he retains the 1.96 given in Eq. (18.2). By substituting, he finds

$$n = \frac{1.96^2 p(1-p)}{w^2} = \frac{3.8416 \times 0.7(1-0.7)}{0.1^2} = 80.7.$$

18.3. The predicted required sample size will be the same as if the r were positive, due to the symmetry property of Table 18.1. In Table 18.1, $r = 0.23$ corresponds to $n = 74$.

18.4. $\pi = 0.18$. As π is not near 0 or 1, the binomial form Eq. (18.5) will be used. The test is one-sided (the training will not increase the number of enhancements), so $z_{1-\alpha} = 1.645$:

$$n = \left[1.645\sqrt{(0.18 \times 0.82)} + 0.84\sqrt{(0.12 \times 0.88)}\right]^2/(0.12 - 0.18)^2$$
$$= 15.0826^2 = 227.5.$$

At least 228 residents would be required, which is too large of a number to evaluate the training device in one medical center in a reasonable period of time; the plan for this study must be either dropped or arranged as a multicenter study.

18.5. $p_m = (0.23 + 0.13)/2 = 0.18$, not near 0 or 1, so the binomial form Eq. (18.8) is used. He believes the laser device can only improve the enhancement rate, so the test is one-sided, using $z_{1-\alpha} = 1.645$. By substituting in Eq. (18.8), he finds

$$\begin{aligned} n_1 &= n_2 \\ &= \left[1.645\sqrt{(2 \times 0.18 \times 0.82)} \right. \\ &\quad \left. + 0.84\sqrt{(0.23 \times 0.77 + 0.13 \times 0.87)}\right]^2 / 0.10^2 \\ &= 181.25. \end{aligned}$$

He would need a minimum of 182 eyes per method. To include a safety factor (see Section 18.2), he should take a few more.

18.6. The posttrauma heart rate can be either greater or less than the healthy rate, so the test will be two-tailed; $z_{1-\alpha/2} = 1.96$ and $z_{1-\beta} = 0.84$. From Eq. (18.11),

$$n = (z_{1-\alpha/2} + z_{1-\beta})^2 \sigma^2 / d^2 = (1.96 + 0.84)^2 (9.1)^2 / 6^2 = 18.0.$$

He needs at least 18 patients. For reasons set forth in Section 18.2, he should choose a few more than 18.

18.7. Either trauma type could evoke a higher heart rate, so the test is two-tailed; $z_{1-\alpha/2} = 1.96$ and $z_{1-\beta} = 0.84$. From Eq. (18.12),

$$n_1 = n_2 = (z_{1-\alpha/2} + z_{1-\beta})^2 (6.13^2 + 6.34^2)/6^2 = 16.9.$$

He needs at least 17 in each group and, by Section 18.2, is advised to choose a few more than 17.

Chapter 19

Modeling and Clinical Decisions

19.1. SUMMARY OF MODELING

DEFINITIONS AND GOALS

In the context of this book, *a model is a quantitative (or geometric) representation of a relationship or process*. Modeling was first introduced in Section 8.1. The example given was an increase in leukocyte count (WBC) with the level of infection. This was modeled (a) as a straight line and (b) only for certain values of the two variables (e.g., for WBC, from the upper limit of normal to a large, but not astronomical, value). The model may not represent the true relationship. Usually biological processes are so complicated that a model can represent only certain aspects of the process and in only certain ranges of the variables. WBC depending on infection might start rather flat and curve upward with infection level in an exponential fashion. Alternatively, it might start that way but then flatten again, approximating a plateau, as in a biological growth curve. The flexibility of model shape is not so much a weakness in modeling as a strength; the model can be changed with increasing knowledge and data and become ever closer to approximating the true event. Via such evolving models, we pass through the sequence of scientific learning from describing a process to testing its causal factors to being able to predict it. When we understand the causes of a process or an event and can predict it reliably, we have considerable knowledge that we can apply to clinical decision making.

TYPES OF MODELING AND CLINICAL DECISION MAKING

Only four types will be exemplified in this book: algebraic models, logical models, recursive partitioning, and outcomes analysis.

Algebraic Models

In algebraic models, the dependent variable, representing the biological event or process, is equal to a mathematical combination of independent variables, the causal factors. This mathematical expression is termed a *function* of the variables. The functional form of the model often may be visualized by a geometric relation among the variables, as the WBC was modeled as a straight line fit to the level of infection. There are various methods of fit, the most common of which and the only one addressed in this book being regression, a method that will be examined in some detail in Chapter 20. An algebraic model is not restricted to a straight line, but may be curved. Curved models are treated in Section 19.3. An algebraic model is not restricted to one dependent and one independent variable, but may have more than one of either. Models having one variable dependent on several independent ones are termed *multivariate* and will be treated in Section 19.5. The name *multivariable* tends to refer to multiple dependent variables, a case too advanced for this book.

Logical Models

Some models arise from the methods of mathematical logic (often combined with probability theory). The simplest forms are the "If A then B, but if not A then C" sort of logical analysis. Screening results and the number needed to treat (NNT) often are of this type, and logical models will be limited to screening and NNT in this book. This subject is addressed in Section 19.6.

Recursive Partitioning

Daily the clinician passes through a logical sequence of questions (decision points) in ruling out potential causes of illness and closing upon a diagnosis. The decision points consist of partitioning information into indicators of one disease but not another. Done repeatedly, or recursively, the partitioning leads to diagnosis or optimal therapy. Whereas the use of this method is second nature in common cases and usually is not even recognized, its formal use sometimes is of assistance in more complicated cases or in developing diagnostic or therapeutic procedures for newly discovered diseases. Clinical decision models using recursive partitioning are treated in Section 19.7, although they are in rather simple forms so that the user may concentrate on the method rather than the subject matter.

Outcomes Analysis

Clinical decisions based on the eventual overall outcome of treatment rather than on a single physiologic measure fall into this class. Outcomes analysis was introduced in Section 8.6 and is treated further in Section 19.8. An overall outcome seldom is based on a single measure, but usually involves a combination of indicators. Finding the nature of relationship among these indicators and combining them into a single measure of effectiveness (MOE) is a form of modeling.

19.2. SUMMARY OF STRAIGHT LINE MODELS

REVIEW OF SECTION 8.2

Let us think of a graph with x as the horizontal axis and y as the vertical axis. A straight line is determined by two pieces of information. A useful form of expressing a straight line relationship between medical variables is a slope β_1 (inclination of the line from horizontal) and a point. In the most commonly seen form, the point is the y intercept $(0, \beta_0)$ (slope–intercept form). However, actual data often place the intercept at an awkward distance, so a form using the x and y means, (m_x, m_y) often is preferable. This form was seen as Eq. (8.1). The algebraic expressions of these two forms follow:

$$\text{slope–intercept form: } y = \beta_0 + \beta_1 x \tag{19.1a}$$

$$\text{slope–means point form: } y - m_y = \beta_1(x - m_x). \tag{19.1b}$$

Straight lines are termed *first degree*, because no x in the expression has an exponent greater than 1. Other common algebraic forms for determining straight lines are a slope and a point anywhere on the line and two points on the line. In mathematics and physics, some variables are related exactly by a straight line and the fit is just a mathematical exercise. In biology and medicine, however, multiple causal factors are usual so that a straight line relationship is only approximate and the quality of a fit must be expressed in probability. Indeed, a straight line relationship may not exist for all values of x and y, but may be useful only in certain ranges. We are familiar with the estimates of m_x and m_y and how they are calculated. The best fit for the slope may be calculated by different criteria of "best," but the most common is named *least squares*: finding the smallest possible sum of squares of vertical distances from the data points to the line. A straight line fit to data subject to variability is a form of *regression*, which was introduced in Section 8.3 and will be examined further in Chapter 20.

19.3. CURVED MODELS

TYPES OF CURVED MODELS

Relationships between x and y may have almost any shape. Only the most common are presented here. Because fitting of functional forms to data is treated in Chapter 20, this section will consist of displaying common shapes in data relationships and noting the algebraic form that may express that relationship. Graphs of medical data are given and the user is asked to recognize the form.

Adding a Squared Term

Let us start with the slope–intercept form of a straight line, $y = \beta_0 + \beta_1 x$, and add a squared term to obtain $y = \beta_0 + \beta_1 x + \beta_2 x^2$. We now have a curved line, part of a parabola. A parabola is shown in Fig. 19.1A for negative β_2; the parabola would be concave upward for a positive β_2. All or any portion of it could be used to model a curved relationship. An example is shown in the box, which is enlarged in Fig. 19.1B. When 2 is the highest power, the expression is termed *second degree*.

Example

In DB3, the effect of azithromycin on serum theophylline level of emphysema patients was shown. Figure 19.2 shows day 10 levels as predicted by baseline levels. What is the shape of the relationship? A case could be made for either a first or second degree fit. Both fits were made using the least squares method and are shown superposed on the data in Fig. 19.2. Evaluation of these fits will be addressed in Chapter 20 on regression.

Method

The shape of a model is best derived from knowing the physiologic forces that generate the relationship. This shape may be verified or "fine-tuned" using curve-fitting methods. Positing a relationship directly from inspection of a data plot is reserved for the data exploration at the very beginning of knowledge acquisition. It is helpful in the interpretation of relationships to recognize general shapes from a data plot. After the general shape is noted and portions of a theoretical curve that are irrelevant to the relationship are deleted, the fit may be adjusted by sliding the curve horizontally or vertically on the axes or by stretching or shrinking the curve horizontally or vertically on the axes. These mechanisms will be examined in the next section.

Common Shapes of Relationship

Aside from a straight line (first degree) and a downward opening parabola (second degree), which were seen in the preceding example, commonly seen curves are illustrated in Figs. 19.3A–F. These include (A) the upward opening parabola (perhaps weight depending on height), (B) a third degree curve (adding an x^3

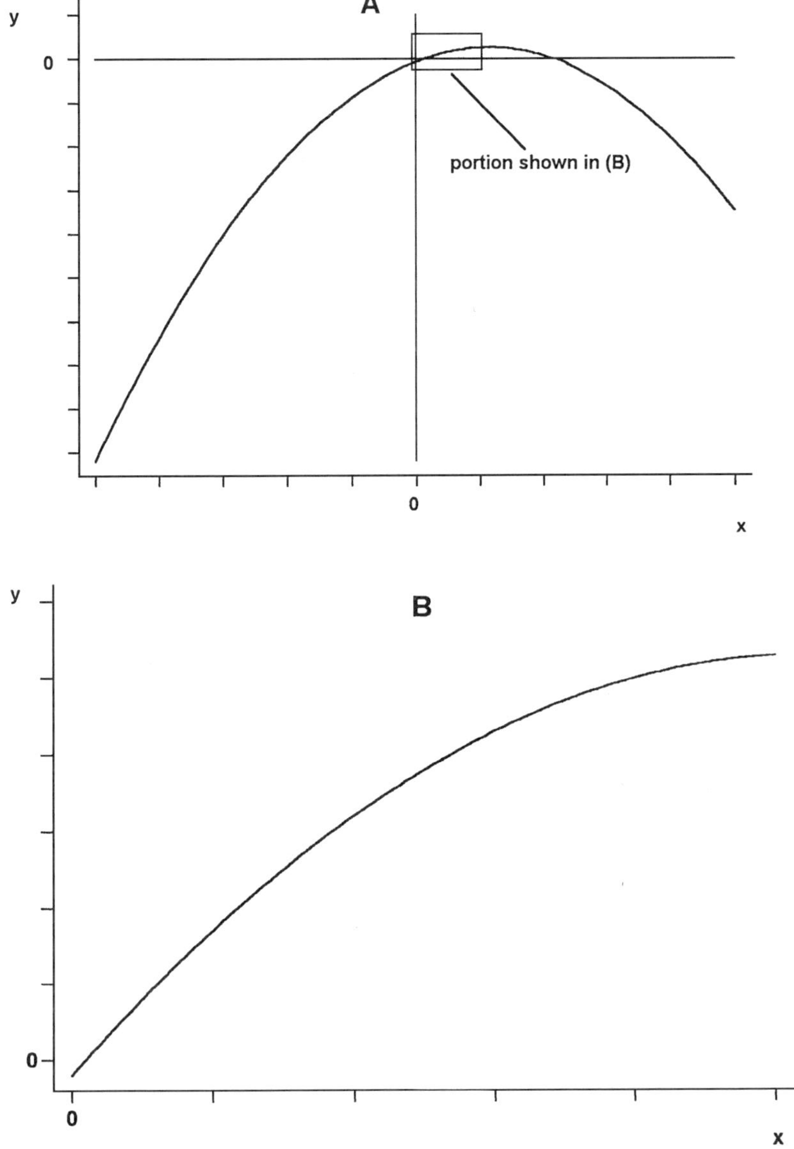

Figure 19.1 A parabola, concave downward as a result of a negative β_2, is shown in part A. A portion of the parabola, useful in the example to follow, is shown in part B.

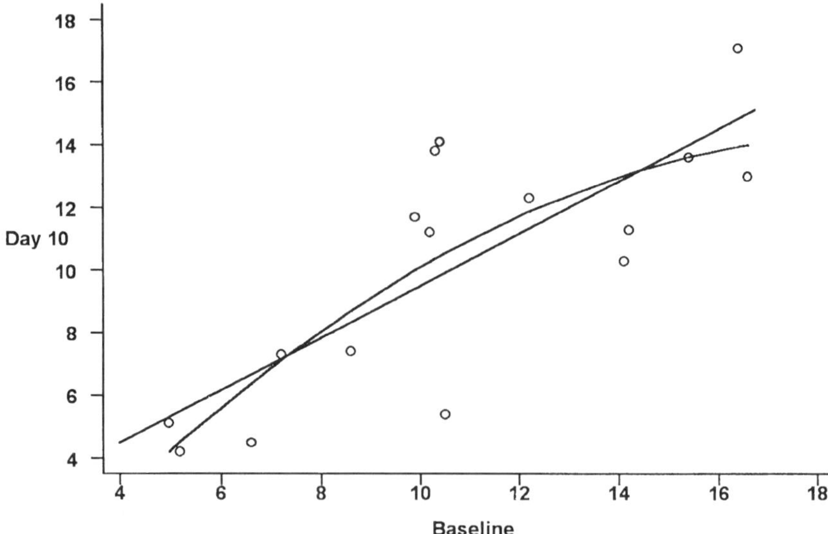

Figure 19.2 Serum theophylline levels at day 10 as predicted by baseline are shown, with straight line and parabolic fits superposed. Note that the curved fit is similar to the portion of the parabola shown in Fig. 19.1B.

term to a parabolic model), (C) a logarithmic curve, (D) an exponential curve, (E) a biological growth curve, and (F) a sine wave. Sign changes will flip the third degree curve top for bottom in shape. The logarithmic curve looks a little like a portion of the downward opening parabola, but it never reaches a maximum as does the parabola, increasing, however, more and more slowly with increasing x. The exponential curve looks a little like a portion of the upward opening parabola, but it increases more rapidly. Growth curves fit many growth patterns, for example, that of animal (and human) weight over time. Periodic curves, of which the sine wave is a simple case, frequently are seen in cardiopulmonary physiology.

Note that (A) and (B) are called *linear models* because they are composed of simple algebraic terms added together even though they are not straight lines. However, (C) through (F) are *nonlinear models* because their terms, not simple algebraic terms, contain logarithms, exponentials, and trigonometric expressions.

Additional Example

In part of the experiment giving rise to DB11, rats infected with malaria were treated with healthy red blood cells (RBCs) and with a placebo (hetastarch), 100 in each sample. Number (same as %) in each sample surviving by day for 10 days is plotted in Figs. 19.4A, B. The RBC curve appears to follow a sequence of plateaus,

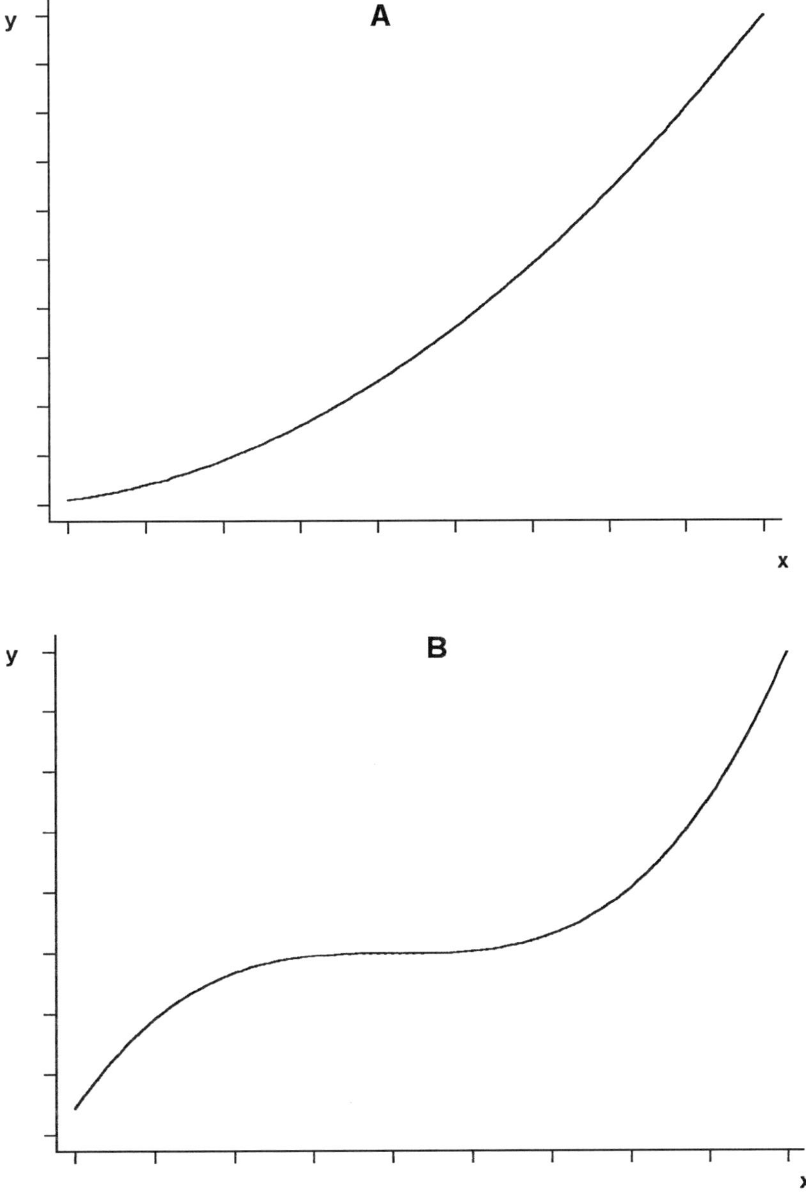

Figure 19.3 Representative portions of the following classes of curve are illustrated: (A) second degree curve (parabola) opening upward; (B) third degree curve; (C) logarithmic curve; (D) exponential curve; (E) biological growth curve; and (F) sine wave.

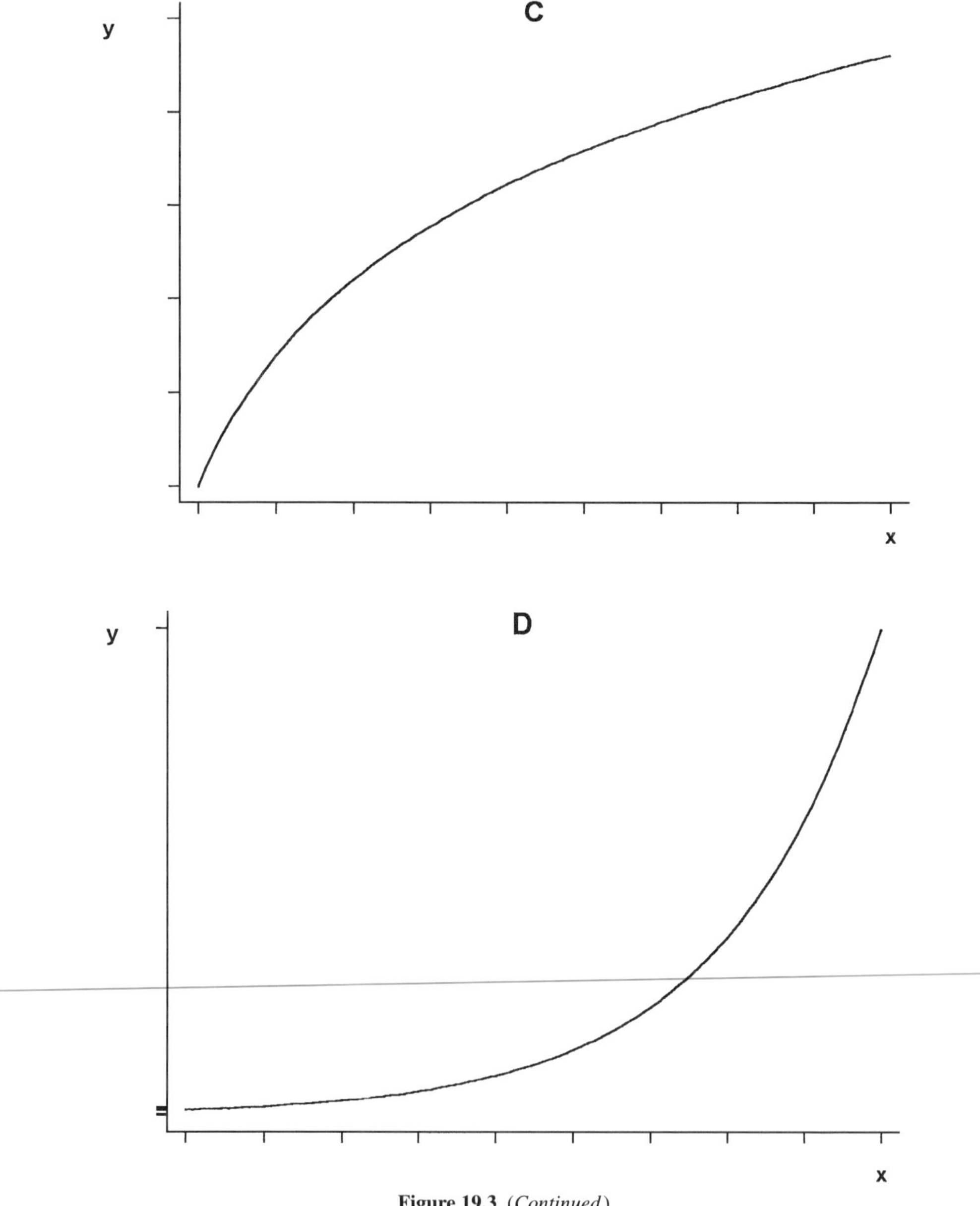

Figure 19.3 (*Continued*)

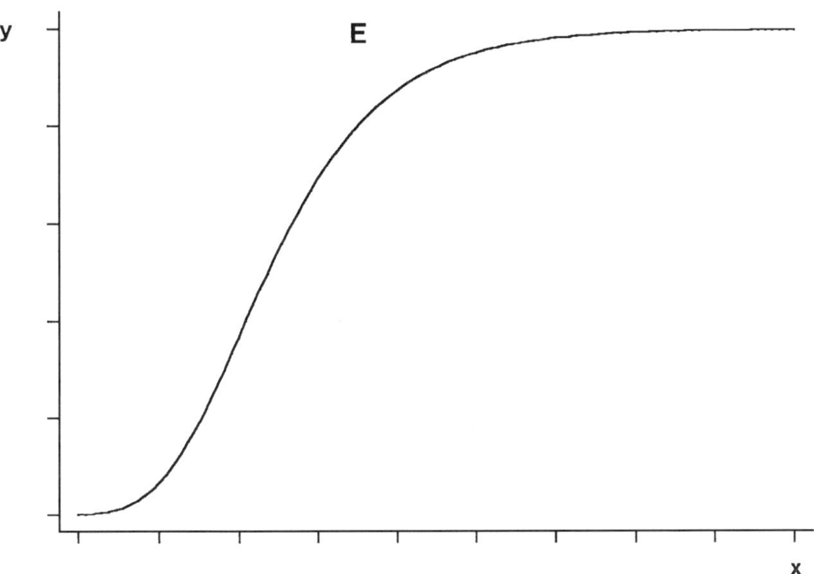

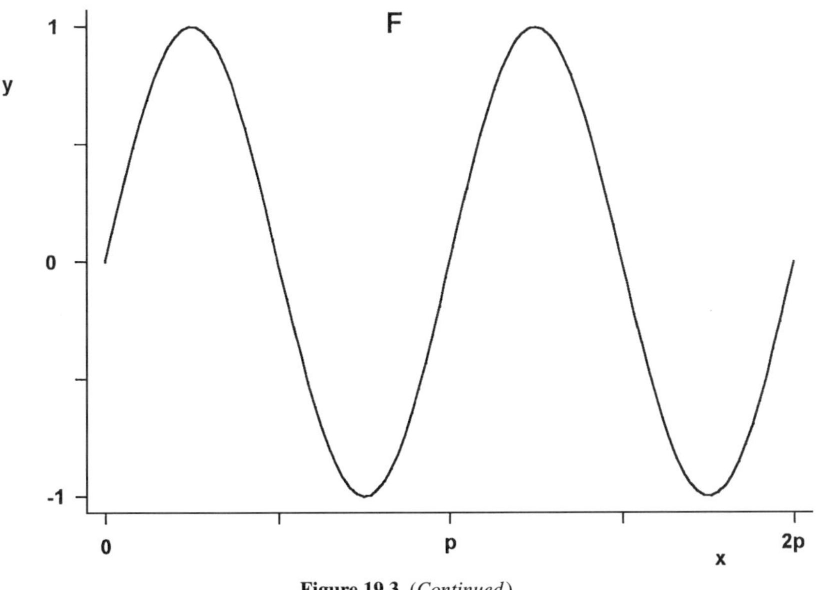

Figure 19.3 (*Continued*)

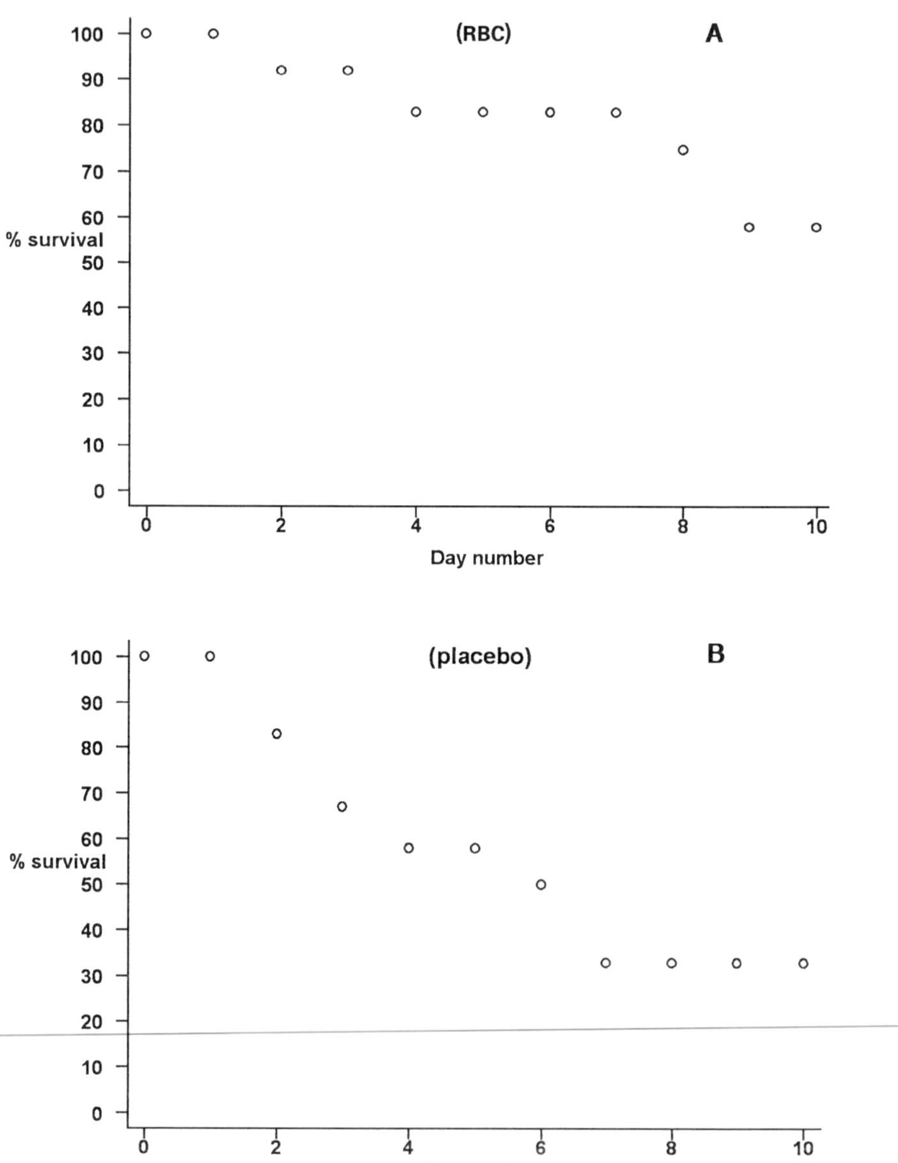

Figure 19.4 Survival percent of malarial rats treated (A) with red blood cells (RBCs) and (B) with a placebo. The combined graph (C) shows a straight line fit to the RBC data and a parabolic fit to the placebo data.

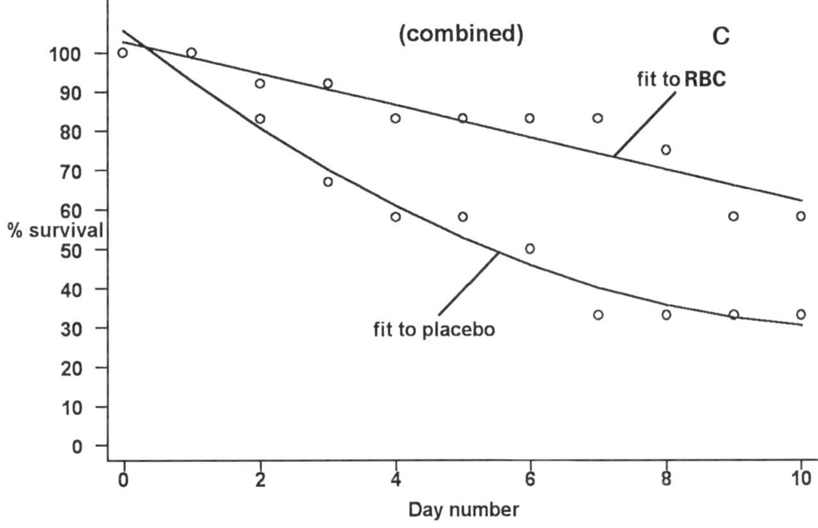

Figure 19.4 *(Continued)*

but is not clearly any common shape other than a straight line. The placebo survival diminishes more rapidly and appears to be approaching a minimum survival percent toward the end of the period, looking more like a segment of an upward opening parabola (second degree expression). These two curves were fit to the data and superposed to form the combined graph in Fig. 19.4C. Under the proper conditions, these fits will follow certain probability distributions, and statistical tests may be made of their shape and their similarity; such methods will be addressed in Chapter 20 on regression.

Exercise 19.1. Using data from DB9, Fig. 19.5A shows transforming growth factor (TGF) plotted depending on platelet count, and Fig. 19.5B shows a similar plot for platelet-derived growth factor (PDGF). Recognize the shape and choose the curve (from those presented earlier in this section) that seems by eye to provide the best fit for each.

19.4. CONSTANTS OF FIT FOR ANY MODEL

Example

In DB3, serum theophylline level 10 days after the beginning of antibiotic treatment would be expected to be related to baseline level, although not exactly on a

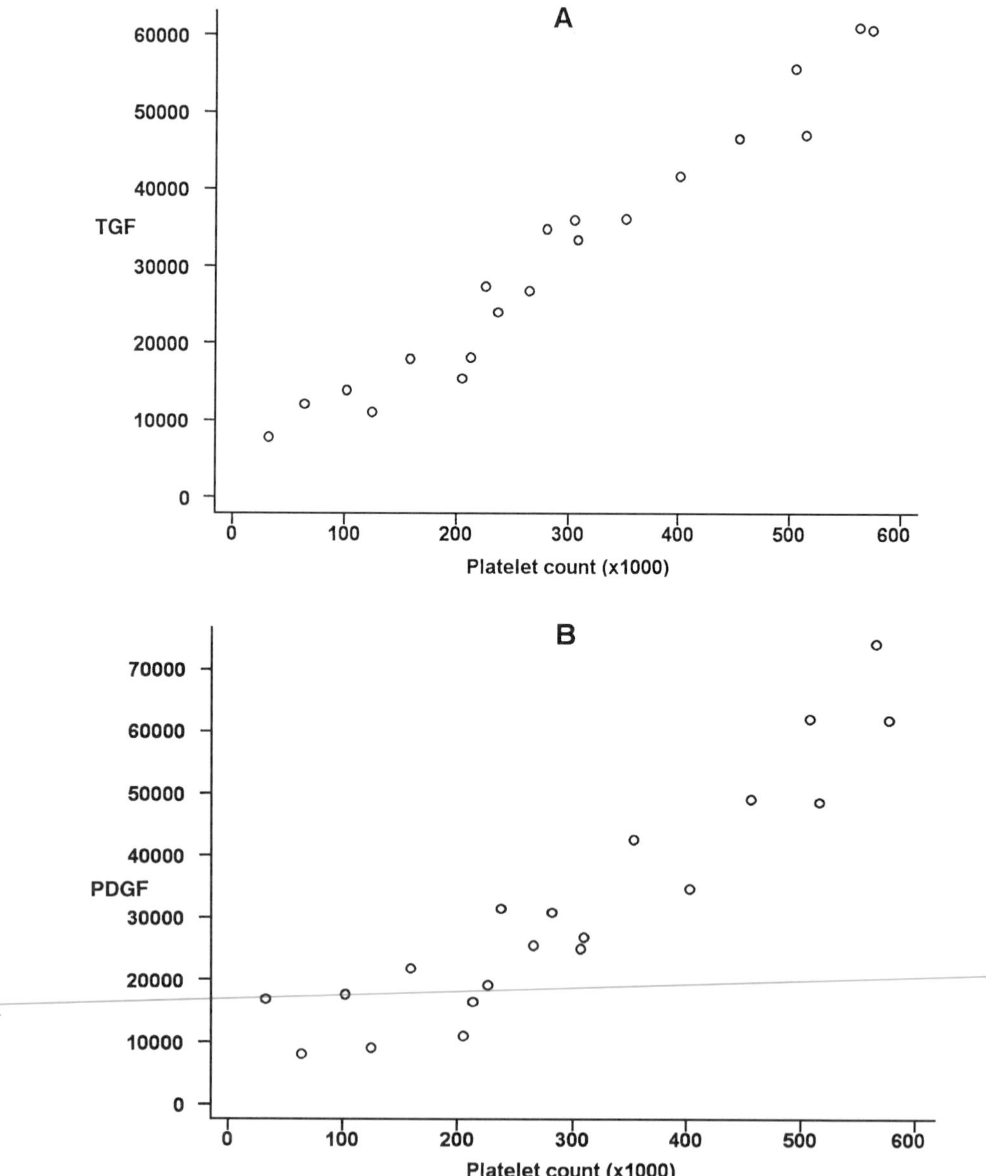

Figure 19.5 Growth factor levels as depending on platelet counts.

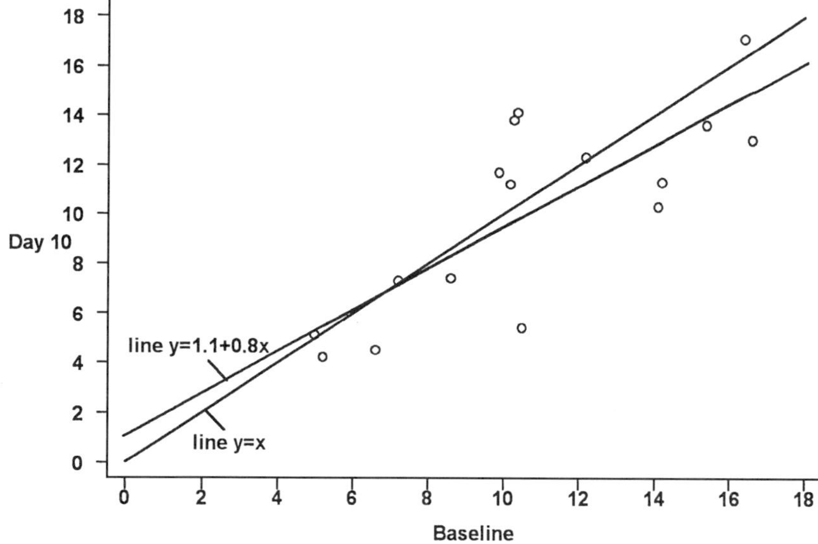

Figure 19.6 Ten-day serum theophylline level as related to baseline level. The line $y = 0 + 1x$ is shown to illustrate the change in equation parameters required for the best fit $y = 1.1 + 0.8x$.

straight line. If we started with the straight line $y = x$, which is a line with slope 1 passing through an intercept of 0, what manipulations would provide a better fit? Figure 19.6 shows that data with the line $y = x$ and with a better fitting line $y = 1.1 + 0.8x$. (The better fit actually is the least squares best fit.) We can see that the slope needs to be less steep. This can be accomplished by stretching the x-axis, which, from Table 19.1, can be done by multiplying x by a constant less than 1. Because the slope needs to be only a bit less steep, we can estimate by eye that a

Table 19.1

Effects of Fit Constants (Parameters) That Change the Function $y = f(x)$ to $y = d + cf(ax + b)$ and Effects of the Values They May Take On

Fit constant	Along which axis	General effect	Detailed effect
a	x	Stretches–shrinks curve	$a < 1$: stretches $a > 1$: shrinks
b	x	Slides curve	$b > 0$: to left $b < 0$: to right
c	y	Stretches–shrinks curve	$c > 1$: stretches $c < 1$: shrinks
d	y	Slides curve	$d > 0$: up $d < 0$: down

multiplier of around 0.8 or 0.9 should suffice. We can see further that the resulting line, which would be parallel to the best fit line, needs to slide up the y-axis by about a unit, which, from Table 19.1, can be done by adding a constant of about 1 to the right side.

Method

When we are faced with a relationship between factors in a physiologic process shown on a plot of data representing this process, we can imagine the relationship as a geometric curve typifying the essence of the dependence of one factor upon the other. We often can see the family of curves by inspection, as we did in Fig. 19.2. But how do we pass from a family of curves to the particular member of that family? In most cases, the family member can be specified by sliding, stretching, or shrinking the general family model on one or both of the axes. This is done by adding or multiplying by one or more of four possible parameters, where the values of these parameters at this stage are estimated roughly by eye.

The Purpose of Such Manipulations

Of course, we do not attempt to fit models to statistical data by manipulating parameters with judgmental values; we use mathematical optimization methods. The use of examining the parameters is two-fold. First, an understanding of the role of the parameters helps us relate the mathematical expression of models to the physiologic processes generating the data. Second, by understanding the roles of the parameters, we can look at a process or at data and often anticipate the functional form of the model. This anticipation also prevents gross errors that sometimes arise by using statistical software without careful thought.

The Four Parameters Are Scale and Position Constants for x and y

Suppose we have a relationship in which the way y depends on x is expressed by $y = f(x)$. This f expresses the form of the relationship and usually is called the *function*. WBC is a straight line function of time. However, the nature of the form does not tell us needed details. We need to select the scales and the starting positions for x and y that will make the relationship realistic. The four constants are termed parameters because they remain constant only for the one member of a family of functions, but vary from member to member. They will specify the horizontal and vertical scales and the horizontal and vertical positions. Say these parameters are a, b, c, and d. Let us attach them to the function so that we have a multiplier and an additive for each of x and y. Conceptually, the multipliers "stretch" or "shrink" the curve in the x or y direction to adjust the scale, and the additives "slide" the curve along the respective scale to adjust the position.

Effect of Fit Parameters

The effects of the four parameters used in fitting a function of the form

$$y = d + cf(ax + b) \tag{19.2}$$

are summarized in Table 19.1.

Additional Example

An allergist suspects from his practice that aspergillosis occurs more in the winter and less in the summer, although that has not been shown previously.[64] He collects numbers of cases for 4 years and averages the incidence by season. If his intuition is correct, average incidence should follow the form of a (portion of a) sine wave, $y = \sin(x)$, illustrated in Fig. 19.7.

Definition of a Sine Wave

The reader probably was exposed to sine waves in lower school. Think of a clock having numbers around a circle with a hand extending from the center to the perimeter. x- and y-axes are superposed on the clock with the x-axis passing through 9 o'clock to 3 o'clock and the y-axis passing through 12 o'clock to

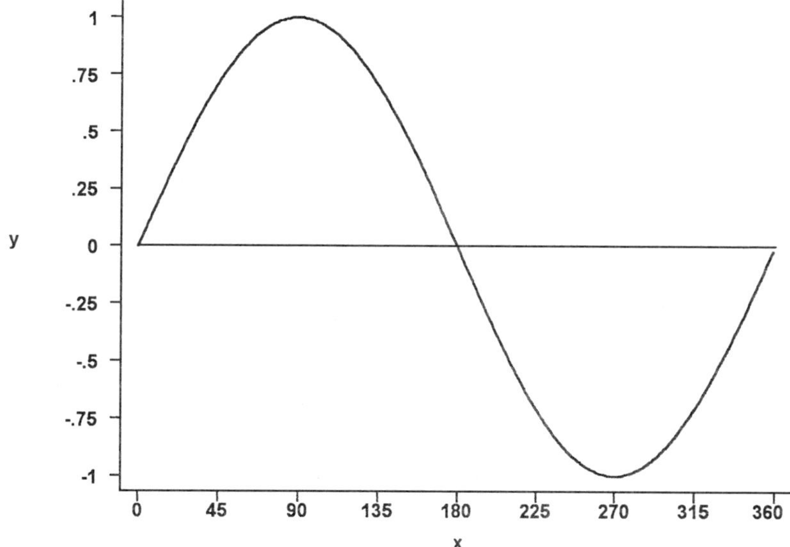

Figure 19.7 The first cycle of a sine wave.

6 o'clock. As the hand travels in a counter-clockwise direction from the rightmost x-axis (3 o'clock) around the 360° of the circle, there is a vertical distance from the x-axis to the end of the hand. The sine is defined as the ratio of this length to the length of the hand.

Aspergillosis Data and Fitting

The allergist finds the mean number of cases he treats by season to be the following: Fall, 3.33; Winter, 7.75; Spring, 4.67; and Summer, 2.33. The overall average is 4.77, as shown in Fig. 19.8.

Relating Observed Data to a Family of Curves

A look at the similarity of form in Figs. 19.7 and 19.8 will show that the data start in the Fall near the mean, increase to a maximum at 90° (Winter), drop through 180° (Spring) to a minimum at 270° (Summer), and finally move back toward the average at 360° (return to Fall). The form of the model, following Eq. (19.2), will be

$$y = d + c\sin(ax + b). \tag{19.3}$$

If the seasonal designations are chosen as Fall at 0°, Winter at 90°, etc., the data follow the sine shape in the horizontal direction; he does not need to adjust the scale or slide the curve on the x-axis to fit, so $a = 1$ and $b = 0$. As for the y-axis, he wants the incidence average to lie at $y = 0$ (on the x-axis), so that the seasonal

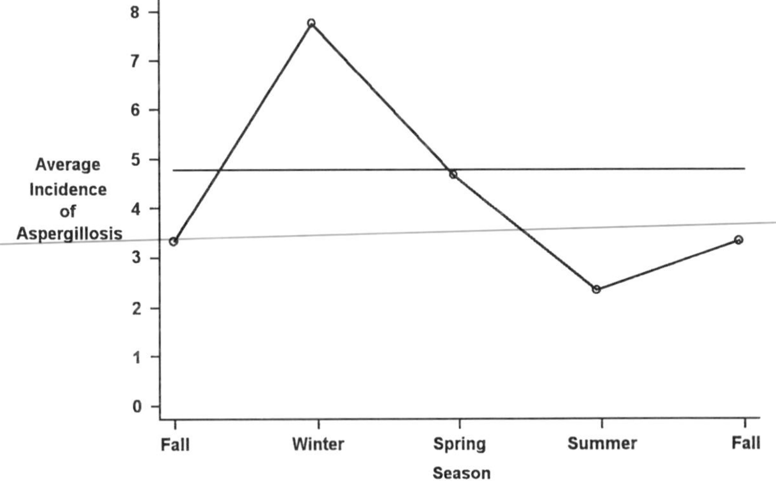

Figure 19.8 Average incidence of aspergillosis by season.

effect deviates from average. He slides the sine curve up to this level by selecting $d = 4.77$, the average. This leaves the model $y = 4.77 + c\sin(x)$, with c to be estimated from the data.

Estimating *c*

Our allergist wants to find a c that will minimize the $\Sigma(\text{obs} - \text{fit})^2/\text{fit}$. Eventually, this will be done mathematically and data substituted in the result. At this stage, the purposes are understanding the process and verifying that the correct family of models has been chosen. In six iterations on a calculator, taking "fit" as $4.77 + (\text{evolving } c)\sin(x)$, he finds that $c = 2.56$, so the model becomes $y = 4.77 + 2.56\sin(x)$. Interestingly, the sum of squares that he minimized is the chi-square goodness-of-fit statistic discussed in Chapter 17 (Eq. 17.2). The 2.56 value of c yields a chi-square of 0.9021 and a p-value of 0.924, indicating that the fit is quite acceptable. Figure 19.9 shows the fitted sine wave superposed on the aspergillosis data.

The Effect of Each Parameter in Table 19.1 on a Sine Wave

The basic $y = \sin(x)$ function is illustrated in Fig. 19.10A, and the effect of altering each of the four parameters of Eq. (19.2) in turn is shown in Figs. 19.10B–E.

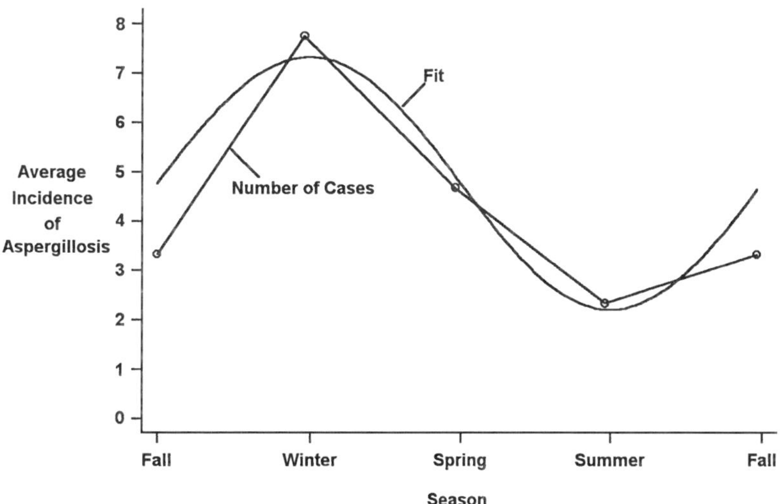

Figure 19.9 Average incidence of aspergillosis by season with the least squares sine wave fit superposed.

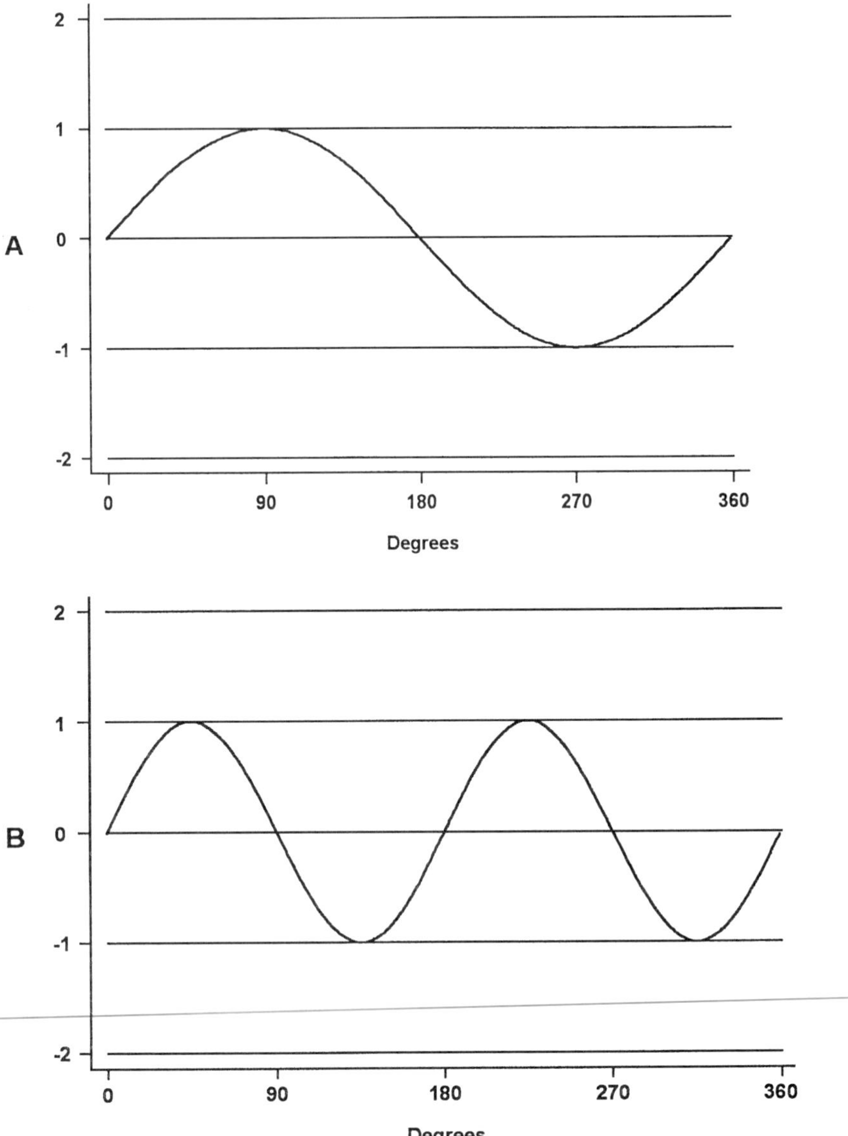

Figure 19.10 Effects of four fit constants. Compare each with (A). (A) Basic sine wave, $y = \sin(x)$. (B) $y = \sin(2x)$; $a = 2$ shrinks curve (A) into $1/a$ of original width. (C) $y = \sin(x + 90^\circ)$; $b = 90^\circ$ (use same units as x) slides curve (A) 90° to the left. (D) $y = 2\sin(x)$; $c = 2$ doubles height of curve (A). (E) $y = 1 + \sin(x)$; $d = 1$ slides curve (A) up one unit.

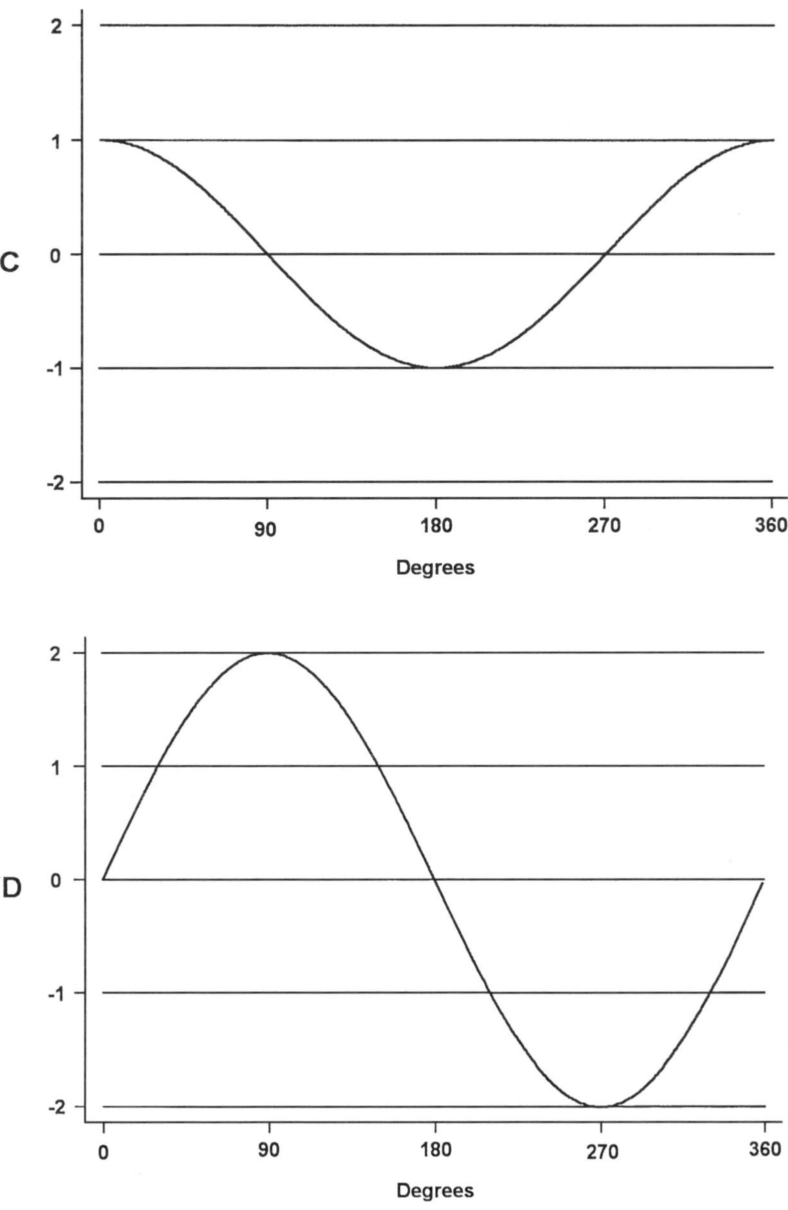

Figure 19.10 *(Continued)*

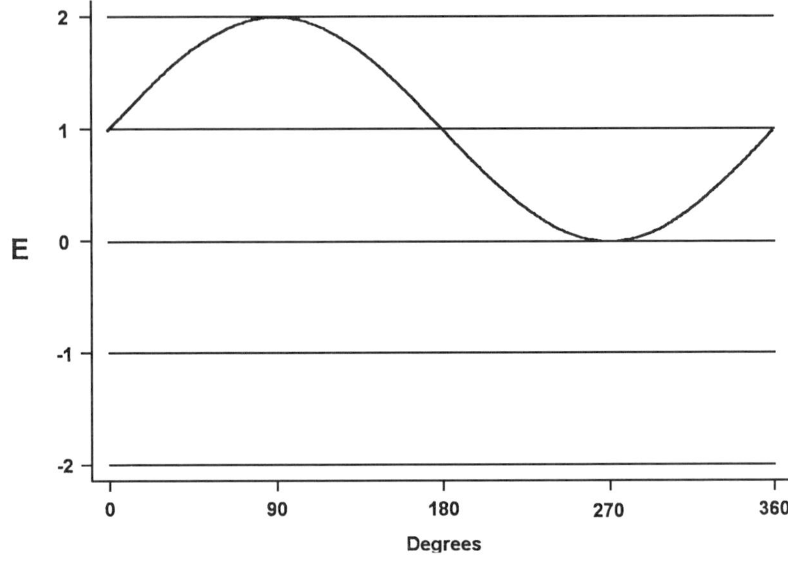

Figure 19.10 (*Continued*)

Exercise 19.2. Using data from DB10, Fig. 19.11 shows a plot of the time to hop as related to the distance hopped. Visualize a straight line passing through the points and choose the parameters a, b, c, and d required to express its equation.

19.5. MULTIPLE-VARIABLE MODELS

Concept

So far, we have looked at models with only two variables, which can be represented by the x- and y-axes; y is thought of as depending on x. We know that y may very well depend on more than one variable, as systolic blood pressure (SBP) depends on physical condition, age, recency of exercise (in minutes), and doubtless other factors. Such a relationship can be expressed algebraically.

Visualizing Three Dimensions

The case of y depending on two x's can be visualized geometrically, as with the expression $y = \beta_0 + \beta_1 x_1 + \beta_2 x_2$. If y is SBP, x_1 might be age in years

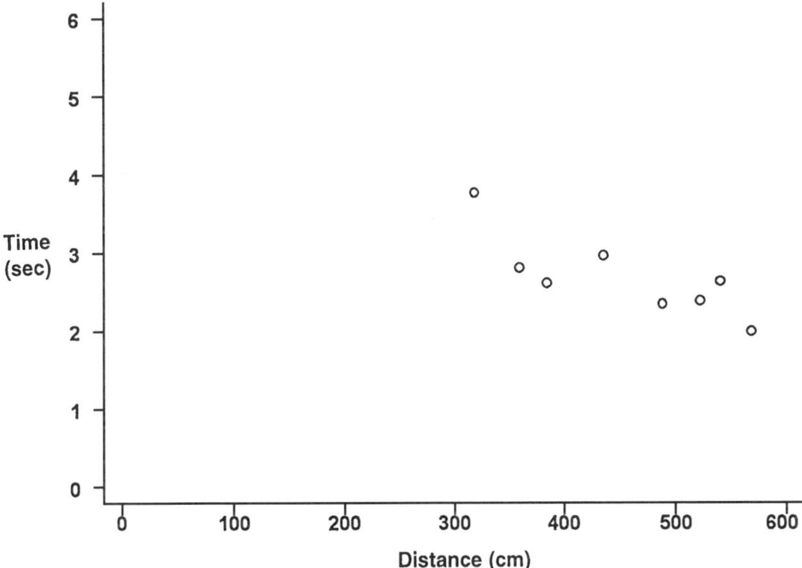

Figure 19.11 Time (seconds) to perform a triple hop on the post-operative leg related to the distance (centimeters) hopped after surgery on hamstrings or quadriceps.

and x_2 might be minutes of vigorous exercise just prior to the measure. The β's are the parameters of fit, which are conceptually similar to those considered in Section 19.4. To visualize the relationship, think of y as the intersection of two walls in the corner of a room and the two x's as the intersections of these walls with the floor. An observation with values (y, x_1, x_2) is represented as a position in the space above and in front of the corner. x_1 and x_2 are readings on the independent variables (e.g., age and minutes of exercise), and y is the reading on the dependent variable (e.g., SBP). Just as a line may be fit to a sample of points in two dimensions, a plane may be fit to a sample of points in three dimensions. Figure 19.12 represents a three-dimensional space showing a single point and a plane that might have been fit to a set of such points.

A Curved Surface in Three Dimensions

Just as the straight line $y = \beta_0 + \beta_1 x$ may be generalized to represent a curve by adding a squared term, as $y = \beta_0 + \beta_1 x + \beta_2 x^2$, the plane $y = \beta_0 + \beta_1 x_1 + \beta_2 x_2$ may be generalized to become a curved surface by adding one or two squared terms, as perhaps $y = \beta_0 + \beta_1 x_1 + \beta_2 x_2 + \beta_3 x_2^2$. A curved surface rather than a flat surface in three dimensions may still be easily visualized.

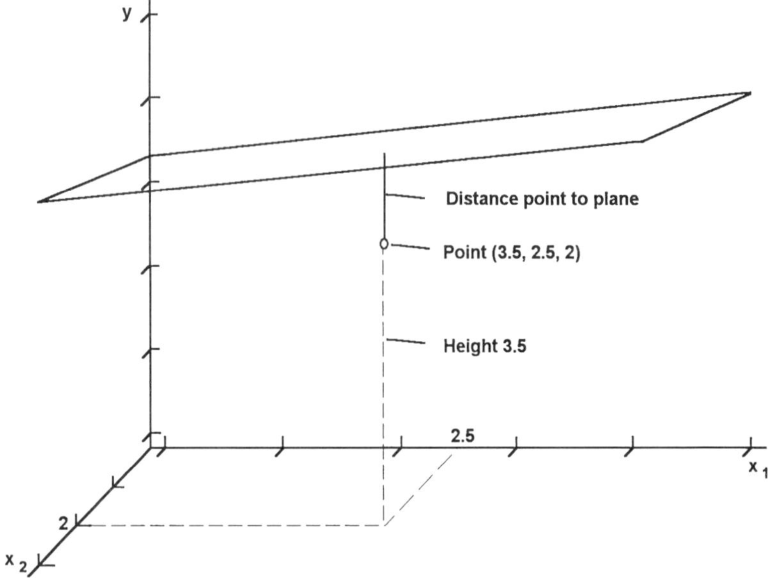

Figure 19.12 Conceptual geometry of a three-dimensional model showing a sample point ($y = 3.5, x_1 = 2.5, x_2 = 2$) and a plane fit to a set of points in the space.

More Than Three Dimensions

Suppose the dependent variable y depends on more than two dimensions, as if we added a measure of general cardiovascular health x_3? Algebraically, we have no problem. We can add as many variables in whatever powers we want, and the model may be readily used in analysis. Visualization of a relationship in four or more dimensions is difficult, if possible at all. Four-dimensional displays have been attempted using time (moving images), colors or shades, and other mechanisms, but with limited success, because depiction of the fourth dimension necessarily is different in nature from that of the first three. The clinician usually will have success at modeling by visualizing variables three at a time and restricting higher dimensionality to algebraic methods. An algebraic expression of a four-dimensional plane would be $y = \beta_0 + \beta_1 x_1 + \beta_2 x_2 + \beta_3 x_3$.

The Term "Linear Model" Often Is Seen in Analyses and Software Packages

A linear model is a model in which the terms are added, such as has been used so far in this section, rather than multiplied or divided. A linear model is not restricted to a straight line or its analogue in higher dimensionality. Sometimes we see a reference to a curved model that is still called linear, which may seem oxymoronic but arises from particular mathematical connotations. The curved shape, $y = \beta_0 + \beta_1 x + \beta_2 x^2$, is a linear model because terms are added and only one variable appears per term. The model $y = \beta_0 x_1/x_2$ is not linear.

The Case of Multiple Dependent Variables

Suppose we are concerned with both SBP and diastolic blood pressure (DBP) as predicted by the several independent variables; we have y_1 and y_2 depending on the several x's. Methods exist to analyze such a situation, but they are more complex and beyond the scope of this book.

Exercise 19.3. In DB10, we anticipate surgery on hamstrings or quadriceps and would like to predict the post-op hop distance. We measure the patient's hop time and distance on the uninjured leg. What are the dependent and independent variables? What is the nature of the geometric picture?

19.6. SCREENING AND NUMBER NEEDED TO TREAT (NNT)

The Primary Issues in Screening Questions

The statistical aspects of screening a population for a disease are issues of efficacy and cost-effectiveness. Does a screening program work? If so, does it provide enough benefit to be worth the resources expended? The first question is one of the number needed to treat (NNT), defined as *estimating the number of people screened in order to detect one case to treat*, and testing this NNT to learn whether it is significantly greater than chance. For example, how many mammograms must be run on randomly chosen women of a certain age in order to find one otherwise undetected case of breast cancer? How many vaccinations for hepatitis C are required to prevent one case? The second question is one of estimating the cost of the resources (time, facilities, personnel, money) expended for one detection and trading off this cost against the gain of treating that patient. The gain usually is intangible, and the cost-effectiveness becomes a matter of comparing events from two different value bases. This might be likened to comparing the value of coins from two different monetary systems: we have to find or develop a medium of exchange, i.e., an MOE that will equate the cost of the NNT and the gain to the patient. MOEs are considered in the next section of this chapter. This section will include only the NNT itself, which can be treated as a logical model.

Example

A catchment is composed of male smokers in Baltimore in 1980.[73] Mortality from lung cancer was 0.0045, taken as p_e (the probability of a randomly chosen member dying from the disease during the year). A total of 10,387 were screened (n_s). $n_d = n_s p_e = 47$, the number of dying members found by the screening. By Eq. (19.4) NNT $= n_s/n_d = 221$ needed to be screened for each catchment member to be found prior to dying from lung cancer.

Method

Number of Patients Screened per Detection

To develop a logical model, we need some explicit definitions to refer unequivocally to logical compartments and symbols to represent these compartments. Let us adopt the following definitions, referring to whatever disease is at issue, perhaps cancer or hepatitis.

n_p: catchment size, i.e., number of people in the population with the potential to be screened.
n_e: number of people having the disease within the catchment, assumed to be distributed randomly.
p_e: probability that a randomly chosen member of the catchment will have the disease, $=n_e/n_p$.
n_s: number of people screened, i.e., sample size.
n_d: number of cases of the disease detected in screening n_s people.

Given these definitions, the number detected by screening will be the number of catchment members screened multiplied by the chance that any randomly chosen member will have the disease, or

$$n_d = n_s p_e = n_s n_e / n_p.$$

The number of people screened in order to detect one case to treat then is

$$\text{NNT} = n_s/n_d. \tag{19.4}$$

(Note that, for truly random distribution and truly random sampling, NNT $= 1/p_e$.) To consider the cost per detection, let us further define

c_s: cost for screening program, i.e., cost to screen n_s people.
c_d: cost per detection.

The cost per detection c_d is simply the cost per screening procedure multiplied by NNT, or

$$c_d = (c_s/n_s)\mathrm{NNT}. \tag{19.5}$$

Number Screened per Detection When Some Cases Would Be Otherwise Detected

The NNT developed in the prior paragraph deals with a screening process to detect disease cases that otherwise would be undetected. Suppose some of the cases would be detected by ordinary health care (patients presenting with complaints about the disease's symptoms) or overlap with another screening program (routine physicals, for example, or a competitive screening capability believed to be less capable). For example, in a screening program proposed for ovarian cancer, some of the cases found by screening would have been found without the program.

n_c: number of cases of disease in the catchment detected by other means.
n_{cd}: number of cases detected by the screening program that would have been found otherwise.

n_{cd} is the number falling in the overlap of n_d and n_c. Perhaps the concept can be seen more clearly in Fig. 19.13, a diagram using what mathematicians term

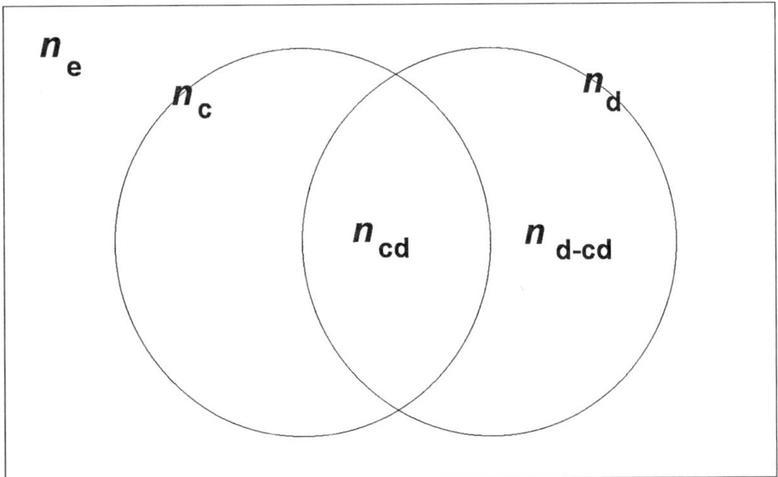

Figure 19.13 Euler circles representing various sets of cases associated with screening. The set of cases detected by the screening that would not have been detected otherwise is shown by the subset n_{d-cd}, that part of n_d that is not also in n_c.

Euler (pronounced "oiler") circles arising from set theory. The box represents n_e, the set of people having the disease. The circles n_d and n_c represent the sets of cases that would have been detected by the screening program and by other means, respectively. The subset of cases that would have been detected by both is shown as the overlap of the two sets, or the area n_{cd}. Then the number of cases detected by the screening program that would not have been found by other means is the subarea of the circle n_d designated by $n_{d-cd} = n_d - n_{cd}$. For this case,

$$\text{NNT} = n_s/n_{d-cd}. \tag{19.6}$$

Costing follows Eq. (19.5) as before, using, however, NNT from Eq. (19.6).

Detection Compared to Other MOEs, Such as Mortality

Is detection the final criterion of screening efficacy? It certainly is not the only one. We already have, in addition to NNT, the number detected by the screening program (n_d) and the cost per detection (c_d). However, even the fact of a statistically significant portion of the population detected by the screening is not evidence that the screening is beneficial. Suppose more diseased patients are detected, but that does not help them. In a German study,[75] 41,532 men born between 1907 and 1932 were screened for lung cancer with chest fluorography every 6 months for 10 years and compared with age-matched men screened similarly every 18 months. No significant reduction in lung cancer mortality or in overall mortality was found. When mortality rather than detection rate was taken as the measure of effectiveness, tripling of the screening rate provided no improvement. An investigator, and certainly a reader of medical articles, should carefully consider the MOE used. MOEs are considered further in the next section.

Additional Example

Oral leukoplakia, which frequently progresses to overt squamous cell carcinoma, was treated with 13-*cis*-retinoic acid (cRA) in $n_s = 44$ patients.[25] $n_d = 24$ patients responded histologically. NNT $= n_s/n_d = 1.83$ patients treated per responder.

Exercise 19.4. In a study[13] on radiographic screening in a correctional facility in New York City, the rate of tuberculosis among entering inmates was 0.00767. A total of 4172 entering inmates were screened. How many were detected by the radiographic screening? Of those detected, 25 had entered with a prior diagnosis of tuberculosis. What is the NNT for those newly diagnosed by the screening?

19.7. CLINICAL DECISION BASED ON RECURSIVE PARTITIONING

EXAMPLE

A set of 20 patients is known clinically to suffer from a myeloma, some from multiple myeloma (designated 0) and some from a syndrome known as mgus (1). Associated measures are immunoglobulin type (IgM, 0; IgG, 1; IgA, 2), sex (f, 0; m, 1), and protlev (protein level of patient divided by the midrange of the healthy protein level range). Part way through the partitioning process, it was noticed that protlev seems to differentiate between preceding partitions at about a level of 2, so protlev then was categorized as protein level category (protlev < 2, 0; protlev ≥ 2, 1). The resulting data appear as Table 19.2.

Logic and Charting

Inspection will show that each outcome appears in each diagnosis, except for Ig type; Ig 0's (IgM) appear only with diagnosis 1 (mgus). Thus, we can start

Table 19.2

Ordering of Myeloma Categories as Related to Immunoglobulin (Ig), Sex, Protein Level Multiple (protlev), and Protein Level Category (protcat)

Myeloma	Ig	Sex	Protlev	Protcat
0	1	0	6.5	1
0	1	0	6.0	1
0	1	0	5.3	1
0	1	1	4.4	1
0	1	1	2.6	1
0	1	1	1.9	0
0	2	0	5.4	1
1	0	0	1.1	0
1	0	0	1.0	0
1	0	0	0.9	0
1	0	1	1.7	0
1	1	0	2.1	1
1	1	0	1.9	0
1	1	0	1.9	0
1	1	0	1.9	0
1	1	0	1.6	0
1	1	0	1.6	0
1	1	0	1.5	0
1	1	0	1.1	0
1	2	0	0.7	0

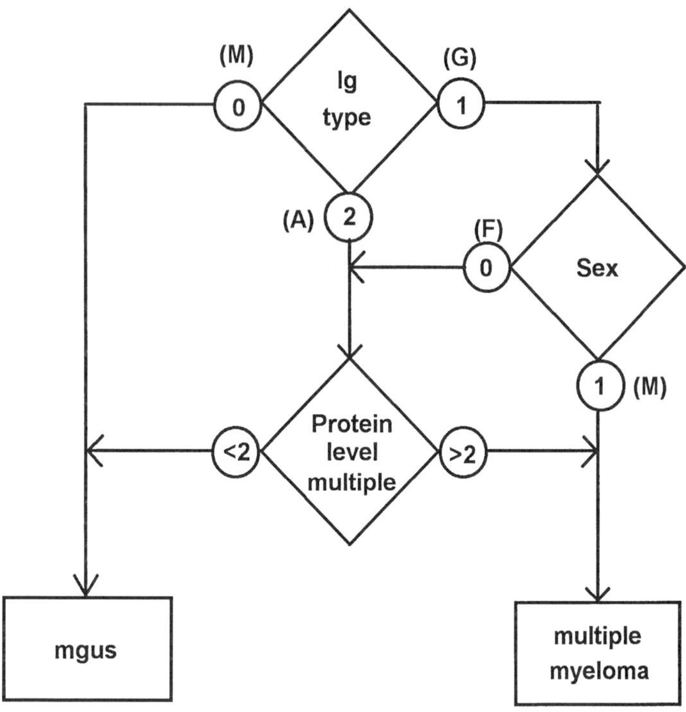

Figure 19.14 Logical sequence of decisions (recursive partitions) leading to myeloma diagnosis.

Fig. 19.14 with a decision box on Ig with an arrow leading to outcome box mgus. We note that Ig 2 falls in both outcomes, but only one sex, so sex will not distinguish between outcomes; however, diagnosis 0 is associated with protlev 1 and diagnosis 1 with protlev 0, so protlev will partition Ig 2 into the diagnoses. We draw another decision box for protlev with arrows passing from the Ig box to the protlev box and from there to the decision boxes. We note that, for Ig 1, all males are associated with diagnosis 0, so we draw a sex box and appropriate arrows. Finally, we note that, for Ig 1 and for females, protlev will distinguish the diagnosis. We connect the final arrows.

Method

Often a set of indicators will diagnose a particular malady or predict the outcome of a particular treatment. A patient having symptoms A, B, and C is suffering from disease 1. However, if the list of indicators is long, the number of possible combinations becomes unwieldy. It works better to pass through a sequence of branchings for each indicator. In mathematics, the selection of the particular branch of an indicator is termed partitioning, so that the sequential process is termed *recursive partitioning*. Given a set of data on a list of indicator signs and symptoms and the illnesses that may be associated, recursive partitioning may identify which indicators are decisive in diagnosis and which are not. It may be able to distinguish the logical sequence through which the indicators should be considered. Finally, it can compare the logical sequence of partitions used successfully in a new set of data with a traditionally used sequence to either reinforce or replace the established mechanism.

Steps to Develop the Decision Process

Small indicator groups and not more than three categories per indicator will be addressed here. Mathematical sorting routines for large sample sizes and more complicated categorizations exist but are beyond the scope of this text. Sort the possible outcomes (diagnoses or result of treatment), listing those alike in adjoining rows. Identify the indicator (symptom, sign, or condition) most consistently related to the outcome, and then the next, etc. Draw a decision box with arrows extending out, depending on initial partitioning. Draw the next decision boxes with appropriate arrows extending to them and more arrows extending out, depending on the next round of partitions. Continue until reaching the final outcomes. The boxes should be ordered such that no looping back can occur and no box is repeated. There may be some trial and error occurring. The best way to perceive the process is to follow one of the examples.

Additional Example

In a sample of 1500 malignant glioma patients, radiotherapy (RT) was found to be useful to some of the patients and not to others. (Inspired by ref 65, but simplified and one datum fabricated to complete the example.) The patients were grouped by possible indicators of RT usefulness, as in Table 19.3. We note that all of the younger patients are in the useful class, which composes the first branching box in Fig. 19.15.

Now we concentrate on the four groups over 50 years of age. One class with high Karnofsky performance status (KPS) and one with low KPS lie in each of RT useful and RT not useful, so KPS is not a helpful discriminant alone. On the other hand, we note that the RT not useful groups have either abnormal neurology or treatment lag, but not both, whereas the RT useful groups have neither. Thus, the logic path passes through branching boxes for these discriminants; if either is "yes," the arrow goes to RT not useful, otherwise it goes to RT useful. We now have a logical recursive partitioning path to use in deciding whether to treat a patient with radiotherapy.

Table 19.3

Ordering of Usefulness of Radiotherapy as Related to Malignant Glioma Patient Categories Age, Karnofsky Performance Status (KPS), Condition of Neurology, and Period between First Symptoms and Initiation of Treatment

Radiotherapy useful	Age over 50	High KPS	Abnormal neurology	Treatment lag >3 months
Yes				
Yes			X	X
Yes		X		
Yes	X			
Yes	X	X		
No	X	X		X
No	X		X	

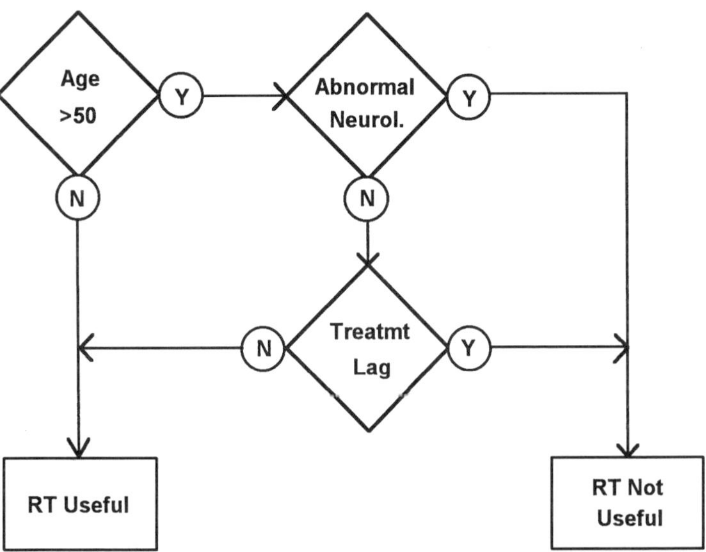

Figure 19.15 Logical sequence of decisions (recursive partitions) leading to decision to treat with radiotherapy.

Exercise 19.5. The disease of patients whose ocular pressure has tested high must be classified as glaucoma, which is damaging to the optic nerve, or ocular hypertension, which is rather benign.[54] The pressure, the angle between the iris and the peripheral cornea, the field of vision, and the disc (optic nerve head) are examined. High pressure coupled with a narrow angle signals glaucoma. If the angle is wide, either a bad field or a bad disc in conjunction with the high pressure indicates glaucoma. Otherwise, ocular hypertension is inferred. Draw a decision chart representing the logical partitioning.

19.8. CLINICAL DECISION BASED ON MOEs: OUTCOMES ANALYSIS

Review of Section 8.6

It was noted that clinical decisions usually are made on the basis of a *measure of effectiveness* (*MOE*), or often more than one; there is no unique MOE. Several commonly used MOEs were listed, including the probability of cure, the probability of cure relative to other treatments, the risk of debilitating side effects, the cost of treatment relative to other treatments, and, for a surgeon, time in surgery, time to heal, and patient survival rate. Patient satisfaction with his physician might be informative. What might be best under one MOE may not be under another. Perhaps the ultimate MOE is patients' satisfaction with their state of health.

Outcomes Analysis

Simple measures often are precise and unequivocal, but the content of information may be shallow. It was noted that MOEs related to the eventual "outcome" of the treatment rather than an interim indicator of progress have come to be termed *outcomes analysis*. Certainly outcomes often are more difficult to quantify and take much longer to obtain, but without doubt are better indicators of the patient's general health and satisfaction.

Example (The reader is encouraged to review the example of Section 8.6 about an elderly stroke patient): Carpal Tunnel Syndrome (CTS)

CTS involves hand paresthesia, pain, weakness, and sometimes sensory loss and wasting as a result of pressure on the median nerve from edema arising from one or more of a variety of causes. In primary or idiopathic CTS, a common surgical treatment is to relieve the pressure by cutting the transverse carpal ligament. A nonsurgical approach is to induce passive traction for some minutes on alternate days for a month by a controlled pneumatic device.* It is claimed that this treatment slightly extends the wrist area thereby reducing the pressure, which allows the edema to be resorbed by the lymphatic system. In a RCT to compare these two treatments,[55] patients are randomized to treatment; blinding is not possible. The issue of this example is the MOE used for comparison. Not only the improvement but also its duration is important; the MOE will be taken at 1 month post-op, 1 year, and 2 years. Individual measures posed are median nerve conduction amplitude (microvolts) and latency (milliseconds), grip and pinch strength (kilograms), pain [visual analogue scale (VAS) 0–100], and percent normality of function (0–100). A single MOE is developed as a weighted sum of nerve conductions (x_1, x_2) and strengths (x_3, x_4) (four scores of maximum 100 each) as percent of normal, pain (x_5) (one score of maximum 100), and normality of function (x_6), which is defined as "percent ability for the hand to carry out its normal functions" (one score of maximum 100). x_2 and x_5 are negative, as smaller values indicate better condition. By denoting weights as respective b's, the MOE becomes $b_1x_1 - b_2x_2 + \cdots + b_6x_6$. What are b values? At this point, the development of the MOE becomes somewhat arbitrary, because judgment of the relative importance of the component measures will vary with the investigator. One set of evaluations follows. Nerve conductions and strengths are taken as equal; $b_1 = b_2 = b_3 = b_4 = 1$. Pain is as important as these four combined; $b_5 = 4$. Normality of function is taken as equal to pain level; $b_6 = 4$. This might engender disagreement, but note that the two are related: pain will impair normality of function. The final measure of effectiveness is

$$\text{MOE} = x_1 - x_2 + x_3 + x_4 - 4x_5 + 4x_6.$$

The MOE is measured for the two treatment groups, and the resulting data are compared using appropriate statistical methods. The larger MOE signals the better treatment.

Method

The First Step

MOEs might be better thought of as being "built" than being discovered. There is no formula to build MOEs. Building an MOE is as much art as technology. Like so many aspects of medicine, an MOE is a matter of thoughtful judgment. The first step is to ask the question, "What are we really trying to accomplish?" Is our

*CTD-Mark I by Para Tech Industries, Dayton, OH.

goal a perfect surgery? Patient survival rate? Minimum pain? Minimum cost? We might think of combining several measures. As with a medical study, we start by clearly and unequivocally defining our goal.

The Second Step

We must identify the components of the MOE that will satisfy the goal. These must be quantifiable variables. We must specify how they will be quantified, in what units, and with what precision.

The Third Step

We must identify the relationship among the components, at first verbally, but eventually quantitatively. We must remember that they are mostly in different units of measurement. We must weight each component to adjust for units. We must note that the precision of the entire MOE is no greater than that of the least precise of its variables.

The Fourth Step

The components of the MOE (the variables) represent different levels of relative importance. A serious question is how relative importances are weighted. A major issue is weighing the cost of treatment against the chance of it being effective. Some weights occur rather naturally, but with others the best an investigator can do is to set forth good judgment and allow readers to accept or reject it for themselves.

Subsequent Steps

Of course, a study having a clearly defined and planned MOE must then follow the usual steps of any good scientific study, addressed in various sections throughout this book.

Different MOEs

Recall that there is no unique MOE for a problem. The MOE is just a window through which we seek the truth. We may see the truth through several different windows, and one is not by definition better than another. This is not to say that all MOEs are acceptable. Each must be evaluated with reasoned judgment and rejected if it is likely to yield spurious information.

Additional Example

In photorefractive keratectomy (PRK), the surface of the cornea is reshaped by laser to alter the angle of light refraction entering the eye. PRK has been shown to be an effective surgical correction for myopia, as measured by post-operative visual acuity. However, some patients complain of glare, especially at night.[62] An outcomes analysis would assess success in terms of overall patient satisfaction with the procedure, rather than using only the single success measure of visual acuity. One possible MOE might be a pre-operative and a post-operative weighted sum of measures of visual correction v (diopters of correction for distance correction), glare g [patient rating from no glare (0) to severe impairment due to glare(4)], and "Would you do it again under the same circumstances?" satisfaction w [patient rating from definitely not (0) to without doubt(4)]. The measures could be made roughly equivalent to be additive by multiplying visual correction by 2 (two diopters of correction should represent moderate dissatisfaction), and willingness to repeat by 2 (twice as important as glare), after reversing the direction of its range so that 0 is desirable by subtracting it from 4. Then the MOE would be $2v + g + 2(4 - w)$. Smaller MOEs are associated with improvement. The pre-op minus post-op MOE is a difference, say d, that would be zero if there were no change due to the surgery, so H_0: $d = 0$ can be tested by a paired t test if d is distributed approximately normally or by the signed-rank test otherwise.

Exercise 19.6. Another ophthalmologic surgical procedure to treat myopia is radial keratotomy (RK), in which corneal incisions radiating around a clear central zone allow a controlled amount of collapse of the cornea, altering the angle of light refraction entering the eye. RK provides almost 20/20 uncorrected visual acuity immediately post-operatively, but the acuity tends to drift afterward, becoming hyperopic over some years, and some patients complain of impaired night vision. What might be a useful MOE to compare the overall outcome of RK with PRK?

ANSWERS TO EXERCISES

19.1. The TGF curve appears to be a straight line fit. The PGDF curve appears to be well fit by a section of a parabola, opening upward. The figures are repeated here with those respective fits.

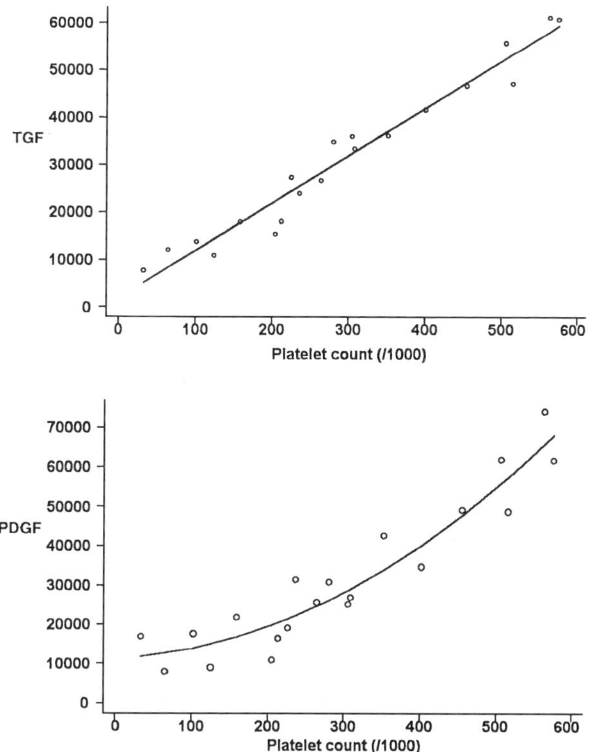

19.2. Although we could use the means of the two variables for the b and d constants, the plot is drawn such that we can see the intercept and need use only d. By drawing a line along a ruler with the edge passing through the points as a rough eye fit, we see that it passes through a value of around 5 on the y-axis. Because the functional form of a straight line $f(x)$ can be taken as just x, either a or c may be used; let us say a. a is the amount of change in y per unit increase in x and is negative, because the line decreases from left to right. The line drawn with the ruler shows a drop of about 1 second per 200 cm increase in distance, or a is approximately 0.005. Thus, the roughly fitted equation is seconds $= 5 - 0.005 \times$ centimeters.

19.3. The dependent variable y is the post-op hop distance. There are two independent variables, x_1 and x_2, hop time and distance on the uninjured leg. The geometric picture would be a plane in three dimensions, much as depicted in Fig. 19.12.

19.4. $p_e = 0.00767, n_s = 4172, n_d = n_s p_e = 32, n_{cd} = 25, n_{d-cd} = 32 - 25 = 7$, NNT $= 4172/7 = 596$ entering inmates screened for every new tuberculosis case discovered.

19.5.

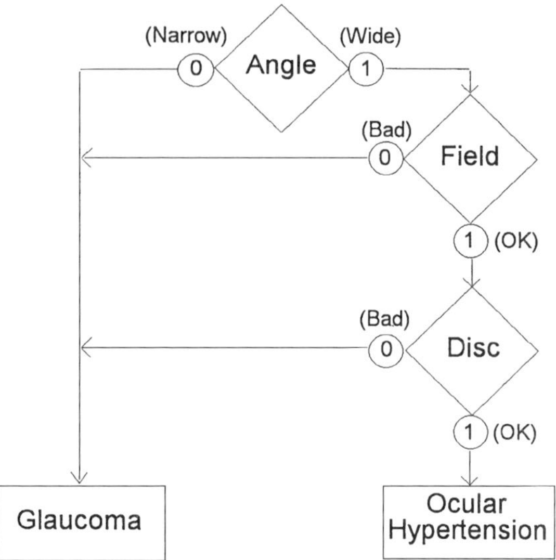

19.6. One possible MOE might be a 10-year post-operative weighted sum of measures of visual correction v, glare g, night vision n [patient rating from no interference (0) to nonfunctional vision at night(4)], and "Would you do it again under the same circumstances?" satisfaction w. The measures could be made roughly equivalent to be additive by multiplying visual correction by 2 (two diopters of correction should represent moderate dissatisfaction) and glare and night vision by 1. Willingness to repeat must have its range reversed in direction so that 0 is desirable by subtracting it from 4, and then it might have a 2 multiplier (twice as important as glare or night vision). Then the MOE is $2v + g + n + 2(4 - w)$. The smaller the MOE, the better the patient's condition. The mean MOE for RK and PRK patient groups could be contrasted by using the two-sample t test if the data distributions are approximately normal in shape with similar standard deviations or using the rank-sum test if these assumptions are not satisfied. The user may not agree with these weightings; they were chosen for illustration.

Chapter 20

Regression and Correlation Methods

20.1. REGRESSION AND CORRELATION CONCEPTS AND ASSUMPTIONS

WHAT IS REGRESSION?

Regression, introduced in Section 8.3, is a statistical tool that describes and assesses the relationship between two or more variables, at least one being an independent variable and at least one being a dependent variable predicted by the independent variable. The description is based on an assumed model of the relationship. This model may describe, or fit, the relationship well or poorly; the method tells us how well the model fits. If the model is inadequate, we may seek a better fitting model. The model may be a straight line (simple regression, Section 20.2), a curved line of any functional form (curvilinear regression, Section 20.6), or a single dependent variable predicted by two or more independent variables (multiple regression, Section 20.7). (The possibility of two or more dependent variables is not addressed in this book.) Model types were discussed in more detail in Chapter 19.

PREDICTIVE VERSUS EXPLORATORY USES OF REGRESSION

Regression is most useful when the model is dictated by an understanding of the underlying physical or physiological factors causing the relationship. In this case, regression allows us to predict the value of the dependent variable that will arise from a particular clinical reading on the independent variable and to measure the quality of this prediction. However, in the absence of this causal understanding between the variables, regression can be used as an exploratory tool suggesting which factors are related and/or the nature of such a relationship. It can serve the sequence of steps in acquiring scientific knowledge: detecting the existence of a relationship between variables, describing this relationship, testing the quality of this description, and, finally, predicting outcome values based on causal values.

Five Assumptions Underlying Regression

(1) There is the usual assumption in statistical methods that *the errors in data values* (i.e., the deviations from average) *are independent from each other*. Four other assumptions remain that are important to note, as they often are not recognized or assessed in day-to-day clinical research. (2) Obviously, *regression depends on the appropriateness of the model used in the fit*. Figure 20.1 shows two fits on a data set. The first-degree model, $y = b_0 + b_1x$, provides a horizontal regression line ($b_1 = 0$), indicating no relationship between x and y. A parabolic (second-degree) model, $y = b_0 + b_1x + b_2x^2$, shows an almost perfect fit.

(3) *The independent* (x) *readings are measured as exactly known values* (measured without randomness). This arises because the least squares method

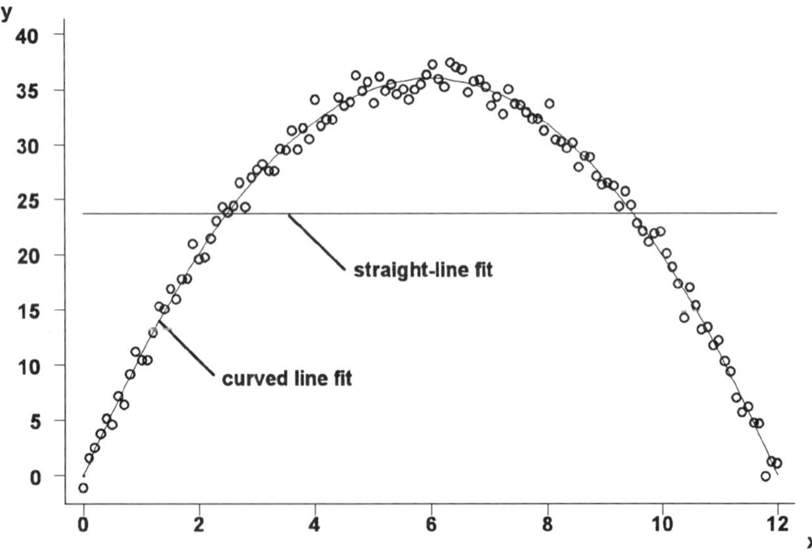

Figure 20.1 A data set showing how one model (here a straight line) can be a useless fit, whereas another model (here a curved model) can be an almost perfect fit.

minimizes the sum of squared errors vertically, i.e., on the y-axis but not on the x-axis. This assumption would be reasonable if we were relating yearly number of illnesses to patient age, as age is recorded rather exactly. However, if we were relating yearly number of illnesses to patient obesity (excess body fat estimated from a height–weight table), this assumption would be violated because this measure of obesity is rather inaccurate. What do we do in the face of a violation? We cannot eliminate the inaccuracies, and refusal to calculate the regression would deny us useful information; we can only proceed and make a careful note that the quality of, and therefore confidence in, the regression is weakened. Figure 20.2 shows a regression line fitted to data with a vertical-only error shown. (Note that this assumption is not required in correlation.)

(4) *The variance of y is the same for all values of x.* As we move from left to right along the regression line, the standard deviation of y about this line is constant.

(5) *The distribution of y is approximately normal for all values of x.* As we move from left to right along the regression line, the distribution of data remains normal for each x with mean at the regression line. Figure 20.3 illustrates assumptions (4) and (5) simultaneously. Regression is reasonably robust to these last two assumptions; one need not worry too much unless the violations are severe.

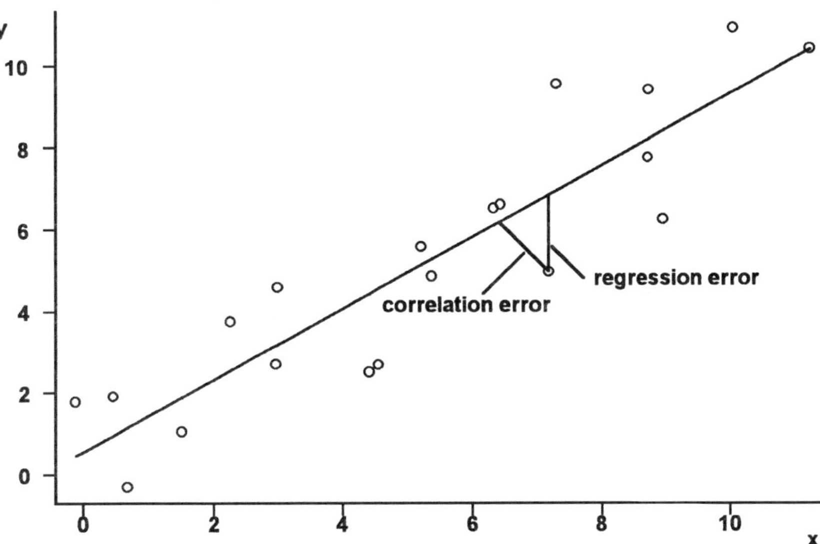

Figure 20.2 A regression or correlation line (data chosen so the line will be either) fitted to a set of data. The deviations, or "errors," between a point and the line as assumed in regression and in correlation are labeled. Note that the regression error is vertical, indicating no x variability, whereas the correlation error allows variability in both x and y.

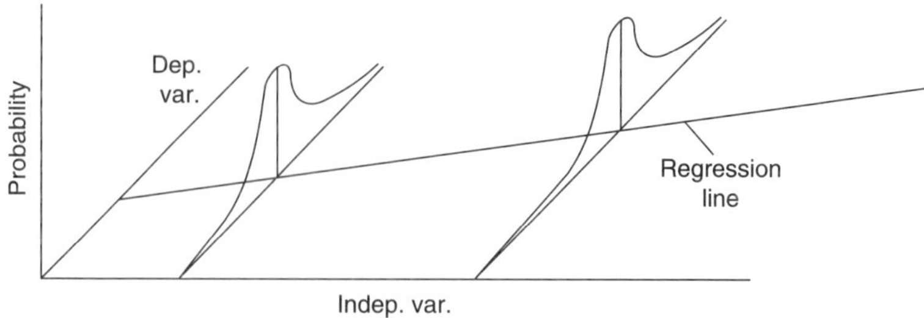

Figure 20.3 A regression line shown on an x,y-plane laid flat with the assumed probability distribution rising vertically for two representative points on the line. Note that the distribution is normal for both and shows the same variability for both.

What Is Correlation?

"Correlation" as a general term implies simply a relationship among events. In statistics, it refers to a quantitative expression of the interrelationship, namely, a *coefficient of correlation*. In the context of statistics, the term correlation usually refers to a correlation coefficient and will be so used here. The correlation coefficient for continuous variables was introduced in Section 3.1, where its calculation was given as the covariance of x and y divided by both standard deviations. This division has the effect of standardizing the coefficient so that it always represents points scattered about a 45° line. In correlation, the level of association is not measured by the slope of the line as in regression, but by how tightly or loosely the x,y observations cluster about the line. Because this coefficient is standardized by dividing by the standard deviations, it lies in the range -1 to $+1$, with 0 representing no relationship at all and ± 1 representing perfect predictability. A positive coefficient indicates that both variables tend to increase or decrease together, whereas with a negative coefficient, one tends to increase as the other decreases. We would agree that a correlation coefficient of 0.10 implies little if any relationship between the two variables and that one of 0.90 indicates a strong relationship. Figure 20.4 shows correlations from three of our data sets, illustrating the relationship between the coefficient and the scatter pattern of data. We might ask the following: What is the value of the correlation coefficient when it passes from probably coincidental (due to chance) to probably associative (the measures vary together)? Such questions will be addressed in Section 20.5.

Assumptions Underlying Correlation

Let us compare assumptions about continuous-variable correlation with the five regression assumptions. (1) Correlation requires the same assumption that *the errors in data values are independent from each other.* (2) *Correlation always requires the assumption of a straight line relationship.* A large correlation coefficient implies that there is a large linear component to the relationship, but not that other components do not exist. In contrast, a zero correlation coefficient only implies that there is not a linear component; there may be curved relationships, as was illustrated in Fig. 20.1. (3) The assumption of exact readings on one axis is *not* required of correlation; *both x and y may be measured with random variability*, as was illustrated in Fig. 20.2. (4) and (5) take on a different form, because x and y vary jointly, so that what is assumed for y relative to x also is assumed for x relative to y. x and y are assumed to follow a bivariate normal distribution, i.e., sort of a hill in three dimensions, where x and y are the width and length and the height is the probability (could be read as relative frequency) of any joint value of x and y. The peak of the hill lies over the point specified by the two means, and the height of the hill diminishes in a normal shape in any direction radiating out from the means point. If the bivariate normal assumption is badly violated, it is possible to calculate a correlation coefficient using rank methods.

Rank Correlation

Sometimes the data to be analyzed consist of ranks rather than continuous measurements. At other times, the assumption of a bivariate normal distribution is violated, requiring that the rankings of the data replace the continuous measurements. In these cases, a measure of correlation based on ranks is required. If the formula for the ordinary correlation coefficient is used with ranks rather than with continuous-type observations, a coefficient emerges that may be interpreted in the same way.

Names for Correlation

The continuous-variable correlation coefficient was originated by Francis Galton. British statistician Karl Pearson (who credits Galton, incidentally), along with Francis Edgeworth and others, did a great deal of the work in developing this form of correlation coefficient, so sometimes it is referred to as Pearson's correlation. Another name sometimes seen is product-moment correlation. Moments are mathematical entities related to the descriptors we use, such as the mean (first moment) and the variance (second moment about the first moment). Moments derived using a product of x and y are called product moments. The covariance used in calculating the correlation coefficient is a form of product moment. These names really are not necessary except in the context of distinguishing correlation coefficients based on continuous variables from those based on ranks. The rank

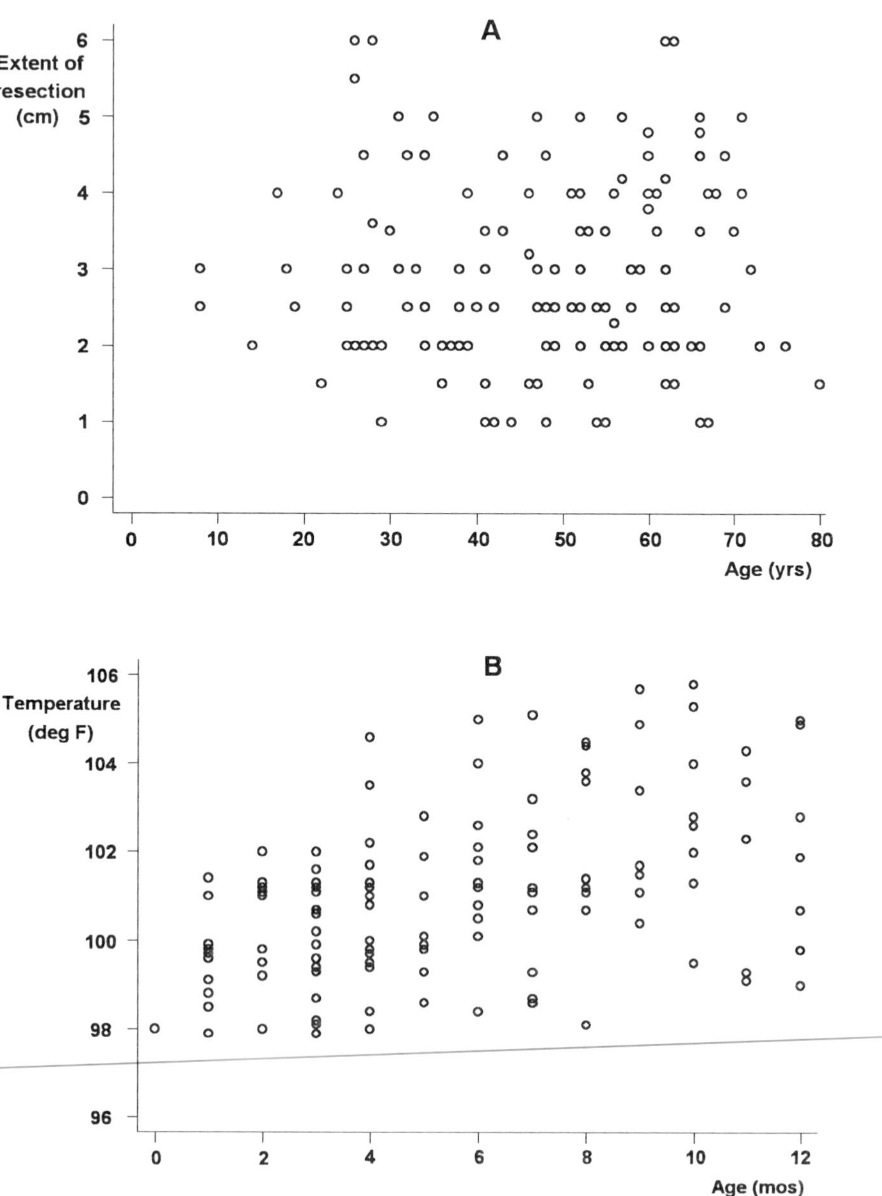

Figure 20.4 Low, moderate, and high correlation coefficients as related to the scatter pattern of data from three sources: (A) $r = 0.02$ for the extent of carinal resection as related to patient age (from DB12); (B) $r = 0.48$ for temperature as related to age for infants with pulmonary complications in their first year (one extreme datum was omitted to facilitate the illustration); (C) $r = 0.98$ for transforming growth factor count as related to platelet count (from DB9).

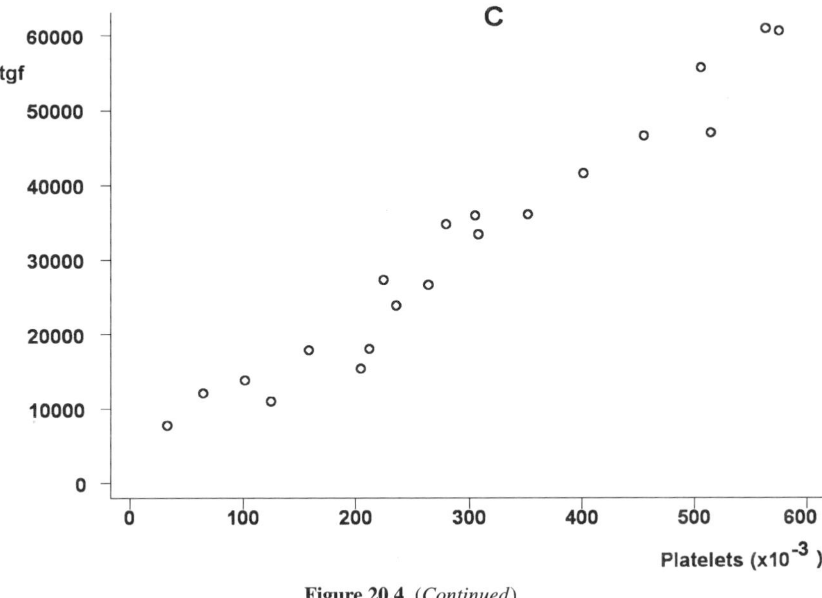

Figure 20.4 *(Continued)*

correlation coefficient was first written about by C. E. Spearman, who also simplified the formula. The subscript s (for Spearman) is attached to the population ρ or sample r to signify this form. (In the early part of the 20th century, before the Greek for population and Roman for sample convention became standard, ρ sometimes was used for the Spearman correlation; if you encounter it, consider it a historical leftover.)

20.2. SIMPLE REGRESSION

Review of Examples of Chapter 8

A regression example of white blood cell (WBC) count depending on level of infection was given in Section 8.3. Mean bacterial culture count m_x was 16.09 ($\times 10^{-9}$), mean WBC count m_y was 40.96 ($\times 10^{-9}$), and the slope b_1 was 0.1585, giving rise to the regression equation $y - 40.96 = 0.1585(x - 16.09)$. The graph was shown in Fig. 8.3. WBC count seems to increase with level of infection. A second example, number of days of hospital treatment for psychiatric patients depending on intelligence quotient (IQ), was given in Section 8.4. Mean number of days m_x was 10.5, mean IQ m_y was 100, and the slope b_1 was 0.3943, giving rise to the regression equation $y - 10.5 = 0.3943(x - 100)$. The graph was shown in Fig. 8.4. Time spent in treatment at a psychiatric hospital seems to increase with IQ.

Example

DB3 contains data on levels of serum theophylline (a vasodilator to treat asthma, emphysema, etc.) just prior to administration of an antibiotic (baseline) and 10 days later. The relationship between the two levels was modeled as a straight line fit in Section 19.4 (Fig. 19.6). The inputs to the equation for this regression line are calculated as $m_x = 10.7988$, $m_y = 10.1444$, $s_{xy} = 11.8282$, and $s_x^2 = 14.1942$, yielding the line [Eq. (20.1)] $y - 10.1444 = 0.8333(x - 10.7988)$. Solution for y yields a simpler form for prediction: $y = 1.1458 + 0.8333x$. The line drawn in Fig. 19.6 was simplified by rounding to $y = 1.1 + 0.8x$. Suppose a patient has a baseline serum theophylline level of 10 and we want to predict the postantibiotic level, $y|x = 10$. We substitute $x = 10$ to obtain $y|10 = 9.4788$, or about 9.5. (Note that substitution of $x = 10$ in the rounded formula yields 9.1, which illustrates the advisability of carrying several decimal places of precision during calculation and rounding afterward.)

Method

The Regression Equation

A straight line, including simple regression, is determined by two pieces of information (Section 8.2). A useful form of a regression line, using the slope β_1 of the line and the mean point (m_x, m_y) in the x, y-plane, was given by Eq. (8.1) as

$$y - m_y = \beta_1(x - m_x). \tag{20.1}$$

Recall that theoretical or population coefficients in models are denoted by β's, whereas sample-based estimates of the β's are denoted by b's. The estimate of β_1, b_1, is the covariance of x and y divided by the variance of x, or s_{xy}/s_x^2. (The formulas for the m's and s's may be found on the summary page for Chapter 3.) This is the best fit by least squares (and also other mathematical criteria) expressing the relationship between x and y.

Predicting y from x

The most likely value of y, that is, its prediction, from a chosen value of x is just the value of y, say $y|x$ (read "y given x"), arising from substituting the x value in Eq. (20.1) and solving for y. If many predicted values are to be calculated, an easier form for substitution is the slope–intercept form, $y = b_0 + b_1x$, in which $b_0 = m_y - b_1m_x$:

$$y|x = b_0 + b_1x. \tag{20.2}$$

It should be noted that a prediction is valid only over the range of existing data. (In the example to be seen in Section 20.6, extending the days after malarial infection far enough will appear to bring dead rats back to life.)

Additional Example

Lung congestion often occurs in illness among infants, but is not verified easily without radiography. Are there indicators that could predict whether lung opacity will appear on an X ray? A study[71] of 234 infants included age (months), respiration rate (breaths/minute), heart rate (beats/minute), temperature (degree Fahrenheit), pulse oximetry (percent), clinical appearance of illness on physical exam, and lungs sounding congested on physical exam. Lung X rays were taken to be "truth" and recorded as clear or opaque. The goal of this study was to predict infants' lung opacity. However, the use of a binary outcome (yes or no, + or −, 0 or 1, etc.) as a dependent variable requires logistic regression and will be addressed in Section 20.8. Until then, relationships between continuous measurements will be used for exemplification.

Predicting Temperature by Age

The following question arises: Is temperature associated solely with illness or is it influenced by age? Let us fit a regression line to temperature as predicted by age. If the line is horizontal, knowledge of the age gives us no ability to predict temperature. However, if the line has a marked slope (testing the slope statistically is treated in Section 20.4), temperature provides some predictive capability and is at least one influencing factor. Regression line inputs from age (taken as x) and temperature (y) were calculated as $m_x = 10.9402$, $m_y = 101.5385$, $s_{xy} = 5.6727$, and $s_x^2 = 45.5329$. $b_1 = s_{xy}/s_x^2 = 0.1246$. The slope–mean form of the regression line, from Eq. (20.1), is $y - 101.5385 = 0.1246(x - 10.9402)$. $b_0 = 100.1754$, leading to the slope–intercept form as $y = 100.1752 + 0.1246x$. If an infant is 20 months of age, the most likely prediction of temperature would be $y|20 = 100.1752 + 0.1246 \times 20 = 102.6674$, or about 102.7°F. The data and the regression line are shown in Fig. 20.5.

Exercise 20.1. As part of a study on circulatory responses to intubation during laryngoscopy,[66] the following question arose: Could changes in systolic blood pressure (SBP, y-axis) due to laryngoscopy be predicted by skin vasomotor reflex amplitude (SVmR, x-axis)? Readings (from a graph; may be off by some decimal units from the authors') were taken on $n = 26$ patients with the following results: $m_x = 0.1771$, $m_y = 25.6538$, $s_{xy} = 2.2746$, and $s_x^2 = 0.0241$. Calculate b_1 and b_0. Write the slope–mean and slope–intercept forms for the regression line. Sketch the SVmR and SBP axes and the regression line. If the SVmR amplitude is measured as 0.3, what is the most likely prediction of change in SBP?

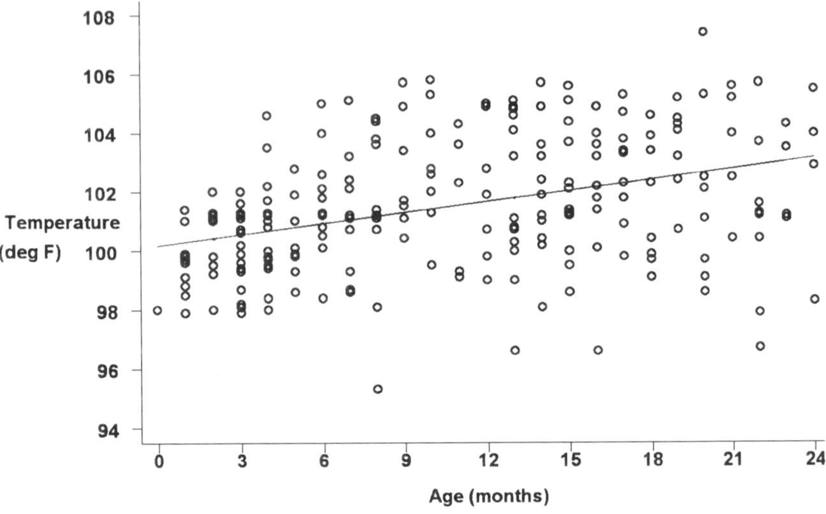

Figure 20.5 Temperature depending on age for 234 infants.

20.3. CORRELATION COEFFICIENTS

EXAMPLE

In the Example of Section 20.2, DB3 data used baseline serum theophylline level to predict the level 10 days after antibiotic treatment. The covariance s_{xy} was given as 11.8282 and the regression line as $y = 1.1458 + 0.8333x$. Additional statistics calculated from the data are the standard deviations $s_x = 3.7675$ and $s_y = 3.9808$. By using the relationship of Eq. (20.3), $r = 11.8282/(3.7675 \times 3.9808) = 0.7887$. Note that the second part of Eq. (20.3) also can be used, yielding $r = 0.8333 \times 3.7675/3.9808 = 0.7887$. This correlation coefficient of about 0.79 is rather high, indicating a close straight line association. Were the assumptions underlying r justified? The frequency distribution of baseline is not far enough from normal to worry us much, but the day 10 readings are. It is preferable to use r_s. Table 20.1 shows the DB3 data with ranks and d_i^2. $n = 16$ and $\sum d_i^2 = 192$. By substituting in Eq. (20.4), we find $r_s = 0.7176$, or about 0.72, which is not far different from $r = 0.79$.

METHOD

When to Use Correlation as Opposed to Regression

Correlation is used when the question of interest is how closely x and y are associated (in a straight line relationship). They are not thought of as dependent

Table 20.1

DB3 Data (Serum Theophylline Levels) for Baseline and 10 Days after Beginning Antibiotic, along with Associated Ranks and d_i^2 (= Squared Difference between Ranks)

Patient no.	Baseline	Rank	10 day	Rank	d_i^2
1	14.1	12	10.3	7	25
2	7.2	4	7.3	5	1
3	14.2	13	11.3	9	16
4	10.3	8	13.8	14	36
5	15.4	14	13.6	13	1
6	5.2	2	4.2	1	1
7	10.4	9	14.1	15	36
8	10.5	10	5.4	4	36
9	5.0	1	5.1	3	4
10	8.6	5	7.4	6	1
11	16.6	16	13.0	12	16
12	16.4	15	17.1	16	1
13	12.2	11	12.3	11	0
14	6.6	3	4.5	2	1
15	9.9	6	11.7	10	16
16	10.2	7	11.2	8	1

and independent variables. There is no intent to predict one from the other. In regression, x is a factor (partially) causing y, or at least is related to causal factors so that it can predict y.

Calculating Correlation

The calculation of the correlation coefficient was given in Section 8.3 as

$$r = \frac{s_{xy}}{s_x s_y}\left(=b_1\frac{s_x}{s_y}\right). \tag{20.3}$$

The first expression, the covariance divided by the standard deviations, usually is used. However, if a regression has already been calculated, the second expression, the regression slope multiplied by the ratio of standard deviations, may be more convenient.

Calculating the Rank Correlation

For each of n pairs of x and y ranks in the sample, find the difference x-rank − y-rank; these are denoted d_i, the difference in x and y ranks for the ith patient. Square and add together these d_i. Spearman's formula (simplified from the formula for the continuous coefficient) is

$$r_s = 1 - \frac{6\sum d_i^2}{n(n^2 - 1)}. \tag{20.4}$$

Additional Example

Continuing the Additional Example of Section 20.2 on infant lung opacity,[71] we posed the following question: Is temperature associated with age? The covariance is $s_{xy} = 5.6727$ and the standard deviations are $s_x = 6.7478$ and $s_y = 2.2557$. $r = 5.6727/(6.7478 \times 2.2557) = 0.3727$. The correlation coefficient is not high, but neither is it negligible. Is it statistically significant, i.e., greater than what is likely to occur by chance? This question is answered in Section 20.5. If we were investigating rather than illustrating, at the beginning of the exercise we would have asked whether the assumptions underlying correlation are satisfied. If we plot quick frequency distributions of temperature and age, we find that temperature is approximately normal in distribution but age is bimodal, although the two modes are rather weak, and is not far from a uniform distribution (nearly the same frequency for all age intervals). The assumptions for age are not satisfied; we should use r_s rather than r. Upon ranking the data, finding, squaring, and adding together the rank differences, and substituting in Eq. (20.4), we find $r_s = 0.3997$. This is rather close to the r of 0.3727, so that the violation of an assumption did not cause a major error in r.

Exercise 20.2. As part of a study on circulatory responses to laryngoscopy and intubation (Exercise 20.1),[66] the relationship between change in systolic blood pressure (SBP) due to laryngoscopy and skin vasomotor reflex amplitude (SVmR) was of interest. Readings were taken on $n = 26$ patients with the following results: $s_{xy} = 2.2746$, $s_x = 0.1553$, and $s_y = 20.0757$. Calculate r. What does this r indicate about the association of SBP change and SVmR? If $\sum d_i^2 = 863$, what is r_s? How does r_s agree with r?

20.4. TESTS AND CONFIDENCE INTERVALS ON REGRESSION PARAMETERS

Example

In the example of Section 20.2 using DB3, serum theophylline level at day 10 was predicted from baseline level by the regression line $y = 1.1458 + 0.8333x$ ($b_1 = 0.8333$). The calculated components we will need are $n = 16$, $m_x = 10.7988$, $s_{xy} = 11.8287$, $s_x = 3.7675$, and $s_y = 3.9808$. From Eq. (20.5), $s_e = 2.5334$.

(1) Are x and y Related?

To test H_0: $\beta_1 = 0$, we need s_b. Substitution in Eq. (20.6) yields $s_b = 0.1736$. We use Table B to find the 5% two-tailed critical value of t for $n - 2 = 14$ *df* as 2.145. From Eq. (20.7), the calculated $t = 4.80$, which is much larger than critical. We conclude that the slope of the line, and therefore the x,y association, is significant. However, is baseline theophylline level the major predictor, i.e., major causal factor?

(2) How Strong Is the x,y Relationship?

Use of Eq. (20.3) yielded $r = 0.7887$ (in Section 20.3), so $R^2 = 0.6220$. We can say that about 62% of the possible capability to predict the day 10 serum theophylline level from baseline level is provided by this straight line model; 38% remains for all other factors combined plus randomness. This certainly is not a perfect predictor, but we can conclude that baseline level is the major predictor. To put a confidence interval on the slope, we substitute b_1, s_b, and critical t in Eq. (20.10) to find the confidence interval:

$$\begin{aligned} &\mathrm{P}[0.8333 - 2.145 \times 0.1736 < \beta_1 < 0.8333 + 2.145 \times 0.1736] \\ &\quad = \mathrm{P}[0.46 < \beta_1 < 1.21] = 0.95. \end{aligned}$$

We can say that the predicted slope is not more than about three-eighths of a unit off in y per unit of x with 95% confidence. Again, the prediction is not perfect, but it is rather good.

(3) What Is the Confidence of the Prediction of Average y for a Given x?

Suppose we have a group of patients with baseline serum level 10. The predicted $m|x$ is, of course, the value of the regression obtained by substituting in that x, in this case 9.479. We want a confidence interval on the mean of this group. Use of Eq. (20.11) yields the standard error of this prediction statistic as $s_{m|x} = 0.6484$. We found the 5% two-tailed critical value of t for 14 *df* to be 2.145. By substituting in Eq. (20.12), we find the confidence interval on mean day 10 level for a baseline level of 10 to be

$$\begin{aligned} &\mathrm{P}[9.479 - 2.145 \times 0.648 < \mu|10 < 9.479 + 2.145 \times 0.648] \\ &\quad = \mathrm{P}[8.089 < \mu|10 < 10.869] = 0.95. \end{aligned}$$

(4) What Is the Confidence of the Regression Prediction of y for an Individual Patient's x?

Suppose we have an individual patient with baseline serum level 10. The predicted $y|x$ is still 9.479. We want a confidence interval on this individual's prediction. Use of Eq. (20.13) yields the standard error of this prediction statistic as $s_{y|x} = 2.615$. The critical value of t remains 2.145. By substituting in Eq. (20.14), we find the confidence interval on the patient's day 10 level for a baseline level of 10 to be

$$\begin{aligned} &P[9.479 - 2.145 \times 2.615 < E(y)|10 < 9.479 + 2.145 \times 2.615] \\ &\quad = P[3.870 < E(y)|10 < 15.088] = 0.95. \end{aligned}$$

The confidence interval on the individual's predicted 10-day level is very much wider than that on the mean.

(5) Are Two Regression Slopes Different?

By using the symbols to distinguish the two samples as in the Method section, we found the regression of 10-day serum level to have slope $b_{1:1} = 0.8333$, $s_1^2 = 14.1942$, and $s_{e:1}^2 = 6.4181$. Let us also consider the regression of the 5-day serum level on baseline. In returning to the data of DB3, we find the slope to be $b_{1:2} = 0.8206$, $s_2^2 = s_1^2$, and $s_{e:2}^2 = 12.5218$. $n_1 = n_2 = 16$. Substitution in Eq. (20.15) yields $s_{b:1-2} = 0.2983$ and in Eq. (20.16) yields $t = 0.0426$. The critical two-tailed 5% α-value of t from Table B with $n_1 + n_2 - 4 = 28$ *df* is 2.048, which is very much larger than the calculated t. (The actual p-value is calculated as 0.966.) There is no evidence that the slopes are different.

Method

Assessing Regression

Five questions might be asked of the regression and will be considered in turn. (1) Does the regression show that x and y are related? (2) How strong is this relation? (3) By using regression methods for prediction, what will be confidence limits on average y for a given value of x? (4) In prediction, what will be confidence limits on the best predicted y for an individual patient's x? (5) Given two samples, are the regression slopes different?

Standard Error Notation

In Part I, the standard error of the mean was symbolized as SEM, which is fairly usual in medicine. However, in regression, we shall have to find the standard errors of other statistics and use them in formulas, and so we need a more succinct and flexible notation. Because a standard error of a statistic is just its standard deviation, it will be convenient to use the standard deviation symbol s with the respective statistic indicated as a subscript. Thus, the SEM becomes s_m. We will need four more standard errors: the standard error of the residual (residuals are the observations' deviations from the regression line), usually denoted s_e in statistics (e for "error"), the standard error of the estimate of the regression slope b_1, s_b, the standard error of the estimate of the mean values of y for each x, $s_{m|x}$, and the standard error of the estimate of the individual predictions of y for each x, $s_{y|x}$. As the residual standard error s_e is used in the others, it is given first. Starting with the sum of squares of deviations from the regression line, we define

$$s_e^2 = \sum (y - b_0 - b_1 x)^2/(n-2)$$

[where $n - 2$ will be degrees of freedom (*df*), because we lost 2 *df* by calculating the two b's]. Some algebra will yield the following forms. Use whichever is easier computationally.

$$s_e = \sqrt{\frac{n-1}{n-2}\left(s_y^2 - b_1^2 s_x^2\right)} = s_y\sqrt{\frac{n-1}{n-2}(1-R^2)}. \tag{20.5}$$

[R^2, the coefficient of determination, introduced in Section 8.4, will be discussed more fully in paragraph (2) on the strength of the x, y relationship.]

(1) Does the Regression Show That x and y Are Related?

If the regression line is horizontal, the predicted y is the same for every x; the x,y relationship has no predictive ability. If the line is sloped, each x yields a different y; there is predictive ability. Is this slope significantly different from horizontal, or could an apparent slope be due only to chance? In a test of this question, $H_0{:}\beta = 0$ versus $H_1{:}\beta \neq 0$ (or <0, or >0 if one tail is impossible or clinically irrelevant). In the hypothesis test of a mean, we asked whether the estimate of the mean was significantly larger than the standard error of that mean, i.e., if the ratio of a statistic to its standard error was larger than a critical t-value. The pattern here is the same. We find the standard error of the slope as

$$s_b = \frac{s_e}{\sqrt{(n-1)}s_x} \tag{20.6}$$

To test H_0, t with $n - 2$ *df* is simply

$$t_{(n-2)df} = b_1/s_b, \tag{20.7}$$

and we reject H_0 if b_1/s_b is farther out in the tails of the t distribution than the critical t. If the calculated t is not rejected, then *either* the relationship is improbable *or* the relationship does not follow a straight line.

Testing against a Theoretical Slope

Suppose the slope is to be compared not to zero slope but to a theoretical slope, say β_1. Situations in which such a β_1 might arise are, for example, when a relationship has been posed on the basis of established physiology or when comparing with previously published results. The standard error s_b remains the same, as does the $n - 2$ *df*. The hypotheses are H_0:$\beta = \beta_1$ versus H_1:$\beta \neq \beta_1$. The t statistic becomes

$$t_{(n-2)df} = \frac{b_1 - \beta_1}{s_b}, \tag{20.8}$$

which is tested and interpreted in the same way as for zero slope.

(2) How Strong Is the x,y Relationship?

The *coefficient of determination*, introduced in Section 8.4, indicates how well the model predicts the dependent variable. It might be defined as the proportion of predictive capability represented by this model. Generally designated R^2, it sometimes is denoted r^2 in the case of a single x predicting y by a straight line, but we shall use R^2 in all cases to be consistent. In the single x straight line case, R^2 is just the square of r, the correlation coefficient. In the case of a curved line or multiple x, it is more complicated. Note that R^2 does not evaluate how well x predicts y, but rather how well *this model of the x,y relationship* predicts y. Sometimes a straight line is a very poor predictor, whereas a curved line such as a parabola is a good one, as was illustrated in Fig. 20.1. In this case, $y = b_0 + b_1x$ yields a very small R^2 (0.002 in the figure), but $y = b_0 + b_1x + b_2x^2$ yields a large one (0.970 in the figure). We know that an r, and therefore R^2, of 0 indicates no (straight line) relationship and that an r of -1 or $+1$, and therefore an R^2 of 1, indicates perfect predictability. At what value of R^2 does the relationship become greater than chance? It turns out that this value is the same as the value at which b_1 becomes significantly greater than 0, as tested by Eq. (20.7). Algebra will permit this form to be rewritten as a test of R^2 (for straight line single x regression only!). The null hypothesis H_0: $\rho^2 = 0$ is tested by

$$t_{(n-2)df} = \sqrt{\frac{(n-2)R^2}{1 - R^2}}. \tag{20.9}$$

Because Eq. (20.9) tells us nothing new over Eq. (20.7), R^2 usually is used in interpreting rather than testing the x,y relationship.

Confidence Interval on the Slope

Sometimes in describing the slope of the regression relationship, a confidence interval on the slope will be informative. The general pattern of confidence intervals was given in Section 4.4. To follow that pattern, we need the estimate of the statistic (sample slope b_1), the critical value of the probability distribution ($t_{1-\alpha/2}$), and the standard error for that statistic (s_b), all of which were given earlier. The confidence interval on the population slope β_1 is

$$\mathrm{P}[b_1 - t_{1-\alpha/2}s_b < \beta_1 < b_1 + t_{1-\alpha/2}s_b] = 1 - \alpha, \tag{20.10}$$

where the critical t has $n - 2$ *df*. A tight confidence interval indicates a strong relationship.

(3) What Is the Confidence of the Regression Prediction of the Average y for a Given Value of x?

Because there is only one regression line, there is only one prediction of y from a given x. The average y for a given x is the same as the most likely y for a given x. However, the confidence interval for a mean y is not the same as that for an individual patient's y, so these confidence intervals are given separately in this and the next paragraph. The confidence interval follows the same pattern as before: the estimated value on the y axis $\pm$ a critical t multiplied by the standard error. The estimate and the critical t are the same as in Eq. (20.10); only the standard error differs. We symbolized the sample mean value of y for a given x as $m|x$, estimating the population mean value μ for a given x, $\mu|x$. Its standard error is

$$s_{m|x} = s_e\sqrt{\frac{1}{n} + \frac{(x - m_x)^2}{(n-1)s_x^2}} \tag{20.11}$$

The $1 - \alpha$ confidence interval, where the critical t's have $n - 2$ *df*, then is

$$\mathrm{P}[m|x - t_{1-\alpha/2}s_{m|x} < \mu|x < m|x + t_{1-\alpha/2}s_{m|x}] = 1 - \alpha. \tag{20.12}$$

(4) What Is the Confidence of the Regression Prediction of y for a Given Patient's Individual x?

The average regression more often is of interest in research. In clinical practice, the predicted value for an individual patient often is of interest. The prediction will be the same; the average is the most likely value and our best guess. However, the standard error is slightly different, leading to an altered confidence statement. We symbolized the most likely value of y for a given x as $y|x$, estimating the population expected value of y for a given x, $E(y)|x$. Its standard error is

$$s_{y|x} = s_e\sqrt{1 + \frac{1}{n} + \frac{(x - m_x)^2}{(n-1)s_x^2}}. \tag{20.13}$$

The $1 - \alpha$ confidence interval, where the critical t's have $n - 2$ *df*, is

$$\mathrm{P}[y|x - t_{1-\alpha/2}s_{y|x} < E(y)|x < y|x + t_{1-\alpha/2}s_{y|x}] = 1 - \alpha. \tag{20.14}$$

(5) Given Two Samples, Are the Regression Slopes Different?

To distinguish the statistics calculated from the two samples, let us denote n as n_1 and n_2 for samples 1 and 2, respectively, b_1 as $b_{1:1}$ and $b_{1:2}$, s_x^2 as s_1^2 and s_2^2, and s_e^2 as $s_{e:1}^2$ and $s_{e:2}^2$. The test of the null hypothesis $\mathrm{H}_0{:}b_{1:1} = b_{1:2}$ is a t test with the usual format, having n_1 and $n_2 - 4$ *df*. The standard error of difference in slopes is

$$s_{b:1-2} = \sqrt{\left(\frac{(n_1 - 2)s_{e:1}^2 + (n_2 - 1)s_{e:2}^2}{n_1 + n_2 - 4}\right)\left(\frac{1}{(n_1 - 1)s_1^2} + \frac{1}{(n_2 - 1)s_2^2}\right)}, \tag{20.15}$$

which yields a t as

$$t = \frac{b_{1:1} - b_{1:2}}{s_{b:1-2}} \tag{20.16}$$

If the calculated t is larger than a two-tailed critical t for n_1 and $n_2 - 4$ *df*, H_0 is rejected.

Additional Example

In the lung congestion study[71] introduced in the Additional Example of Section 20.2, we asked whether temperature could be predicted by infant age. The regression line was calculated to be $y = 100.1752 + 0.1246x (b_1 = 0.1246)$. The regression prediction for a 20-month-old infant was 102.6674°F. The interim statistics we need are $n = 234$, $m_x = 10.9402$, $s_{xy} = 5.6727$, $s_x = 6.7478$, and $s_y = 2.2557$. From Eq. (20.5), $s_e = 2.0979$.

(1) Are x and y Related?

To test $\mathrm{H}_0{:}\mathrm{H}\ \beta_1 = 0$, we need s_b. Substitution in Eq. (20.6) yields $s_b = 0.0204$. We interpolate in Table B to find a 5% two-tailed critical value of t for $n - 2 = 232$ *df* as about 1.97. From Eq. (20.7), the calculated $t = 6.1174$, which is much larger than the critical t. We conclude that the slope of the line, and therefore the x,y association, is significant. This tells us that age is a real causal factor in temperature, but not whether it is a major or a minor cause.

(2) How Strong Is the x,y Relationship?

Use of Eq. (20.3) yielded $r = 0.3727$ (in Section 20.3), so $R^2 = 0.1389$. We can say that about 14% of the possible capability to predict temperature from age is provided by this straight line model, with the remaining 86% arising from other causal factors and randomness. This tells us that temperature is a minor causal factor. To put a confidence interval on the slope, we substitute b_1, s_b, and critical t in Eq. (20.10) to find the confidence interval:

$$\begin{aligned}&\mathrm{P}[0.1246 - 1.97 \times 0.0204 < \beta_1 < 0.1246 + 1.97 \times 0.0204]\\&\quad = \mathrm{P}[0.08 < \beta_1 < 0.16] = 0.95.\end{aligned}$$

(3) What Is the Confidence of the Prediction of Average y for a Given x?

Let us consider a group of 20-month-old infants. The predicted $m|x$ is the value of the regression obtained by substituting that x, in this case 102.6674. We want a confidence interval on the mean of this group. Use of Eq. (20.11) yields the standard error of this prediction statistic as $s_{m|x} = 0.2299$. We found the 5% two-tailed critical value of t for 232 *df* to be 1.97. By substituting in Eq. (20.12), we find the confidence interval on mean temperature of 20-month-old infants to be

$$\begin{aligned}&\mathrm{P}[102.6674 - 1.97 \times 0.2299 < \mu|20 < 102.6674 + 1.97 \times 0.2299]\\&\quad = \mathrm{P}[102.2 < \mu|20 < 103.1] = 0.95.\end{aligned}$$

(4) What Is the Confidence of the Regression Prediction of y for an Individual Patient's x?

Suppose we have an individual infant at age 20 months. The predicted $y|x$ is still 102.6674. We want a confidence interval on this individual's prediction. Use of Eq. (20.13) yields the standard error of this prediction statistic as $s_{y|x} = 2.1104$. The critical value of t remains 1.97. By substituting in Eq. (20.14), we find the confidence interval on the 20-month-old infant to be

$$\begin{aligned}&\mathrm{P}[102.6674 - 1.97 \times 2.1104 < E(y)|20 < 102.6674 + 1.97 \times 2.1104]\\&\quad = \mathrm{P}[98.5 < E(y)|20 < 106.8] = 0.95.\end{aligned}$$

Whereas the confidence interval on the mean might be useful in research, the confidence interval on temperature as predicted by age for an individual infant is useless, encompassing almost the entire range of the data set. If we want to predict temperature for clinical use, we will have to incorporate more important causal factors in our model, probably going to a multiple regression.

Exercise 20.3. In Exercise 20.1,[66] the question posed was the following: Could change in SBP (y) due to laryngoscopy be predicted by SVmR (x)? Required interim statistics are $n = 26, m_x = 0.1771, s_{xy} = 2.2744, s_x = 0.1553$, and $s_y = 20.0757$. Find s_e and s_b. Look up the 95% critical t. Test $H_0{:}\beta_1 = 0$. Is the slope significantly greater than 0? Find R^2 and the 95% confidence interval on β_1. Is SVmR a major predictor? What percent of the predictive capability remains for other predictors and randomness? For SVmR $= 0.3$, calculate $s_{m|x}$ and $s_{y|x}$ and find the 95% confidence intervals on $m|x$ and $y|x$.

20.5. TESTS AND CONFIDENCE INTERVALS ON CORRELATION COEFFICIENTS

EXAMPLE

Let us continue the emphysema example of relating serum theophylline level 10 days after beginning an antibiotic to the baseline level. In Section 20.3, r was found to be 0.7887. In Section 20.4, we tested $H_0{:}\beta_1 = 0$ using Eq. (20.7), which we noted is the same as testing $H_0{:}\rho = 0$ using Eq. (20.17); we concluded that the t of 4.80 showed the x,y association to be significant.

Test of Two Correlation Coefficients

Returning to the data of DB3, we find the correlation coefficient between baseline and the 5-day serum level to be 0.6707. Are the 5- and 10-day correlations the same, differing only due to random fluctuations, or do we have probabilistic evidence that they are different? First, we must note that we have only $n = 16$ in our sample, which is too small for a proper approximation; we shall carry out the calculations only for illustration, not for a legitimate medical conclusion. Substitution of 0.7887 and 0.6707 in turn in Eq. (20.18) yields $m_1 = 1.0189$ and $m_2 = 0.8120$. From Eq. (20.20), both variances are 1/13 = 0.0769, yielding a pooled standard deviation of 0.3922. By substituting in Eq. (20.22), we find $z = 0.5275$. A critical z, using two-tailed $\alpha = 0.05$, is the familiar 1.96. The calculated z is far less than the critical z; we cannot reject the null hypothesis of no difference. We have no evidence that the two correlation coefficients are different.

Confidence Interval on the Correlation Coefficient

Using the estimated correlation coefficient $r = 0.7887$, what are 95% confidence limits on the population ρ? By substituting r, $z_{1-\alpha/2} = 1.96$, and $n = 16$ in Eq. (20.23), we find $P[0.7004 < \rho < 0.8242] = 0.95$.

METHOD

The sample correlation coefficient, r, introduced in Section 20.3, estimates the population correlation coefficient, ρ. It indicates how closely a scattergram of x, y points cluster about a 45° straight line. A tight cluster (see Fig. 20.4) implies a high degree of association. The coefficient of determination, R^2, introduced in Section 20.4, indicates the proportion of variability in y that can be attributed to the model from independent variables. In this case, with one x and that in a straight line relationship, R^2 is just the square of r. It was noted that Eq. (20.9) provides a test of the hypothesis that R^2, and therefore r, is 0, i.e., that x and y are independent of each other. Rewritten using r, the test of H_0:$\rho = 0$ is

$$t_{(n-2)\,df} = \sqrt{\frac{(n-2)r^2}{1-r^2}}. \tag{20.17}$$

If the calculated t is greater than a critical t from Table B, H_0 is rejected.

A Test for ρ Other Than 0

Suppose the correlation coefficient between two blood test measures for repeated samples of healthy people has proven to be some ρ_0, a theoretical correlation coefficient other than 0, perhaps 0.6, for example. Now we have a sample of ill patients and want to know whether the correlation coefficient between the blood tests is different. The (unknown) population coefficient from the ill patients is ρ. The null hypothesis becomes H_0:$\rho = \rho_0$. It has been shown mathematically that the expression

$$m = \frac{1}{2}\ln\left(\frac{1+r}{1-r}\right) \tag{20.18}$$

is distributed approximately normal (for larger samples, $n > 50$) with mean

$$\mu = \frac{1}{2}\ln\left(\frac{1+\rho_0}{1-\rho_0}\right) \tag{20.19}$$

and standard deviation

$$\sigma = \frac{1}{\sqrt{n-3}}. \tag{20.20}$$

The test is just the usual z test on the standardized normal

$$z = \frac{m-\mu}{\sigma}. \tag{20.21}$$

If the calculated z from Eq. (20.21) is larger than a critical z found from Table A, H_0 is rejected.

A Test of Two Correlation Coefficients

Suppose we have large-sample correlation coefficients between blood test measures for type 1 and type 2 diseases; we want to compare two sample correlation coefficients, r_1 and r_2. We test the null hypothesis that the two ρ's, the correlation coefficients for the populations of all patients with these diseases, are equal, i.e., $H_0{:}\rho_1 = \rho_2$. We calculate m_1 and σ_1 for sample 1 and m_2 and σ_2 for sample 2 in the forms of Eqs. (20.18) and (20.20). The test is a z test conducted as Eq. (20.21), where

$$z = \frac{m_1 - m_2}{\sqrt{\sigma_1^2 + \sigma_2^2}}. \tag{20.22}$$

No good tests have been developed for these cases for small samples.

A Confidence Interval on ρ

Given a sample r, we can find a confidence interval for the population ρ from which r was drawn, as introduced in Section 12.9. However, the expression and calculation are somewhat bothersome. It is preferable to use a confidence interval on the regression β_1 if appropriate, but, if not, a few minutes with a capable calculator will provide the confidence interval using Eq. (20.23):

$$\mathrm{P}\left[\frac{1+r-(1-r)e^{\frac{2z_{1-\alpha/2}}{\sqrt{n-3}}}}{1+r+(1-r)e^{\frac{2z_{1-\alpha/2}}{\sqrt{n-3}}}} < \rho < \frac{1+r-(1-r)e^{-\frac{2z_{1-\alpha/2}}{\sqrt{n-3}}}}{1+r+(1-r)e^{-\frac{2z_{1-\alpha/2}}{\sqrt{n-3}}}}\right] = 1-\alpha. \tag{20.23}$$

Additional Example

Let us continue the example of lung opacity in infants.[71] The correlation coefficient between temperature and age was found to be 0.3727. In Section 20.4, we tested $H_0{:}\beta_1 = 0$ using Eq. (20.7), which we noted is the same as testing $H_0{:}\rho = 0$ using Eq. (20.17); we concluded that the t of 6.11 showed the x,y association to be significant.

Test of Two Correlation Coefficients

Of the 234 infants, 78 proved to have lung opacity on radiography (sample 1) and 156 did not (sample 2). The correlation coefficients between temperature and age for these groups were $r_1 = 0.4585$ and $r_2 = 0.3180$. By substituting in Eq. (20.18), we find $m_1 = 0.4954$ and $m_2 = 0.3294$. Similarly, by using Eq. (20.20), $\sigma_1^2 = 0.0133$ and $\sigma_2^2 = 0.0065$. Substitution of these values in Eq. (20.22) yields $z = 0.5386$, which is very much smaller than the 5% two-tailed critical t for 230 df of about 1.97. There is no evidence of a difference between correlation coefficients.

Confidence Interval on the Correlation Coefficient

What is the 95% confidence interval on the population ρ? The sample $r = 0.3727$, $z_{1-\alpha/2} = 1.96$, and $n-3 = 231$. Substitution of these values in Eq. (20.23) yields $P[0.3654 < \rho < 0.3800] = 0.95$.

Exercise 20.4. Let us continue with the SVmR example,[66] in which the correlation between SVmR and SBP was 0.7295 for 26 patients. In Exercise 20.3, the hypothesis $H_0{:}\beta_1 = 0$ was tested. Repeat the test in the form of Eq. (20.17) to test $H_0{:}\rho = 0$. Suppose physiological theory posed a ρ of 0.5. Does this sample agree with the theory or differ from it?

20.6. CURVED REGRESSION

Example

DB11 presented data on percent survival of malaria-infected rats (placebo group) as dependent on day number. The data plot (shown in Fig. 19.4) is redisplayed as Fig. 20.6A. We want to fit a regression curve expressing the general pattern of survival over time.

Choosing the Model

The goal is to describe and assess the pattern of survival over time. Survival drops over time, but the drop rate seems to diminish. The data suggest a second-degree model, opening upward. We select the model $y = \beta_0 + \beta_1 x + \beta_2 x^2$, where y is percent survival and x is day number.

Data Input

We select regression with its appropriate model in whatever statistical software package we choose. We enter percent survival into the y position and day number into x. We square day number and enter these values into x^2.

Results Output

Different packages use different result display formats, but most are labeled well enough to select the values we need. We can perform a check on the correctness of our selection by anticipating a gross approximation to the values we desire. In this

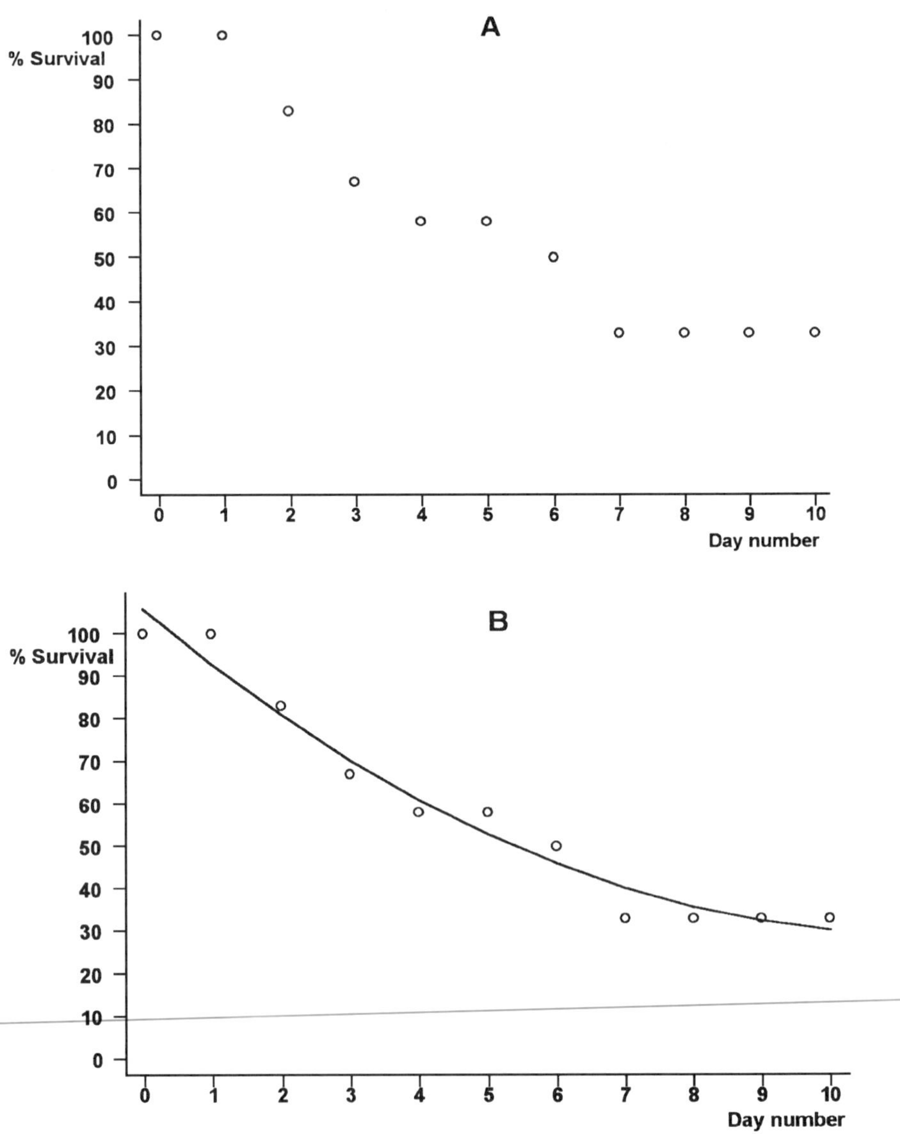

Figure 20.6 Percent survival by day of rats infected with malaria: (A) data; (B) parabolic regression curve fitted to the data.

example, we find the sample estimates of the β's to be $b_0 = 105.77$, $b_1 = -13.66$, and $b_2 = 0.61$. Substitution in the model yields the equation representing the prediction of percent survival by day number as $y = 105.77 - 13.66x + 0.61x^2$. The curve given by this equation is shown superposed on the data in Fig. 20.6B. By looking further at the results, we find the p-value for the F test of the model to be <0.001 and the R^2 to be about 0.97.

Interpretation

The significant p-value indicates that a real (curved) predictive relationship of percent survival by day number does exist. The very large R^2 indicates that survival percent can be predicted quite well by this model, with only 3% of the survival variability left for randomness and other causal factors.

An Admonition

This prediction is valid up to the modeled 10 days only; if we extend the model to periods outside the experiment, the model will claim that the rats come back to life and the percent survival begins to increase. This nonsensical result illustrates the necessity of inferring conclusions only within the limits modeled.

Method

Concept

The concept of curved (more exactly, curvilinear) regression is the same as simple regression throughout, except that the form of the model is not restricted to a straight line. We now can generally refer to the regression curve, which includes the straight line as a subordinate case. Model forms were considered at some length in Section 19.3. The most frequently used curves are the parabola, which is like a simple regression with an x^2 term added, and the logarithmic and exponential curves, which are like a simple regression with the x term replaced by a $\log x$ or e^x term. However, any mathematical function may be appropriate.

Choosing the Model

The method of choosing the model varies with the goals of the study. If the study is being used to assess a theoretical relationship (physiology, etc.), the form of the model will arise from the theory and the regression significance will be used to validate the theory. If the study is being used to develop the predictor of an established form, that form dictates the model and the regression is used to identify the parameters (constants) used in the prediction. If the study is used to explore relationships, the form of the model will be suggested by shape and pattern in the data plot. The model must be appropriate only within the range of existing data (see **Admonition**, two paragraph above).

Data Input

The model that is chosen dictates the inputs. Basically, we have a y depending on some function of x. We just substitute x- and y-values in the forms given by the model. Where y appears, y-values are put in; where x^2 appears, x-values are squared and those squares put in; where $\ln(x)$ appears, logarithms of x-values are found and put in; and so forth.

Solution

The regression curve calculated is the best fit curve according to various mathematical criteria of "best," as appropriate to the form and assumptions. In simple regression, the criterion was least squares used for linear models (see Section 19.3). Other criteria are maximum likelihood (used more for nonlinear models), unbiasedness, minimum variance, etc., or combinations of these. For simple regression, the least squares solutions gave rise to relatively simple formulas, seen earlier in this chapter. However, for more complicated models, sets of linear equations derived using calculus must be solved by methods of matrix algebra, which is not easily done by hand. These now have come to be solved using computer programs contained in statistical software packages. It is reasonable to assume that any investigator using curvilinear regression will have access to such a package. Sections 20.6–20.8 do not attempt to present solutions, but will concentrate on choosing the model, entering the data, and interpreting the results.

Results to Select and Their Interpretation

Statistical software packages usually display a number of results, many of which are needed only occasionally. The user must select what is needed. The following types of results are the most likely to be of use: (1) In validating a model or exploring data to identify relationships, the p-value of a test of the model (usually an F test) tells us whether the relationship between x and y is probably real or probably just due to sampling fluctuations. For relationships that test significant, the coefficient of determination R^2 (no longer the same as r^2) tells us whether the predictive capability is clinically useful. The value $1 - R^2$ tells us the proportion of predictive capability attributable either to causal factors not contained in the model or to the x factor in a different model form and to random effects. Thus, in a computer display of regression results, we seek the p-value of a test of the model and R^2. (2) In evaluating the contribution of model components, p-values of t tests on model components tell us whether to retain them in the model. (3) In developing a prediction equation, coefficients for the model equation can be identified.

ADDITIONAL EXAMPLE

Let us consider again the dependence of temperature on age in infants with pulmonary complications,[71] introduced in the Additional Example of Section 20.2. At that time, our simple regression fit was $y = 100.1752 + 0.1246x$. Further, in Section 20.4, we found that the p-value for a t test on the model was <0.001 and that $R^2 = 0.1389$.

Choosing the Model

By looking at Fig. 20.5, we can see that the line seems to be centered on the data in the right part of the plot, but lies a bit above center on the left. That causes us to conjecture that temperature, which we showed by simple regression to increase with age, increases rapidly with age in newborns and slows its increase as the infant grows older. This suggests a logarithmic fit. We want to determine whether we obtain a better fit by using the model $y = \beta_0 + \beta_1 \ln(x)$.

Data Input

We enter our model into the software package. We calculate the (natural) logarithm of x for each x and enter them and the y-values. We instruct the computer to calculate the regression of temperature on log age. The calculations are carried out just as in simple (straight line) regression, but use log age rather than age.

Results Output

The p-value for the F test on the model and coefficient of determination R^2 for the two models are shown in Table 20.2, and the log fit on the data is shown in Fig. 20.7.

Table 20.2
p-Value and R^2 for Straight Line and Logarithmic Fits to Infant Pulmonary Data

Model	p-value for F test	R^2
Straight line	<0.001	0.1389
Logarithmic	<0.001	0.1651

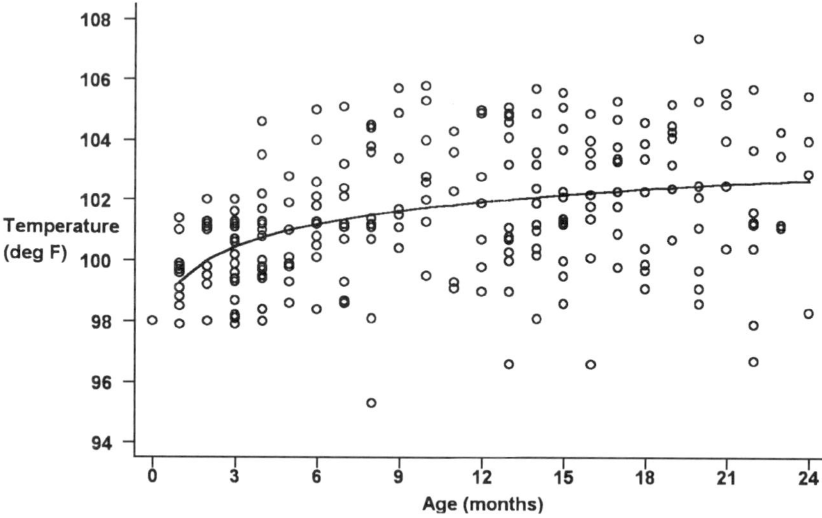

Figure 20.7 Temperature depending on age for 234 infants with pulmonary complications, with logarithmic regression fit shown.

Interpretation

We can see from the relatively low R^2 in both cases that, whereas age is a significant predictor, it is not very important clinically. However, R^2 has increased from about 14% to about 17%; the log fit better describes the physiologic process at work.

Exercise 20.5. To continue the question of circulatory response to intubation during laryngoscopy,[66] we found that a simple regression of SBP on SVmR gave the fit $y = 8.9388 + 94.3817x$, that the p-value of a significance test on the model was <0.001, and that $R^2 = 0.5322$.

Choosing the model: Figure 20.8 shows the data. Although the simple regression fit seems to be useful, a case certainly can be made for curvature, opening downward. Write the equation for a parabolic fit using SBP and SVmR rather than y and x.

Data input: What data would be entered into the computer?

Results output: The outputs are read as $b_0 = -2.92$, $b_1 = 289.00$, $b_2 = -414.41$, p-value on the model test is <0.001, and $R^2 = 0.6822$.

Interpretation: Write the final predictive equation. Is the relationship between SBP and SVmR significant in both models? Is the modeled SVmR a major predictor in both models? Which model provides a better fit?

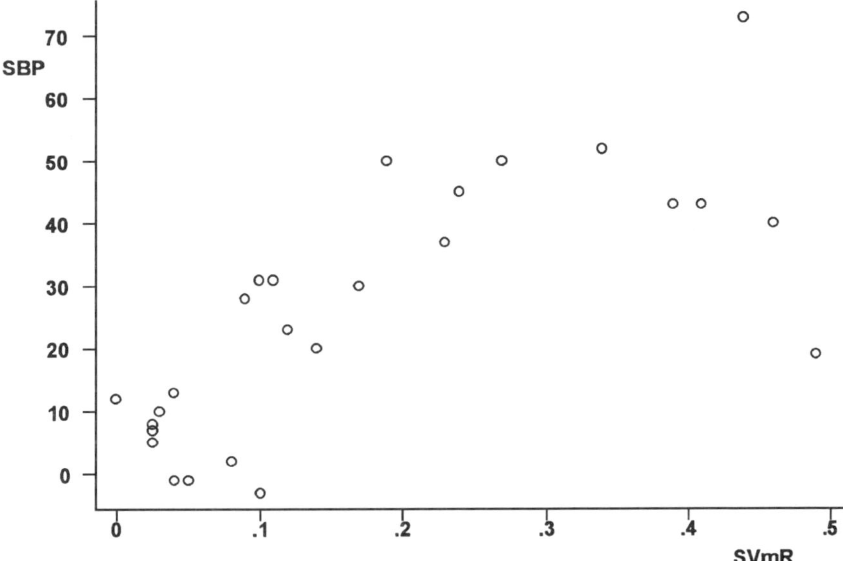

Figure 20.8 Change in SBP as depending on SVmR amplitude in intubated patients.

20.7. MULTIPLE REGRESSION

EXAMPLE

A psychologist wants to be able to predict length of hospital stay (days in) for inpatients at time of admission.[17] Information available prior to seeing the patient is intelligence quotient (IQ, mean = 100, standard deviation = 10), age (years), and sex (0,1). Data are available for $n = 50$ inpatients.

Choosing the Model

The dependent variable days in is y. The others are x_1, x_2, and x_3, respectively. The model becomes $y = \beta_0 + \beta_1 x_1 + \beta_2 x_2 + \beta_3 x_3$. With three variable-containing terms in the model, $df = n - k - 1 = 50 - 3 - 1 = 46$.

Data Input

In the software package, enter the data for days in into the y position, the data for IQ into the x_1 position, age into the x_2 position, and sex into the x_3 position.

Results to Select and Their Interpretation

(1) The computer result gives the p-value of the F test to be 0.030. We conclude that the predictive ability of the model is real and not due to chance. (2) $R^2 = 0.175$. This tells us that, even though the model is significant as a predictor, it represents less than 18% of the predictive capability; 82% remains for other predictors and the influence of randomness. (3) The values of t calculated for the independent portion of each x are IQ 2.258, age 1.624, and sex 0.244. Sex produced the smallest t and does not appear to be a useful predictor. Let us delete sex and recalculate the multiple regression using the new model $y = \beta_0 + \beta_1 x_1 + \beta_2 x_2$. (1) The p for the F test is 0.011, which is actually somewhat improved. (2) $R^2 = 0.174$. We lost nothing by dropping sex; it is not clinically useful. (3) The values of t calculated for the independent portion of each x are IQ 2.312 and age 1.688. IQ is shown to be significant alone ($p = 0.025$), but age is not ($p = 0.098$). We question whether age contributes to the prediction, even though it is not significant by itself. We delete age and recalculate the regression, using the reduced model $y = \beta_0 + \beta_1 x_1$. The significance of the model is little changed ($p = 0.012$), but $R^2 = 0.124$, which is a 5% drop in predictive ability. We conclude that we should retain age for predictive purposes, even though it is not of significant use. We return to the model $y = \beta_0 + \beta_1 x_1 + \beta_2 x_2$. (4) The computer output lists the estimates of the β's as: $b_0 = -32.5938$ (constant), $b_1 = 0.3576$ (coefficient of IQ), and $b_2 = 0.1686$ (coefficient of age). The resulting predictive model is days in $= -32.5938 + 0.3576(\text{IQ}) + 0.1686(\text{age})$. Patient number 10 remained 4 days in the hospital. His IQ was 90.4 and his age was 24. His predicted days in was $-32.5938 + 0.3576 \times 90.4 + 0.1686 \times 24 = 3.8$.

Method

Concept

Multiple regression is the term applied to the prediction of a dependent variable by several, rather than one, independent variables. For example, in an investigation of cardiovascular syncope, no one sign would be sufficient to predict its occurrence. The investigator would begin with, at least, SBP, DBP, and HR and extend the list of predictors to include perhaps the presence–absence of murmurs, clicks, vascular bruits, etc. The concept of multiple regression is similar to that of simpler regression, in that the dependent variable is related to the independent variables by a best fit. However, the geometry is extended from an x-axis to an x_1,x_2-plane or to what is called an $x_1,x_2,x_3,\ldots$-hyperplane, which is a plane extended to more than three dimensions. A hyperplane can be treated similarly to a plane mathematically, although it cannot be visualized. A multiple regression model with two independent variables is $y = \beta_0 + \beta_1 x_1 + \beta_2 x_2$. Models of this sort were considered in Section 19.5 and visualized in Fig. 19.12. More generally, we are not even restricted to a plane, i.e., to first-degree terms. The model can contain second-degree or other terms of curvature, which leads to a curved surface or, in several dimensions, a curved hypersurface. An example of such a model might be $y = \beta_0 + \beta_1 x_1 + \beta_2 x_2 + \beta_3 x_2^2$. The foregoing conceptualizations may be more confusing than enlightening to some readers. If so, it is sufficient to remember that several independent variables combine to predict one dependent variable.

Choosing the Model

We can consider each predictor x one at a time and enter its relationship to the dependent variable y as if it were alone. If y is related to that x, say x_1, in a straight line, we add $\beta_1 x_1$ to the model. If y is related to x_1 in a second-degree curve, we add $\beta_1 x_1 + \beta_2 x_1^2$ to the model. Then we proceed with x_2, etc. (Components combining variables in the same term are possible but form nonlinear models, which are unusual and outside the realm of this book.)

Setting up the Predictor Variables

Independent variables used to predict the dependent variable may be used just as recorded if they are continuous measurements or can be put in order, e.g., small to large. The only type of variable that must be altered for use in multiple regression is nominal data that cannot be ordered, e.g., ethnic group or disease type. A dichotomy, perhaps malignant versus benign, would not require special treatment due to symmetry. However, a categorization with three or more classes cannot be used as is. A racial heritage categorization classified as European, African, or Asian, for example, if assigned recording codes 1, 2, or 3, respectively, would predict a disease state differently than if assigned 1, 3, or 2. In this case, a strategy to use such classes as predictors is to reduce them to a set of dichotomies, i.e., to create "dummy variables." One class is chosen as a baseline or reference variable and given all 0 values. The remaining classes are coded "that class" (=1) versus "not that class" (=0). Thus, we would replace the ethnic variable with three dichotomous variables, say, European (all entries 0), African (yes = 1, no = 0), and Asian (yes = 1, no = 0). After this change is made, all variables then are used as predictor variables in the usual way.

Data Input

Data are entered into the computer software model just as in simpler regressions. Where x_1 appears in the model, we enter the x_1 data; where x_1^2 appears, we square each datum and enter the squares; and so forth.

Solution

As in curved regression, to estimate the β's that provide a best fit, we have to solve a set of linear equations simultaneously. This process is better done by statistical software on a computer. A little more detail on the reason for this may be found in the curvilinear regression section. After the best fit is calculated, the significance of the model is tested by F and the associated p-value given. For a model with k terms (which are the variable-containing components added together to form the model), F has $n - k - 1$ *df*. A regression with model $y = \beta_0 + \beta_1 x_1 + \beta_2 x_2$ for 50 patients would have $50 - 2 - 1 = 47$ *df*. Also, for each predictor, that part of its contribution that is not also provided by another predictor is tested by t and the associated p-value is given. These results conceptually are not very different from the equivalent results in simpler regressions. The coefficient of determination R^2 also is given. R^2 is 1−(residual variance/total variance), where total variance is s_y^2 and residual variance is the variance of differences of data from the model.

Results to Select and Their Interpretation

As with other regression forms, the software packages often provide a variety of results; the user must select those that answer the questions being asked of the data. As with curvilinear regression, the following types of results are the most likely to be of use: (1) In validating a model or exploring data to identify relationships, the p-value of a test of the model (usually an F test) tells us whether the relationship between y and the model is probably real or probably just due to sampling fluctuations. (2) For relationships that test significant, the coefficient of determination R^2 tells us whether the predictive capability is clinically useful. The value $1 - R^2$ tells us the proportion of predictive capability attributable to causal factors not contained in the model, to a different model form, and to random effects. (3) In evaluating the contribution of model components, p-values of t tests on model components tell us how to rank the clinical usefulness of the components in the model. (4) R^2 also helps to identify the clinically useful predictors. For a model with k components, note its R^2. Remove a component that you suspect may not be useful (perhaps that with the smallest t test p-value) and recalculate the regression. Note R^2 for the reduced model. The reduction in R^2 evoked by removing the variable indicates how useful that variable is as a predictor. (5) In developing a prediction equation, coefficients for the model equation can be identified so that its predictive equation can be written down.

An Admonition

The b's estimating the β's used in the model depend on the units chosen. Temperature measured in degrees Fahrenheit will yield different coefficients from that measured in degrees Celsius. However, the statistical results, F's, t's, and R^2's, will not change.

Additional Example

Let us consider again the prediction of temperature in infants with pulmonary complications,[71] first used in the Additional Example of Section 20.2. We found age to be a significant predictor. Data on heart rate (HR) and pulse oximetry had also been recorded. Are they useful predictors?

Choosing the Model

The model for age (x_1) as a predictor of temperature (y) was $y = \beta_0 + \beta_1 x_1$. Addition of terms for HR (x_2) and pulse oximetry (x_3) gives the model $y = \beta_0 + \beta_1 x_1 + \beta_2 x_2 + \beta_3 x_3$. There are $n = 234$ patients. The number of variable-containing terms is $k = 3$. The model has $n - k - 1 = 234 - 3 - 1 = 230$ *df*.

Data Input

In the software package, the sample's temperature values are selected to enter in the y position, age value in the x_1 position, etc.

Results to Select and Their Interpretation

(1) The computer result gives the p-value of the F test to be <0.001. We conclude that the predictive ability of the model is real and not due to chance. (2) $R^2 = 0.289$. This tells us that even though the model is significant as a predictor, it represents only about 29% of the predictive capability; 71% remains for other predictors and the influence of randomness. (3) The values of t calculated for the independent portion of each x are age 7.117, HR 6.895, and pulse oximetry 0.111. Pulse oximetry produced the smallest t and does not appear to be a useful predictor. Let us delete pulse oximetry and recalculate the multiple regression using the new model $y = \beta_0 + \beta_1 x_1 + \beta_2 x_2$. (1) The p for the F test is still <0.001. (2) $R^2 = 0.284$. We lost a negligible amount of the predictive ability by dropping pulse oximetry; it is not clinically useful. (3) The values of t calculated for the independent portion of each x are age 7.117 and HR 6.895. Both are significantly large, so we conclude that both are clinically useful predictors. (4) The computer output lists the estimates of the β's as $b_0 = 94.4413$ (constant), $b_1 = 0.1333$ (coefficient of age), and $b_2 = 0.0354$ (coefficient of HR). The resulting predictive

model is temperature $= 94.4413 + 0.1333$(age) $+0.0354$(HR). Infant number 1 had an observed temperature of 101.4°F. Her age was 1 month and HR was 180. Her predicted temperature was $94.4413 + 0.1333 \times 1 + 0.0354 \times 180 = 100.9$°F, which is half a degree off.

Exercise 20.6. By using the data of DB10, we may be able to predict the strength of hamstring or quadriceps muscles or tendons following surgery by using the strength and control of the unoperated leg.

Choosing the Model: Strength following surgery is measured by the distance covered in a triple hop on the operated leg. Possible predictors are the equivalent on the unoperated leg (x_1) and the time to perform the hop (x_2). Write down the equation of the model.

Data Input: What are the data to be entered into a software package?

Results to Select and their Interpretation: F's $p < 0.001.R^2 = 0.974$. t-values are 11.617 for x_1 and 1.355 for x_2. By omitting x_2, the F test's $p < 0.001$, $R^2 = 0.965$, and $t = 12.832$. For the simple regression of y on x_1, $b_0 = -300.868$ and $b_1 = 1.466$. Is the predictive ability of the model using both x's real? Is it clinically useful? Judging from the t-values of each x, should we consider dropping x_2? If we do, is the reduced model significant? Clinically useful? What is the predictive equation for the reduced model? If the triple hop distance for a particular patient is 504 cm, what is the predicted distance for the operated leg? How does this agree with an observed distance of 436 cm from DB10 data?

20.8. LOGISTIC REGRESSION

EXAMPLE

The data of DB12 arose from a study on resection of the tracheal carina. A patient who dies is recorded with a data code of 1; one who survives the operation, a code of 0. Independent variables on which survival may depend are age at surgery (years), whether patient had prior tracheal surgery (1) or not (0), extent of resection (centimeters), and whether intubation was required at the end of surgery (1) or not (0).

Choosing the Model

The left side of the model is the log odds ratio form as in Eq. (20.24). The right side of the model is a four-variable multiple regression, $\beta_0 + \beta_1 x_1 + \beta_2 x_2 + \beta_3 x_3 + \beta_4 x_4$, where x_1 is age, x_2 is prior surgery, x_3 is extent of resection, and x_4 is intubation.

Data Input

The survival or dying 0 or 1 codes are entered into the statistical software package in the position for the left side of the model; the recordings for age, prior surgery, extent, and intubation are in the positions for the right side of the model.

Results to Select and Their Interpretation

(1) From the χ^2 test of the model, $p < 0.001$, which tells us that the relationship between y and the model is probably real and not due to sampling fluctuations. (2) The coefficient of determination, R^2, is about 0.34, which tells us that these predictors account for about one-third of the predictive ability; this set of predictors is important and likely useful, but by no means is completely decisive. (3) The variables' p-values, ranked by size, are intubation, <0.001; extent, 0.031; prior surgery, 0.244; and age, 0.947. Clearly, intubation and extent are significant and age contributes almost nothing. Prior surgery is far from significant and likely contributes little. Let us assess its contribution by recalculating the regression with prior surgery and age removed. (1) The new logistic regression based on intubation and extent retains the $p < 0.001$ of the model's χ^2 test. These variables are real rather than chance predictors. (2) The new R^2 is about 33%, still indicating useful but not perfect prediction. (3) The p-values for tests on the predictors are intubation, <0.001; extent, 0.044. Both are still significant. (4) The R^2 of 33% shows that the regression has lost only about 1% of its predictive ability by omitting prior surgery and age. The χ^2 statistic, 34.5 for the four variables, is now 33.2, a negligible reduction. We conclude that prior surgery and age are not predictive and we can do as well without them. (5) The coefficients for the model equation are identified as constant, −4.6171; intubation, 2.8714; and extent, 0.5418. The right side of the final model is $b_0 + b_1x_1 + b_2x_2 = -4.6171 + 2.8714(\text{intubation}) + 0.5418(\text{extent})$. A prediction may be made for any one patient by substituting this expression in Eq. (20.25). For example, the expression for a patient who was intubated (substitute 1 for x_1) following a 2-cm resection (substitute 2 for x_2) is −0.6621. Substitution of this for the exponent of e in Eq. (20.25) yields

$$p_m = e^{-0.6621}/(1 + e^{-0.6621}) = 0.3403.$$

The chance of this patient dying is predicted by this model to be about 34%.

METHOD

Concept

In medicine, a large number of situations arise in which we want to predict a binary outcome (survival or not; a patient heals faster than usual or not; a disease is present or not), which can be coded 1 or 0 for numerical treatment. If we set the binary outcome y equal to a regression line, $\beta_0 + \beta_1 x_1$, we get nonsensical results, usually anything except 0 or 1. By returning to basics, we note that, for a continuous y, the ordinary regression prediction yields the expected y (most likely value of y). For a binary y, the expected value is the probability that a code of 1 (a survival, etc.) occurs, estimated by the proportion of 1's in the sample. Appropriately, this proportion is the mean of the sample, that is, the sum of the 0 and 1 codes divided by the number in the sample. Let us affix the subscript m for mean so that the population probability is denoted π_m and the sample proportion p_m. Note that $p_m/(1 - p_m)$ gives the odds that a code of 1will occur in the sample on any one opportunity. If we take the logarithm of this expression, we have the *log odds ratio*, introduced in Chapter 13. Because the probability distribution of the log odds ratio is known, it can be used in the statistical tests needed for regression. Thus, rather than the simple regression model $y = \beta_0 + \beta_1 x_1$, when we face binary outcomes we will use the model

$$\ln\left(\frac{p_m}{1 - p_m}\right) = \beta_0 + \beta_1 x. \tag{20.24}$$

Logistic regression is just a transformation of the dependent variable to the log odds ratio, after which the usual regression procedures are followed. Curvilinear and multiple logistic regression are used just the same as in ordinary regression, with the dependent variable transformed. The right side of Eq. (20.24) may be extended to include whatever terms are required.

Choosing the Model

We choose the right side of the model just as in simple, curvilinear, or multiple regression. If unorderable nominal variables, e.g., three or more ethnic groups, are to be used, see the paragraph setting up the predictor variables in Section 20.7.

Data Input

Independent variable data are entered into the computer software model just as in ordinary regressions. The 0 or 1 binary codes are entered as are the y values in ordinary regression; we are ready for the computer package to make the transformation to the log odds ratio.

Solution

Because of the transformation to the log odds ratio, as well as solving simultaneous linear equations in cases more complicated than a single first-degree x, the computation process is better done by statistical software on a computer. This software provides a best fit (where the appropriate mathematical criterion of "best" is maximum likelihood for logistic regression). The fitting process estimates the β's, the parameters of fit. The estimates are denoted as b's. The right side of Eq. (20.24) becomes $b_0 + b_1 x$. To provide a regression prediction, one step more than that for continuous regression is required. The prediction desired is the estimate of the probability of survival, patient improvement, or treatment success, i.e., of a code of 1. We have denoted this estimate as m_{p}. When the observed x-values for a particular patient or case are substituted in the right side of the model, the log odds ratio results and must be solved to provide p_m. If we take the antilogarithm (exponential) of both sides of Eq. (20.24) and solve for p_m, we obtain

$$p_m = \frac{e^{b_0 + b_1 x}}{1 + e^{b_0 + b_1 x}}. \tag{20.25}$$

For any model other than $b_0 + b_1 x$, the $b_0 + b_1 x$ of Eq. (20.25) is replaced by the right side of that model.

Results to Select and Their Interpretation

As with other regression forms, the software packages often provide a variety of results; the user must select those that answer the questions being asked of the data. The following types of results are the most likely to be of use: (1) In validating a model or exploring data to identify relationships, the p-value of a test of the model (in logistic regression, a χ^2 rather than an F) tells us whether the relationship between y and the model is probably real or probably just due to sampling fluctuations. (2) For relationships that test significant, the coefficient of determination R^2 would be useful to tell us whether the predictive capability is clinically useful. However, due to the transformation, the usual R^2 cannot be calculated in the same way. Most software packages provide an approximate equivalent to R^2 or to an R that can be squared, which can be interpreted in much the same fashion. We can use the value $1 - R^2$ to indicate the proportion of predictive capability attributable to causal factors not contained in the model, to a different model form, and/or to random effects. (3) In evaluating the contribution of model components, p-values of tests on model components, in this case normal (z) tests, tell us how to rank the clinical usefulness of the components in the model. (4) The R^2 equivalent also helps to identify the clinically useful predictors by noting changes when the model is changed. In the absence of a legitimate R^2, the value of the χ^2 statistic used to test the model can be used in much the same way. (5) In developing a prediction equation, coefficients for the model equation can be identified. A prediction may then be made using Eq. (20.25) (or its equivalent with a more sophisticated model substituted for the $b_0 + b_1 x$).

Additional Example

It would be useful to predict the presence or absence of lung congestion in infants with respiratory problems[71] without resorting to X rays. In a study of 234 infants, variables recorded were age (months), respiration rate (RR), heart rate (HR), temperature (temp), % pulse oximetry (pulsox), clinical appearance of illness on physical examination (physex) (1, appeared ill; 0, did not), and sound of congestion in lungs on physical examination (lungex) (1, sounded congested; 0, did not). Pulmonary X rays were taken to be "truth" and recorded as clear (0) or opaque (1).

Choosing the Model

The left side of the model is the log odds ratio form as in Eq. (20.24). The right side of the model is a seven-variable multiple regression, $\beta_0 + \beta_1 x_1 + \beta_2 x_2 + \beta_3 x_3 + \beta_4 x_4 + \beta_5 x_5 + \beta_6 x_6 + \beta_7 x_7$, where x_1 is age, x_2 is RR, x_3 is HR, x_4 is temp, x_5 is pulsox, x_6 is physex, and x_7 is lungex.

Data Input

The 0 or 1 codes denoting clear or opaque X rays are entered in the position for the left side of the model; the recordings for age, RR, HR, temp, pulsox, physex, and lungex in the positions for the right side of the model.

Results to Select and Their Interpretation

(1) From the χ^2 test of the model, $p = 0.001$, which tells us that the relationship between y and the model is probably real and not due to sampling fluctuations. (2) The coefficient of determination, R^2, is about 0.09, which tells us that these variables, although significantly related to lung opacity, are rather poor predictors and unlikely to be of great help clinically. (3) The variables' p-values, ranked by size, are RR 0.005, lungex 0.022, age 0.118, plusox 0.186, physex 0.228, temp 0.273, and HR 0.855. Recall that these p-values are calculated for that portion of each variable that does not overlap in predictive capability with another variable, i.e., the independent portions of the variables. (For example, we saw in earlier sections that temperature was related to age. We would expect that the predictive ability of the two combined would be less than the sum of that for each alone.) We decide to retain only the first three variables, due to the larger p-values of the others. We retain age despite its not being significant, because we suspect its independent portion might become so when the

correlated temperature is removed. Now we have the right side of the model $\beta_0 + \beta_1 x_1 + \beta_2 x_2 + \beta_3 x_3$, where x_1 is RR, x_2 is lungex, and x_3 is age. (1) The p-value for the χ^2 test of the model is <0.001. These are significant predictors. (2) R^2 is a little over 7%. The prediction will not be very useful clinically. (3) The p-values for the tests on the individual variables are 0.002, 0.018, and 0.008, respectively. The age did indeed become significant. (4) R^2 dropped from its previous 9% to a little over 7%, and the χ^2 statistic for the model test dropped from 25.1 to 20.7. Although these are noticeable reductions, the bulk of the predictive ability remains. (5) The coefficients to be used in a prediction are $b_0 = -3.3591$, $b_1 = 0.0410$, $b_2 = 0.7041$, and $b_3 = 0.0607$, leading to the right side of the model as $-3.3591 + 0.0410(\text{RR}) + 0.7041(\text{lungex}) + 0.0607(\text{age})$. Suppose an 8-month-old infant with respiratory problems has a respiration rate of 30 and its lungs sound congested. The model's right side becomes $-3.3591 + 0.0410 \times 30 + 0.7041 \times 1 + 0.0607 \times 8 = -0.9394$. Substitution of this value for the exponent of e in Eq. (20.25) yields $p_m = e^{-0.9394}/(1 + e^{-0.9394}) = 0.6417$. The chance that this infant's lungs will appear opaque on X ray is predicted by this model to be about 64%. However, we have little faith in this prediction, because about 93% of the ability to predict lung opacity lies with other factors and with randomness.

Exercise 20.7. DB1 includes several variables related to prostate cancer (CaP). The "truth" indicator is positive or negative biopsy (coded 1 or 0, respectively). We try to predict biopsy result on the basis of PSA, volume, TRU (1 for indicated CaP, 0 not), DRE (1 for indicated CaP, 0 not), and age. What is the right side of the model? (1) The p-value of the test of the model is <0.001. Is the model a significant predictor? (2) $R^2 = 0.1513$. Is the prediction clinically useful? (3) The individual p-values are PSA <0.001, volume 0.002, TRU 0.014, DRE 0.336, and age 0.794. What should be dropped from the model? (3) The reduced model retains $p < 0.001$ and has $R^2 = 0.1488$. Is the reduced model satisfactory? (4) Was much predictive ability lost by the reduction? (5) The coefficients to be used in a prediction are $b_0 = -0.8424$, $b_1 = 0.1056$ (PSA), $b_2 = -0.0315$ (vol), and $b_3 = 0.7167$ (TRU). One of the patients had PSA = 9.6, a volume of 62, and a positive TRU. What does this model predict the probability of CaP to be?

ANSWERS TO EXERCISES

20.1. $b_1 = 94.3817$ and $b_0 = 8.9388$. The slope–mean form is $y - 25.6538 = 94.3817(x - 0.1771)$ and the slope–intercept form is $y = 8.9388 + 94.3817x$. If SVmR = 0.3, the change in SBP is predicted to be 37.2533. The axes and regression are shown on the accompanying graph along with the data.

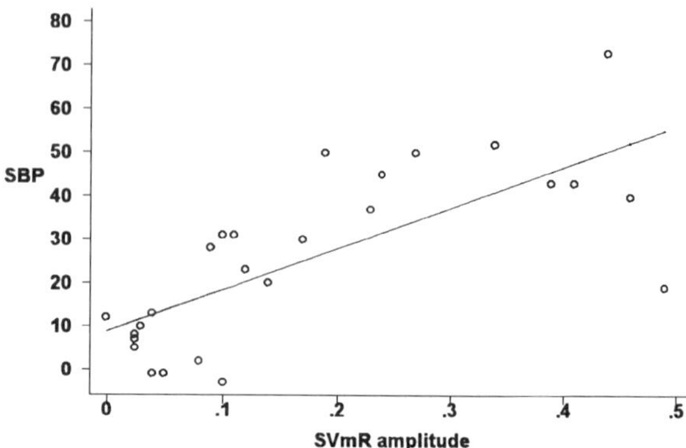

20.2. $r = 2.2746/(0.1553 \times 20.0757) = 0.7295$. A correlation coefficient of about 0.73 is rather high; clearly there is an association between the variables. $r_s = 0.7050$, which is close to r.

20.3. $s_e = 14.0072$ and $s_b = 18.0389$. The two-tailed 95% critical t for 24 *df* is 2.064. Calculated t to test the slope is 5.2321, which is significantly greater than the critical t; the association between SVmR and SBP is greater than chance. $R^2 = 0.5322$. $P[57 < \beta_1 < 132] = 0.95$. SVmR is a major predictor. 47% of the predictive capability remains for other predictors and randomness. $s_{m|0.3} = 3.5306$ and $s_{y|0.3} = 14.4453$. $P[30 < \mu|0.3 < 45] = 0.95$. $P[7.4 < E(y)|0.3 < 67.1] = 0.95$.

20.4. $r^2 = 0.5322$. The two-tailed 95% critical t for 24 *df* is 2.064. The calculated t is $\sqrt{(24 \times 0.5322/0.4678)} = 5.2253$, which is much larger than the critical t. The population correlation coefficient is probably greater than 0. (The slight difference from the other form appearing in the answer to Exercise 20.3 is due to rounding.) Denote ρ_s as the correlation coefficient of the population from which the sample was drawn. To test the null hypothesis $H_0{:}\rho_s = 0.5$, substitute the appropriate values in Eqs. (20.18) through (20.21). $m = 0.9277$, $\mu = 0.5493$, $\sigma = 0.2085$, and $z = 1.81$. The critical $z = 1.96$. The calculated z is less, so we must conclude that there is inadequate evidence to reject H_0. The correlation has not been shown to be different from the theoretical value.

20.5. *The model:* $\text{SBP} = b_0 + b_1(\text{SVmR}) + b_2(\text{SVmR})^2$. *Data*: The square of SVmR would be calculated. SBP, SVmR, and SVmR^2 would be entered. *Interpretation*: The final predictive equation is $\text{SBP} = -2.92 + 289.00(\text{SVmR}) - 414.42(\text{SVmR})^2$. The fit is shown in the figure. The p-values for tests of both models are <0.001, which is significant. The modeled prediction accounts for the majority of variability in both models; SVmR is a major predictor in either model. Moving from the simple model to the parabolic model increases the R^2 from about 53% to about 68%, indicating that the curved model is the better fit.

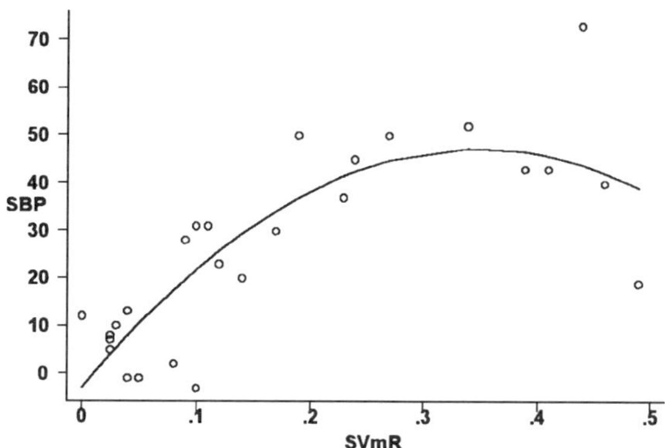

20.6. *Model:* $y = \beta_0 + \beta_1 x_1 + \beta_2 x_2$. *Data:* Enter data for the triple hop distance using the operated leg into the y position, the same using the unoperated leg into the x_1 position, and the time to hop using the unoperated leg into the x_2 position. *Interpretation.* The predictive ability using both x's is real and clinically useful. Dropping x_2 should be considered. The reduced model also is significant and very nearly as clinically useful. The predictive equation is $y = -300.868 + 1.466x_1$. For a nonoperated leg hop distance of 504cm, the predicted distance on the operated leg is 438 cm, which agrees very well with the observed 436 cm.

20.7. $\beta_0 + \beta_1 x_1 + \beta_2 x_2 + \beta_3 x_3 + \beta_4 x_4 + \beta_5 x_5$. (1) Yes. (2) Not very. (3) Drop DRE and age. Reduced model: (1 and 2) The model still is a significant predictor and not a very useful one. (4) The resultant R^2 is still about 15%. No predictive capability was lost by the reduction. (5) The right side of the model becomes $-0.8424 + 0.1056 \times 9.6 - 0.0315 \times 62 + 0.7167 \times 1 = -1.0649$. Substitution for the exponent of e in Eq. (20.25) yields $p_m = 0.5262$. The probability is just over 0.5 that this patient's biopsy is positive. (Of possible interest: it was not.)

Chapter 21

Survival and Time-Series Analysis

21.1. TIME-DEPENDENT DATA

Time-Dependent Data Are Used Daily in Medicine

Time-dependent data are shown on monitors in surgery, including a variety of cardiac and pulmonary measures. Cardiac stress measures are time-dependent data. Electroencephalograms are time-dependent data. Many epidemiological measures are time-dependent, including survival.

Time Series

A large number of observations through time on the same variable usually are called a time series in statistics. Although taken literally, time-dependent data would include before-and-after observations and post-treatment follow-up, data sets such as these are not considered time series. To be susceptible to time-series analysis, a sequence of observations should number on the order of multiples of 10. Survival data sets usually have fewer observations than a true time series. However, both share a focus on a process through time rather than on a specific event and so are included together in this chapter.

21.2. SURVIVAL CURVES: ESTIMATION

Survival Data Record the Proportion of a Cohort's Survival through Time

The historic life table was introduced in Section 9.6. This table gives the proportion of a cohort (demographic group) surviving to the end of each time interval.

Recall that survival is not restricted to remaining alive, but may be surviving without the onset of illness or functioning without failure. However, we shall use the remaining alive connotation for convenience. If no patients are lost to follow-up, the proportion surviving simply is surviving number divided by initial number. A patient lost to follow-up before dying is termed *censored*. The method given in Section 9.6 included the treatment of censored data: using them while they are known to be alive and removing them from the data base when they are lost.

Data and Calculations Required for a Life Table

A sample life table is given as Table 21.1. As described in Section 9.6, basic data for a life table on n patients are the following: time intervals; *begin*, the number at the beginning of each time interval; *died*, the number dying in each time interval; and *lost*, the number lost to follow-up in each time interval. The rest of the table is calculated from these basic data. It was pointed out that the method used here is the simplest, assuming that the time of death or loss occurs at the end of the time interval. Other methods giving sophisticated adjustments exist. For convenience, a second line is entered for a time interval having censored data. Calculation for a column 5 entry is $end = begin - died - lost$. Calculation for a column 6 entry is S (the proportion surviving) $= S$ for last period $\times$ (*end* for this period $\div$ *end* for last period). The reason for this comes from a basic law of probability: the probability that two independent events occur together is the product of their probabilities. Thus, the chance of two heads on two coin tosses is the chance of heads on one toss multiplied by that on the other, or $\frac{1}{2} \times \frac{1}{2} = \frac{1}{4}$. Similarly, the chance of surviving to the end of the current interval is the chance of surviving to the beginning of the interval multiplied by the chance of surviving during the interval.

Table 21.1

Survival Data of 319 Men in Rochester, MN, Having Adult-Onset Diabetes Mellitus Who Were Greater than 45 Years at Onset during 1989–1990

Interval (years)	Begin	Died	Lost	End	S (survived)
0 (outset)	319	0	0	319	1.0000
>0–2	319	16	0	303	0.9498
>2–4	303	19	0	284	0.8902
>4–6	284	19	0	265	0.8306
>6–8	265	8	0	257	0.8055
	257	0	2	255	
>8–10	255	6	0	249	0.7866

Life Table for Men with Diabetes Mellitus

Table 21.1 provides basic and calculated data for a life table on the survival of 319 men.[35] The equivalent table for women was seen as Table 9.3 in Section 9.6. In the first period (>0–2 years), *died* = 16 and *lost* = 0, so *end* = 319 − 16 − 0 = 303 and $S = 1.00 \times (303/319) = 0.9498$. In the second period, $S = 0.9498 \times (284/303) = 0.8902$. In the third period, $S = 0.8902 \times (265/284) = 0.8306$. In the fourth period, eight died and two were lost to follow-up, which were separated on two lines, died first. S for that period is $0.8306 \times (257/265) = 0.8055$. At the end of that period, we subtracted the two *lost*, leaving 255. Because we assumed that they remained alive to the end of the period they did not reduce the survival, but they are removed for calculating survival in the next period. At the end of 10 years, about 79% of the men remain alive. This also may be interpreted as the probability that a man chosen randomly at the outset will remain disease-free longer than 10 years is estimated to be 0.79.

Survival Curves

The graphical display of survival information was introduced in Section 9.6. It was mentioned that a method of estimating survival functions developed by E. L. Kaplan and P. Meier in 1958, is more accurate than a life table and should be used when statistical software is available. Lacking that, or for the purpose of understanding the concepts, a simple mode of display is just to graph the survival data from the life table against the time intervals. A survival datum stays the same for the period of an interval, dropping at the end, which produces a stepped pattern. The survival curve for Table 21.1 is shown as Fig. 21.1. Note that the number lost to follow-up (censored) is shown as a small integer over the line for the period in which they were lost, distinguishing those lost from those dying.

Confidence Intervals

The survival curve shows estimates of a population's survival pattern based on the data from a sample. How confident of that estimate are we? As with many other estimates, we can find confidence intervals. In this case, there will be a confidence interval on each survival proportion, which leads to confidence curves enclosing the survival curve. The confidence curves have a similar stepped appearance. Different methods exist to calculate the confidence intervals on survival proportions. The most general are evolved from a method originated by M. Greenwood in 1926, but these are difficult to calculate. They are fine to use if statistical computer software offers the capability. Otherwise, a much simpler method by Peto *et al.*[51]

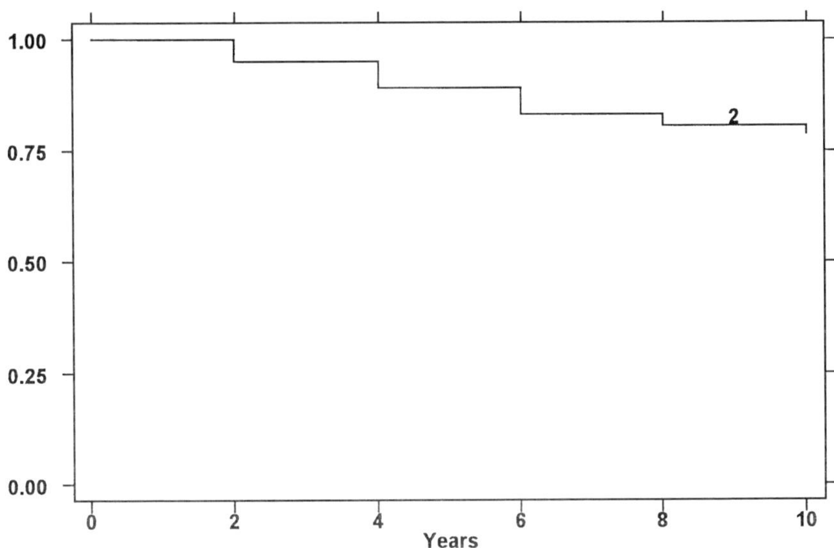

Figure 21.1 A survival curve for the diabetic men's data of Table 21.1.

may be used, as long as the user remembers that they are rougher approximations. The pattern of a confidence expression is the same for confidence intervals on other types of estimates, namely, that given as Eq. (4.2). (The probability that a population statistic from a distribution of estimates of that statistic is contained in a specified interval is given by the area of the distribution over that interval.) It was stated in Section 13.6 that a proportion is distributed approximately normal for moderate to large samples. If S_i denotes the estimate of the proportion survival at the end of interval i and SEE denotes the standard error of the estimate, the probability is $1 - \alpha$ that the true proportion survival is bracketed by $S_i \pm z_{1-\alpha/2} \times$ SEE. For 95% confidence, $z_{1-\alpha/2} = 1.96$. SEE, for proportions discussed in Section 13.6, depends only on S_i and the number at the beginning of each time period, let us say n_{i-1} (n_{i-1} replaces *begin* in order to keep track of the interval involved)

$$\text{SEE} = S_i\sqrt{\frac{1 - S_i}{n_{i-1}}}. \tag{21.1}$$

The 95% confidence interval on the true survival proportion for each time period becomes

$$S_i \pm 1.96 \times \text{SEE} = S_i \pm 1.96 S_i\sqrt{\frac{1 - S_i}{n_{i-1}}}. \tag{21.2}$$

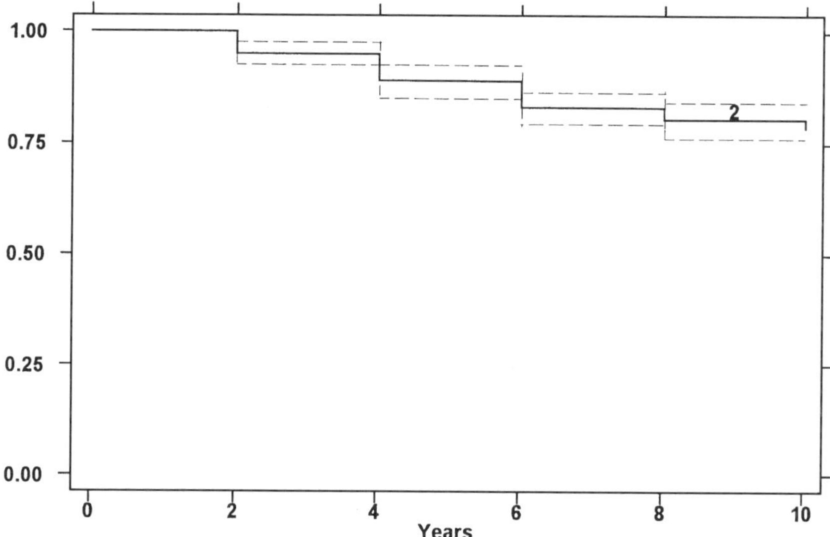

Figure 21.2 Survival curve of Fig. 21.1 enclosed by confidence curves as calculated in Table 21.2.

Because these confidence intervals are not very exact, we have to use common sense to avoid letting them exceed 1 or fall below 0 in reporting or graphing them.

EXAMPLE

Table 21.2 shows confidence intervals calculated using Eq. (21.2) for the 319 diabetic men of Table 21.1. Figure 21.2 shows the survival curve of Fig. 21.1 with the confidence intervals calculated in Table 21.2. The user may note that the confidence limits associated with a particular period in Table 21.2 are drawn about

Table 21.2

Survival Data of Table 21.1 with Confidence Intervals Calculated

Period (years)	Begin (n_{i-1})	S_i	SSE	Confidence interval	
0 (outset)	319	1.0000			
>0–2	319	0.9498	0.0119	0.9264	0.9731
>2–4	303	0.8902	0.0169	0.8570	0.9234
>4–6	284	0.8306	0.0203	0.7908	0.8704
>6–8	265	0.8055	0.0218	0.7627	0.8483
>8–10	255	0.7866	0.0228	0.7420	0.8312

the succeeding period in Fig. 21.2. The reason is that the proportion survival is related to the end of the period and is maintained until the next death figure, at the end of the following period. If we had data giving the exact time of death rather than a period during which it occurred, this pictorial lag would not occur.

Exercise 21.1. Life table data for survival of diabetic women[35] in period 1970–1980 is shown in Table 21.3. Complete the life table. Graph a survival curve. Calculate and graph the 95% confidence intervals on this survival curve.

21.3. SURVIVAL CURVES: TESTING

EXAMPLE

Figure 21.3 superposes the survival curves for 319 men (Fig. 21.1) and 370 women (Fig. 9.2 in Answers to Exercises of Part I) with diabetes mellitus during the 1980–1990 decade.[35] We see a difference by inspection, but is this difference significant? From Table C giving χ^2 values, the critical χ^2 for 1 degree of freedom (*df*) is 3.84. The log-rank test yields $\chi^2 = 7.2$, which is greater than 3.84. We conclude that men have significantly better survival than women. (The actual log-rank p-value $= 0.007$.)

METHOD

Are Two Survival Curves Different?

One statistical procedure that answers this question is the *log-rank test*. This test uses a chi-square statistic based on the difference between the observed survival and the survival that would be expected if the curves were not different, in the

Table 21.3

Survival Data of 274 Women in Rochester, MN, Having Adult-Onset Diabetes Mellitus Who Were Older Than 45 Years at Onset during 1970–1980

Interval (years)	Begin (n_{i-1})	Died	Lost	End (n_i)	S_i (survived)	Confidence interval
0 (outset)	274	0	0	274	1.0000	
>0–2	274	14	0			
>2–4	260	13	0			
>4–6	247	14	0			
>6–8	233	18	0			
	215	0	1			
>8–10	214	19	0			

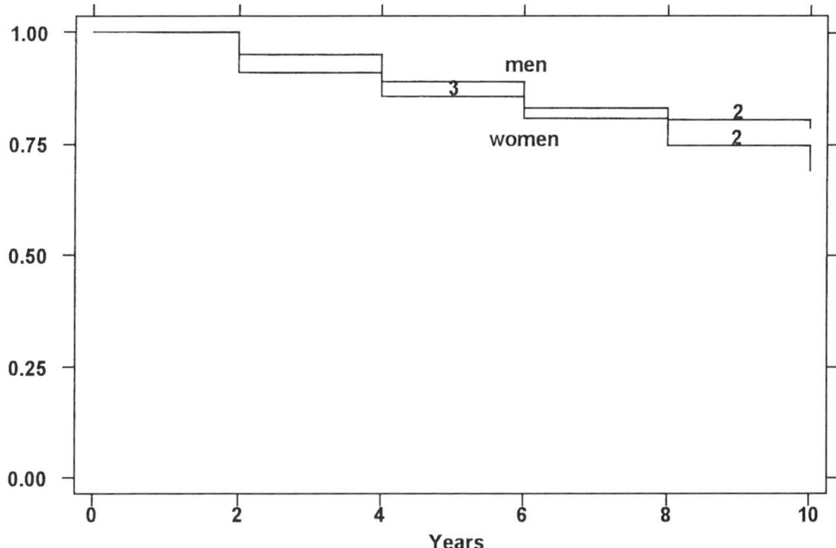

Figure 21.3 Survival curves for 370 women and 319 men in Rochester, MN, having adult-onset diabetes mellitus who were older than 45 years at onset during the decade 1980–1990.

same way that a chi-square goodness of fit [Eq. (17.2) of Section 17.2] uses the sum of squares of weighted differences between the observed and expected curves. However, the log-rank test's χ^2 is more complicated to calculate. It uses matrix algebra, multiplying vectors of differences for the time periods and the matrix of variances and covariances. A statistical software package should be used for this calculation. The result of the calculation is a χ^2 statistic, which may be compared with a χ^2 critical value from Table C for df = number of survival curves − 1. When the two curves of Fig. 21.3 are tested, $df = 1$. If the calculated statistic is greater than the critical value, the curves are significantly different.

The Log-Rank Test Compared to Other Tests of Survival Curves

Two alternative tests that might be considered for use are the Mantel–Haenszel test and the Cox proportional hazards test. The Mantel–Haenszel test is almost the same as the log-rank test. Indeed, both Mantel and Haenszel contributed to the theory of the log-rank test. However, the Mantel–Haenszel test is restricted to two curves, whereas the log-rank test may use more than two. Therefore, the log-rank test is recommended. The Cox proportional hazards test allows the risk of death to vary within the model, whereas the log-rank test assumes it to be the same throughout. The Cox assumption leads to rather complicated mathematics, and the methods must be used carefully and exactly to avoid a number of potential criticisms. The user is advised to seek a biostatistician if the death rates vary within the data set.

Additional Example

Figure 21.4 shows survival curves for patients with advanced cancer simulated for classroom use by a radiation oncologist.[28] In this example, treatment 0 implies that no treatment was given to the patient, and treatments 1 and 2 refer to experimental treatments of unknown efficacy. Because three curves are being compared in the log-rank test, $df = 2$. The critical χ^2 for 2 *df* from Table C is 5.99. A software package yields $\chi^2 = 6.35$. Because the calculated χ^2 is larger than the critical χ^2, the null hypothesis of no difference is rejected. (The actual p-value $= 0.042$.) It appears that treatment 1 is worse for survival than no treatment and treatment 2 is better.

Exercise 21.2. The survival data[35] for 370 diabetic women during the decade 1980–1990 was given as Table 9.4 in the answer to Exercise 9.6. The equivalent data on 274 women for the decade 1970–1980 were found in the table in the answer to Exercise 21.1. A log-rank test of the difference between the two curves yields

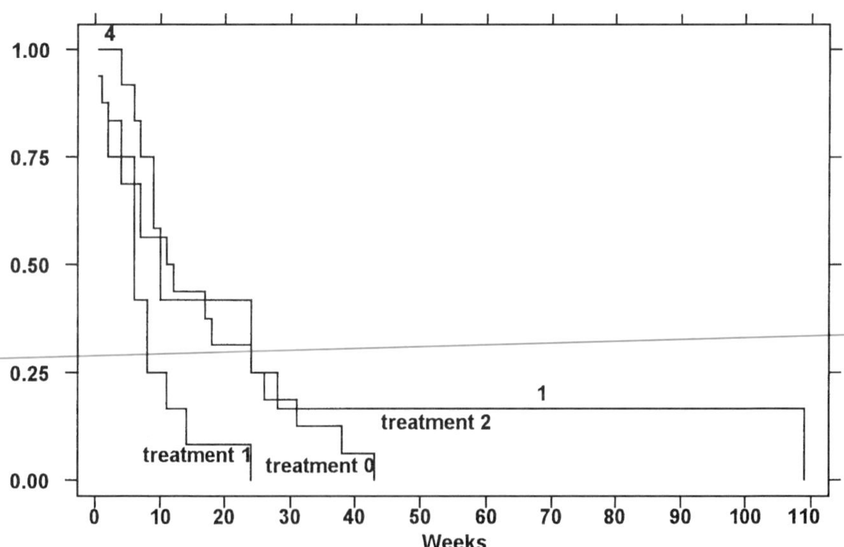

Figure 21.4 Survival curves of 44 patients with advanced cancer. Treatment 0 implies no treatment. Treatments 1 and 2 are experimental treatments of unknown efficacy. Note that five patients in treatment 2 are lost to follow-up.

$\chi^2 = 0.63$. Look up the critical value in Table C for 1 *df*, compare the χ^2 values, and interpret the resulting decision.

21.4. SEQUENTIAL ANALYSIS

INTRODUCTION

Suppose you were advising Ignaz Semmelweis in Vienna in 1847 on an experiment showing the effect on patient mortality of hand washing between patients.[57] You plan to randomize 1000 patients into two arms, one treated by physicians who wash between patients and the other not, and compare the mortality rates. After 100 patients in each arm, you have found only 1 death from sepsis in the wash arm, but 18 deaths in the nonwash arm. The probability that such a difference would occur by chance is less than 1 in 10,000. If you allow the experiment to continue at these rates, 68 additional patients in your study will die that can be saved if you immediately institute hand washing between patients for all physicians. The ethical challenge is obvious. In addition to mortality, carrying studies past clear decision points may cause unnecessary morbidity or inconvenience to patients, study costs, demand on facilities, and delay in reporting the useful information. In sequential analysis, a decision is made after acquiring each datum as to whether to (1) accept the null hypothesis, (2) accept the alternate hypothesis, or (3) continue sampling. This method, however, has been available at least since Wald's pioneering 1947 book[74] and has hardly proved to be a panacea. Limitations exist and will be examined along with the method after an example.

EXAMPLE

Sequential analysis might have helped Semmelweis had he done the study just posed. Of course, we have no idea what the actual sequence of outcomes was, but let us suppose it was as in Table 21.4. As in the preceding paragraph, we suppose

Table 21.4

A Table of Possible Outcomes from Semmelweis' Experiment, Shown with Associated Probabilities under the Two Hypotheses and the Decision Statistic[a]

k (Obs. no.)	1	2	3	4	5	6–29	30	31	32
Outcome	0	0	0	1	0	All 0	0	0	0
D_k	1.2073	1.4576	1.7597	0.0978	0.1179	...	13.1040	15.8204	19.1000

[a] Observation outcome is 0 for survival and 1 for death of the patient.

that one death resulted in the first hundred patients of the experimental group For illustration, we let this death occur early on, as the fourth patient in the sequence. (1) The null hypothesis states that the probability of a patient dying is no different from the old procedure, or H_0:population death rate = 0.18. The alternate hypothesis poses the new value, or H_1:population death rate = 0.01. (2) We select α, the risk of rejecting H_0 when it is true, as 0.05 and β, the risk of accepting H_0 when it is false, as 0.10. The two critical values are calculated from Eq. (21.4) as $\beta/(1-\alpha) = 0.10/0.95 = 0.1053$ and $(1-\beta)/\alpha = 0.90/0.05 = 18$. (3) We designate a patient surviving as 0 and one dying as 1. The first patient survived, so $D_1 = P(0|H_1)/P(0|H_0) = [1 - P(1|H_1)]/[1 - P(1|H_0)] = 1.2073$. (4) The multiplying probability ratios used to find the succeeding D_k will be $P(1|H_1)/P(1|H_0) = 0.01/0.18 = 0.0556$ when the patient died and $P(0|H_1)/P(0|H_0) = 0.99/0.82 = 1.2073$ when the patient survived. We enter D_k in Table 21.4 using calculations from Eq. (21.3). Bythe rule of Eq. (21.4), we will accept H_0 the first time the decision statistic D_k becomes less than 0.1053 or will reject H_0 the first time D_k becomes greater than 18. In Table 21.4, D_1 is 1.2073. After that, D_k starts to increase, drops dramatically with the death of patient number 4, and then starts to build again. With patient number 32, D_{32} exceeds 18 and we reject H_0; hand washing has proved beneficial. We note that the number of patients required is far less than first planned, but also that much of this small sample requirement is due to the dramatic difference in the old and new death rates.

METHOD

α, β, and n in Traditional Hypothesis Tests

A hypothesis test compares a decision statistic, for example, a sample mean Hct or proportion of surgical patients having complications, with a pair of hypotheses about the population value of this statistic and selects the appropriate hypothesis on the basis of the size of the risk of being wrong. The relationship among risks and probability distributions in making this selection was illustrated in Fig. 5.2, which is reproduced here as Fig. 21.5. A critical value divides possible outcomes of a decision statistic into acceptance and rejection regions. The outcome of the test is controlled by three quantities: α, the risk of selecting H_1 when H_0 is true; β, the risk of selecting H_0 when H_1 is true; and n, the sample size. In traditional hypothesis testing, β cannot be calculated because the alternate value of the population parameter being tested (a mean or proportion, for example) is unknown, so α and n are selected and β falls where it may. In the rare case in which a specific alternate value of the decision statistic is known, both α and β are selected and the minimum value of n may be calculated. (This is, in fact, the basis of minimum sample size estimation, the so-called "power analysis," in which a clinically relevant alternate hypothesis value of the decision statistic is conjectured.)

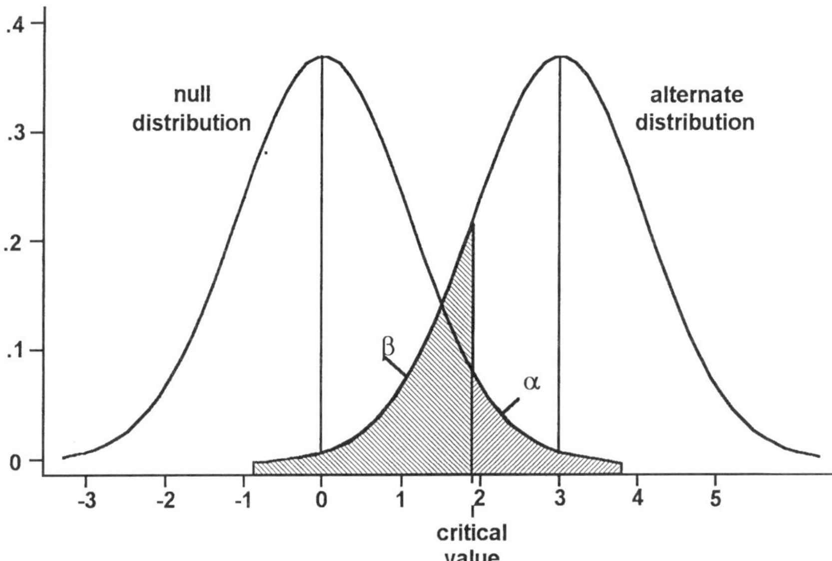

Figure 21.5 Reproduction of Fig. 5.2. A critical value of a decision statistic divides the horizontal axis into two regions. If the sample value of the decision statistic falls to the right of the critical value, H_0 is rejected. Otherwise, H_0 is accepted.

Concept of Sequential Analysis

Sequential analysis requires the alternative hypothesis value to be known. In this case, α and β can be specified and the sample size depends on them. Two critical values are chosen and the test's outcome is assigned to one of three regions, one region for each of the three decisions: accept H_0, accept H_1, or continue sampling. The relation among risks and probability regions is illustrated in Fig. 21.6, which is Fig. 21.5 altered to allow the third decision. Now, because the sample size is not an input but depends on α and β, it may be treated as a variable. Let us designate this increasing sample size as k in order to distinguish it from a fixed n. The decision is made for a k. If the decision is to continue sampling, k is increased and the decision is made again. This continues until the decision statistic falls into either the acceptance or rejection region, as is illustrated in Fig. 21.7. The dots show possible outcomes of the decision statistic for increasing k. When a value of the statistic falls outside the continue-sampling corridor, the final decision is made and sampling stopped.

The Issue of Accumulating Risk in Repeated Testing

We have noted before that testing using repeated samples on the same decision statistic leads to an accumulating probability of error. For example, if five tests,

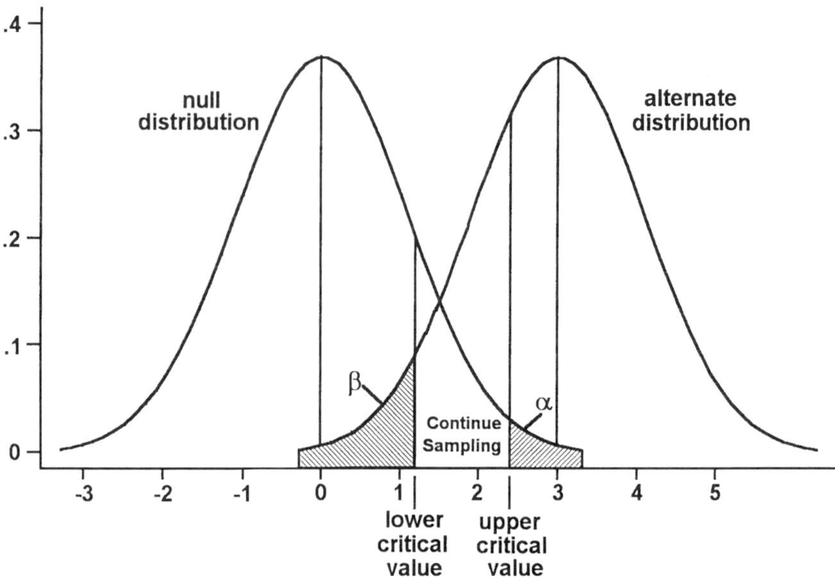

Figure 21.6 Diagram of probability distributions associated with the null and alternate hypotheses with α and β error risks shown. As long as the decision statistic (calculated from the sample of increasing size) falls between the shaded areas, sampling continues.

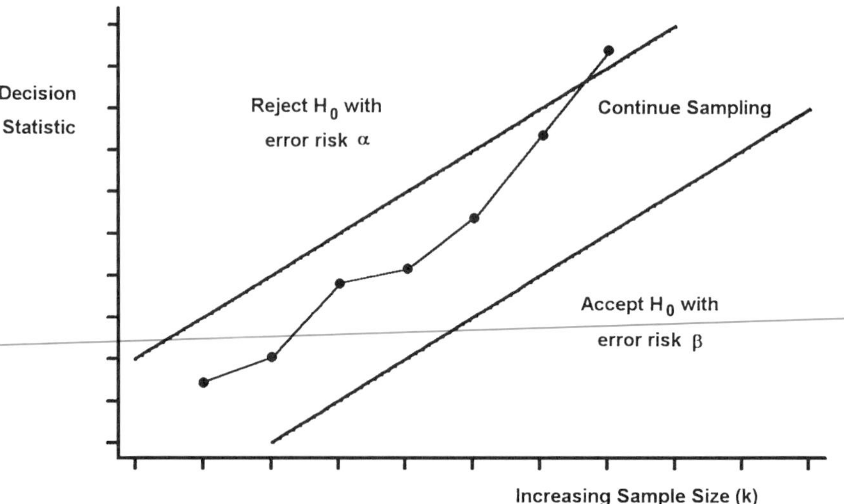

Figure 21.7 A graph of the decision statistic against k, the increasing sample size. As long as the statistic falls between the lines, sampling continues. If the statistic falls above the upper line, H_0 is rejected with risk α of making the wrong decision. If the statistic falls below the lower line, H_0 is accepted with risk β of making the wrong decision.

each with probability $\alpha = 0.05$ of a spurious rejection of H_0, are conducted, the probability that at least one will be spurious becomes $1 - (0.95)^5 = 0.226$, which is nearly 1 in 4, no longer an acceptable risk. Sequential sampling does not involve testing different samples in this way, as the same sample augmented by new observations is used, but the problem persists. To solve this problem, Wald developed the test using a theoretical basis different from the least squares we have seen in many tests. Because k could be expressed depending on the error risks, the solution was developed for a general k, whatever value it might take on. Thus, the sequential test is based on a fixed α and β for any k.

Probability of a Particular Sequence Occurring

Suppose a form of surgery led to complications (C) one-quarter of the time. The probability of complications, say P, on any randomly chosen patient is 0.25. The probability of no complication (N) is, of course, $1 - P$. The probability of two randomly chosen surgeries resulting in no complications on the first and complications on the second, i.e., in the sequence NC, is $(1 - P) \times P = 0.75 \times 0.25 = 0.1875$. For four patients, the sequence NCNN has probability $(1 - P) \times P \times (1 - P) \times (1 - P) = P \times (1 - P)^3 = 0.25 \times 0.75^3 = 0.1055$. In this fashion, we can calculate the probability for any particular sequence. Note well that the probability is for this particular sequence, not for any other positioning of the patients' outcomes in the sequence.

Test of a Binary Sequence

Now suppose we are studying a new type of surgery that we believe to have the lower complication rate 0.10. We pose H_0:the rate of the new surgery is still 0.25 and H_1:the new rate is 0.10. We record 1 as the outcome when a complication appears and 0 if it does not. Thus, the probability of a complication is 0.25 if H_0 is true, or $P(1|H_0) = 0.25$. Similarly, $P(1|H_1) = 0.10$. As usual, we assign α, the risk of accepting H_1 when H_0 is true, and β, the risk of accepting H_0 when H_1 is true. The sequential test's decision statistic, say D, is based on the ratio of likelihoods for H_1 being true over H_0 being true for a given sequence of observations. For the first patient, the ratio of probabilities that complications occur is $P(1|H_1)/P(1|H_0) = 0.10/0.25 = 0.4$, and the ratio of probabilities that complications do not occur is $[1 - P(1|H_1)]/[1 - P(1|H_0)] = 0.90/0.75 = 1.2$. For a sequence of k patients, we can calculate the ratio D_k of probabilities for any particular sequence of outcomes using

$$D_k = D_{k-1} \times P(1|H_1)/P(1|H_0) \text{ if the complications occur or}$$
$$D_k = D_{k-1} \times [1 - P(1|H_1)]/[1 - P(1|H_0)] \text{ if the complications do not occur.} \tag{21.3}$$

Thus, the increasing sequences N, NC, NCN, NCNN have decision statistics $D_1 = 1.2$, $D_2 = D_1 \times 0.4 = 0.48$, $D_3 = D_2 \times 1.2 = 0.576$, and $D_4 = D_3 \times 1.2 = 0.6912$. The critical values used to decide which decision region the D_k is in have been shown theoretically to be approximately the following:

$$\begin{aligned} &\text{Accept } H_0 \text{when} \quad D_k \frac{\beta}{1-\alpha}, \\ &\text{Reject } H_0 \text{when} \quad D_k \geq \frac{1-\beta}{\alpha} \\ &\text{Continue sampling otherwise.} \end{aligned} \tag{21.4}$$

One of these three choices is selected after each observation.

Test of a More General Sequence

For binary data (success–failure, occur–not, die–survive, etc.), the calculations of the basic probabilities usually are as simple as counting the number of complications, because there are only two outcomes. In the case of a test on continuous data, such as means or standard deviations, the probability ratio used to multiply D_{k-1} to find D_k varies with each sampling and must be recalculated for each additional observation. For a test on means, we know that means are distributed approximately normal (Central Limit Theorem, Section 2.8), so we use the normal distribution in calculations. For a test on standard deviations (actually on variances), we would use the chi-square or F distribution. More detail is required than is given in the tables of this book. We need electronic tables or very complete printed tables.

Steps to Conduct a More General Sequential Test

The sequential test procedure, extended to include continuous statistics, may be easier to follow step by step. Let us denote by x_k the observation on the kth patient. This will be the reading on whatever is being studied, such as Hct, PSA, died: 1 or survived: 0, etc. Denote by $P(x_k|H_0)$ the probability of x_k occurring if H_0 is true and by $P(x_k|H_1)$ the probability of x_k occurring if H_1 is true.

(1) Pose the null and alternate hypotheses.
(2) Assign error risk values to α and β and calculate the critical values.
(3) Find the probability ratio $D_1 = P(x_1|H_1)/P(x_1|H_0)$.
(4) Fill in Table 21.5, calculating

$$D_k = D_{k-1} \times P(x_k|H_1)/P(x_k|H_0). \tag{21.5}$$

(5) After each patient, make a decision using the criteria of Eq. (21.4). If H_0 is accepted or rejected, stop, if not, sample another patient and repeat steps (4) and (5).

Table 21.5

Sequence of Observations with Associated Decision Statistic Values

k (Obs. no.)	1	2	3	4	5	6	...
Obs. outcome							
D_k							

Step (4) Specified for a Test of Proportions

If the observation is binary, x_k can be expressed as either a 0 or a 1. The calculation of D_k will be as in Eq. (21.3).

Step (4) Specified for a Test of Means

Denote the mean under the null hypothesis as μ_0 and that under the alternate as μ_1; denote the variance as σ^2. Simplification of the ratio of two normal probabilities yields the multiplying increment in Eq. (21.5) as

$$\exp\left\{-\frac{1}{2\sigma^2}[(x_k - \mu_1)^2 - (x_k - \mu_0)^2]\right\}, \tag{21.6}$$

where $\exp\{\cdots\}$ implies $e^{\{\cdots\}}$.

A Graphical Solution

If the user wishes, it is possible to solve the expressions in Eq. (21.4) for a general k number of observations, which results in two straight line equations, and set up a graph as in Fig. 21.7. It is more work for binary data, but often less for continuous data, as equations can be derived for drawing the critical value lines.

The Average Sample Size Will Be Smaller in the Long Run

We want to know what the average sample size using sequential analysis would be and how it would compare to fixed sample size methods. However, the average sample size depends on the population's value of the decision statistic, and we have only an estimate that is changing with each new sample element. It is possible to find the average sample size based on a conjecture of what the population value would be, but the resulting size then would be a conjecture itself. Suffice to say that, in the long run, sample sizes from sequential sampling techniques are smaller than those from fixed sample size techniques.

Disadvantages of Sequential Analysis

If the sample size generally will be smaller with sequential analysis, why is it not used more frequently? The primary drawback is the requirement to specify the alternate hypothesis value of the decision statistic, which seldom is known. Why would Semmelweis have believed that hand washing would have reduced the mortality rate to 1% as opposed to 5% or 10%? Additionally, the method is demanding computationally, but has not found its way into many statistical software packages.

Additional Example

In DB5, the change in plasma silicone was measured on 30 women after silicone breast implants. Mean difference was 0.0073, with standard deviation 0.1222. A quick plot of the data shows approximate normality. A one-sample t test on the difference with a null hypothesis of no difference yielded $p = 0.745$. The mean difference is far from significant, and most investigators would conclude that implantation did not change the plasma silicone level. However, did we need $n = 30$? Let us conduct a sequential test following the five steps. (1) Hypotheses: μ is the population mean difference, $H_0{:}\mu = 0$. The alternate hypothesis is a problem, as we have no idea what the population mean difference is if it is not 0. Let us conjecture $H_1{:}\mu = 0.1$. We can make a test and come to a conclusion, but it is a test of only *this* alternate, not any other. Furthermore, we do not know σ^2. Suppose we find some published data from prior studies indicating that the standard deviation is about 0.2. (2) Let us choose $\alpha = 0.05$, as is common in medicine. The implication of a Type I error is to say that women receive no increase in plasma silicone from implantation when in fact they do; this would encourage implantation. A Type II error would be to say that women do receive an increase in silicone level from implantation when they do not; this would discourage implantation. As the decision about breast implants more often is cosmetic than medical, a quantification of the difference in loss from the two types of error is not clear-cut; let us choose β to be the same as α. From Eq. (21.4), the two critical values are $\beta/(1-\alpha) = 0.05/0.95 = 0.0526$ and $(1-\beta)/\alpha = 0.95/0.05 = 19$. When the accumulating D_k falls below 0.0526 or above 19, the test is concluded. (3) By substituting μ_0, μ_1, and σ in Eq. (21.6) and simplifying, we find that expression to be $\exp[-12.5(0.01 - 0.2x_k)]$. From the data of DB5, the first difference is -0.06. $D_1 = 0.7595$. The second difference is -0.11. The multiplying probability ratio is 0.6703. $D_2 = 0.7595 \times 0.6703 = 0.5092$. The progress through the sequence can be seen in Table 21.6, varying up and down until dropping below 0.0526 for D_{18}. On the 18th patient, the test results in accepting $H_0{:}\mu = 0$; the silicone level is not changed by the implantation.

Table 21.6

DB5 Data Showing Sequence of Plasma Silicone Differences before Minus after Implantation, Multiplying Probability Ratio, and Decision Statistic D_k[a]

k (patient no.)	Plasma silicone difference	Multiplying probability ratio	D_k (decision statistic)
1	−0.06		0.7596
2	−0.11	0.6703	0.5092
3	0.29	1.8221	0.9277
4	0.08	1.0779	1.0000
5	0.11	1.1618	1.1618
6	0.17	1.3499	1.5683
7	0.02	0.9277	1.4549
8	−0.03	0.8187	1.1912
9	−0.11	0.6703	0.7984
10	0.04	0.9753	0.7787
11	−0.12	0.6538	0.5091
12	−0.13	0.6376	0.3246
13	−0.23	0.4966	0.1612
14	−0.26	0.4607	0.0743
15	0.04	0.9753	0.0724
16	0.06	1.0253	0.0743
17	−0.07	0.7408	0.0550
18	−0.04	0.7985	0.0439

[a] H_0 is accepted when D_k drops below 0.0526 or rejected when D_k exceeds 19. H_0 is accepted with patient no. 18.

Exercise 21.3. From the data of DB12, 5.2% of nonintubated carinal resection patients die. Through experience, the surgeon believes that intubated patients have a much higher death rate, seeming to have a 50:50 chance. You want to test this belief. Take intubated patients from the data set one by one and decide from a sequential test whether their death rate is the same as that for nonintubated patients or is 50%.

21.5. LONG-SERIES DATA: REVEALING PATTERNS

Where Long-Series Data Appear

Long series most often appear as a sequence of data through time, or a time series, and most analysis of long-series data is found under a *time-series* heading. Types of long sequences other than time-dependent ones also are important and will be illustrated by examples, but time will be referred to for convenience. Some examples of time-dependent data from literature are incidence of nosocomial infection in a hospital, waveform analysis of neurologic potentials in infants, the course of Meniere's disease through time, course of opioid use during bone marrow transplantation, seasonal variation in hospital admissions for specific diseases, critical care monitoring, analysis of respiratory cycles, velocity of eye movements during locomotion, trends in juvenile rheumatoid arthritis, movement effects in MRI, and assessing the level of anesthesia. Indeed, time series are encountered in almost every field of medicine.

What Questions Can Be Answered by Analysis of Long-Series Data on an Event

(1) Is there a trend in the event through time? Identification of the best-fit regression curve will give a view of trend through time (Chapters 8 and 20). (2) Is the event cyclic through time? Autocorrelation, introduced in Section 9.7, may detect cycles and describe their nature. (3) Is the event correlated with other events in time? Cross correlation, also introduced in Section 9.7, may detect other events that follow related patterns through time. (4) Is there a point in time at which the event changes its pattern? Change-point estimation will be addressed in Section 21.6.

Time-Series Methods Introduced Here Are Basic

As with much of statistics, more sophisticated methods than will be met here exist. For example, a term sometimes encountered in contemporary medical articles is autoregressive moving average (ARMA), a weighted moving mean adjusted for the influence of autoregression. This book will have accomplished its purpose if the user understands the basic ideas and can appreciate what can be done.

The Need for Smoothing Processes

Very often, a potential pattern of a sequential event is obscured by variability and is better discerned if the variability about the pattern is reduced, or "smoothed." Smoothing is unnecessary for very small samples, because patterns cannot be seen anyway, whatever the method. Smoothing becomes useful when used on sequences with dozens, or better hundreds, of data.

Example

Sequential data from DB1 are shown in Figs. 21.8 and 21.9. In addition to the major ideas, this first example illustrates long-series data that are not time series.

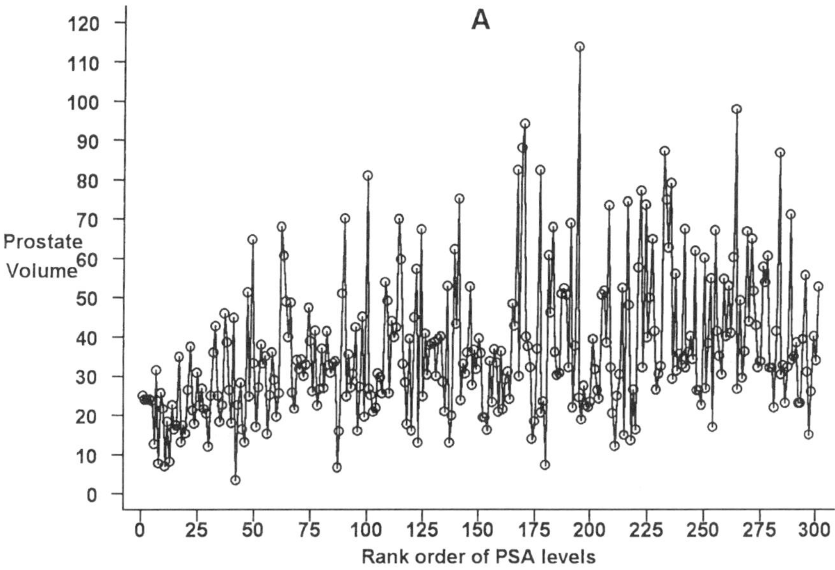

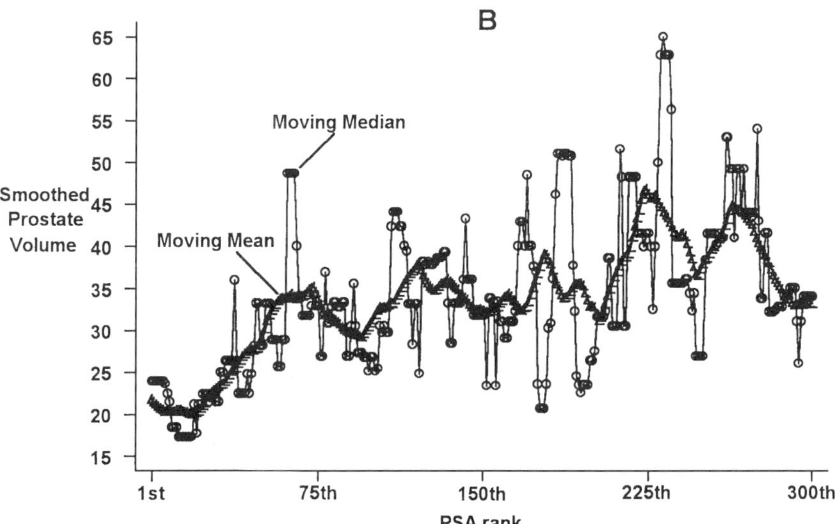

Figure 21.8 Prostate volume of 301 men as depending on increasing levels of PSA: (A) original data; (B) moving medians and moving means of prostate volumes.

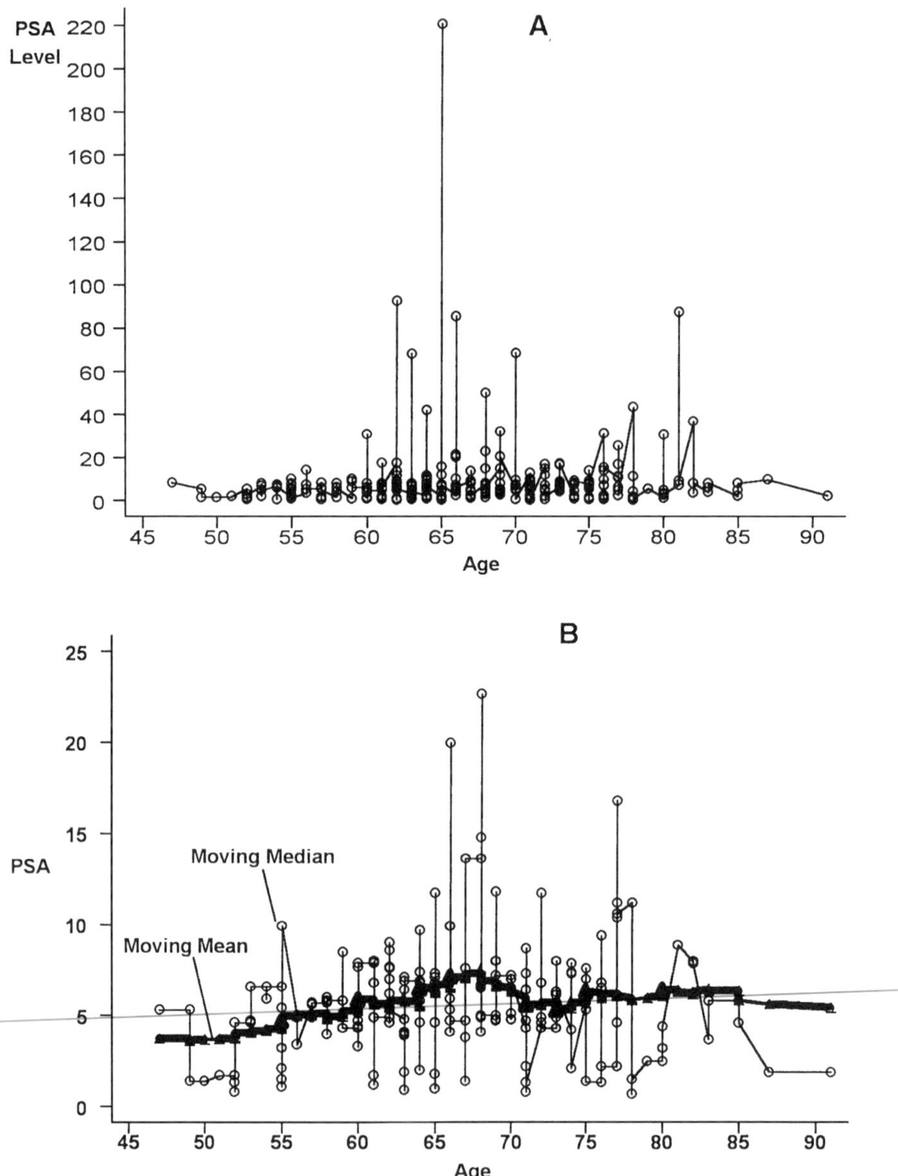

Figure 21.9 (A) PSA levels of 301 men as depending on increasing age. (B) Moving medians and moving means of PSA plotted against age.

Relation of Prostate Volume to PSA

Figure 21.8A shows the prostate volumes of 301 men presenting with urological problems related to the rank order of PSA levels in increasing sequence. Any pattern of change in volume with PSA is rather well obscured by the variability. We first use a moving median of $k = 7$ to replace some of the most extreme volumes by their neighbors. (Seven is chosen because there are some cases in which two or three nearly adjacent cases need to be subdued.) The graph of the moving medians of volume is shown in Fig. 21.8B. Note that the vertical axis is now a different scale, showing the reduced variability. We then use a moving mean of $k = 51$ to smooth the moving medians. (Fifty-one is chosen because a k smaller than 50 leaves too much variability and a larger one leaves too few observations; an odd number is easier to program.) The graph of that moving mean is superposed on the moving medians in Fig. 21.9. The resulting graph still varies up and down in what seem to be random cycles, but a pattern begins to emerge. The prostate volume certainly is increasing with PSA, but not quite in a straight line; it seems to be slightly curved, concave downward. We fit a second-degree regression curve to it (see Chapter 21 on regression), using the model $y = \beta_0 + \beta_1 x + \beta_2 x^2$ (see Chapter 19 on models). The resulting F statistic is 1101.57 (!), yielding $p < 0.001$ and $R^2 = 0.881$ and indicating that the second-degree model of PSA rank accounts for 88% of the predictive ability of the smoothed volume data. This is a very good fit. We conclude that prostate volume increases with PSA, more rapidly at first, declining with larger PSA, and finally perhaps ceasing to increase.

Relation of PSA to Age

In Fig. 21.9A, PSA levels from the same men are shown in the sequence of the men's age. Is there a pattern of change in PSA level with increasing age? A number of single observations of very large levels obscures any pattern that might be there. Some investigators might suggest deleting the large levels, but doing so would no longer leave the same data set; we might even be obscuring the pattern that we want to see. Can we mute the large values without destroying the pattern? We apply a moving median of three, which is a wide enough moving sample to reduce the most extreme levels because most large levels do not occur next to each other. Then we apply a moving mean of 51 as before. The moving median and moving mean are shown superposed in Fig. 21.9B. Note that the vertical axis has a very much smaller scale, allowing the local variations to be perceived. Inspection of the shape of the smoothed PSA by age reveals that it is not far from a straight line, but is curved slightly, opening downward. Upon fitting a second-degree regression model as with volume, we find the F statistic $= 401.93$, $p < 0.001$, and $R^2 = 0.730$, which again is a good fit. We might interpret the result as age predicting the typical (smoothed average) PSA, but not able to account for its variability.

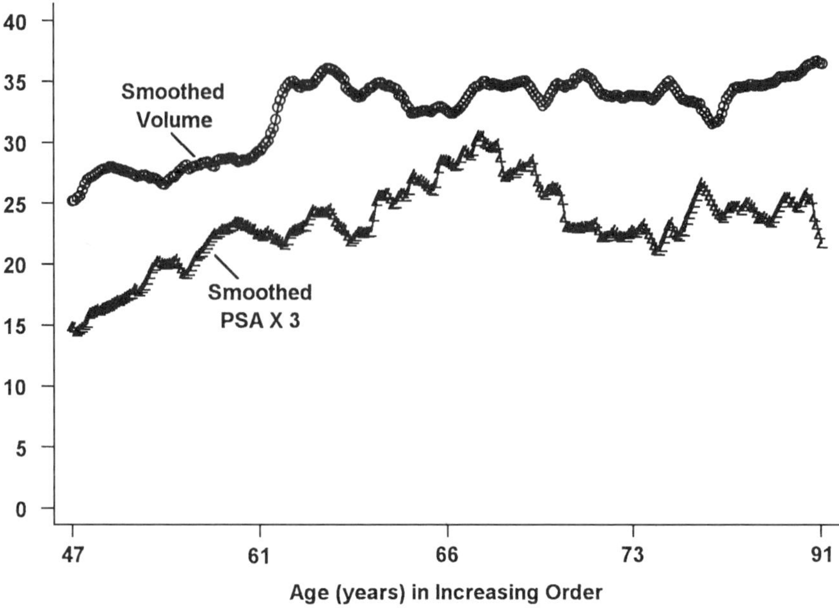

Figure 21.10 Smoothed series of volume and 3 × PSA (to assist visual comparison). Cross-correlation coefficient is 0.681. Both appear to increase until the mid-60s and then level out.

Cross Correlation of PSA and Prostate Volume Depending on Age

We noted that smoothed volume appears to depend on PSA, smoothed PSA appears to depend on age, and both dependencies follow similar models. If we consider both smoothed PSA and smoothed volume against age, do they have similar patterns of behavior as age increases? Figure 21.10 shows a plot of the smoothed paths of volume and PSA (multiplied by three in order to make it visually comparable to the volume curve) plotted against ranked values of age, i.e., patient ages placed in increasing order at equal distances apart. Both curves seem to increase at first, until age reaches the mid-60s, and then level out. The cross correlation between these curves is calculated to be 0.681, indicating that the perceived similarity of pattern is real.

Method

Moving Samples

Smoothing is based on the concept of a moving sample. Consider a sequence composed of n data, perhaps 100, and a subset of k data, say 10. We take the first

10 data and calculate some statistic, perhaps an average. Then we drop off the 1st datum, add the 11th datum, and recalculate the average. We continue, dropping the 2nd and adding the 12th, dropping the 3rd and adding the 13th, etc. We have a sample moving through the sequence, always with size k, providing a statistic moving through the sequence. We may name this sequence of samples a *moving sample* and also apply "moving" to the statistic, as a *moving average*. The moving average mutes the variability that obscures patterns.

Moving Averages

There are two relevant moving averages: the moving mean and the moving median. The moving mean subdues the variability, bringing extremes closer to the overall path through time, but allowing them some influence. In a moving mean of 20 in a sequence of 1000 visual evoked potential readings, a "hump" of 50 beats due to a stimulus image being presented will still appear, although it will be somewhat muted. However, a single extreme reading due to a blink also will appear as a slightly enlarged mean. The moving median, even one as small as three, completely eliminates single outliers, as the greatest reading in the three will always be replaced by the middle one. Thus, we would think of a moving mean to smooth but not eliminate causal influences and of a moving median to remove single outliers. Other more subtle uses will appear to the user with practice.

Calculation

A moving mean or median is just the ordinary mean or median of the moving sample. However, because the sample drops the left-most reading and adds one to the right end, most of the last calculated average will be the same; it only needs to be adjusted for the two readings changed. If a moving sample of readings x is of width k and its first element is i (it is composed of readings $x_i, x_{i+1}, \ldots, x_{i+k-1}$), and we denote its mean by m_i, m_{i+1} will be $m_i + (x_{i+k} - x_i)/k$. If we had readings 2, 4, 3, 5, 1, and 6 and wanted a moving mean of three, m_1 would be $(2+4+3)/3 = 3$. m_2 would be $3 + (5 - 2)/3 = 4$. The values of a moving median of three would be 3, 4, 3, 5. There are missing elements at the beginning and end unless they are supplied by specially defined values. For example, in the moving mean of three from the sequence just illustrated, the first mean might be twice the first value plus the second value divided by 3, or $(2 \times 2 + 4)/3 = 2.67$.

Serial Correlation

Other types of patterns we might want to discern may be detectable using serial correlation. A relationship between two variables through time may be identified by cross correlation, and the repetition of a pattern, or periodicity, by autocorrelation.

These concepts were introduced in connection with epidemiology in Chapter 9, but they may also be useful in clinical medicine.

Cross Correlation

If the matching data sets are taken sequentially through time, the correlation between them is termed cross correlation. It tells us how closely related the two variables are through time. Blood pressure and cardiac output through a sequence of exercise and rest would be expected to be cross-correlated. The correlation is based on the relationship between them and not on their individual behavior through time. Thus, if they both rise and fall together, the correlation is high whatever the time-dependent pattern may be. The calculation may be understood easily if we think of lining the two data sets in adjacent columns of a table and calculate the ordinary correlation coefficient between the columns. Cross correlation also can be calculated with one of the sets lagged behind the other. For example, the appearance of symptoms of a disease having a 2-week incubation period can be correlated with exposure to the disease, where exposure observations are paired with the symptom observations that occurred 2 weeks later. By varying the lag, we may be able to find the incubation period. For example, bacterial vaginosis has been found to facilitate AIDS infection. We would expect to see a cross correlation between incidences of the two diseases, although not a high one because each occurs alone. The issue is not the size of the coefficient but the lag at which it is maximum, which might provide insight into the nature and timing of exposures. The calculation again may be thought of as finding the ordinary correlation coefficient between variables listed in two columns of a table, but now one column is slid down the table a number of rows equal to the desired lag.

Autocorrelation

Observations through time may be correlated with a lagged version of themselves. If the autocorrelation coefficient retreats from 1.00 as the lag increases but then returns to nearly 1.00, we know that we have a periodically recurring disease. If that lag is 12 months, the disease is seasonal. In the additional example of Section 19.4, we looked at aspergillosis as a seasonal phenomenon and found that mean incidence by season fitted a sine wave with a period of 1 year. We ask whether older patients are more susceptible in winter. If we calculate the autocorrelation of mean age of infected patients per season with mean age 1 year later, we find the coefficient to be −0.22, which tells us that age of infected patient is not seasonal. We also ask whether percent infection by sex is seasonal, which we do not expect. The autocorrelation for percent male with a 1-year lag yields an autocorrelation coefficient of −0.14, telling us that sex is not seasonal. Interestingly, the cross correlation coefficient of age and percent male is 0.58, telling us that older patients tend to be male.

Additional Example

A large dental clinic was concerned about the purity of water being used to wash drilled teeth and small open wounds. Dental unit water tubing harbors bacteria-laden biofilms, which often contain pathogens. Although technicians are instructed to use purified water and purge the lines with compressed air at scheduled intervals, they do not always follow these procedures with sufficient care. A 12-week study compared eight technician groups.[43] The level of contamination of water ejected from the spray head was examined by a pathologist and rated according to the number of colony-forming bacterial units found. Technician group and date were recorded. Figure 21.11 shows data smoothed by a moving mean of 9 (initial data overlapped too much to perceive any process) in the order recorded (part A) and further smoothed by a moving mean of 21 (part B). Examination of the data in the vicinity of the peaks shows that group seven was using tap water, a discovery that might not have been made from the raw data. In addition, it appears that the curve would average a constant level at first, but begins a steady rise about halfway through the study. This will be examined further in the exercise of Section 21.6.

Autocorrelation

The tap-water peaks look as if they might be periodic rather than haphazard. The autocorrelation coefficient was calculated for various lags. The greatest coefficient, appearing at a lag of about 50, was 0.18. We conclude that tap-water usage is not periodic.

Exercise 21.4. The systolic time ratio (STR) indicates the strength and efficiency of the heart. Does STR relate to heart rate (HR)? Figure 21.12A displays STR graphed against 228 patients' HRs in increasing order.[61] A linear regression shows no relationship, which just says that a straight line fit does not have a significant slope, not that no pattern of relationship exists. Perhaps a smoothing process will reveal some relationship. A moving mean of 51 is superposed on the raw data. Figure 21.12B shows the moving mean with the vertical axis enlarged so that the pattern can be perceived. What hypothesis for further testing may be posed from part (B)?

21.6. LONG-SERIES DATA: TESTING

What Constitutes a Test

In long series, testing is mostly concerned with change points. If a change point is established, we know that the form of the series is different from that before the change point, so a change-point test is equivalent to a test on a difference in the

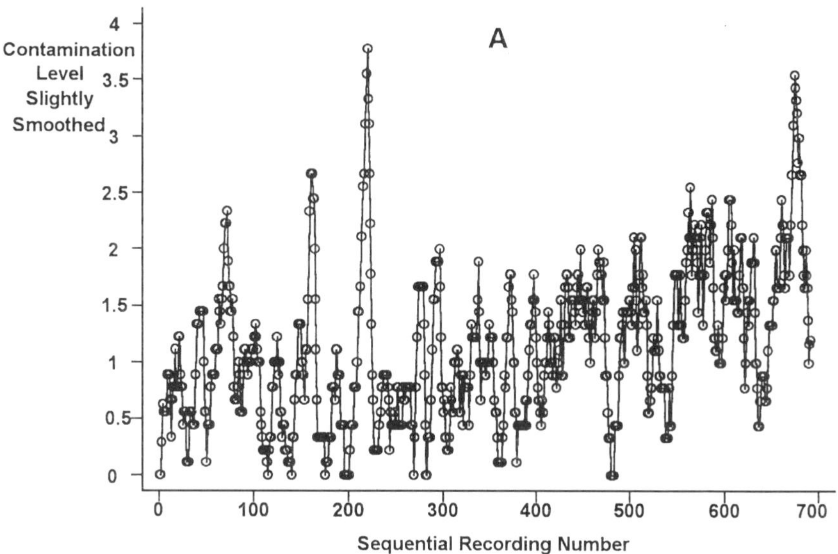

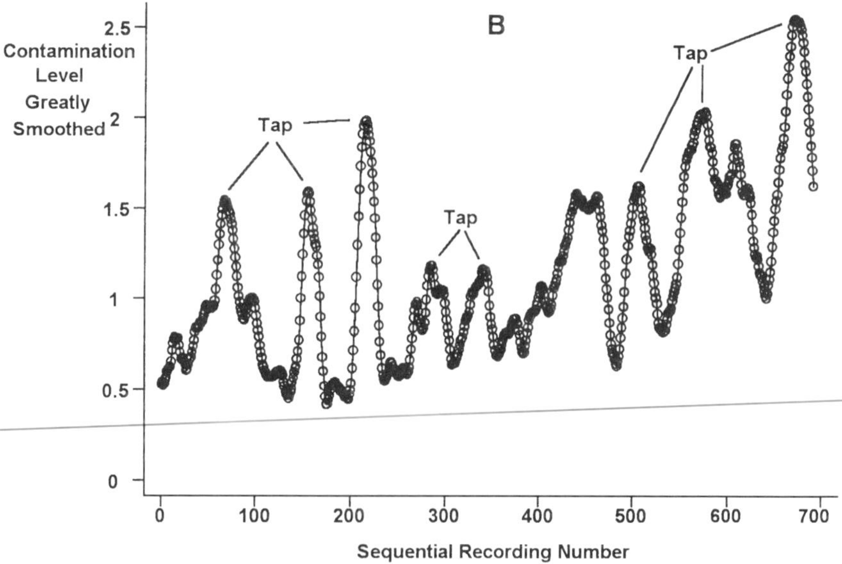

Figure 21.11 Contamination level of water for eight procedures over 12 weeks. Rating ≤ 2 satisfies ADA standards. (A) Data smoothed by a moving mean of 9. (B) Data further smoothed by a moving mean of 21. A technician group using tap water was discovered.

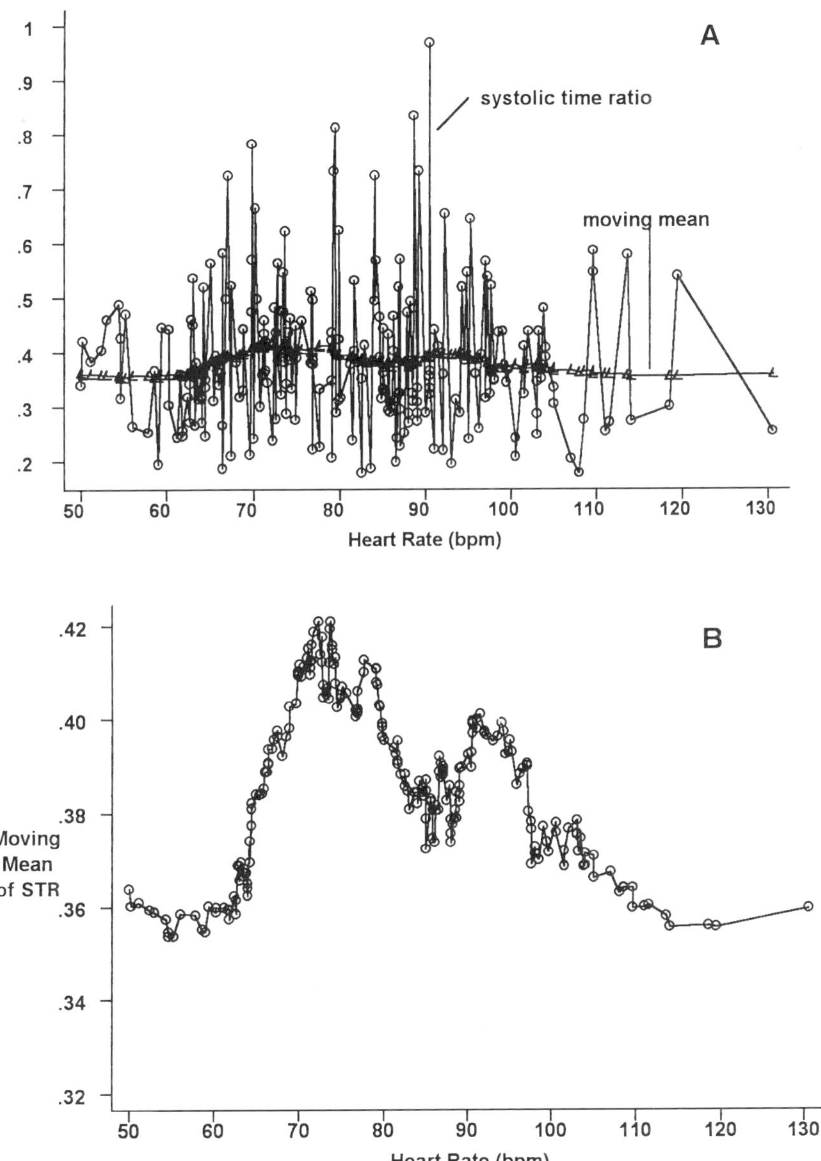

Figure 21.12 (A) Systolic time ratio against heart rate for 228 patients with a moving mean of 51 superposed. (B) Moving mean with vertical axis scale enlarged to perceive effect.

series at two locations. A number of change point tests exist, but most are rather complicated. One rather simple test that seems to work well will be given here. In this test, the variance of a moving sample is divided by a baseline sample variance, creating a moving F statistic. The point at which this moving F first exceeds a critical value as it moves through time is a change point, and the time series is different from baseline as long as the moving F remains significant.

Example

The U.S. Navy Hospital Corps is composed of enlisted technicians who support the Medical Corps (physicians), the Dental Corps, the Nurse Corps, and the Medical Service Corps (other scientific disciplines). Corpsmen provide basic medical service aboard ships, to Marines in land action, and at on-shore bases. The size of the Hospital Corps through time presents an interesting commentary on the politicomilitary history of the United States. Figure 21.13A shows the strength of the Corps during this century.[18] Growth spurts can be seen at the times of World War I, World War II, and the Korean War, after each of which the Corps was maintained at higher staffing than before. We hardly need tests. However, were the seeming increases at the times of the Vietnam War, the military buildup of the 1980s (what might be thought of as an economic war against the Soviet Union), and the Gulf War significant? If not, we would model post-Korean War staffing level as a constant. The 7-year mean level for 1955–1961 is taken as baseline (6 *df*). Its mean is 23,310 and standard deviation is 676.3215 (variance 457,410.8). We begin a moving sample of 7 (6 *df*) with 1962, dividing its variance by the baseline variance to create a moving F statistic. From Table E, we see that a critical value of F at $\alpha = 0.05$ and 6,6 *df* is 4.28. Figure 21.13B shows the moving F for the years 1962–1998. The increase in staffing level becomes significant in 1964. The course of the Vietnam War can be followed year by year: support of "advisors," open warfare buildup, and swift decline. Staffing level returns to baseline for 1979–1984. It rises in 1985, becoming significant in 1986 and remaining so until the end of the arms race with the Soviet Union. With the collapse of the Soviet Union, it returns to baseline. It does not rise to significance with the Gulf War.

Method

Moving Sample Designations

A moving sample is composed of a sequence of (mostly overlapping) values, say x-values. We need to keep track of the member of the sequence of samples with which we are dealing at any moment. As in the last section, let us designate by

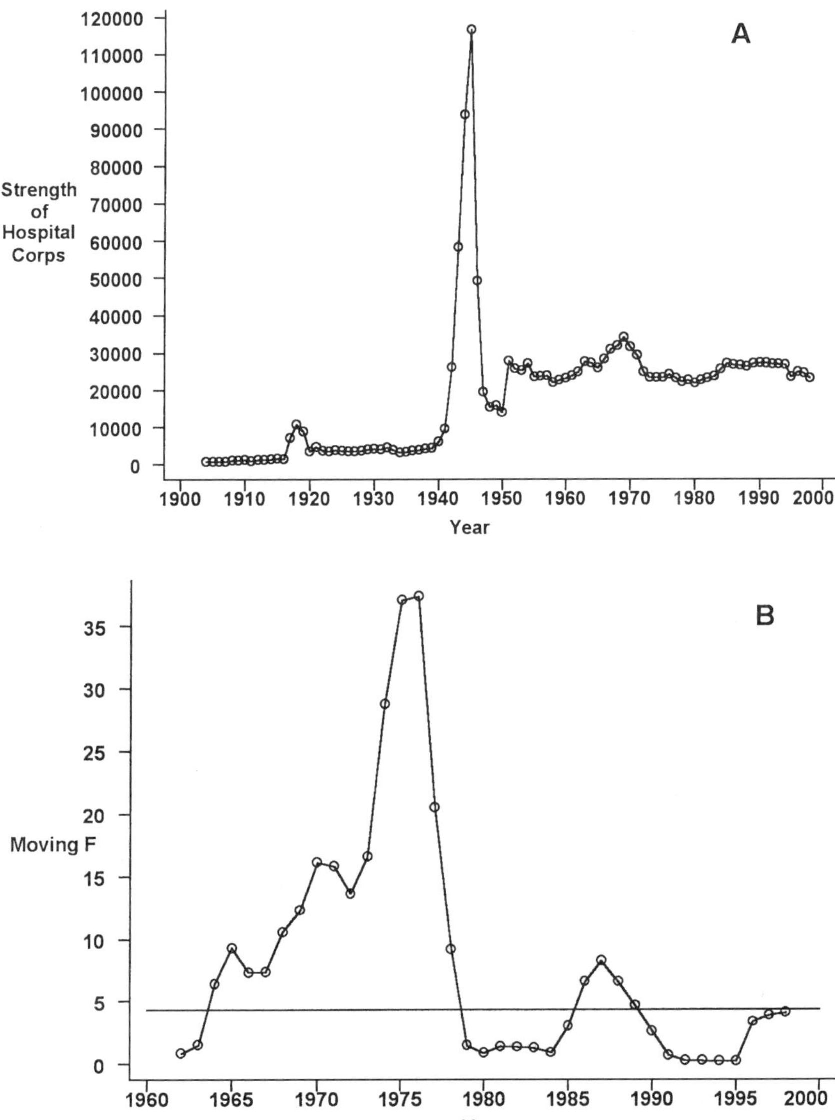

Figure 21.13 (A) Strength of Navy Hospital Corps. (B) Post-Korean War pattern of moving F, showing variance of moving sample of seven in ratio to baseline for 1955–1961.

a general indicator i the first value in a moving sample of size k, so that the sample elements are $x_i, x_{i+1}, \ldots, x_{i+k-1}$. The moving mean became $(x_i + x_{i+1} + \cdots + x_{i+k-1})/k = m_i$. The first moving mean was m_1, the second m_2, etc. m_i is just the mean of k data starting with number i. Similarly, we could think of a moving variance s_i^2 as just the sample variance of the same k data.

Position in the Time Interval Associated with a Moving Sample

A moving statistic does not occur at a point on the time axis, but is calculated from an interval. Until now, a statistic associated with the interval $x_i, x_{i+1}, \ldots,$ x_{i+k-1} has been designated by i, that is, named for the first element in the interval. A plot of a statistic so designated against time might associate the impact of the entire interval with the beginning of the interval. We might be better advised to associate the impact of the interval with the median position of the interval, although that requires the awkward subscript $i + (k-1)/2$ to identify the statistic for the $x_i, x_{i+1}, \ldots, x_{i+k-1}$ interval.

The Concept of a Simple Moving Test

Suppose we start a time series with a stable baseline of k values, perhaps a critical care blood pressure monitor. This baseline has variance $s_{(k+1)/2}^2$ (associating it with the center of the first interval). Recall that an F test is just the ratio of two variances (assuming the data are approximately normal). If we start with datum $k+1$ and calculate the set of moving variances, dividing each by $s_{(k+1)/2}^2$, we have a moving F statistic traveling through the time series. Upon comparing this with a critical value of F from Table E for $df(k-1, k-1)$, perhaps for $\alpha = 0.05$, we can see where the variability exceeds baseline variability so much that it is unlikely to have occurred by chance. This is a moving F test. It will detect a sudden increase in blood pressure. (The monitor example is given to aid conceptualization; it is not suggested that a moving F test is needed to perceive a clinically crucial change in BP.)

Graphing a Moving F Test

If the moving F is plotted against the time-series axis and a horizontal line drawn at the critical F-value, the time-series values for which the variability is significantly greater than baseline will be clearly visible. If the moving F were displayed on a blood pressure monitor, a sudden increase would be visible immediately.

A Two-Tailed Test

We may be concerned not only with an increase in blood pressure, but also a decrease. We could split the α, for example, 5%, into two 2.5% areas and identify an upper and a lower critical F, the value having 97.5% of the F distribution to the right and the value having 2.5% to the right. (A more complete F table than that given in this book would be required.) Then we could detect both significant increases and decreases.

Multiple Causes of Variability Are Possible

The moving F considered to this point will test for any combination of changes in the process: a change in the shape of the process, a shift in the average, and/or the process becoming more variable. Often we need to identify which influence is causing the significant F. Consider an electronic monitoring instrument. Its readings could just have become more variable. Alternatively, it could have shifted its setting while maintaining the same variability about the setting. Either event would trigger an increase in F in comparison with the baseline. How are these different sources of variability separated and identified? The numerator of the moving sample's variance is the sum of squares (SS) of deviations of x-values from the baseline mean, say m_b for simplicity, or $SS_i = \Sigma(x - m_b)^2$. We can add and subtract the moving mean value m_i from x to obtain $\Sigma(x - m_i + m_i - m_b)^2$, which mathematically can be shown to be $\Sigma(x - m_i)^2 + k(m_i - m_b)^2$, a component due to randomness at the moving sample's position in the time series and a component due to the difference between the baseline mean and the mean at the moving sample's position. When divided by *df*, they become variances. Taken in ratio to the baseline variance, we have a moving F due to mean shift and one due to random variability. Each may be compared with critical F-values to form a test. (It also is possible to separate out and test a component due to the shape of the process, but that subtlety will not be pursued here.)

Additional Example

Morphine given intravenously (IV) to a severely injured patient with extensive blood loss impairs the already traumatized vascular system. It was hypothesized that intrathecal (IT) administration of morphine (injection under the nerve-covering sheath) would mitigate that impairment. An experiment[56] used a sample of two pigs, one assigned to IV and the other to IT injection. A number of variables were measured for a 30-min baseline and a 60-min simulated hemorrhage. The hemorrhage was stopped and morphine injected. Measurements were continued for an additional 180 min. Figure 21.14A shows heart rate (HR) for the two pigs during this period. The variance of the first 15 prehemorrhage HRs averaged for the two pigs was taken as baseline. The moving sample also was taken as size 15. From Table E (interpolated), the 95% critical value of F for 14,14 *df* is 2.48. Figure 21.14B shows the plots of moving F for IV and IT treatments. Whereas both

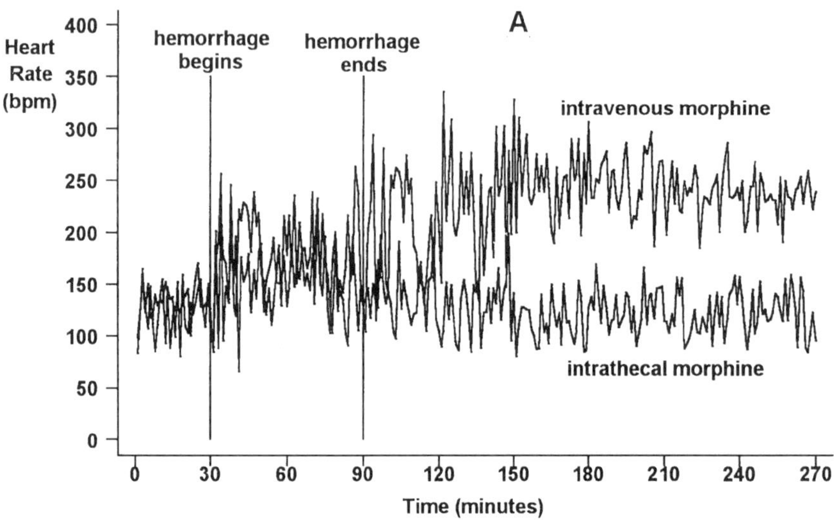

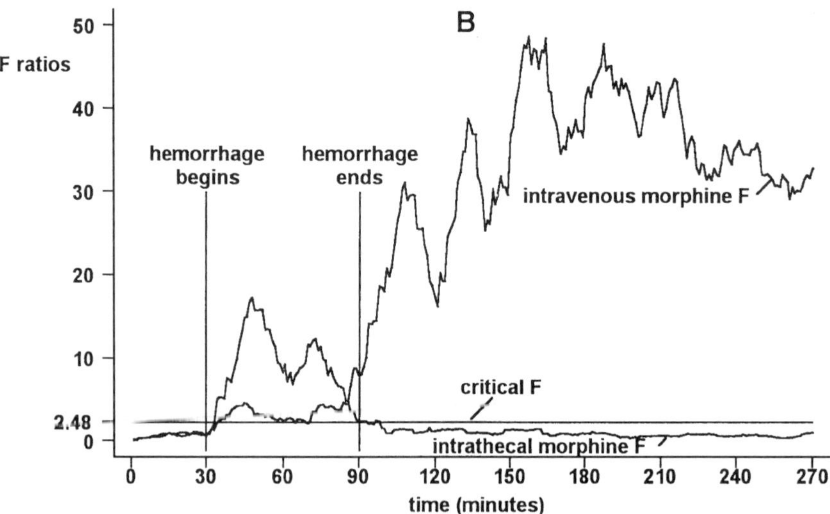

Figure 21.14 (A) Heart rates for IV and IT morphine at baseline, during hemorrhage, and post-hemorrhage. (B) Moving *F* of HR for IV and IT morphine over the same periods. Both subjects show significantly increased HR during hemorrhage, but IV morphine at the end of hemorrhage exacerbates HR even further, whereas IT morphine allows HR to return to normal.

curves rise above the critical value during hemorrhage, the F for IV morphine rises even further after the end of hemorrhage and the F for IT morphine drops back to the vicinity of baseline, losing significance. The evidence indicates that IT morphine is better for the vascular system of trauma patients following hemorrhage.

Exercise 21.5. In the Additional Example of Section 21.5, Fig. 21.11B showed a smoothing of the contaminated dental water data.[43] The contamination level appeared to be constant at first, such as indicated by the conjecture lines on Fig. 21.15, and then turn to an upward slope somewhere in the vicinity of the question mark on the figure, between recordings 300 and 400. Knowledge of when this change occurred might help identify its cause. The mean of the beginning horizontal pattern is 0.86. From a moving sample of 21 on the moving mean data (denoted for the moment as x) shown in Fig. 21.15, a moving variance was calculated as $\Sigma(x - 0.86)^2/20$. The first moving variance, serving as baseline, was 0.000731. The moving F was calculated as (moving variance)/0.000731. The critical F for $\alpha = 0.05$ and 20,20 *df* from Table E is 2.12. A fragment of the data appears as Table 21.7. Complete the missing data and identify the recording number at which the change point occurs. The moving sample results were recorded for the middle of the sample (10 pre- and 10 postrecording position). To find the moving variance, say V_{i+1} for position $i+1$, calculate $[20V_i - (x_{i-10} - 0.86)^2 + (x_{i+10} - 0.86)^2]/20$. The moving F_{i+1} is $V_{i+1}/0.000731$.

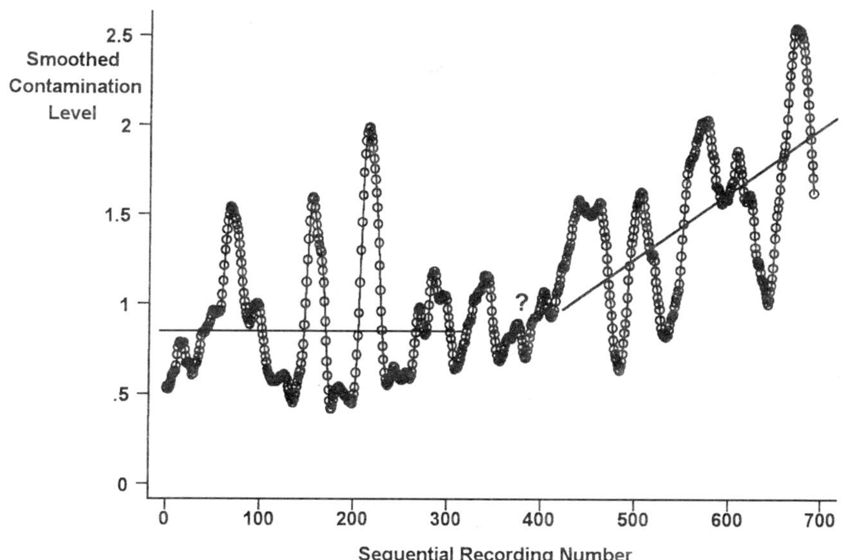

Figure 21.15 Smoothed contamination levels of dental water with initial constant mean prior to recording number 300 and conjectured sloped mean after about 400.

Table 21.7

Data Required to Calculate Values of the Moving Variance and the Moving F Statistic for Recording Numbers 334 and 335[a]

Recording no.	x (smoothed level)	Moving variance	Moving F
323	0.9104	...	...
324	0.9111	...	...
...	...	...	...
331	0.9172	...	1.605
332	0.9183	...	1.749
333	0.9196	0.001398	1.912
334	0.9210		
335	0.9225		
336	0.9242	...	...
...	...	...	...
343	0.9412	...	...
344	0.9443	...	...

[a] The recording number at which F becomes significant can be seen.

ANSWERS TO EXERCISES

21.1. See Table 21.8 and Fig. 21.16.

21.2. The critical χ^2 value for $\alpha = 0.05$ for 1 *df* is 3.84. The calculated 0.63 is much less than 3.84. Conclusion: No difference between the survival patterns has been shown. (Actual p-value = 0.428.)

21.3. (1) H_0:population death rate = 0.052. H_1:population death rate = 0.50. (2) Any difference found will not be used in clinical decisions, but will tell

Table 21.8

Completion of Table 21.3, Survival Data of 274 Women in Rochester, MN, Having Adult-Onset Diabetes Mellitus Who Were Older Than 45 Years at Onset during 1970–1980

Interval (years)	Begin (n_{i-1})	Died	Lost	End (n_i)	S_i (survived)	Confidence interval	
0 (outset)	274	0	0	274	1.0000		
>0–2	274	14	0	260	0.9489	0.9235	0.9743
>2–4	260	13	0	247	0.9015	0.8671	0.9359
>4–6	247	14	0	233	0.8504	0.8094	0.8914
>6–8	233	18	0	215	0.7844	0.7376	0.8312
	215	0	1	214			
>8–10	214	19	0	195	0.7147	0.6636	0.7658

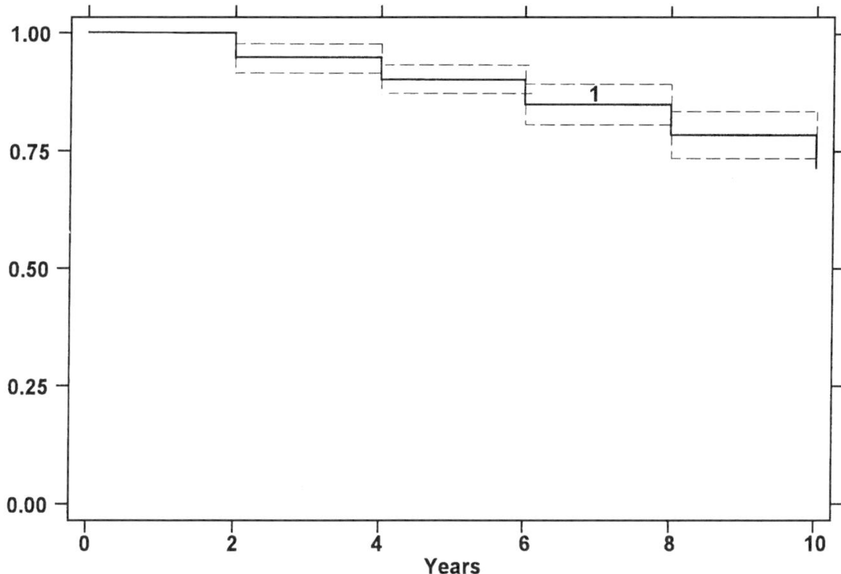

Figure 21.16 Survival curve with confidence limits derived from Table 21.8.

the investigator that a different baseline death rate should be calculated for intubated patients. Thus, there is no clinical reason for different α and β; they both are chosen as 0.05. From Eq. (21.4), the critical values are $0.05/0.95 = 0.0526$ and $0.95/0.05 = 19$. (3) The first intubated patient is no. 32, who survived. $D_1 = [1 - P(1|H_1)]/[1 - P(1|H_0)] = [1 - 0.50]/[1 - 0.052] = 0.5274$. This also will be the multiplying increment in Eq. (21.5) for each surviving patient, and $[P(1|H_1)]/[P(1|H_0)] = [0.50]/[0.052] = 9.6154$ will be the multiplying increment for each dying patient. (4) Table 21.5 is filled in as Table 21.9. The upper critical value is surpassed on observation eight. The test indicates that H_1 should be accepted: the population death rate for intubated patients is 50%.

Table 21.9

Completion of Table 21.5

Patient no.:	32	54	65	68	71	83	85	95
k (Obs. no.)	1	2	3	4	5	6	7	8
Obs. outcome	0	0	1	0	0	1	0	1
D_k	0.5274	0.2782	2.6750	1.4108	0.7441	7.1548	3.7734	36.2828

21.4. It appears that the heart exhibits greater efficiency when the HR is in the normal range of about 70–80 bpm, with inferior efficiency below 65 bpm and efficiency diminishing gradually as the HR increases above 80 bpm. This pattern revealed by time-series analysis is unlikely to be detected with regression or other curve-fitting techniques.

21.5. Table 21.10 reproduces Table 21.7 with the missing data included. Figure 21.17 shows the moving *F* statistic with critical value 2.12. The statistic crosses the critical line at recording number 335, which is taken as the point of change from a horizontal mean to a sloped mean. Following identification of the change point, the investigator examined adherence to the scientific protocol and concluded that the technician teams began to become bored with the study as it neared the halfway mark and thereafter became increasingly less careful.

Table 21.10

Completion of Table 21.7

Recording no.	*x* (smoothed level)	Moving variance	Moving *F*
323	0.9104	...	...
324	0.9111	...	...
...	...	...	...
331	0.9172	...	1.605
332	0.9183	...	1.749
333	0.9196	0.001398	1.912
334	0.9210	0.001601	2.190
335	0.9225	0.001826	2.498
336	0.9242	...	...
...	...	...	...
343	0.9412	...	...
344	0.9443	...	...

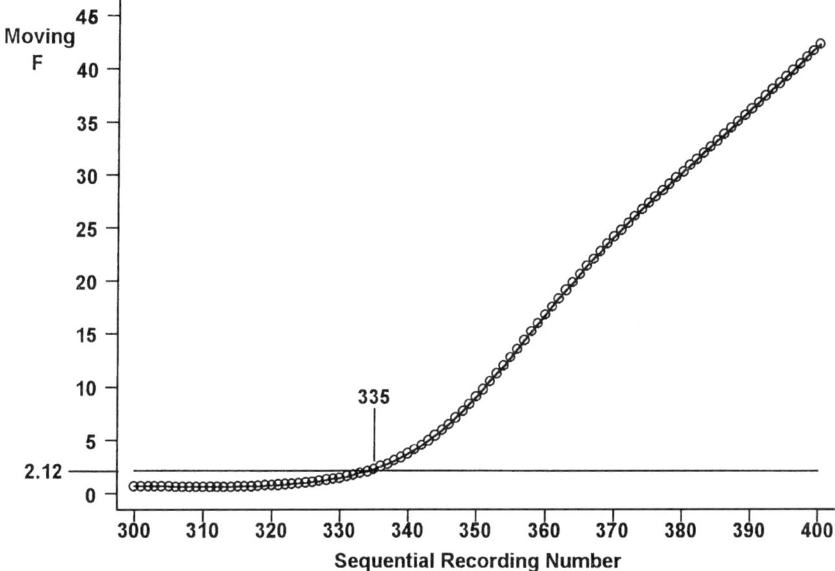

Figure 21.17 Plot of the moving *F* statistic in the 300–400 range.

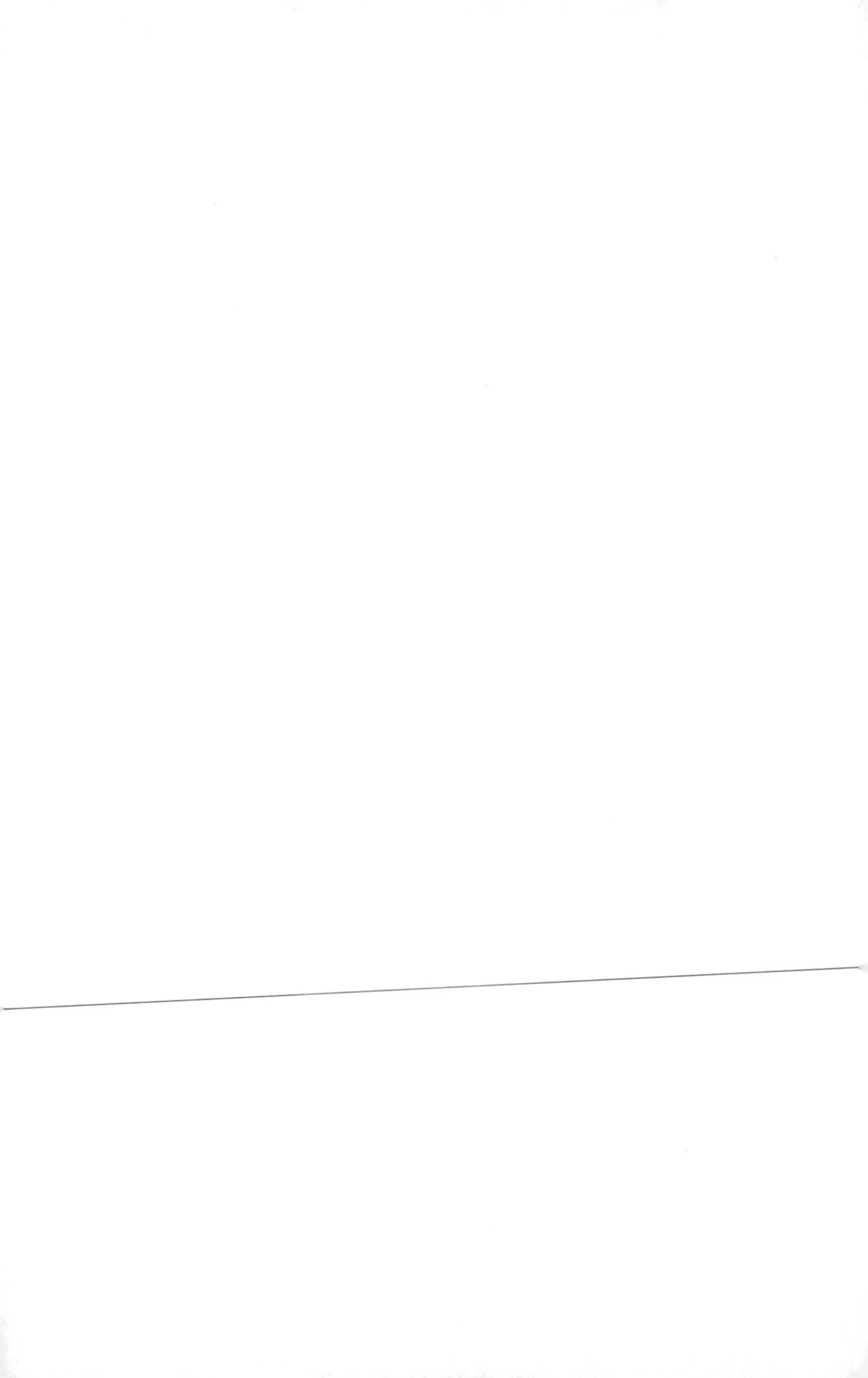

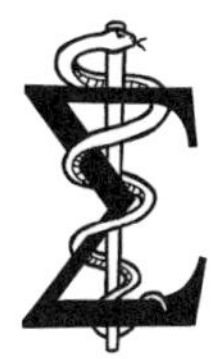

Chapter Summaries

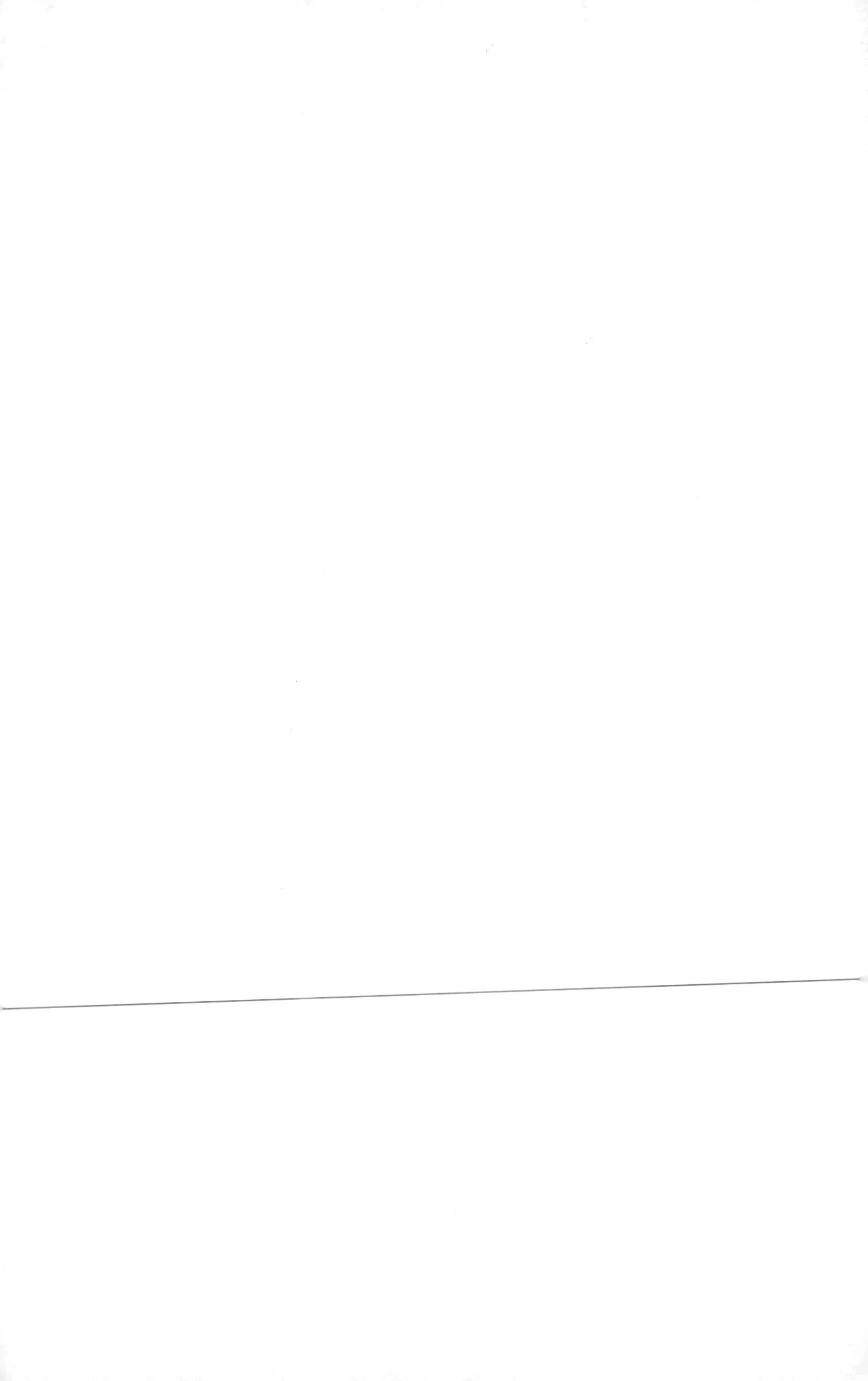

Chapter Summaries

SUMMARY OF DATA AND NOTATION FROM CHAPTER 1

DATA TYPES

Continuous data are positions on a scale, which may be as close to one another as the user can discern and record. Example: blood clotting time. *Discrete data* are a subset of continuous data that are recorded only as distinct values; there is a required distance between adjacent data. Example: age in years.

Rank-order data are indicators of the positions of data that can be positioned according to some ordering characteristic of the subject, such as magnitude of each datum. Example: ordered lengths of surgery on six patients, shortest (rank 1) to longest (rank 6).

Categorical (or nominal) data are indicators of type or category and may be thought of as counts. Example: number of patients undergoing a type of surgery with and without complications.

Ratings may be of any form, depending on the indicator being rated. Ratings are based only on the subject being rated; they are not ranks, which are based on the subject's position relative to other subjects. Example: cancer stage.

SYMBOLS

Name symbols behave like family names, indicating to which family the thing or event symbolized belongs. Example: x or μ. *Subscripts* behave like first names, indicating which member of the family is being considered. Example: *1* in x_1 or *postop* in $\text{Hct}_{\text{postop}}$.

Operator (or command) symbols represent an instruction to act rather than a thing. Example: ÷ ("divide what appears before by what appears after") or Σ ("add together the elements that follow").

Relationship symbols express a relationship between two families or two members of a family. Example: = ("what appears before is the same as what appears after") or > ("what appears before is greater than what appears after").

Indicator symbols denote a member of a family without specifying which member. Example: i in x_i could be x_1, x_5, or x_{332}.

Terms

Population. The entire set of subjects about whom (or which) we want information.

Sample. A subset of the population. The usual goal in statistics is to decribe the characteristics of a sample and generalize them to the population from which the sample was drawn.

Representativeness and Bias. The generalization from sample to population is valid only if the sample represents the population in the characteristics being generalized. If the sample does not represent the population, it is termed biased.

Random. The physical or mathematical mode of choosing a datum based solely on probability so that no organized bias may influence the choice.

Control Group. A sample group having all the characteristics of the experimental group except the treatment under study.

Placebo. An apparent treatment, given so that the subject and/or investigator cannot distinguish control subjects from experimental subjects.

Variable. An observation or reading giving information used in answering the study question.

Independent Variable. A variable that, for the purposes of the study question to be answered, occurs independently of other influences.

Dependent Variable. A variable that depends on or is influenced by an independent variable.

Types of Study

Registry. An accumulation of data from an uncontrolled sample.

Case–Control. A type of study in which an experimental group of patients is chosen for being characterized by some outcome factor, such as having acquired a disease, and a control group lacking the factor is matched patient-for-patient. Control is exerted over the selection of cases but not over the acquisition of data within these cases. Often, but not always, a case–control study is based on prior records and therefore sometimes is loosely termed a *retrospective study*.

Cohort. A type of study that starts by choosing groups that have already been assigned to study categories, such as diseases or treatments, and follows these groups forward in time to assess the outcomes.

Prospective. A descriptor indicating that a study is planned prior to observing data and then is followed forward in time.

Randomized Controlled Trial (RCT). The soundest type of study, often called a *clinical trial*. An RCT is a true experiment in which patients prospectively are assigned randomly to study categories, such as clinical treatment.

SUMMARY OF DISTRIBUTION CONCEPTS FROM CHAPTER 2

Tally. A collection of tick marks, one for each datum marked in its respective interval within the range of possible occurrences of variable values. The shape of a completed tally approximates the shape of the frequency distribution.

Frequency Distribution. The pattern in which the data are distributed along the scale (or axis) of the variable of interest. A sample frequency distribution appears as a sequence of bars of varying height, having the tally intervals as width.

Relative Frequency Distribution. A frequency distribution in which the height of the bar over each respective interval represents the proportion of the sample falling into that interval.

Probability. The relative frequency with which an event occurs when all events in a population are given equal opportunity to occur. As the sample size increases, tending toward the population size, the relative frequency distribution tends toward the population probability distribution.

Mean. An average; the center of gravity of a distribution, denoted μ for a population's probability distribution and m for a sample's relative frequency distribution.

Median. An average; the value of the variable for which half the sample or population is smaller and half is larger.

Mode. An average; the value of the variable having greatest relative frequency.

Midrange. An average; the midpoint between the smallest and greatest values of a variable that occur. (A probability distribution with one or both tails extending without bound, e.g., the normal distribution, has no midrange.)

Variance. A measure of variability; the average (mean) of squared deviations from the sample or population mean.

Standard Deviation. A measure of variability; the square root of the variance. The purpose is to put the measure of variability in the same units as the observations and mean.

Skewness. A measure of asymmetry of a distribution. If one tail is stretched out more than the other, the distribution is skewed (e.g., right tail stretched out, right skew).

Inference. Concluding characteristics of a population on the basis of a sample. (This is an oversimplification, but is the kernel of a complicated concept.)

Robust. A characteristic of a statistic (a summarizing calculation from a sample) in which the statistic is little affected by moderate violation of the assumptions under which the statistic was formed.

Normal Distribution. A family of bell-shaped probability distributions.

Standard Distribution. A probability distribution or relative frequency distribution that has been transformed so that it has mean 0 and standard deviation 1. This transformation is achieved by subtracting the mean from each data element and dividing by the standard deviation. The most frequent use is in the standard normal distribution.

Central Limit Theorem (CLT). Data from any distribution (whatever its form) have means distributed approximately normal.

t Distribution. A bell-shaped distribution, slightly wider than the normal, that arises when the standard normal divisor is the sample standard deviation rather than that of the population. ("Student": the nom-de-plume of W. S. Gossett, who derived the distribution.)

Degrees of Freedom (df). An integer related to sample size that determines which member of a family of probability distributions is appropriate in a particular case. The standard normal has only one member and does not use *df*, but the *t* has many members and does use *df*.

Chi-Square (χ^2) Distribution. A right-skewed family of probability curves arising from the variance. The statistic: sample variance $\times$ *df* $\div$ population variance is distributed χ^2.

F Distribution. A right-skewed family of probability curves arising from the ratio of two sample variances. It depends on two *df* values, one for each sample variance.

Binomial Distribution. A discrete probability distribution of the relative likelihood of outcomes of a two-category event, e.g., the heads or tails of a coin flip, survival or death of a patient, or success or failure of a treatment.

Poisson Distribution. A discrete probability distribution of the relative likelihood of outcomes of a two-category event when one of the events is very rare, e.g., a citizen of a developed nation contracting bubonic plague.

Standard Error of the Mean (SEM). The standard deviation of the sample mean. In most cases, it is the standard deviation of the sample observations divided by the square root of the sample size.

Joint Frequency Distribution. The pattern in which the data are distributed in the two-dimensional plane of two simultaneous scales (or axes) of two variables of interest. Each variable has a mean and standard deviation, as it would alone, but there also is a covariance (or correlation: covariance divided by the two standard deviations) between the two variables representing the strength of their relationship.

FORMULAS FOR DESCRIPTIVE STATISTICS FROM CHAPTER 3

Mean. μ (population mean) and m (sample mean). (m is sometimes seen as the variable from which it is calculated with an overbar, as $\bar{x}$.)

$$\mu \text{ or } m = \sum x/n. \tag{3.1}$$

Median. Algorithm for the *median* (sometimes *md*) in words rather than in symbols:

- Put the n observations in order of size.
- *Median* is the middle observation if n is odd.
- *Median* is the halfway between the two middle observations if n is even.

Mode. Algorithm for approximate *mode* (sometimes *mo*) in words rather than in symbols (n must be large), depending on the bar chart's interval widths and start point:

- Make a bar chart of the data.
- *Mode* is the center value of the highest bar.

Variance. Population:

$$\sigma^2 = \frac{\sum x^2 - n\mu^2}{n}. \tag{3.2}$$

Variance. Sample:

$$s^2 = \frac{\sum x^2 - nm^2}{n-1}. \tag{3.3}$$

Standard Deviation σ or s. Square roots of the respective variance.

Standard Error of the Mean (SEM). Population (where σ appears) or sample (where s appears):

$$\sigma_m = \sigma/\sqrt{n} \quad \text{or} \quad s_m = s/\sqrt{n}. \tag{3.4}$$

Covariance between x and y. Population:

$$\sigma_{xy} = \frac{\sum xy - n\mu_x\mu_y}{n}. \tag{3.5}$$

Covariance between x and y. Sample:

$$s_{xy} = \frac{\sum xy - nm_x m_y}{n-1}. \tag{3.6}$$

Correlation Coefficient between x and y. Population (where ρ appears) or sample (where r appears):

$$\rho_{xy} = \frac{\sigma_{xy}}{\sigma_x\sigma_y} \quad \text{or} \quad r_{xy} = \frac{s_{xy}}{s_x s_y}. \tag{3.7}$$

Standard Error of the Mean (SEM) for Two Samples from the Same Population. Population standard deviation (σ) known:

$$\sigma_m = \sigma\sqrt{\frac{1}{n_1} + \frac{1}{n_2}}. \tag{3.8}$$

Population standard deviation unknown; sample standard deviations s_1 and s_2:

$$s_p = \sqrt{\frac{(n_1 - 1)s_1^2 + (n_2 - 1)s_2^2}{n_1 + n_2 - 2}} \tag{3.9}$$

and

$$s_m = s_p\sqrt{\frac{1}{n_1} + \frac{1}{n_2}}. \tag{3.10}$$

SUMMARY OF CONFIDENCE INTERVALS AND PROBABILITY FOR CHAPTER 4

General Forms for Confidence Intervals

Confidence Interval on an Individual Observation. The probability that a randomly drawn observation from a given probability distribution is contained in a specified interval is given by the area of the distribution under the curve over that interval.

Confidence Interval on a Statistic. The probability that a population statistic from a distribution of estimates of that statistic is contained in a specified interval is given by the area of the distribution over that interval. The common format for a confidence interval on a statistic is P[lower critical value < population statistic < upper critical value] $= 1 - \alpha$.

CONFIDENCE INTERVAL ON A MEAN, KNOWN σ

A mean from a normal distribution uses the standard normal distribution, arising from $z = (x - \mu)/\sigma$.

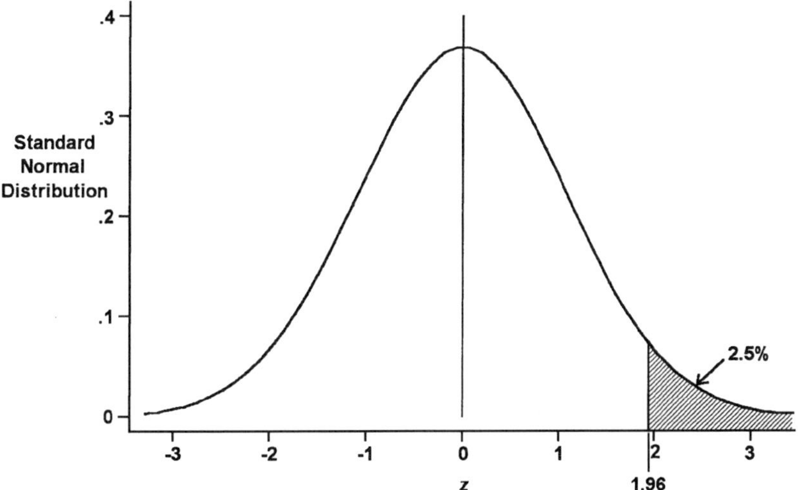

Figure 4.1 A standard normal distribution shown with a 2.5% α and its corresponding $z = 1.96$. The α shown is the area under the curve to the right of a given or calculated z. For a two-tailed computation, α is doubled in order to include the symmetric opposite tail. A two-tailed $\alpha = 5\%$ lies outside the ± 1.96 interval, leaving 95% of the area under the curve between the tails.

Form of a confidence interval on a mean, known σ:

$$\mathrm{P}[m - z_{1-\alpha/2}\sigma_m < \mu < m + z_{1-\alpha/2}\sigma_m] = 1 - \alpha. \tag{4.5}$$

CONFIDENCE INTERVAL ON A MEAN, σ ESTIMATED BY s

A mean with σ estimated by s uses the t distribution, arising from $z = (x - \mu)/s$ (see overleaf). Form of a confidence interval on a mean, σ estimated by s:

$$\mathrm{P}[m - t_{1-\alpha/2}s_m < \mu < m + t_{1-\alpha/2}s_m] = 1 - \alpha. \tag{4.6}$$

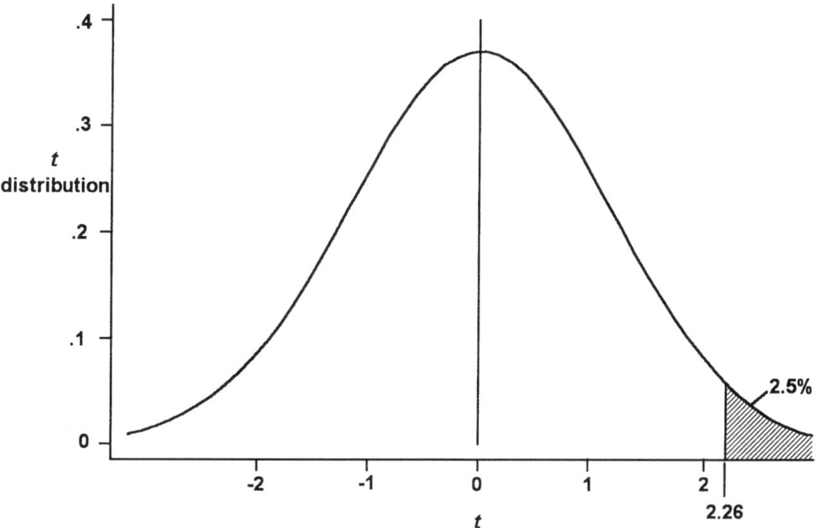

Figure 4.2 A t distribution shown with $\alpha = 2.5\%$ and its corresponding t for 9 *df*. The α shown is the area under the curve to the right of a given or calculated t. For a two-tailed computation, α is doubled in order to include the symmetric opposite tail. As pictured for 9 *df*, 2.5% of the area lies to the right of $t = 2.26$. For a two-tailed use, the frequently used $\alpha = 5\%$ lies outside the interval $\pm t$, leaving 95% of the area under the curve between the tails.

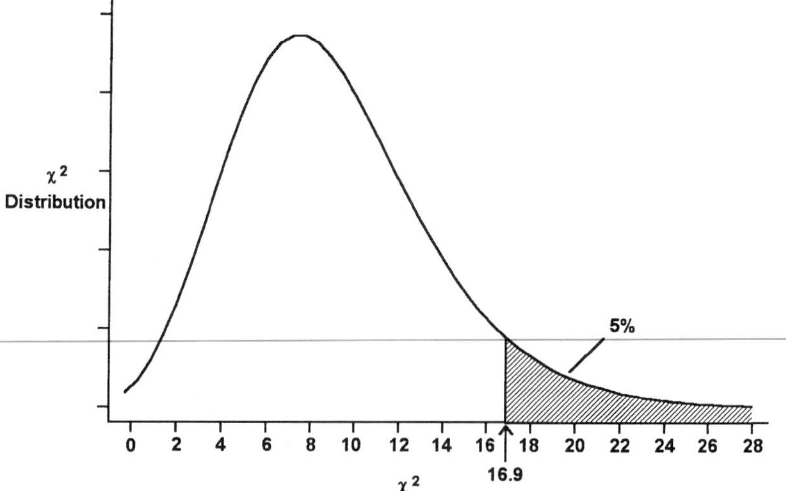

Figure 4.3 The χ^2 (chi-square) distribution for 9 *df* with a 5% α and its corresponding chi-square value of 16.9. The α probability is shown as the shaded area under the curve to the right of a critical chi-square, in this case representing a 5% probability that a value drawn randomly from the distribution will exceed a critical chi-square of 16.9.

Confidence Interval on a Variance or Standard Deviation

A variance uses the chi-square distribution, arising from $\chi^2 = s^2 \times df/\sigma^2$. Form of a confidence interval on σ^2:

$$P\left[s^2 \times df/\chi^2_R < \sigma^2 < s^2 \times df/\chi^2_L\right] = 1 - \alpha, \tag{4.7}$$

where χ^2_R is the right tail critical value (use Table C) and χ^2_L the left (use Table D). Form of a confidence interval on σ: Same as Eq. (4.7) but with square roots of components within the brackets.

CONCEPTS AND PROCEDURES IN HYPOTHESIS TESTING FROM CHAPTER 5

Common Assumptions in Hypothesis Testing

The Assumption of Independence. All tests assume that "errors" (understood as "deviations from typical") in sample data are independent one from each other. This is a major reason for random sampling.

The Assumption of Normality of Errors. Many, but not all, tests also assume that these errors are drawn from a normal distribution. A major exception is rank-order tests.

The Assumption of Equality of Variability. A third assumption made frequently in tests comparing two or more sample statistics is that the standard deviations (or variances) of the errors are the same.

Types and Probabilities of Error

Here, "error" is used in the more traditional sense: making the wrong decision.

Type I (α) Error, the p-Value. The null hypothesis is rejected when it should not have been, occurring with probability α. After the acceptance-or-rejection decision is made, this error is termed a *false positive* and the data-dependent estimate of α is the *p-value*.

Type II (β) Error, Power of a Test. The null hypothesis is accepted when it should have been rejected, occurring with probability β. After the acceptance-or-rejection decision is made, this error is termed a *false negative*. $1 - \beta$ is termed the *power* of the test.

Table 5.1

Relationships among Types of Error and Their Probabilities as Dependent on the Decision and the Truth

		Decision	
		H_0 true	H_0 false
Truth	H_0 true	Correct decision True negative (probability $1 - \alpha$)	Type I error False positive (probability α)
	H_0 false	Type II error False negative (probability β)	Correct decision True positive (probability $1 - \beta$)

Steps in Setting up a Test

(1) Write down the question you will ask of your data. (Does treating my infected patients with a particular antibiotic make them healthy again?)

(2) Select the variable(s) on which you can obtain data that you believe best highlight the contrasts in the question. (I think WBC will best show the state of health.)

(3) Select the descriptor of the distribution of the variable that will furnish the contrast, e.g., mean, standard deviation. (Mean WBC will furnish the most telling contrast.)

(4) Write down the null and alternate hypotheses indicated by the contrast. (H_0: $\mu_a = \mu_h$; H_1: $\mu_a \neq \mu_h$, where a represents patients treated with antibiotics and h, healthy patients.)

(5) Write down a detailed, comprehensive sentence describing the population(s) measured by the variable involved in that question. (The healthy population is the set of people who have no current or chronic infections affecting their WBC. The treated population is the set of people who have the infection being treated and no other current or chronic infection affecting their WBC.)

(6) Write down a detailed, comprehensive sentence describing the sample(s) from which your data on the variable will be drawn. [My sample is selected randomly from patients presenting to my clinic passing my exclusion screen (other infections, etc.).]

(7) Ask yourself what biases might emerge from any distinctions between the makeup of the sample(s) and the population(s). Could this infection be worse for one age, sex, cultural origin, etc., of patient than another? Are the samples representative of the populations with respect to the variable being recorded? (I have searched and found studies that show that mortality and recovery rates, and

therefore probably WBC, are the same for different sexes and cultural groups. One might infer that the elderly have begun to compromise their immune systems, so I stratify my sample to assure that my sample reflects the age distribution at large.)

(8) Recycle steps 1–7 until you are satisfied that all steps are fully consistent one with one another.

(9) In terms of the variable descriptors and hypotheses being used, choose the most appropriate statistical test and select the α level you will accept.

(10) Verify that you have an adequate sample size to answer the question.

CONCEPTS AND PROCEDURES IN HYPOTHESIS TESTING FROM CHAPTER 6

CONTINGENCY TESTS ON 2 × 2 TABLES

Contingency Table of Prediction versus Truth Showing *n* Symbols for Cell Counts, Marginal Totals, and Grand Total

		Prediction		
		Yes	No	Totals
Truth	Yes	n_{11}	n_{12}	$n_{1\cdot}$
	No	n_{21}	n_{22}	$n_{2\cdot}$
	Totals	$n_{\cdot 1}$	$n_{\cdot 2}$	n (or $n_{\cdot\cdot}$)

Chi-Square Test of Contingency to Test Independence. The expected value of a cell is

$$e_{ij} = \frac{n_{\cdot i} n_{\cdot j}}{n} \tag{6.1}$$

The chi-square statistic with one degree of freedom is calculated by

$$\chi^2 = \sum_i^2 \sum_i^2 \frac{(|n_{ij} - e_{ij}| - 0.5)^2}{e_{ij}}, \tag{6.2}$$

where the 0.5 term is a continuity correction. The critical value of χ^2 is found for the chosen α from the $df = 1$ line of Table C. If χ^2 is larger than the critical value, reject H_0.

Risks and Odds in Medical Decisions

Table 6.6

Truth Table Showing Counts of the Prediction of Presence or Absence of a Malady as Related to the Truth of That Presence or Absence

		Prediction (Exposure or test result)		
		Have disease	Do not have	
TRUTH	Have disease	n_{11} True positive	n_{12} False negative	$n_{1\cdot}$ (Yes)
	Do not have	n_{21} False positive	n_{22} True negative	$n_{2\cdot}$ (No)
		$n_{\cdot 1}$ (Predict yes)	$n_{\cdot 2}$ (Predict no)	n (or $n_{\cdot\cdot}$)

Table 6.8 (Reduced)

Concepts of False Positive and Negative, Sensitivity, Specificity, Accuracy, and Odds Ratio Based on Sample Error Rates Arising from the Format of Table 6.6[a]

Values found from a sample truth table		Population definitions of probabilities and odds of values being estimated	
Names of estimates	Sample computing formulas	Definitions	Relationships
False positive sample rate (p-value)	$n_{21}/n_{2\cdot}$	Probability of a false positive (α)	P(predict yes|no)
False negative sample rate	$n_{12}/n_{1\cdot}$	Probability of a false negative (β)	P(predict no|yes)
Sensitivity	$n_{11}/n_{1\cdot}$	Probability of a true positive: *power* $(1-\beta)$	P(predict yes|yes)
Specificity	$n_{22}/n_{2\cdot}$	Probability of a true negative $(1-\alpha)$	P(predict no|no)
Accuracy	$(n_{11}+n_{22})/n_{\cdot\cdot}$	Overall probability of a correct decision	P(predict no|no or yes|yes)
Odds ratio (OR)	$\frac{n_{11}/n_{21}}{n_{12}/n_{22}}$ or $n_{11}n_{22}/n_{12}n_{21}$	Odds of a disease when predicted in ratio to odds of the disease when not predicted	$\frac{\text{Ratio(yes/no\|predicted yes)}}{\text{Ratio(yes/no\|predicted no)}}$

[a] The third and fourth columns show the population entities these values are estimating.

Rank-Sum Test to Compare Two Samples

Steps in Rank-Sum Test Using Table I.

1. Sample sizes are n_1 and n_2; n_1 is the smaller. If $n_2 > 8$, use the normal approximation.
2. Rank combined data, keeping track of the sample from which each datum arose.
3. Add up the ranks of the data from the smaller sample and name it T.
4. Calculate $U = n_1 n_2 + n_1(n_1 + 1)/2 - T$.
5. Look up p-value from Table I and use it to accept or reject the null hypothesis.

Normal Approximation to Rank-Sum Test.

1. Follow steps 1–3.
2. Calculate $\mu = n_1(n_1 + n_2 + 1)/2$, $\sigma^2 = n_1 n_2(n_1 + n_2 + 1)/12$, and $z = (T - \mu)/\sigma$.
3. Find the normal critical value from Table A. If z is larger than the critical value, reject H_0.

Normal or *t* Test to Compare Two Sample Means

If σ is known or estimated from a large sample, use the normal test. If σ is estimated by s from a small sample, use the t test with $n_1 + n_2 - 2$ degrees of freedom. Calculate

$$z = (m_1 - m_2)/\sigma_d,$$

where

$$\sigma_d = \sigma\sqrt{\frac{1}{n_1} + \frac{1}{n_2}},$$

or

$$t = (m_1 - m_2)/s_d,$$

where

$$s_d = \sqrt{\left(\frac{1}{n_1} + \frac{1}{n_2}\right)\left[\frac{(n_1 - 1)s_1^2 + (n_2 - 1)s_2^2}{n_1 + n_2 - 2}\right]}.$$

Reject H_0 if z or t is larger than the critical z from Table A or the critical t from Table B.

CONCEPTS AND FORMULAS FOR SAMPLE SIZE FROM CHAPTER 7

Concept of Choosing Sample Size for a Means Test

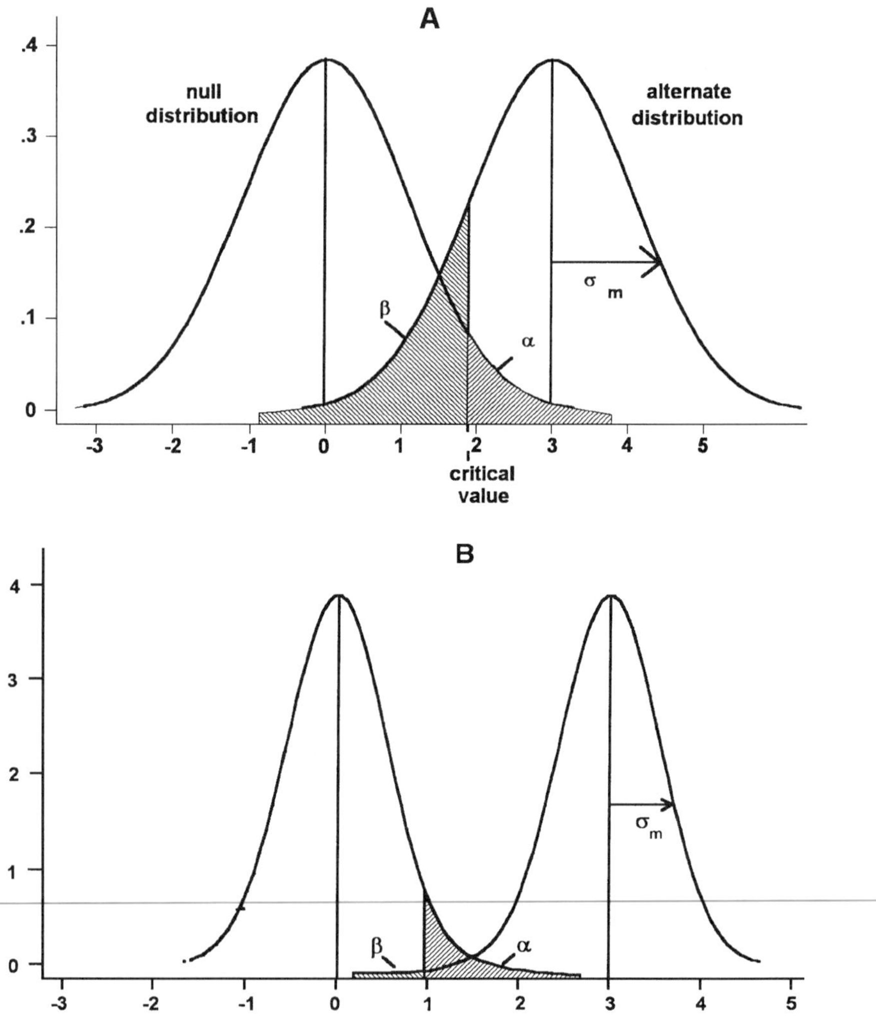

Figure 7.1 Distributions for null and alternate hypotheses in a test of means (A) with sizes of associated error probabilities indicated by shaded areas (see Section 5.2). If the sample size is quadrupled, $\sigma_m = \sigma/\sqrt{n}$ shrinks to half the size, yielding an equivalent diagram (B) with more slender curves. Note how much β has shrunk for a fixed α. The method of estimating a minimum sample size to yield specified error sizes for detecting a given distance between means is to start with those error sizes and that distance and "back-solve" the relationships to find the associated n.

Formula to Calculate Minimum Required Sample Size for a Test of Means

Substitute error risks α and β, estimated standard deviation σ^2, and clinically important deviation d of sample mean m from theoretical mean μ in the equation to solve for n:

$$n = \frac{(z_{1-\alpha/2} + z_{1-\beta})^2 \sigma^2}{d^2}.$$

For two means, substitute α, β, the two standard deviation estimates, and $d = m_1 - m_2$ in

$$n_1 = n_2 = \frac{(z_{1-\alpha/2} + z_{1-\beta})^2 \left(\sigma_1^2 + \sigma_2^2\right)}{d^2}.$$

FORMULAS AND RELATIONSHIPS OF STATISTICAL PREDICTION FROM CHAPTER 8

Regression

The purpose is to predict a dependent variable y from an independent variable x. From analytic geometry, the point–slope form for a point (x_1, y_1) and slope b_1 is $y - y_1 = b_1(x - x_1)$. We choose the joint mean (m_x, m_y) as the point, and the best fit slope is shown to be

$$b_1 = \frac{s_{xy}}{s_x^2} = \frac{\text{cov}(x, y)}{sd(x)sd(x)}.$$

This yields a straight line regression fit as

$$y - m_y = \frac{s_{xy}}{s_x^2}(x - m_x).$$

Assumptions: Errors in y are independent from each other; x is measured without error; and the standard deviation in y is the same for all x.

Correlation as Related to Regression

Because the sample correlation coefficient r is

$$r = \frac{s_{xy}}{s_x s_y} = \frac{\text{cov}(x, y)}{sd(x)sd(y)},$$

the relationship between the slope of the regression line and the correlation coefficient is

$$r = b_1 \frac{s_x}{s_y}.$$

The implication is as follows. The closer the slope of the regression line is to 45°, the greater the relationship between x and y. The tighter the envelope of data points about the plot of the correlation, the greater the relationship between x and y.

Also, the square of the correlation coefficient, r^2, indicates the proportion of the possible causal influence on y by x; the closer r^2 is to 1.0, the better x is as a predictor of y. This statistic is termed the *coefficient of determination*. It usually is written R^2 because it largely is used with multiple independent variables.

Outcomes Analysis

The concept of examining the total impact of a treatment on a patient (is the patient's quality of life improved?) rather than a single clinical indicator (is platelet count increased?) is termed *outcomes analysis*. The approach is to find a *measure of effectiveness (MOE)*, usually a combination of indicators, that represents a total influence on the patient.

DEFINITIONS AND FORMULAS FOR EPIDEMIOLOGY FROM CHAPTER 9

Incidence rate of a disease: the rate at which new cases of the disease occur.

Prevalence rate: the proportion having that disease at a point in time.

Mortality rate: the rate at which the population is dying rather than becoming ill.

If n denotes the number of individuals in the epidemiological population,
n_{new} denotes the number of new cases in a specified interval,
$n_{present}$ denotes the number of cases present at any one point in time, and
n_{dying} denotes the number dying during the specified interval, then

Incidence rate is

$$I = 1000 \times \frac{n_{new}}{n}.$$

Prevalence rate is

$$P = 1000 \times \frac{n_{present}}{n}.$$

Mortality rate is

$$M = 1000 \times \frac{n_{dying}}{n}.$$

Odds ratio (OR) is

$$\frac{\text{Odds of a disease given a characteristic}}{\text{Odds of the disease given not the characteristic}}.$$

Life tables provide the proportion surviving at the end of an associated interval. (Also, the probability that any randomly chosen member alive at the outset will survive longer than the end of that interval.)

The first six lines of an infant malaria morbidity table are shown to illustrate the format:

Interval (weeks)	Begin	Died	Lost	End	S (survival)
0 (outset)	155	0	0	155	1.0000
>0–13	155	14	0	141	0.9097
>13–26	141	23	0	118	0.7613
	118	0	3	115	
>26–39	115	17	0	98	0.6488

A survival curve shows numbers survived and lost to follow up (censored) by interval. A survival curve for infant malaria morbidity data is shown to illustrate the format:

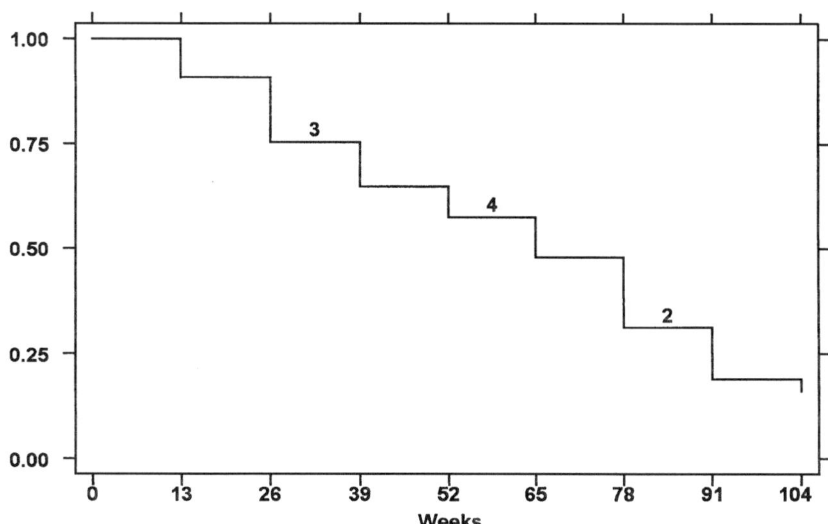

Criteria of evidence supporting causality:

(1) Size of effect. Relative risk >2.0.
(2) Strength of association. p-value <0.05.

(3) Consistency of association. Reproducible effect.
(4) Specificity of association. Effect from a single cause.
(5) Temporality. Cause precedes effect.
(6) Biologic gradient. Evidence of dose–response effect.
(7) Biologic plausibility. Reasonable explanatory model.

STEPS IN READING ARTICLES AND PLANNING STUDIES FROM CHAPTER 10

FINDING AND ORGANIZING MEDICAL INFORMATION FROM AN ARTICLE

Ways to Improve Efficiency in Reading Medical Articles:

(1) Allow enough time to *think* about the article.
(2) Identify the central question and read with this in mind.
(3) Think about how you would have attacked the problem posed.
(4) Verify that the author has specified goals, selected variables and descriptive statistics that satisfy the goals, chosen null and alternate hypotheses and error risks, described population, sample, and how biases were avoided, demonstrated that sample size was adequate, used appropriate statistical methods, and logically passed from goals through data and analyses to conclusions.
(5) Read the article repeatedly.
(6) Plan a revision to the study that would avoid any flaws you find.

SOME BIOSTATISTICAL ASPECTS OF ARTICLES TO WATCH FOR

(1) Confusion of statistical and clinical significance.
(2) Violation of assumptions upon which statistical methods are based.
(3) Generalization from a biased or poorly behaved sample to the population.
(4) Failure to define data formats, symbols, or statistical terms not obvious from the context.
(5) Use of multiple related tests leading to a cumulative p-value.

META-ANALYSIS

A Meta-analysis Should Be Developed as Follows:

(1) Define the inclusion–exclusion criteria for admitting articles.

(2) Search exhaustively and locate all articles addressing the issue.
(3) Assess the articles against the criteria.
(4) Quantify the admitted variables on common scales.
(5) Aggregate the admitted data bases through an organized scheme.

Biases That May Infiltrate an Integrative Literature Review:

(1) Data on which conclusions are based are not given or even summarized.
(2) Some of the studies were carried out with insufficient scientific rigor.
(3) No-result findings are absent, leading to overestimation of the success of an approach.

Criteria for an Acceptable Meta-analysis:

(1) The study objectives were identified clearly.
(2) Inclusion criteria of articles and data were established prior to selection.
(3) An active effort was made to find and include all relevant articles.
(4) An assessment of publication bias was made.
(5) Specific data used were identified.
(6) Assessment of article comparability (controls, circumstances, etc.) was made.
(7) The meta-analysis was reported in enough detail to allow replication.

Planning a Study

(1) Start with objectives. Do not start with the abstract.
(2) Develop the background from prior studies and relevance. (What will it contribute?)
(3) Plan your materials, methods, and data and their integration in conducting the study.
(4) Define your population. Verify representative sampling. Assure adequate sample size.
(5) Anticipate what statistical analysis will yield results that will satisfy your objectives.
(6) Plan the bridge from results to conclusions (the discussion).
(7) Anticipate the form in which your conclusions will be expressed.
(8) Now write the abstract, summarizing all of the foregoing in half a page or so.
(9) After drafting this terse summary, review steps 1–8 and revise as required.

Some Mechanisms to Facilitate Study Planning

(1) *Work backward through the Logical Process.* (a) What conclusions are needed to answer these questions? (b) What data results and how many data will I need to reach these conclusions? (c) What statistical methods will I need to obtain these results? (d) What is the nature and format of the data I need to apply these statistical methods? (e) What is the design and conduct of the study I need to obtain these data? (f) And, finally, what is the ambiance in the literature that leads to the need for this study in general and this design in particular?

(2) *Analyze Dummy Data.* Make up representative numbers and analyze them.

(3) *Play the Role of Devil's Advocate.* Criticize your work as if you were a reviewer.

A First-Step Guide to Choosing Tests

Table 10.1 Appears inside the Back Cover. It provides "first-aid" in selecting a statistical test for a given set of conditions. The method of selection is explained in the table's caption.

Ethics in Study Design

Keep the Patient in Mind. The design of studies affects not only scientific knowledge but also patients. A study affects two groups of patients: those used in the study and the future patient who will be affected by the study results.

What Affects the Patient. (a) The choice of the clinically important difference δ between a sample and a population characteristic (e.g., a mean) or between that of two samples. (b) The choice of α, the risk of a false positive. (c) The choice of β, the risk of a false negative. (d) The ratio of α to β. (e) The sidedness of the test chosen. (f) The sample size chosen.

Verify That the Study Will Not Affect Patients in Unanticipated Ways. After the study is planned to satisfy scientific and statistical design criteria, review the study design with both current and future patients in mind. If the design will affect either group in an undesirable way, revise the design as necessary to eliminate undesirable aspects.

REFERENCE FOR TABLES FROM CHAPTER 11

The distributions from which Tables A–G are obtained appear here. (Tables H and I are specialty tables from Chapter 14 on rank-order methods.)

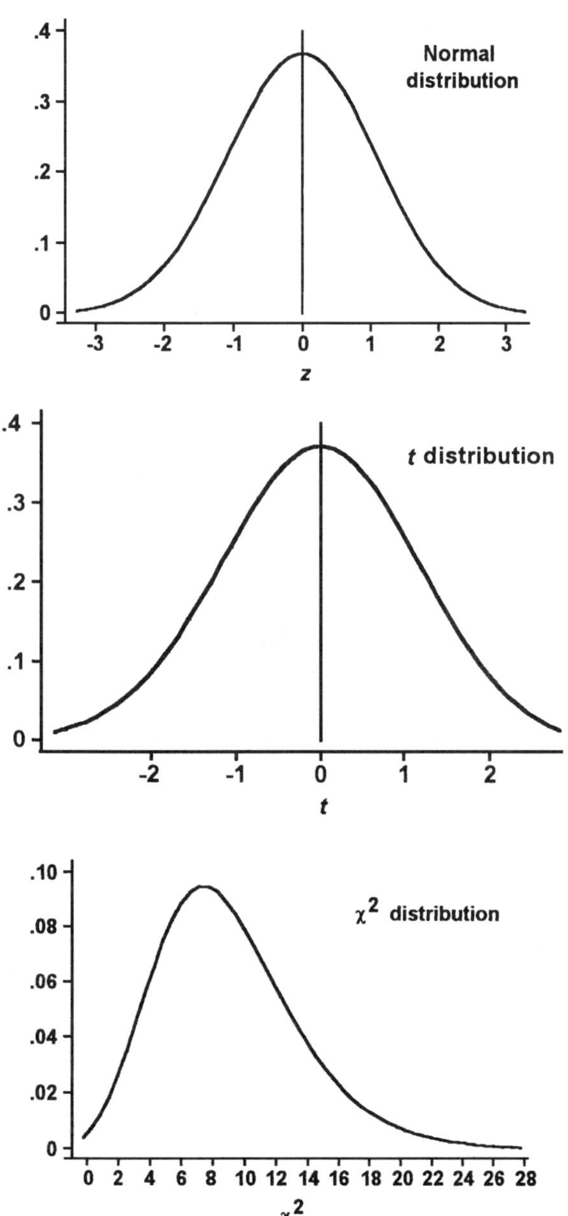

Normal distribution
.4
.3
.2
.1
0
-3 -2 -1 0 1 2 3
z
t distribution
.4
.3
.2
.1
0
-2 -1 0 1 2
t
χ^2 distribution
.10
.08
.06
.04
.02
0
0 2 4 6 8 10 12 14 16 18 20 22 24 26 28
χ^2

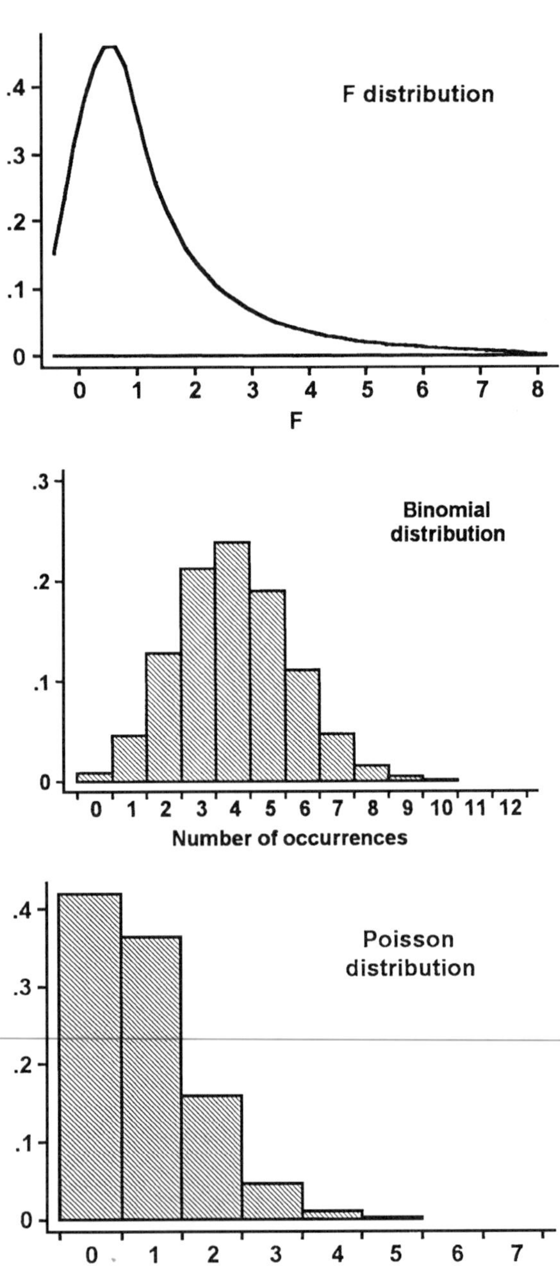
F distribution
.4
.3
.2
.1
0
0 1 2 3 4 5 6 7 8
F
Binomial distribution
.3
.2
.1
0
0 1 2 3 4 5 6 7 8 9 10 11 12
Number of occurrences
Poisson distribution
.4
.3
.2
.1
0
0 1 2 3 4 5 6 7
Number of occurrences

FORMULAS FOR CONFIDENCE INTERVALS FROM CHAPTER 12

General Form of Confidence Interval on a Statistic:

The probability
that a population statistic
from a distribution of estimates of that statistic
is contained in a specified interval
is given by
the area of the distribution over that interval (12.1)

or

$$P[\text{lower critical value} < \text{population statistic} < \text{upper critical value}] = 1 - \alpha. \quad (12.2)$$

$1 - \alpha$ *Confidence Interval on a Mean, Known (Population) Standard Deviation* σ:

$$P[m - z_{1-\alpha/2}\sigma_m < \mu < m + z_{1-\alpha/2}\sigma_m] = 1 - \alpha. \quad (12.3)$$

Above Interval for 95% Confidence:

$$P[m - 1.96\sigma_m < \mu < m + 1.96\sigma_m] = 0.95. \quad (12.4)$$

$1 - \alpha$ *Confidence Interval on a Mean, Estimated (Sample) Standard Deviation* s:

$$P[m - t_{1-\alpha/2}s_m < \mu < m + t_{1-\alpha/2}s_m] = 1 - \alpha. \quad (12.7)$$

$1 - \alpha$ *Confidence Interval on a Variance or Standard Deviation:*

$$P\left[s^2 \times df/\chi^2_R < \sigma^2 < s^2 \times df/\chi^2_L\right] = 1 - \alpha, \quad (12.8)$$

where χ^2_R is Table C area under right tail of chi-square and χ^2_L is Table D area under left tail. For a confidence interval on the standard deviation, take the square root of each component within the brackets in Eq. (12.8).

Confidence Interval on a Proportion: If π, the unknown population proportion, is not near 0 or 1, calculate the sample proportion p and $\sigma = \sqrt{[p(1-p)/n]}$ and substitute to obtain

$$P[p - 1.96\sigma - 1/2n < \pi < p + 1.96\sigma + 1/2n] = 0.95. \quad (12.9)$$

If π is near 0 or 1, substitute p and $\sigma = \sqrt{(p/n)}$ to obtain

$$P[p - 1.96\sigma < \pi < p + 1.96\sigma] = 0.95. \quad (12.10)$$

If confidence other than 95% is desired, replace 1.96 as appropriate from Table A.

Confidence Interval on a Correlation Coefficient: The normal-transformed correlation coefficient has mean and standard deviation

$$m = \frac{1}{2}\ln\left(\frac{1+r}{1-r}\right) \tag{12.11}$$

and

$$\sigma = \frac{1}{\sqrt{n-3}}. \tag{12.12}$$

A $1-\alpha$ (e.g., 95%) confidence interval is

$$\mathrm{P}\left[\frac{1+r-(1-r)e^{\frac{2z_{1-\alpha/2}}{\sqrt{n-3}}}}{1+r+(1-r)e^{\frac{2z_{1-\alpha/2}}{\sqrt{n-3}}}} < \rho < \frac{1+r-(1-r)e^{-\frac{2z_{1-\alpha/2}}{\sqrt{n-3}}}}{1+r+(1-r)e^{-\frac{2z_{1-\alpha/2}}{\sqrt{n-3}}}}\right] = 1-\alpha. \tag{12.13}$$

FORMULAS FOR TESTS OF CATEGORIES FROM CHAPTER 13

TRUTH TABLE, SHOWING FREQUENCIES n_{ij}

		Prediction		
		Yes	No	
Truth	Yes	n_{11} (Correct decision)	n_{12} (Type II error)	n_1 (Truly yes)
	No	n_{21} (Type I error)	n_{22} (Correct decision)	n_2 (Truly no)
		n_1 (Predict yes)	n_2 (Predict no)	n (or $n_{..}$)

CONTINGENCY TABLES, $r \times c$ (FISHER–IRWIN AND CHI-SQUARE TESTS)

A 2×2 table is a special case for $r = c = 2$. $\mathrm{H_0}$:Row variable independent of column variable. The Fisher–Irwin (Fisher's exact) test and its p-value are calculated by a statistical software package for small r and c. If $r + c > 7$, every $e_{ij} \geq 1$, and every $n_{ij} \geq 5$, Table C gives the p-value (looked up like α) from a chi-square statistic with $(r-1)(c-1)$ *df*, where $e_{ij} = n_{i\cdot} \times n_{\cdot j} \div n$, using

$$\chi^2 = \sum_i^r \sum_j^c \frac{(|n_{ij} - e_{ij}| - 0.5)^2}{e_{ij}}. \tag{13.3}$$

Risks and Odds in Medical Decisions

Names of sample estimates	Sample formulas	Population definitions of parameters being estimated	Relationships (Y: yes; N: no)
False positive rate (p-value)	$n_{21}/n_{2\cdot}$	P(false positive): α	P(predict Y|N)
False negative rate	$n_{12}/n_{1\cdot}$	P(false negative): β	P(predict N|Y)
Sensitivity	$n_{11}/n_{1\cdot}$	P(true positive): $1-\beta$	P(predict Y|Y)
Specificity	$n_{22}/n_{2\cdot}$	P(true negative): $1-\alpha$	P(predict N|N)
Accuracy	$(n_{11}+n_{22})/n$	Overall P(correct decision)	P(predict N|N or Y|Y)
Positive predictive value	$n_{11}/n_{\cdot 1}$	P(positive prediction is correct)	P(Y|predicted Y)
Negative predictive value	$n_{22}/n_{\cdot 2}$	P(negative prediction is correct)	P(N|predicted N)
Relative risk (RR)	$n_{11}n_{\cdot 2}/n_{12}n_{\cdot 1}$	P(disease predicted) in ratio to P(disease not)	$\frac{\text{P(Y\|predicted Y)}}{\text{P(Y\|predicted N)}}$
Odds ratio (OR)	$n_{11}n_{22}/n_{12}n_{21}$	Odds of a disease predicted in ratio to odds of the disease not predicted.	$\frac{\text{ratio(Y/N\|predicted Y)}}{\text{ratio(Y/N\|predicted N)}}$
Likelihood ratio (LR)	$n_{11}n_{2\cdot}/n_{21}n_{1\cdot}$	P(correctly predicting disease) in ratio to P(incorrectly predicting)	$\frac{\text{P(predictY\|Y)}}{\text{P(predictY\|N)}}$

ROC Curves. A receiver operating characteristic (ROC) curve displays rate of true positive (vertical axis) against rate of false positive (horizontal axis). It can help choose the best (weighted if desired) critical value for a medical decision (sensitivity-to-specificity trade-off). It can help choose the better predictor of two risk factors.

Tests of Association

Log Odds Ratio (L) Test. H_0:L = a hypothesized log odds ratio λ ($\lambda = 0$ if the category types are independent) is tested by

$$\chi^2 = [(L-\lambda)/\text{SEL}]^2, \tag{13.6}$$

where

$$L = \ln[(n_{11}+0.5)(n_{22}+0.5)/(n_{12}+0.5)(n_{21}+0.5)] \tag{13.4}$$

with standard error

$$\text{SEL} = \sqrt{[(1/(n_{11}+0.5)) + (1/(n_{12}+0.5)) + (1/(n_{21}+0.5)) + (1/(n_{22}+0.5))]}. \tag{13.5}$$

Table C using 1 *df* gives the p-value (looked up like α).

Attributable Risk. $(n_{11}/n_{21}) - (n_{12}/n_{22})$ estimates clinical relevance as the increased probability in predicting the outcome characteristic from a positive risk factor over a negative risk factor.

Test of a Proportion π Not close to 0 (π Estimated by Sample Proportion $p_s = n_s/n$)

Small Sample (Binomial Calculation). $H_0{:}p_s = \pi$. Table F gives the p-value, the probability that $p_s > \pi$ by chance alone.

Large Sample (Normal Approximation). $H_0{:}p_s = \pi, n \geq 5/\pi$. Table A gives the two-tailed p-value (looked up as if it were α) for

$$z = \frac{|p_s - \pi| - \frac{1}{2n}}{\sqrt{\pi(1-\pi)/n}}. \tag{13.8}$$

Test of a Proportion π near 0 (π Estimated by Sample Proportion $p_s = n_s/n$)

Small Sample (Poisson Approximation). $H_0{:}p_s = \pi, \pi$ is near $0, n \gg n\pi \gg \pi$. $\lambda = n\pi$. Table G gives probability that $p_s > \pi$ by chance alone (p-value), given n_s and λ.

Large Sample (Normal Approximation). $\lambda > 9$. $H_0{:}p_s = \pi, \pi$ near $0, n \gg n\pi \gg \pi$. $\lambda = n\pi$. Table A gives p-value (looked up as if it were α) for

$$z = (p_s - \pi)\sqrt{(n/\pi)}. \tag{13.9}$$

Matched Pair Sample (McNemar's Test)

To test a certain characteristic for association with a disease, pair n diseased and n control patients. b = number of cases with disease yes but control no and c = number of cases with disease no but control yes. Calculate chi-square with 1 *df*. Table C gives the p-value (looked up like α).

$$\chi^2_{1\,df} = (|b-c| - 1)^2/(b+c). \tag{13.10}$$

FORMULAS FOR TESTS OF RANKS FROM CHAPTER 14

Single or Paired Small Samples: The Signed-Rank Test

Hypothesis: median difference = 0. It may test (1) observations deviating from a hypothetical common value or (2) pairs on the same individuals, as before-and-after data.

1. Calculate the differences of the observations as in (1) or (2).
2. Rank the magnitudes (i.e., the differences without signs).
3. Reattach the signs to the ranks.
4. Add up the positive and negative ranks.
5. Denote by T the unsigned value of the smaller sum of ranks.
6. Look up the p-value for the test in Table H. If $n > 12$, use the normal approximation.

Two Small Samples: The Rank-Sum Test

Think of it informally as testing whether the two distributions have the same median.

1. Name the sizes of the two samples n_1 and n_2; n_1 is the smaller.
2. Combine the data, keeping track of the sample from which each datum arose.
3. Rank the data.
4. Add up the ranks of the data from the smaller sample and name it T.
5. Calculate $U = n_1 n_2 + n_1(n_1 + 1)/2 - T$.
6. Look up the p-value from Table I and use it to accept or reject the null hypothesis. (Table I gives two-tailed error probabilities.)

Three or More Independent Samples: The Kruskal–Wallis Test

Just the rank-sum test extended. Think of it informally as testing whether the distributions have the same median. The χ^2 approximation requires five or more members per sample.

1. Name the number of samples m (3 or 4 or ...).
2. Name the sizes of the several samples $n_1, n_2, \ldots, n_m$; n is the grand total.

3. Combine the data, keeping track of the sample from which each datum arose.
4. Rank the data.
5. Add up the ranks of the data from each sample separately.
6. Name the sums $T_1, T_2, \ldots, T_m$.
7. Calculate the Kruskal–Wallis H statistic, which is distributed as chi-square, by

$$H = \frac{12}{n(n+1)}\left(\frac{T_1^2}{n_1} + \frac{T_2^2}{n_2} + \cdots + \frac{T_m^2}{n_m}\right) - 3(n+1) \qquad (14.1)$$

Obtain the p-value (as if it were α) from Table C (χ^2 right tail) for $m - 1$ degrees of freedom.

THREE OR MORE "PAIRED" SAMPLES: THE FRIEDMAN TEST

An extension of the paired-data concept. In the example, a dermatologist applied three skin patches to test for an allergy to each of eight patients. Hypothesis: the several treatments have the same distributions. Requires five or more patients.

1. Name the number of treatments k (3 or 4 or ...) and of blocks (e.g., patients) n.
2. Rank the data within each block (e.g., rank the treatment outcomes for each patient).
3. Add the ranks for each treatment separately; name the sums $T_1, T_2, \ldots, T_k$.
4. Calculate the Friedman F_r statistic, which is distributed as chi-square, by

$$F_r = \frac{12}{nk(k+1)}\left(T_1^2 + T_2^2 + \cdots + T_k^2\right) - 3n(k+1) \qquad (14.2)$$

5. Obtain the p-value (as if it were α) from Table C (χ^2 right tail) for $k - 1$ degrees of freedom.

SINGLE LARGE SAMPLES: THE NORMAL APPROXIMATION TO THE SIGNED-RANK TEST

Hypothesis: median difference = 0. It may test (1) observations deviating from a hypothetical common value or (2) pairs on the same individuals, as before-and-after data.

1. Calculate the differences of the observations as in (1) or (2).

2. Rank the magnitudes (i.e., the differences without signs).
3. Reattach the signs to the ranks.
4. Add up the positive and negative ranks.
5. Denote by T the unsigned value of the smaller; n is sample size (number of ranks).
6. Calculate $\mu = n(n+1)/4$, $\sigma^2 = (2n+1)\mu/6$, and then $z = (T - \mu)/\sigma$.
7. Obtain the p-value (as if it were α) from Table A for a two- or one-tailed test as appropriate.

Two Large Samples: The Normal Approximation to the Rank-Sum Test

Think of it informally as testing whether the two distributions have the same median.

1. Name the sizes of the two samples n_1 and n_2; n_1 is the smaller.
2. Combine the data, keeping track of the sample from which each datum arose.
3. Rank the data.
4. Add up the ranks of the data from each sample separately.
5. Denote by T the sum associated with n_1.
6. Calculate $\mu = n_1(n_1 + n_2 + 1)/2$, $\sigma^2 = n_1 n_2(n_1 + n_2 + 1)/12$, and $z = (T - \mu)/\sigma$.
7. Obtain the p-value (as if it were α) from Table A for a two- or one-tailed test as appropriate.

FORMULAS FOR TESTS OF MEANS FROM CHAPTER 15

Single or Paired Near-Normal Samples: Normal and t Tests

Paired data: change to single data by subtraction, e.g., before observation minus after. Assume that data are distributed normal. H_0:$\mu_0 = \mu$. Choose H_1:$\mu_0 \neq \mu$, $\mu_0 < \mu$, or $\mu_0 > \mu$. Choose α. If σ_m is known or sample is large, calculate z and use Table A:

$$z = (m - \mu)/\sigma_m = (m - \mu)/\left(\sigma/\sqrt{n}\right). \qquad (15.1)$$

If n is small, calculate t and use Table B with $n - 1$ *df*.

$$t = (m - \mu)/s_m = (m - \mu)/\left(s/\sqrt{n}\right) \tag{15.2}$$

Two Near-Normal Samples: Normal and *t* Tests

Assume that data are distributed normal. $H_0{:}\mu_1 = \mu_2$. Choose $H_1{:}\mu_1 \neq \mu_2$, $H_1{:}\mu_1 < \mu_2$, or $H_1{:}\mu_1 > \mu_2$. Choose α. Method depends on variances equal or not, according to following table:

Total sample size	Subgroup sample size	Variances about equal	Variances somewhat different	Variances extremely different
Large size *or* σ's known	About equal	(1) Normal test, equal variances	(1) Normal test, equal variances	Rank-sum test
	Very different		(3) Normal test, unequal variances	Rank-sum test
Small size	About equal	(2) t test, equal variances	(2) t test, equal variances	Rank-sum test
	Very different		(4) t test, unequal variances	Rank-sum test

If σ's composing σ_d are known or samples are large, calculate z and use Table A:

$$z = (m_1 - m_2)/\sigma_d. \tag{15.3}$$

If n's are small, calculate t and use Table B:

$$t = (m_1 - m_2)/s_d. \tag{15.4}$$

Standard error, case 1. Equal variances, known σ:

$$\sigma_d = \sigma\sqrt{\frac{1}{n_1} + \frac{1}{n_2}}. \tag{15.5}$$

For large n, unknown σ_d is approximated by Eq. (15.6), but normal form Eq. (15.3) is still used. Standard error, case 2. Equal variances unknown, small n's, $df = n_1 + n_2 - 1$ in Table B:

$$s_d = \sqrt{\left(\frac{1}{n_1} + \frac{1}{n_2}\right)\left[\frac{(n_1 - 1)s_1^2 + (n_2 - 1)s_2^2}{n_1 + n_2 - 2}\right]}. \tag{15.6}$$

Standard error, case 3. Unequal variances, known σ_1 and σ_2:

$$\sigma_d = \sqrt{\frac{\sigma_1^2}{n_1} + \frac{\sigma_2^2}{n_2}}. \tag{15.7}$$

For large n_1 and n_2, unknown σ_d approximated by Eq. (15.8), but normal form Eq. (15.3) is still used. Standard error, case 4. Unequal variances unknown, small n's:

$$s_d = \sqrt{\frac{s_1^2}{n_1} + \frac{s_2^2}{n_2}} \tag{15.8}$$

with *df* rounded to the integer next smaller than

$$\text{approx}(df) = \frac{\left(\frac{s_1^2}{n_1} + \frac{s_2^2}{n_2}\right)^2}{\frac{\left(\frac{s_1^2}{n_1}\right)^2}{n_1-1} + \frac{\left(\frac{s_2^2}{n_2}\right)^2}{n_2-1}}. \tag{15.9}$$

Three or More Near-Normal Samples: One-Way ANOVA with Multiple Comparisons

Assume: (a) distributed approximately normal and (b) variances approximately equal. H_0: No differences among means. H_1: One or more differences among means. Choose α and find the associated critical value of F in Table E for $k - 1$ and $n - k$ *df*. Total sample has n observations, mean m, and variance s^2, divided into k groups having $n_1, n_2, \ldots, n_k$ observations with group means $m_1, m_2, \ldots, m_k$.

Source of variability	Sum of squares			Variances or mean squares	
	Designation	Formula	*df*	Designation	Formula
Mean	SSM	$\sum n_i(m_i - m)^2$	$k - 1$	s_m^2 (or MSM)	SSM/$(k - 1)$
Error	SSE	SST − SSM	$n - k$	s_e^2 (or MSE)	SSE/$(n - k)$
Total	SST	$(n - 1)s^2$	$n - 1$	s^2 (or MST)	SST/$(n - 1)$

Calculate $F = \text{MSM}/\text{MSE} = s_m^2/s_e^2$ and compare with critical value from Table E.

Multiple comparisons using statistical software: Outcomes are p-values adjusted so that each may be compared with chosen overall α while retaining this overall α. If statistical software is not available, make two-sample t tests on each pair, but choose the critical t from Table B using $2\alpha/k(k - 1)$ rather than α, interpolating as required. Bonferroni results.

FORMULAS FOR TESTS OF VARIANCES FROM CHAPTER 16

Single Samples

Assume that data are distributed normal. Identify the theoretical σ. Choose α. $\text{H}_0{:}\sigma_0^2 = \sigma^2$. $\text{H}_1{:}\sigma_0^2 > \sigma^2$ (Table C), $\text{H}_1{:}\sigma_0^2 < \sigma^2$ (Table D), or $\text{H}_1{:}\sigma_0^2 \neq \sigma^2$ (both).

$$\chi^2 = \frac{df \times s^2}{\sigma^2}.$$

Use critical value of χ^2 (with $n - 1$ *df*) or find the p-value using a computer to reject H_0 or not.

Two Samples

Assume normality. s_1^2 is the larger variance. $\text{H}_0{:}\sigma_1^2 = \sigma_2^2$. $\text{H}_1{:}\sigma_1^2 > \sigma_2^2$. Choose α:

$$F = s_1^2 / s_2^2$$

Use critical value of F(with $n_1 - 1, n_2 - 1$ *df*) or find p-value with a computer to reject H_0 or not.

Three or More Samples

Assume normality in all samples. $\text{H}_0{:}\sigma_1^2 = \sigma_2^2 = \cdots = \sigma_k^2$. H_1: not H_0. Choose α. i denotes sample number, 1 to k. n is total number. n_i is number of data x_i in ith sample. Find usual variance s_i^2 for each sample:

$$s_i^2 = \frac{\sum x_i^2 - n_i m_i^2}{n_i - 1}.$$

Pool the k sample variances to find the overall variance s^2:

$$s^2 = \frac{\sum (n_i - 1) s_i^2}{n - k}.$$

The test statistic, Bartlett's M, is given by

$$M = \frac{(n-k)\ln(s^2) - \sum (n_i - 1)\ln\left(s_i^2\right)}{1 + \frac{1}{3(k-1)}\left(\sum \frac{1}{n_i - 1} - \frac{k}{n-k}\right)}.$$

Use the critical value of χ^2 (with $k - 1$ *df*) or find the p-value using a computer to reject H_0 or not.

FORMULAS FOR TESTS OF DISTRIBUTION SHAPE FROM CHAPTER 17

TESTS OF NORMALITY OF A DISTRIBUTION

Table 171

Guide to Selecting a Test of Normality of a Distribution

	Prefer less conservative test	Prefer more conservative test
Small sample (5–50)	Shapiro–Wilk test	Kolmogorov–Smirnov test (one-sample)
Medium to large sample (>50)	Shapiro–Wilk test	Chi-square goodness-of-fit test

Details of the method are given next to explain what the tests do and how they do it.

KOLMOGOROV–SMIROV (KS) TEST (ONE-SAMPLE FORM)

Format of Table Providing Calculations Required for the Kolmogorov–Smirnov (KS) Test of Normality

Data	x	k	$F_n(x)$	z	$F_e(x)$	$\lvert F_n(x) - F_e(x) \rvert$
⋮	⋮	⋮	⋮	⋮	⋮	⋮

Hypotheses are H_0: Sample distribution not different from specified normal distribution, and H_1: Sample distribution is different. Choose α.

1. Arrange the n sample values in ascending order.
2. Let x denote the sample value each time it changes. Write x's in a column in order.
3. Let k denote the number of sample members less than x. Write k's next to x's.

4. List each $F_n(x) = k/n$ in the next column corresponding to the associated x.
5. Calculate $z = (x - \mu)/\sigma$ for each x to test against an *a priori* distribution or $z = (x - m)/s$ for each x to test for a normal shape but not a particular normal.
6. For each z, find an expected $F_e(n)$ as the area under the normal distribution to the left of z. This area can be found using a statistical software package or from a very complete table of normal probabilities. If neither of these sources is available, interpolate from Table A. Write down these $F_e(x)$ next to the corresponding $F_n(x)$.
7. Write down next to these the differences $|F_n(x) - F_e(x)|$.
8. The test statistic is the largest of these differences, say L.
9. Calculate the critical value. For a 5% α, use $1.36/\sqrt{n} - 1/4.5n$. Critical values for $\alpha = 1\%$ and 10% are given in the text. If L is greater than the critical value, reject H_0. Otherwise, do not reject H_0.

Large-Sample Test of Normality of a Distribution: Chi-Square Goodness-of-Fit Test

Format of Table of Values Required to Compute the Chi-Square Goodness-of-Fit Statistic

Interval	Standard normal z to end of interval	Probability	Expected frequencies (e_i)	Observed frequencies (n_i)
⋮	⋮	⋮	⋮	⋮

1. Choose α. Define k data intervals as in forming a histogram of the data.
2. Standardize interval ends by subtracting mean and dividing by standard deviation.
3. Find the area under the normal curve to the end of an interval from a table of normal probabilities and subtract the area to the end of the preceding interval.
4. Multiply normal probabilities by n to find expected frequencies e_i.
5. Tally the number of data n_i falling into each interval.
6. Calculate χ^2 value: $\chi^2 = \Sigma n_i^2/e_i - n$.
7. Find critical χ^2 from Table C. If calculated χ^2 is greater than critical χ^2, reject H_0; otherwise, do not reject H_0.

Test of Equality of Two Distributions

Format for Values Required for the Two-Sample KS Test of Equality of Distribution

Ordered data	k_1	k_2	F_1	F_2	$\lvert F_1 - F_2 \rvert$
⋮	⋮	⋮	⋮	⋮	⋮

Two-Sample KS Test. H_0: The population distributions from which the samples arose are not different; H_1: They are different. The sample sizes are n_1 and n_2; n_1 is the larger. Choose α.

1. Combine the two data sets and arrange in ascending order; use format of Table 17.7 (shown just above).
2. For each sample one datum different from the datum above it, record for k_1 the number of data in sample 1 preceding it. Repeat the process for sample 2, recording entries for k_2.
3. For every k_1, list $F_1 = k_1/n_1$. Repeat for sample 2. In all blanks, list F from line above.
4. Calculate and record $|F_1 - F_2|$ for every datum.
5. The test statistic is the largest of these differences; call it L.
6. Calculate critical value. For 5% α, it is $1.36\sqrt{(n_1 + n_2)/n_1 n_2}$; for 1% and 10%, see text. If L is greater than the critical value, reject H_0. Otherwise, do not reject H_0.

FORMULAS FOR REQUIRED SAMPLE SIZES FROM CHAPTER 18

Sample Size for Confidence Intervals

Confidence Interval on a Mean

For a $1-\alpha$ confidence interval on a theoretical mean μ, find $z_{1-\alpha/2}$ from Table A, choose the desired difference $m - \mu$ between the observed and theoretical means, estimate σ from other sources, and substitute these values in

$$n = \frac{z_{1-\alpha/2}^2 \sigma^2}{(m - \mu)^2}. \tag{18.1}$$

Confidence Interval on a Proportion

For a $1 - \alpha$ confidence interval on a theoretical proportion π, find $z_{1-\alpha/2}$ from Table A, choose the desired difference $p - \pi$ between the observed and theoretical proportions, and estimate p from other sources. If π is not near 0 or 1, substitute these values in Eq. (18.2). If π is near 0 or 1, substitute in Eq. (18.3):

$$n = \frac{z_{1-\alpha/2}^2 p(1-p)}{(p-\pi)^2} \tag{18.2}$$

or

$$n = \frac{z_{1-\alpha/2}^2 p}{(p-\pi)^2}. \tag{18.3}$$

Confidence Interval on a Correlation Coefficient

Sample sizes for 95% confidence intervals on a theoretical correlation coefficient ρ for various values of a sample correlation coefficient r are given in Table 18.1. Some representative values from Table 18.1 are given here:

r	0.05	0.10	0.15	0.20	0.25	0.30	0.35	0.40	0.45	0.50
n	1538	385	172	97	63	44	32	25	20	16

Sample Size for Tests on Categorical Data

Case 1: Test of a Sample Proportion against a Theoretical Proportion

Theoretical proportion is π, calculated is p. Look up z-values in Table A for $z_{1-\alpha/2}$ and $z_{1-\beta}$. Substitute in Eq. (18.5) for π not near 0 or 1 (binomial) or in Eq. (18.6) for π near 0 or 1 (Poisson) to find n, the minimum sample size required.

$$n = \left[\frac{z_{1-\alpha/2}\sqrt{\pi(1-\pi)} + z_{1-\beta}\sqrt{p(1-p)}}{p-\pi}\right]^2; \tag{18.5}$$

$$n = \left[\frac{z_{1-\alpha/2}\sqrt{\pi} + z_{1-\beta}\sqrt{p}}{p-\pi}\right]^2. \tag{18.6}$$

Case 2: Two Proportions

Sample proportions are p_1 and p_2; $p_m = (p_1 + p_2)/2$. Look up z-values in Table A for $z_{1-\alpha/2}$ and $z_{1-\beta}$. Substitute in Eq. (18.8) for p_m not near 0 or 1 (binomial) or in Eq. (18.9) for p_m near 0 or 1 (Poisson) to find n, the minimum sample size required:

$$n_1 = n_2 = \left[\frac{z_{1-\alpha/2}\sqrt{2p_m(1-p_m)} + z_{1-\beta}\sqrt{p_1(1-p_1)+p_2(1-p_2)}}{p_1 - p_2}\right]^2 \qquad (18.8)$$

$$n_1 = n_2 = \left[\frac{(z_{1-\alpha/2} + z_{1-\beta})\sqrt{p_1 + p_2}}{p_1 - p_2}\right]^2. \qquad (18.9)$$

Case 3: Contingency Tables

Use Case 2, calculating proportions from cell entries.

Sample Size for Tests on Means

Case 1: One Mean, Normal Distribution (Population or Large-Sample σ Known)

Is m different from μ? Choose a clinically meaningful difference $d = m - \mu$ to detect. Look up z-values from Table A for $z_{1-\alpha/2}$ and $z_{1-\beta}$. Substitute in Eq. (18.11) to find n, the minimum sample size required.

$$n = \left(z_{1-\alpha/2} + z_{1-\beta}\right)^2 \sigma^2 / d^2 \qquad (18.11)$$

Case 2: Two Means, Normal Distributions

Is μ_1 (estimated by m_1) different from μ_2 (estimated by m_2)? Choose a clinically meaningful difference $d = m_1 - m_2$ to detect. Find σ_1^2 and σ_2^2 (estimated by s_1^2 and s_2^2, if necessary). Look up z-values from Table A for $z_{1-\alpha/2}$ and $z_{1-\beta}$. Substitute in Eq. (18.12) to find $n_1 (= n_2)$, the minimum sample size required in *each* sample.

$$n_1 = n_2 = \left(z_{1-\alpha/2} + z_{1-\beta}\right)^2 \left(\sigma_1^2 + \sigma_2^2\right) / d^2 \qquad (18.12)$$

Case 3: Poorly Behaved or Unknown Distributions (Population or Large-Sample σ Known)

The sample size is a conservative overestimate, usually more than required. Is m different from μ? Choose a clinically meaningful difference $d = m - \mu$ to detect, expressed as a number of σ. Choose α. Substitute in Eq. (18.14) to find the minimum sample size required.

$$n = \sigma^2/\alpha k^2 \tag{18.14}$$

Case 4: No Objective Prior Data

For your variable, guess the smallest and largest values you have noticed. σ is estimated as ¼(largest − smallest). Use this value of σ in *Case* 1. Clearly, this "desperation" estimate is of extremely low confidence, but may be better than picking a number out of the air.

FORMULAS AND STEPS FOR MODELING AND DECISION FROM CHAPTER 19

A Model Is a Quantitative (or Geometric) Representation of a Relationship or Process

(1) Algebraic Models

One or more equations. The dependent variable, representing a biological event or process, is a *function* (of any shape) of one or more independent variables.

Straight Line Models. Slope–intercept: $y = \beta_0 + \beta_1 x$. Slope–mean point: $y - m_y = \beta_1(x - m_x)$.

Curved Models. Adding a squared term provides a (portion of a) parabola: $y = \beta_0 + \beta_1 x + \beta_2 x^2$.

Commonly seen curves are illustrated in Figs. 19.3A–F. These include (A) the upward opening parabola, (B) a third degree curve (adding an x^3 term to a parabolic model), (C) a logarithmic curve, (D) an exponential curve, (E) a biological growth curve, and (F) a sine wave.

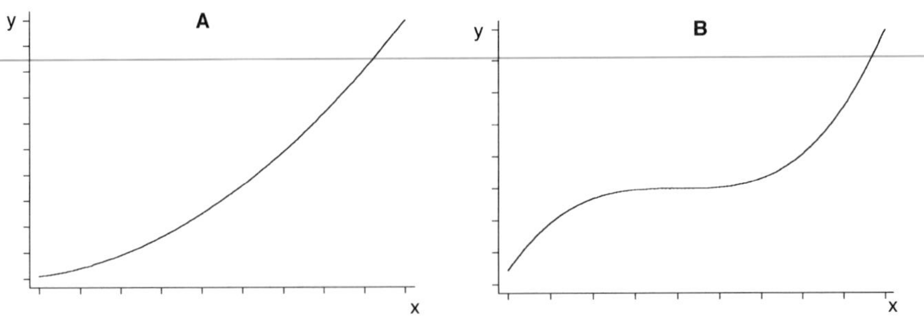

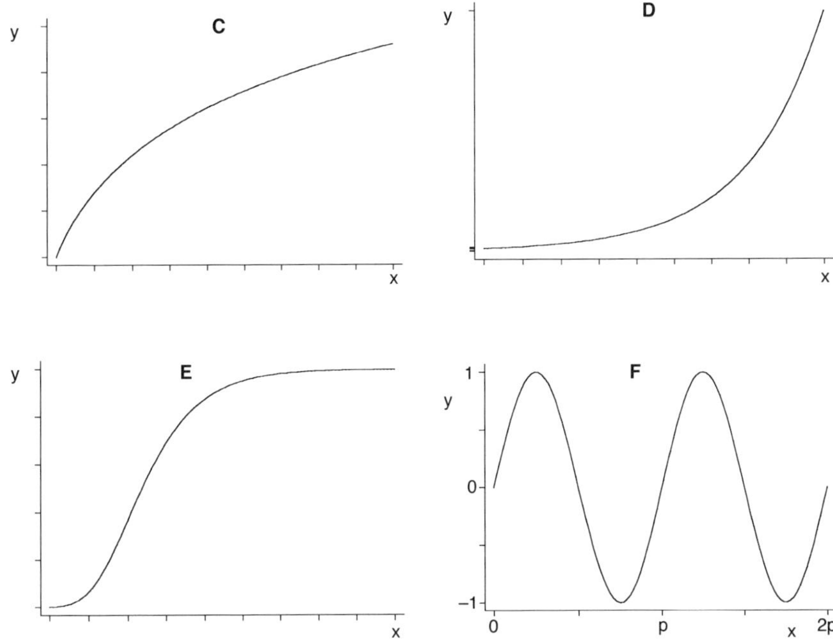

Constants of Fit for Any Model. Specify a particular member of a family of curves by choosing the four constants of scale and position for x and for y. For a family $y = f(x)$, the constants and their location in the equation are $y = d + cf(ax + b)$.

Table 19.1

Effects of Fit Constants (Parameters) That Change the Function $y = f(x)$ to $y = d + cf(ax + b)$ and Effects of the Values They May Take On

Fit constant	Along which axis	General effect	Detailed effect
a	x	Stretches–shrinks curve	$a < 1$: stretches $a > 1$: shrinks
b	x	Slides curve	$b > 0$: to left $b < 0$: to right
c	y	Stretches–shrinks curve	$c > 1$: stretches $c < 1$: shrinks
d	y	Slides curve	$d > 0$: up $d < 0$: down

Multiple-Variable Models. The three-dimensional case of y depending on two x's can be visualized geometrically, as with the expression $y = \beta_0 + \beta_1 x_1 + \beta_2 x_2$. A sample point is $(y = 3.5, x_1 = 2.5, x_2 = 2)$.

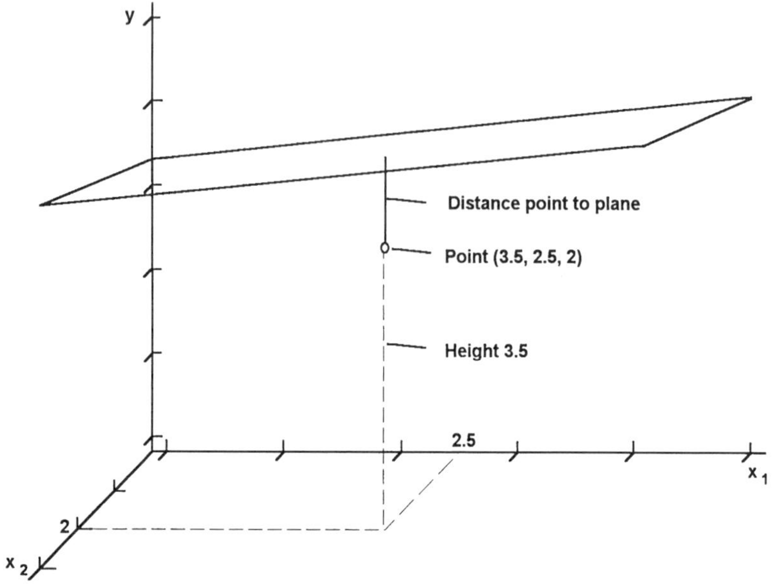

A curved surface in three dimensions is possible (perhaps $y = \beta_0 + \beta_1 x_1 + \beta_2 x_2 + \beta_3 x_2^2$), as is more than three dimensions. Add as many variables in whatever powers as desired. An algebraic expression of a four-dimensional plane would be $y = \beta_0 + \beta_1 x_1 + \beta_2 x_2 + \beta_3 x_3$.

(2) Logical Models, Exemplified by Screening Results and the Number Needed to Treat (NNT)

NNT: an estimate of the number of people that must be screened in order to detect one case to treat.

Number Screened per Detection When Screening Is the Only Detection Mechanism: p_e, probability that a randomly chosen member of the catchment will have the disease ($=n_e/n_p$); n_s, number of people screened, i.e., sample size; n_d, number of cases of the disease detected in screening n_s people; $n_d, = n_s p_e = n_s n_e/n_p$; NNT $= n_s/n_d$; c_s, cost for screening program, i.e., cost to screen n_s people; c_d, cost per detection, $c_d = (c_s/n_s)$NNT.

Number Screened per Detection When Some Cases Would Be Otherwise Detected: n_c, number of cases of disease in the catchment detected by other means; n_{cd}, number of cases detected by the screening program that would have been found otherwise; $n_{d-cd} = n_d - n_{cd}$; NNT $= n_s/n_{d-cd}$.

(3) Clinical Decision Based on Recursive Partitioning Models

Steps to Develop the Decision Process. Sort the possible outcomes (diagnoses or result of treatment), listing those alike in adjoining rows. Identify the indicator (symptom–sign or condition) most consistently related to the outcome, and then the next, etc. Draw a decision box with arrows extending out, depending on initial partitioning. Draw the next decision boxes with appropriate arrows extending to them and more arrows extending out, depending on the next round of partitions. Continue until reaching the final outcomes. The boxes should be ordered such that no looping back can occur and no box is repeated. There usually is some trial and error.

(4) Clinical Decision Based on Outcome-Related MOE Models: Outcomes Analysis

Steps:

(1) Clearly and unequivocally define the goal.
(2) Identify the (quantifiable) components of the MOE that will satisfy the goal.
(3) Express algebraically the relationship among the components. Weight each component to adjust for different units systems.
(4) Weight the components of the MOE (the variables) by their relative importance.

FORMULAS AND ASSUMPTIONS FOR REGRESSION AND CORRELATION FROM CHAPTER 20

Assumptions Underlying Regression:

(1) The errors (i.e., the deviations from average) are independent one from each other.
(2) Regression depends on the appropriateness of the model used in the fit.
(3) The independent (x) readings are measured as exact values (without randomness).
(4) The variance of y is the same for all values of x.
(5) The distribution of y is approximately normal for all values of x.

Assumptions Underlying Correlation:

(1) The errors in data values are independent one from each other.
(2) Correlation always requires the assumption of a straight line relationship.
(3) x and y are assumed to follow a bivariate normal distribution.
(4) Rank correlation assumes only (1) and (2).

Simple Regression Equation: $y - m_y = b_1(x - m_x)$ or $y = b_0 + b_1 x$.
Correlation Coefficients. Continuous variables:

$$r = \frac{s_{xy}}{s_x s_y} \left(= b_1 \frac{s_x}{s_y} \right).$$

Ranked variables:

$$r_s = 1 - \frac{6 \sum d_i^2}{n(n^2 - 1)}.$$

Tests and Confidence Intervals on Regression Parameters. Standard error of residuals:

$$s_e = \sqrt{\frac{n-1}{n-2}\left(s_y^2 - b_1^2 s_x^2\right)} = s_y \sqrt{\frac{n-1}{n-2}(1 - R^2)}.$$

Standard error of slope:

$$s_b = \frac{s_e}{\sqrt{(n-1)} s_x}.$$

t test on slope, $H_0{:}\beta = 0$:

$$t_{(n-2)df} = b_1 / s_b.$$

t test on slope, $H_0{:}\beta = \beta_1$:

$$t_{(n-2)df} = \frac{b_1 - \beta_1}{s_b}.$$

Confidence interval on the slope:

$$P[b_1 - t_{1-\alpha/2} s_b < \beta_1 < b_1 + t_{1-\alpha/2} s_b] = 1 - \alpha.$$

Standard error of mean prediction:

$$s_{m/x} = s_e \sqrt{\frac{1}{n} + \frac{(x - m_x)^2}{(n-1)s_x^2}}.$$

Confidence interval on mean prediction:

$$P[m|x - t_{1-\alpha/2} s_{m|x} < \mu|x < m|x + t_{1-\alpha/2} s_{m|x}] = 1 - \alpha.$$

Standard error of individual prediction:

$$s_{y|x} = s_e \sqrt{1 + \frac{1}{n} + \frac{(x - m_x)^2}{(n-1)s_x^2}}.$$

Confidence interval on individual prediction:

$$P[y|x - t_{1-\alpha/2}s_{y|x} < E(y)|x < y|x + t_{1-\alpha/2}s_{y|x}] = 1 - \alpha.$$

Standard error on slope difference:

$$s_{b:1-2} = \sqrt{\left(\frac{(n_1 - 2)s_{e:1}^2 + (n_2 - 1)s_{e:2}^2}{n_1 + n_2 - 4}\right)\left(\frac{1}{(n_1 - 1)s_1^2} + \frac{1}{(n_2 - 1)s_2^2}\right)}.$$

t test on slope difference:

$$t = \frac{b_{1:1} - b_{1:2}}{s_{b:1-2}}.$$

Tests and Confidence Intervals on Correlation Coefficients. t test on correlation, $H_0{:}\rho^2 = 0$:

$$t_{(n-2)df} = \sqrt{\frac{(n-2)r^2}{1 - r^2}}.$$

z test on correlation, $H_0{:}\rho = \rho_0$:

$$z = \frac{m - \mu}{\sigma},$$

where

$$m = \frac{1}{2}\ln\left(\frac{1+r}{1-r}\right), \quad \mu = \frac{1}{2}\ln\left(\frac{1+\rho_0}{1-\rho_0}\right), \quad \sigma = \frac{1}{\sqrt{n-3}}.$$

z test on two coefficients:

$$z = \frac{m_1 - m_2}{\sqrt{\sigma_1^2 + \sigma_2^2}}.$$

A confidence interval on ρ:

$$P\left[\frac{1 + r - (1 - r)e^{\frac{2z_{1-\alpha/2}}{\sqrt{n-3}}}}{1 + r + (1 - r)e^{\frac{2z_{1-\alpha/2}}{\sqrt{n-3}}}} < \rho < \frac{1 + r - (1 - r)e^{-\frac{2z_{1-\alpha/2}}{\sqrt{n-3}}}}{1 + r + (1 - r)e^{-\frac{2z_{1-\alpha/2}}{\sqrt{n-3}}}}\right] = 1 - \alpha.$$

Logistic Regression. Model:

$$\ln\left(\frac{p_m}{1 - p_m}\right) = \beta_0 + \beta_1 x.$$

Prediction of proportion "successes:"

$$p_m = \frac{e^{b_0+b_1x}}{1+e^{b_0+b_1x}}.$$

METHODS FOR SURVIVAL AND TIME-SERIES ANALYSIS FROM CHAPTER 21

LIFE TABLES AND SURVIVAL CURVES

See summary page for Chapter 9.

CONFIDENCE INTERVALS ON SURVIVAL CURVES

The 95% confidence interval on the true survival proportion for each time period, where S_i is the estimated survival proportion for that period and S_{i-1}, for the prior period, is

$$S_i \pm 1.96 S_i \sqrt{\frac{1-S_i}{n_{i-1}}}.$$

LOG-RANK TEST OF TWO OR MORE SURVIVAL CURVES

Use a statistical software package on a computer.

SEQUENTIAL ANALYSIS

Definitions: x_k, the observation on the kth patient; $\mathrm{P}(x_k|\mathrm{H}_0)$, the probability of x_k occurring if H_0 is true; $\mathrm{P}(x_k|\mathrm{H}_1)$, the probability of x_k occurring if H_1 is true.

Steps:

(1) Pose the null and alternate hypotheses.
(2) Assign error risk values to α and β and calculate the critical values.
(3) Find the probability ratio $D_1 = \mathrm{P}(x_1|\mathrm{H}_1)/\mathrm{P}(x_1|\mathrm{H}_0)$.
(4) Fill in Table 21.5, calculating $D_k = D_{k-1}\mathrm{P}(x_k|\mathrm{H}_1)/\mathrm{P}(x_k|\mathrm{H}_0)$.

For a test of proportions: If the observation is binary, x_k can be expressed as either a 0 or a 1. The calculation of D_k will be $D_k = D_{k-1}\mathrm{P}(1|\mathrm{H}_1)/\mathrm{P}(1|\mathrm{H}_0)$ if event 1 occurs or $D_k = D_{k-1}[1 - \mathrm{P}(1|\mathrm{H}_1)]/[1 - \mathrm{P}(1|\mathrm{H}_0)]$ if event 1 does not occur.

For a test of means: Mean under the null hypothesis is μ_0; that under the alternate is μ_1. Variance is σ^2. The multiplying increment is $\exp\{-\frac{1}{2\sigma^2}[(x_k - \mu_1)^2 - (x_k - \mu_0)^2]\}$.

(5) After each patient, make a decision using the following criteria:

$$\text{Accept H}_0 \text{ when } D_k \leq \frac{\beta}{1-\alpha}.$$

$$\text{Reject H}_0 \text{ when } D_k \geq \frac{1-\beta}{\alpha}.$$

Continue sampling otherwise.

If H_0 is accepted or rejected, stop; if not, sample another patient and repeat steps (4) and (5).

Moving Samples: Estimation

Consider a moving sample of readings x of width k with first element i (x_i, $x_{i+1}, \ldots, x_{i+k-1}$). A moving mean, median, or variance is just the ordinary mean, median, or variance of the k elements of the moving sample. Because the sample drops the leftmost reading and adds one to the right end as it moves, a moving statistic only needs to be adjusted for the two readings changed.

Serial Correlation

A serial correlation coefficient is just the ordinary correlation coefficient of two columns of data, except that the data are ordered in sequence through time. A serial correlation may have a lag in time, which is equivalent to sliding one column down the number of elements in the lag and then calculating the correlation coefficient on the column pairs.

Cross Correlation

A cross correlation is a serial correlation in which the two columns of data arise from two different variables. A cross correlation may or may not be lagged.

Autocorrelation

An autocorrelation coefficient is a lagged serial correlation coefficient in which the second column of data is a repetition of the first.

Moving Samples: Testing

Consider a moving sample in which the beginning sample represents a baseline period (measurements prior to treatment or onset of disease). A moving variance in ratio to the baseline variance provides a moving F statistic, which can be compared for significance with a critical F-value. The baseline variance is an estimate of pre-event random variability. The moving F ratio tests whether succeeding moving variances are increased by a change in the mean, by larger random variability, or by a change in the model of the path through time, or some combination of these. The moving F may be graphed against the time values to identify the points of change and the periods during which differences persist.

References and Data Sources

The data used for examples in this book arose from real medical studies. In many cases data were edited to better illustrate the statistical method, so that the treatment in this book may not represent the true study results or the intent of the investigator. Most were studies on which I advised, some of which were published and are so referenced and some of which are still in progress or in press. Other data arose from studies published in the medical literature and are so referenced.

The terms, prose, and interpretations are mine, not necessarily attributable to the investigator referenced. In cases of misstatement, I beg the reader's indulgence. We will both be better served if you look to the statistical method being illustrated rather than to the medical nuance.

1. Bailar, J. C., and Mosteller, F., eds. (1992). *Medical Uses of Statistics, 2nd Ed.* Boston: NEJM Books.
2. Battaglia, Michael J., MD (LT, MC, USN), Orthopedics Department, Naval Medical Center, San Diego, CA.
3. Blanton, Christopher L., MD, Ophthalmologist, Inland Eye Institute, Glendale, CA.
4. Blanton, C. L., Schallhorn S., and Tidwell, J. (1998). Radial keratotomy learning curve using the American technique. *Journal of Cataract and Refractive Surgery* **24**, 471–476.
5. Choplin, Neil, MD (CAPT, MC, USN), Chairman, Ophthalmology Department, Naval Medical Center, San Diego, CA, and Clinical Assoc. Professor of Surgery, U.S. University of the Health Sciences.
6. Crum, Nancy F., MD (LT, MC, USN), Internal Medicine Department, Naval Medical Center, San Diego, CA.
7. Cupp, Craig, MD (CDR, MC, USN), Otolaryngology Department, Naval Medical Center, San Diego, CA.
8. Curtis, K. M., Savitz, D. A., and Arbuckle, T. E. (1997). Effects of Cigarette smoking, caffeine consumption, and alcohol intake on fecundability. *American Journal of Epidemiology* **146**, 32–41.
9. Daly, Karen A., MD (CDR, MC, USN), Mental Health Department, Naval Medical Clinic, Pearl Harbor, HI.
10. Devereaux, Asha, MD (LCDR, MC, USN), Pulmonary Medicine Department, Naval Medical Center, San Diego, CA.

11. Elsas T., and Johnsen, H. (1991). Long-term efficacy of primary laser trabeculoplasty. *British Journal of Ophthalmology* **75**, 34–37.
12. Freilich, Daniel, MD (LCDR, MC, USN), Infectious Diseases Division, Naval Medical Center, San Diego, CA.
13. Gilmore, D. M., and Frieden, T. R. (1997). Universal radiographic screening for tuberculosis among inmates upon admission to jail. *American Journal of Public Health* **87**(8), 1335–1337.
14. Goldberg, M. A. (1995). Erythropoiesis, erythropoietin, and iron metabolism in elective surgery: Preoperative strategies for avoiding allogeneic blood exposure. *American Journal of Surgery* **170**(Dec), 37S–43S.
15. Grau, Kriste J., RN (LCDR, NC, USN), Nurse Practitioner, Naval Hospital Naples, Napoli, Italia.
16. Greason, Kevin, MD, Cardiac and Vascular Surgery Department, Mayo Clinic, Rochester, MN.
17. Grossman, Ira, Ph.D., Supervisor, Psychology Services, Sharp Mesa Vista Hospital, San Diego, CA.
18. Hacala, M. T. (1998). U.S. Navy Hospital Corps: A century of tradition, valor, and sacrifice. *Navy Medicine* **89**(3), 12–26.
19. Hedges, L. V., and Olkin, I. (1985). *Statistical Methods for Meta-Analysis*. San Diego: Academic Press.
20. Hennekens, C. H., and Buring, J. E. (1987). *Epidemiology in Medicine*. Boston: Little, Brown and Company.
21. Hennrikus, W., Simpson, B., Klingelberger, C., and Reis, M. (1994). Self-administered nitrous oxide analgesia for pediatric fracture reductions. *Journal of Pediatric Orthopedics* **14**, 538–542.
22. Hennrikus, W., Shin, A., and Klingelberger, C. (1995). Self-administered nitrous oxide and a hematoma block for analgesia in the outpatient reduction of fractures in children. *Journal of Bone and Joint Surgery* **77A**, 335–339.
23. Hennrikus, W., Mapes, R., Lyons, P., and Lapoint, J. (1996). Outcomes of the Chrisman–Snook and modified Bostrom procedures for chronic lateral ankle instability. *American Journal of Sports Medicine* **24**, 400–404.
24. Hoffer, Michael E., MD (LCDR, MC, USN), Co-Director, Defense Spatial Orientation Center, Naval Medical Center, San Diego, CA.
25. Hong, W. K., *et al.* (1986). 13-*cis*-Retinoic acid in the treatment of oral leukoplakia. *New England Journal of Medicine* **315**, 1501–1505.
26. Howe, Steven C., MD (LT, MC, USN), General Surgery Department, Naval Medical Center, San Diego, CA.
27. Huisman, Thomas, MD, Urologist, Chiaramonte and Associates Urology, Clinton, MD.
28. Johnstone, Peter A. S., MD, MA (CDR, MC, USN), Chairman, Radiation Oncology Department, Naval Medical Center, San Diego, CA.
29. Johnstone, P. A. S., Powell, C. R., Riffenburgh, R. H., Bethel, K. J., and Kane, C. J. (1998). The fate of 10-year clinically recurrence-free survivors after definitive radiotherapy for $T_{1-3}N_0M_0$ prostate cancer. *Radiation Oncology Investigations* **6**, 103–108.
30. Johnstone, P. A. S., and Sindela, W. S. (1996). Radical reoperation for advanced pancreas carcinoma. *Journal of Surgical Oncology* **61**, 7–13

31. Kelso, John M., MD (CDR, MC, USN), Allergy–Immunology Department, Naval Medical Center, San Diego, CA.
32. Klein, H. G. (1995). Allogeneic transfusion risks in the surgical patient. *American Journal of Surgery* **170**, 21S–26S.
33. Last, J. M., ed. (1988). *A Dictionary of Epidemiology, 2nd Ed.* New York: Oxford University Press.
34. Le Hesran, J. Y., *et al.* (1997). Maternal placental infection with *Plasmodium falciparum* and malaria morbidity during the first 2 years of life. *American Journal of Epidemiology* **146**, 826–831.
35. Leibson, C. L., *et al.* (1997). Relative contributions of incidence and survival to increasing prevalence of adult-onset diabetes mellitus: A population-based study. *American Journal of Epidemiology* **146**, 12–22.
36. Leivers, David, MD (CAPT, MC, USN), Chairman, Anesthesiology Department, Naval Medical Center, San Diego, CA.
37. Lilienfeld, D. E., and Stolley, P. D. (1994). *Foundations of Epidemiology, 3rd Ed.* Oxford University Press. (This is a revision of the original book by Lilienfeld, A. M.)
38. Lyons, A. S., and Petrucelli, R. J. (1978). *Medicine, An Illustrated History*, 1987 ed. New York: Harry N. Abrams.
39. Mausner, J. S., and Kramer, S. (1985). *Mauser and Bahn Epidemiology—An Introductory Text.* Philadelphia: W. B. Saunders Company.
40. McNulty, P. A. F. (1997). Prevalence and contributing factors of eating disorder behaviors in a population of female Navy nurses. *Military Medicine* **162**, 703–706.
41. Meier, P. (1974). *Introductory Lecture Notes on Statistical Methods in Medicine and Biology*. University of Chicago.
42. Missing sources. The sources of a few examples could not be found despite a strong effort to locate them. Such data that could not be referenced were altered slightly so as not to reflect on any investigator appearing later.
43. Mitchell, Jan, DDS (CAPT, DC, USN), Dental Clinic, Naval Hospital Camp Pendleton, Camp Pendleton, CA.
44. Mitchell, John D., MD (LCDR, MC, USN), Staff Cardiothoracic Surgeon, Naval Medical Center, San Diego, CA.
45. Mitts, Kevin G., MD (LCDR, MC, USN), Head, Orthopaedic Surgery Department, Naval Hospital Okinawa, Okinawa, Japan.
46. Muldoon, Michael, MD (CDR, MC, USN), Orthopedics Department, Naval Medical Center, San Diego, CA.
47. Murray, James, MD (CDR, MC, USN), Staff Vascular Surgeon, Naval Medical Center, San Diego, CA.
48. O'Leary, Michael, MD (CAPT, MC, USN), Otolaryngology Department, Naval Medical Center, San Diego, CA.
49. Panos, Reed G., MD (LCOL, MC, USAF), Staff Plastic Surgeon, Naval Medical Center, San Diego, CA.
50. Pekarske, William, MD (LT, MC, USN), Anesthesia Department, Naval Medical Center, San Diego, CA.
51. Peto, R., *et al.* (1977). Design and analysis of randomized clinical trials requiring prolonged observation of each patient. *British Journal of Cancer* **35**, 1–39.

52. Poggi, Matthew, MD, Military Sick Call, Marine Corps Air Station El Toro, Santa Ana, CA.
53. Rao, P. M., Rhea, J. T., Novelline, R. A., Mostafavi, A. A., and McCabe, C. J. (1998). Effect of computed tomography of the appendix on treatment of patients and use of hospital resources. *New England Journal of Medicine* **338**(3), 141–146.
54. Riffenburgh, Ralph S., MD, MA, Ophthalmologic Surgeon, Pasadena, CA.
55. Riffenburgh, Robert H., PhD, Clinical Investigation Department, Naval Medical Center, San Diego, CA.
56. Riffenburgh, R. H. (1994). Detecting a point of any change in a time series. *Journal of Applied Statistical Sciences*, **1**, 487–488.
57. Riffenburgh, R. H. (1996). Reverse gullibility and scientific evidence. *Archives of Otolaryngology Head and Neck Surgery* **122**, 600–601.
58. Riffenburgh, R. H., Olson, P. E., and Johnstone, P. A. (1997). Association of schistosomiasis with cervical cancer: Detecting bias in clinical studies. *East African Medical Journal* **74**, 14–16.
59. Ross, E. Victor, MD (CDR, MC, USN), Dermatology Department, Naval Medical Center, San Diego, CA.
60. Rothman, K. J. (1986). *Modern Epidemiology*. Boston: Little, Brown and Company.
61. Sageman, W. Scott, MD (CAPT, MC, USN), Head, Pulmonary Critical Care Medicine, Naval Medical Center, San Diego, CA.
62. Schallhorn, Stephen, MD (CDR, MC, USN), Ophthalmology Department, Naval Medical Center, San Diego, CA.
63. Schellenberg, G. (1994). Apo-E4: A risk factor, not a diagnostic test. *Science News* **145**, 10.
64. Schnepf, Glenn, MD (CDR, MC, USN), Primary Investigator, Seasonal Aspergillosis in COPD Patients Study, Naval Medical Clinic, Camp Pendleton, CA.
65. Scott, C. B. (1998). Validation and predictive power of Radiation Therapy Oncology Group RTOG recursive partitioning analysis classes for malignant glioma patients: A report using RTOG 90-06. *International Journal of Radiation Oncology, Biology, Physics* **40**(1), 51–55.
66. Shimoda, O., *et al.* (1998). Skin vasomotor reflex predicts circulatory responses to laryngoscopy and intubation. *Anesthesiology* **88**, 297–304.
67. Silverman, M. K., Kopf, A. W., Grin, C. M., Bart, R. S., and Levenstein, M. J. (1991). Recurrence rates of treated basal cell carcinomas, part 2: Curettage–Electrodessication. *Journal of Dermatologic Surgery and Oncology* **17**, 720–726.
68. Smith, Stacy, MD, Dermatologist, San Diego, CA.
69. Student [pseud.] (1908). The probable error of a mean. *Biometrika* **6**, 1–25.
70. Sutherland, J. C. (1968). Cancer in a mission hospital in South Africa. *Cancer* **22**, 372–378. Child/adult ratios were inferred from other sources for larger African areas.
71. Tanen, David, MD, Department of Medical Toxicology, Good Samaritan Regional Medical Center, Phoenix, AZ.
72. Tasker, S. A., O'Brien, W. A., Treanor, J. J., Weiss, P. J., Olson, P. E., Kaplan, A. H., and Wallace, M. R. (1998). Effects of influenza vaccination in HIV-infected adults: A double-blinded placebo-controlled trial. *Vaccine* **16**, 1039–1042.

73. Tockman, M. S. (1996). Progress in the early detection of lung cancer. In *Comprehensive Textbook of Thoracic Oncology* (Aisner, J., *et al.*, eds.) Baltimore: Williams and Wilkins.
74. Wald, A. (1947). *Sequential Analysis*. New York: John Wiley and Sons.
75. Wilde, J. (1989). A 10-year follow-up of semi-annual screening for lung cancer in Erfurt County, GDR. *European Respiratory Journal* **2**, 656–662.
76. Wright, L. (1962). Postural hypotension in late pregnancy. *British Medical Journal* **17**, 760–762.
77. Zilberfarb, J., Hennrikus, W., Reis, M., Larocco, A., and Ungersma, J. (1992). Treatment of acute septic bursitis. *Surgical Forum* **XLIII**, 577–579.

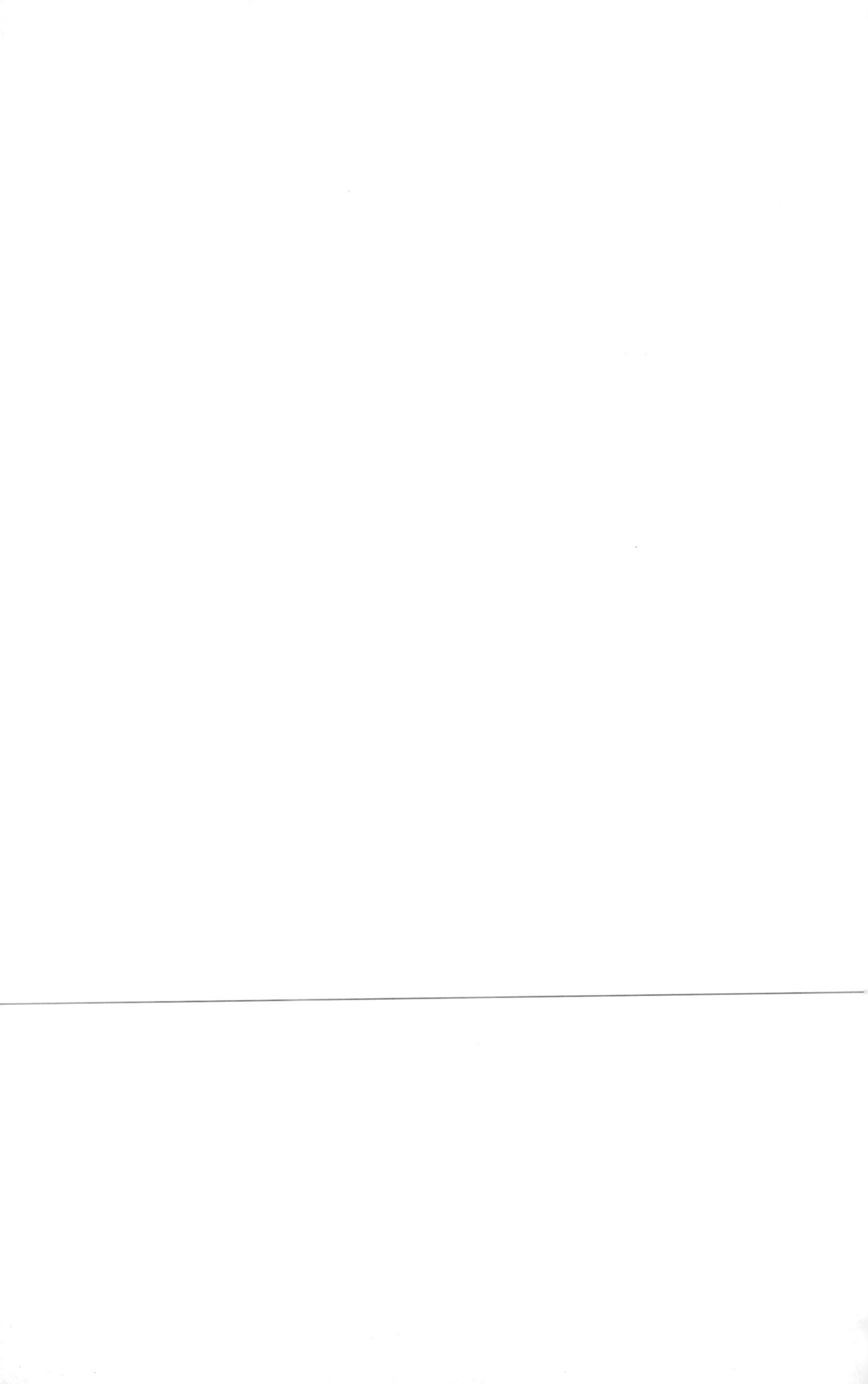

Tables of Probability Distributions

Table A
Normal Distribution[a]

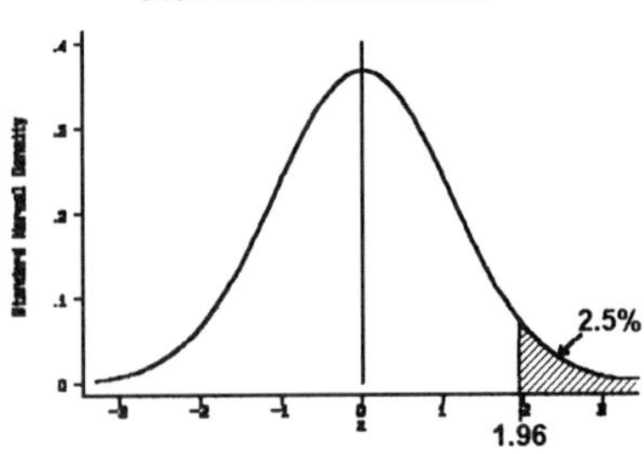

z (no. std. deviations to right of mean)	One-tailed applications: One-tailed α (area in right tail)	One-tailed applications: 1−α (area except right tail)	Two-tailed applications: Two-tailed α (area in both tails)	Two-tailed applications: 1−α (area except both tails)
0	.500	.500	1.000	.000
.10	.460	.540	.920	.080
.20	.421	.579	.842	.158
.30	.382	.618	.764	.236
.40	.345	.655	.690	.310
.50	.308	.692	.619	.381
.60	.274	.726	.548	.452
.70	.242	.758	.484	.516
.80	.212	.788	.424	.576
.90	.184	.816	.368	.632
1.00	.159	.841	.318	.682
1.10	.136	.864	.272	.728
1.20	.115	.885	.230	.770
1.281	*.100*	*.900*	*.200*	*.800*
1.30	.097	.903	.194	.806
1.40	.081	.919	.162	.838
1.50	.067	.933	.134	.866
1.60	.055	.945	.110	.890
1.645	*.050*	*.950*	*.100*	*.900*
1.70	.045	.955	.090	.910
1.80	.036	.964	.072	.928
1.90	.029	.971	.054	.946
1.960	*.025*	*.975*	*.050*	*.950*
2.00	.023	.977	.046	.934
2.10	.018	.982	.036	.964
2.20	.014	.986	.028	.972
2.30	.011	.989	.022	.978
2.326	*.010*	*.990*	*.020*	*.980*
2.40	.008	.992	.016	.084
2.50	.006	.994	.012	.088
2.576	*.005*	*.995*	*.010*	*.990*
2.60	.0047	.9953	.0094	.9906
2.70	.0035	.9965	.0070	.9930
2.80	.0026	.9974	.0052	.9948
2.90	.0019	.9981	.0038	.9962
3.00	.0013	.9987	.0026	.9974
3.100	*.0010*	*.9990*	*.0020*	*.9980*
3.20	.0007	.9996	.0014	.9986
3.300	*.0005*	*.9995*	*.0010*	*.9990*
3.40	.0003	.9997	.0006	.9994
3.50	.0002	.9998	.0004	.9996

[a] For selected distances (z) to the right of the mean are given (a) one-tailed α, the area under the curve in the positive tail; (b) one-tailed $1-\alpha$, the area under all except the tail; (c) two-tailed α, the areas combined for both positive and negative tails; and (d) two-tailed $1-\alpha$, the area under all except the two tails. Entries for the most commonly used areas are italicized.

Table B

t Distribution[a]

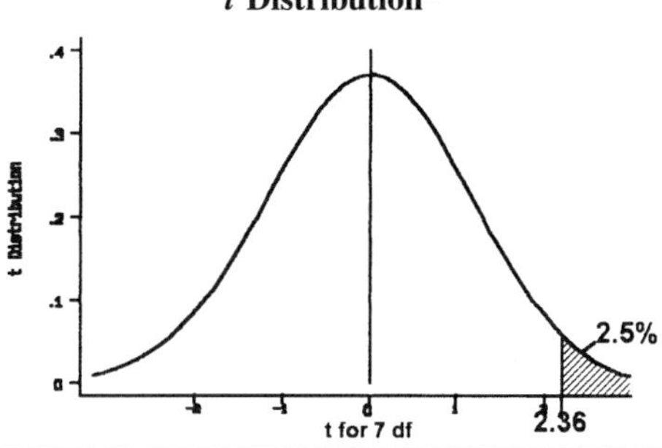

One tailed α (right tail area)	.10	.05	.025	.01	.005	.001	.0005
One tailed 1−α (except right tail)	.90	.95	.975	.99	.995	.999	.9995
Two-tailed α (area both tails)	.20	.10	.05	.02	.01	.002	.001
Two-tailed 1−α (except both tails)	.80	.90	.95	.98	.99	.998	.999
df = 2	1.886	2.920	4.303	6.965	9.925	22.327	31.598
3	1.638	2.353	3.182	4.541	5.841	10.215	12.941
4	1.533	2.132	2.776	3.747	4.604	7.173	8.610
5	1.476	2.015	2.571	3.365	4.032	5.893	6.859
6	1.440	1.943	2.447	3.143	3.707	5.208	5.959
7	1.415	1.895	2.365	2.998	3.499	4.785	5.405
8	1.397	1.860	2.306	2.896	3.355	4.501	5.041
9	1.383	1.833	2.262	2.821	3.250	4.297	4.781
10	1.372	1.812	2.228	2.764	3.169	4.144	4.587
11	1.363	1.796	2.201	2.718	3.106	4.025	4.437
12	1.356	1.782	2.179	2.681	3.055	3.930	4.318
13	1.350	1.771	2.160	2.650	3.012	3.852	4.221
14	1.345	1.761	2.145	2.624	2.977	3.787	4.140
15	1.341	1.753	2.131	2.602	2.947	3.733	4.073
16	1.337	1.746	2.120	2.583	2.921	3.686	4.015
17	1.333	1.740	2.110	2.567	2.898	3.646	3.965
18	1.330	1.734	2.101	2.552	2.878	3.610	3.922
19	1.328	1.729	2.093	2.539	2.861	3.579	3.883
20	1.325	1.725	2.086	2.528	2.845	3.552	3.850
21	1.323	1.721	2.080	2.518	2.831	3.527	3.819
22	1.321	1.717	2.074	2.508	2.819	3.505	3.792
23	1.319	1.714	2.069	2.500	2.807	3.485	3.767
24	1.318	1.711	2.064	2.492	2.797	3.467	3.745
25	1.316	1.708	2.060	2.485	2.787	3.450	3.725
26	1.315	1.706	2.056	2.479	2.779	3.435	3.707
27	1.314	1.703	2.052	2.473	2.771	3.421	3.690
28	1.313	1.701	2.048	2.467	2.763	3.408	3.674
29	1.311	1.699	2.045	2.462	2.756	3.396	3.659
30	1.310	1.697	2.042	2.457	2.750	3.385	3.646
40	1.303	1.684	2.021	2.423	2.704	3.307	3.551
60	1.296	1.671	2.000	2.390	2.660	3.232	3.460
100	1.290	1.660	1.984	2.364	2.626	3.174	3.390
∞	1.282	1.645	1.960	2.326	2.576	3.090	3.291

[a] Selected distances (t) to the right of the mean are given for various degrees of freedom (df) and for (a) one-tailed α, area under the curve in the positive tail; (b) one-tailed $1 - \alpha$, area under all except the tail; (c) two-tailed α, areas combined for both positive and negative tails; and (d) two-tailed $1 - \alpha$, area under all except the two tails.

Table C
Chi-Square Distribution, Right Tail[a]

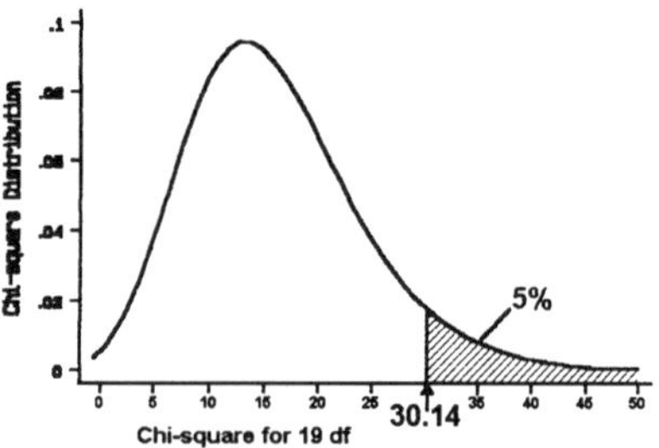

α (area in right tail)	.10	.05	.025	.01	.005	.001	.0005
1−α (except right tail)	.90	.95	.975	.99	.995	.999	.9995
df= 1	2.71	3.84	5.02	6.63	7.88	10.81	12.13
2	4.61	5.99	7.38	9.21	10.60	13.80	15.21
3	6.25	7.81	9.35	11.34	12.84	16.26	17.75
4	7.78	9.49	11.14	13.28	14.86	18.46	20.04
5	9.24	11.07	12.83	15.08	16.75	20.52	22.15
6	10.64	12.59	14.45	16.81	18.54	22.46	24.08
7	12.02	14.07	16.01	18.47	20.28	24.35	26.02
8	13.36	15.51	17.53	20.09	21.95	26.10	27.86
9	14.68	16.92	19.02	21.67	23.59	27.86	29.71
10	15.99	18.31	20.48	23.21	25.19	29.58	31.46
11	17.28	19.68	21.92	24.72	26.75	31.29	33.13
12	18.55	21.03	23.34	26.22	28.30	32.92	34.80
13	19.81	22.36	24.74	27.69	29.82	34.54	36.47
14	21.06	23.69	26.12	29.14	31.32	36.12	38.14
15	22.31	25.00	27.49	30.57	32.81	37.71	39.73
16	23.54	26.30	28.84	32.00	34.27	39.24	41.31
17	24.77	27.59	30.19	33.41	35.72	40.78	42.89
18	25.99	28.87	31.53	34.80	37.16	42.32	44.47
19	27.20	30.14	32.85	36.19	38.58	43.81	45.97
20	28.41	31.41	34.17	37.57	39.99	45.31	47.46
21	29.62	32.67	35.48	38.94	41.40	46.80	49.04
22	30.81	33.92	36.78	40.29	42.80	48.25	50.45
23	32.01	35.17	38.08	41.64	44.19	49.75	52.03
24	33.20	36.41	39.36	42.97	45.56	51.15	53.44
25	34.38	37.65	40.65	44.31	46.93	52.65	51.93
26	35.56	38.88	41.92	45.64	48.30	54.05	56.43
27	36.74	40.11	43.20	46.97	49.65	55.46	57.83
28	37.92	41.34	44.46	48.28	51.00	56.87	59.24
29	39.09	42.56	45.72	49.59	52.34	58.27	60.73
30	40.26	43.77	46.98	50.89	53.68	59.68	62.23
35	46.06	49.80	53.20	57.34	60.27	66.62	69.26
40	51.80	55.76	59.34	63.69	66.76	73.39	76.11
50	63.17	67.51	71.42	76.16	79.50	86.66	89.56
60	74.40	79.08	83.30	88.38	91.96	99.58	102.66
70	85.53	90.53	95.02	100.43	104.22	112.32	115.66
80	96.58	101.88	106.63	112.32	116.32	124.80	128.32
100	118.50	124.34	129.56	135.81	140.16	149.41	153.11

[a] Selected χ^2 values (distances above zero) are given for various degrees of freedom (*df*) and for (a) α, the area under the curve in the right tail, and (b) $1 - \alpha$, the area under all except the right tail.

Table D
Chi-Square Distribution, Left Tail[a]

α (area in left tail)	.0005	.001	.005	.01	.025	.05	.10
1−α (area except left tail)	.9995	.999	.995	.99	.975	.95	.90
df = 1	.0000004	.0000016	.000039	.00016	.00098	.0039	.016
2	.00099	.0020	.010	.020	.051	.10	.21
3	.015	.024	.072	.12	.22	.35	.58
4	.065	.091	.21	.30	.48	.71	1.06
5	.16	.21	.41	.55	.83	1.15	1.61
6	.30	.38	.68	.87	1.24	1.64	2.20
7	.48	.60	.99	1.24	1.69	2.17	2.83
8	.71	.86	1.34	1.65	2.18	2.73	3.49
9	.97	1.15	1.73	2.09	2.70	3.33	4.17
10	1.26	1.48	2.16	2.56	3.25	3.94	4.87
11	1.58	1.83	2.60	3.05	3.82	4.57	5.58
12	1.93	2.21	3.07	3.57	4.40	5.23	6.30
13	2.31	2.61	3.57	4.11	5.01	5.89	7.04
14	2.70	3.04	4.07	4.66	5.63	6.57	7.79
15	3.10	3.48	4.60	5.23	6.26	7.26	8.55
16	3.54	3.94	5.14	5.81	6.91	7.96	9.31
17	3.98	4.42	5.70	6.41	7.56	8.67	10.09
18	4.44	4.90	6.26	7.01	8.23	9.39	10.86
19	4.92	5.41	6.84	7.63	8.91	10.12	11.65
20	5.41	5.92	7.43	8.26	9.59	10.85	12.44
21	5.89	6.45	8.03	8.90	10.28	11.59	13.24
22	6.42	6.99	8.64	9.54	10.98	12.34	14.04
23	6.92	7.54	9.26	10.20	11.69	13.09	14.85
24	7.45	8.09	9.89	10.86	12.40	13.85	15.66
25	8.00	8.66	10.52	11.52	13.12	14.61	16.47
26	8.53	9.23	11.16	12.20	13.84	15.38	17.29
27	9.10	9.80	11.81	12.88	14.57	16.15	18.11
28	9.68	10.39	12.46	13.57	15.31	16.93	18.94
29	10.24	10.99	13.12	14.25	16.05	17.71	19.77
30	10.81	11.58	13.79	14.95	16.79	18.49	20.60
35	13.80	14.68	17.19	18.51	20.57	22.46	24.80
40	16.92	17.93	20.71	22.16	24.43	26.51	29.05
50	23.47	24.68	27.99	29.71	32.36	34.76	37.69
60	30.32	31.73	35.53	37.49	40.48	43.19	46.46
70	37.44	39.02	43.28	45.44	48.76	51.74	55.33
80	44.82	46.49	51.17	53.54	57.15	60.39	64.28
100	59.94	61.92	67.32	70.07	74.22	77.93	82.36

[a] Selected χ^2 values (distances above zero) are given for various degrees of freedom (*df*) and for (a) α, the area under the curve in the left tail, and (b) $1 - \alpha$, the area under all except the left tail.

Table E

F Distribution[a]

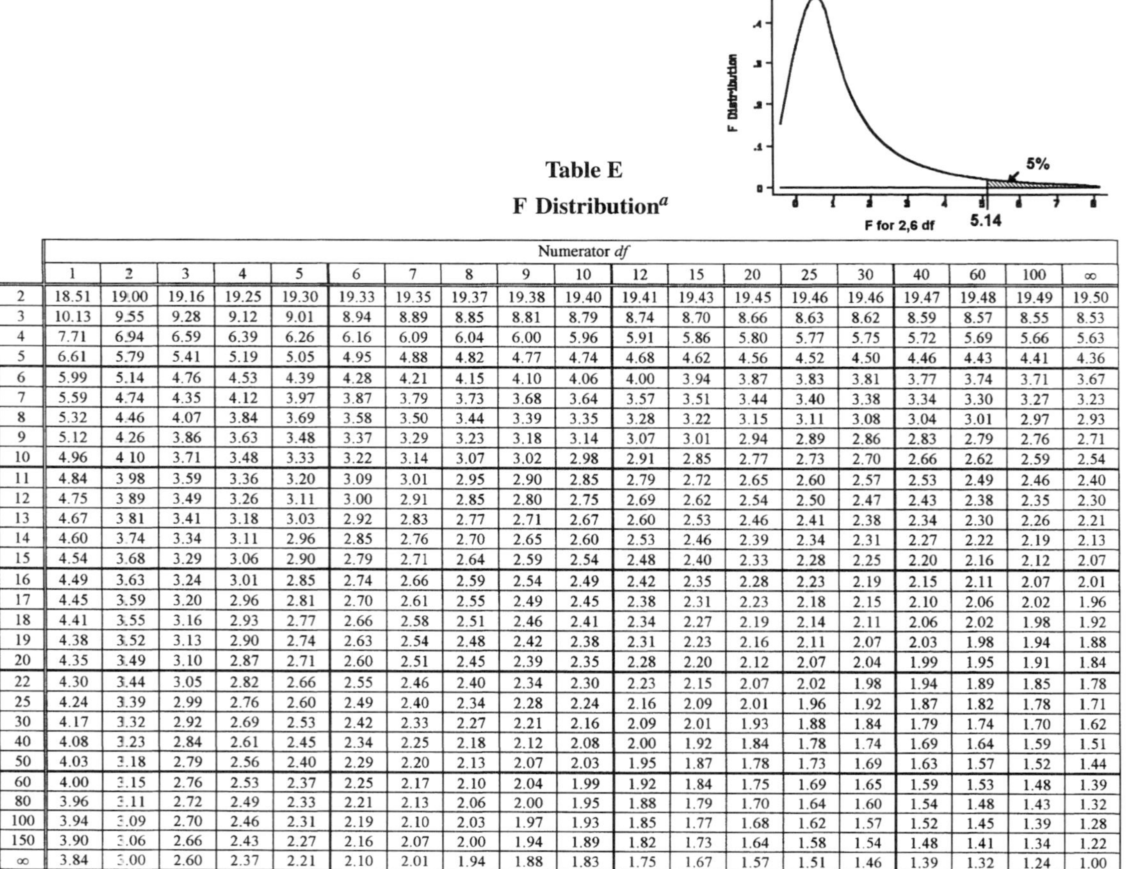

Denominator df	Numerator df 1	2	3	4	5	6	7	8	9	10	12	15	20	25	30	40	60	100	∞
2	18.51	19.00	19.16	19.25	19.30	19.33	19.35	19.37	19.38	19.40	19.41	19.43	19.45	19.46	19.46	19.47	19.48	19.49	19.50
3	10.13	9.55	9.28	9.12	9.01	8.94	8.89	8.85	8.81	8.79	8.74	8.70	8.66	8.63	8.62	8.59	8.57	8.55	8.53
4	7.71	6.94	6.59	6.39	6.26	6.16	6.09	6.04	6.00	5.96	5.91	5.86	5.80	5.77	5.75	5.72	5.69	5.66	5.63
5	6.61	5.79	5.41	5.19	5.05	4.95	4.88	4.82	4.77	4.74	4.68	4.62	4.56	4.52	4.50	4.46	4.43	4.41	4.36
6	5.99	5.14	4.76	4.53	4.39	4.28	4.21	4.15	4.10	4.06	4.00	3.94	3.87	3.83	3.81	3.77	3.74	3.71	3.67
7	5.59	4.74	4.35	4.12	3.97	3.87	3.79	3.73	3.68	3.64	3.57	3.51	3.44	3.40	3.38	3.34	3.30	3.27	3.23
8	5.32	4.46	4.07	3.84	3.69	3.58	3.50	3.44	3.39	3.35	3.28	3.22	3.15	3.11	3.08	3.04	3.01	2.97	2.93
9	5.12	4.26	3.86	3.63	3.48	3.37	3.29	3.23	3.18	3.14	3.07	3.01	2.94	2.89	2.86	2.83	2.79	2.76	2.71
10	4.96	4.10	3.71	3.48	3.33	3.22	3.14	3.07	3.02	2.98	2.91	2.85	2.77	2.73	2.70	2.66	2.62	2.59	2.54
11	4.84	3.98	3.59	3.36	3.20	3.09	3.01	2.95	2.90	2.85	2.79	2.72	2.65	2.60	2.57	2.53	2.49	2.46	2.40
12	4.75	3.89	3.49	3.26	3.11	3.00	2.91	2.85	2.80	2.75	2.69	2.62	2.54	2.50	2.47	2.43	2.38	2.35	2.30
13	4.67	3.81	3.41	3.18	3.03	2.92	2.83	2.77	2.71	2.67	2.60	2.53	2.46	2.41	2.38	2.34	2.30	2.26	2.21
14	4.60	3.74	3.34	3.11	2.96	2.85	2.76	2.70	2.65	2.60	2.53	2.46	2.39	2.34	2.31	2.27	2.22	2.19	2.13
15	4.54	3.68	3.29	3.06	2.90	2.79	2.71	2.64	2.59	2.54	2.48	2.40	2.33	2.28	2.25	2.20	2.16	2.12	2.07
16	4.49	3.63	3.24	3.01	2.85	2.74	2.66	2.59	2.54	2.49	2.42	2.35	2.28	2.23	2.19	2.15	2.11	2.07	2.01
17	4.45	3.59	3.20	2.96	2.81	2.70	2.61	2.55	2.49	2.45	2.38	2.31	2.23	2.18	2.15	2.10	2.06	2.02	1.96
18	4.41	3.55	3.16	2.93	2.77	2.66	2.58	2.51	2.46	2.41	2.34	2.27	2.19	2.14	2.11	2.06	2.02	1.98	1.92
19	4.38	3.52	3.13	2.90	2.74	2.63	2.54	2.48	2.42	2.38	2.31	2.23	2.16	2.11	2.07	2.03	1.98	1.94	1.88
20	4.35	3.49	3.10	2.87	2.71	2.60	2.51	2.45	2.39	2.35	2.28	2.20	2.12	2.07	2.04	1.99	1.95	1.91	1.84
22	4.30	3.44	3.05	2.82	2.66	2.55	2.46	2.40	2.34	2.30	2.23	2.15	2.07	2.02	1.98	1.94	1.89	1.85	1.78
25	4.24	3.39	2.99	2.76	2.60	2.49	2.40	2.34	2.28	2.24	2.16	2.09	2.01	1.96	1.92	1.87	1.82	1.78	1.71
30	4.17	3.32	2.92	2.69	2.53	2.42	2.33	2.27	2.21	2.16	2.09	2.01	1.93	1.88	1.84	1.79	1.74	1.70	1.62
40	4.08	3.23	2.84	2.61	2.45	2.34	2.25	2.18	2.12	2.08	2.00	1.92	1.84	1.78	1.74	1.69	1.64	1.59	1.51
50	4.03	3.18	2.79	2.56	2.40	2.29	2.20	2.13	2.07	2.03	1.95	1.87	1.78	1.73	1.69	1.63	1.57	1.52	1.44
60	4.00	3.15	2.76	2.53	2.37	2.25	2.17	2.10	2.04	1.99	1.92	1.84	1.75	1.69	1.65	1.59	1.53	1.48	1.39
80	3.96	3.11	2.72	2.49	2.33	2.21	2.13	2.06	2.00	1.95	1.88	1.79	1.70	1.64	1.60	1.54	1.48	1.43	1.32
100	3.94	3.09	2.70	2.46	2.31	2.19	2.10	2.03	1.97	1.93	1.85	1.77	1.68	1.62	1.57	1.52	1.45	1.39	1.28
150	3.90	3.06	2.66	2.43	2.27	2.16	2.07	2.00	1.94	1.89	1.82	1.73	1.64	1.58	1.54	1.48	1.41	1.34	1.22
∞	3.84	3.00	2.60	2.37	2.21	2.10	2.01	1.94	1.88	1.83	1.75	1.67	1.57	1.51	1.46	1.39	1.32	1.24	1.00

[a] Selected distances (F) are given for various degrees of freedom (*df*) for $\alpha = 5\%$, the area under the curve in the positive tail, and $1 - \alpha = 95\%$, the area under all except the tail. Numerator *df* appears in column headings, denominator *df* in row headings, and F at the intersection of row and column in the table body.

Table F

Binomial Distribution[a]

		π									
n	n_0	.05	.10	.15	.20	.25	.30	.35	.40	.45	.50
2	1	.098	.190	.278	.360	.438	.510	.578	.640	.698	.750
	2	.003	.010	.023	.040	.063	.090	.123	.160	.203	.250
3	1	.143	.271	.386	.488	.578	.657	.725	.784	.834	.875
	2	.007	.028	.061	.104	.156	.216	.282	.352	.425	.500
	3	.000	.001	.003	.008	.016	.027	.043	.064	.091	.125
4	1	.186	.344	.478	.590	.684	.760	.822	.870	.909	.938
	2	.014	.052	.110	.181	.262	.348	.437	.525	.609	.688
	3	.001	.004	.012	.027	.051	.084	.127	.179	.242	.313
	4	.000	.000	.001	.002	.004	.008	.015	.026	.041	.063
5	1	.226	.410	.556	.672	.763	.832	.884	.922	.950	.969
	2	.023	.082	.165	.263	.367	.472	.572	.663	.744	.813
	3	.001	.009	.027	.058	.104	.163	.235	.317	.407	.500
	4	.000	.001	.002	.007	.016	.031	.054	.087	.131	.188
	5		.000	.000	.000	.001	.002	.005	.010	.019	.031
6	1	.265	.469	.629	.738	.822	.882	.925	.953	.972	.984
	2	.033	.114	.224	.345	.466	.580	.681	.676	.836	.891
	3	.002	.016	.047	.099	.169	.256	.353	.456	.559	.656
	4	.000	.001	.006	.017	.038	.071	.117	.179	.255	.344
	5		.000	.000	.002	.005	.011	.022	.041	.069	.109
	6				.000	.000	.001	.002	.004	.008	.016
7	1	.302	.522	.679	.790	.867	.918	.951	.972	.985	.992
	2	.044	.150	.283	.423	.555	.671	.766	.841	.898	.938
	3	.004	.026	.074	.148	.244	.353	.468	.580	.684	.773
	4	.000	.003	.012	.033	.071	.126	.200	.290	.392	.500
	5		.000	.001	.005	.013	.029	.056	.096	.153	.227
	6			.000	.000	.001	.004	.009	.019	.036	.063
	7					.000	.000	.001	.002	.004	.008
8	1	.337	.570	.728	.832	.900	.942	.968	.983	.992	.996
	2	.057	.187	.343	.497	.633	.745	.831	.894	.937	.965
	3	.006	.038	.105	.203	.322	.448	.572	.685	.780	.856
	4	.000	.005	.021	.056	.114	.194	.294	.406	.523	.637
	5		.000	.003	.010	.027	.058	.106	.174	.260	.363
	6			.000	.001	.004	.011	.025	.050	.089	.145
	7				.000	.000	.001	.004	.009	.018	.035
	8						.000	.000	.001	.002	.004
9	1	.370	.613	.768	.866	.925	.960	.979	.990	.995	.998
	2	.071	.225	.401	.564	.700	.804	.879	.930	.962	.981
	3	.008	.053	.141	.262	.399	.537	.663	.768	.851	.910
	4	.001	.008	.034	.086	.166	.270	.391	.517	.639	.746
	5	.000	.001	.006	.020	.045	.099	.172	.267	.379	.500
	6		.000	.001	.003	.010	.025	.054	.099	.166	.254
	7			.000	.000	.001	.004	.011	.025	.050	.090
	8					.000	.000	.001	.004	.009	.020
	9							.000	.000	.001	.002

(*Continued*)

Table F

(Continued)

		π									
n	n_0	**.05**	**.10**	**.15**	**.20**	**.25**	**.30**	**.35**	**.40**	**.45**	**.50**
10	**1**	.401	.651	.803	.893	.944	.972	.987	.994	.998	.999
	2	.086	.264	.456	.624	.756	.851	.914	.954	.977	.989
	3	.012	.070	.180	.322	.474	.617	.738	.833	.900	.945
	4	.001	.013	.050	.121	.224	.350	.486	.618	.734	.828
	5	.000	.002	.010	.033	.078	.150	.249	.367	.496	.623
	6		.000	.001	.006	.020	.047	.095	.166	.262	.377
	7			.000	.001	.004	.011	.026	.055	.102	.172
	8				.000	.000	.002	.005	.012	.027	.055
	9						.000	.001	.002	.005	.011
	10							.000	.000	.000	.001
11	**1**	.431	.686	.833	.914	.958	.980	.991	.996	.999	.999
	2	.102	.303	.508	.678	.803	.887	.939	.970	.986	.994
	3	.015	.090	.221	.383	.545	.687	.800	.881	.935	.967
	4	.002	.019	.069	.161	.287	.430	.574	.704	.809	.887
	5	.000	.003	.016	.050	.115	.210	.332	.467	.603	.726
	6		.000	.003	.012	.034	.078	.149	.247	.367	.500
	7			.000	.002	.008	.022	.050	.099	.174	.274
	8				.000	.001	.004	.012	.029	.061	.113
	9					.000	.001	.002	.006	.015	.033
	10						.000	.000	.001	.002	.006
	11								.000	.000	.001
12	**1**	.460	.718	.858	.931	.968	.986	.994	.998	.999	1.000
	2	.118	.341	.557	.725	.842	.915	.958	.980	.992	.997
	3	.020	.111	.264	.442	.609	.747	.849	.917	.958	.981
	4	.002	.026	.092	.205	.351	.508	.653	.775	.866	.927
	5	.000	.004	.024	.073	.158	.276	.417	.562	.696	.806
	6		.001	.005	.019	.054	.118	.213	.335	.473	.613
	7		.000	.001	.004	.014	.039	.085	.158	.261	.387
	8			.000	.001	.003	.010	.026	.057	.112	.194
	9				.000	.000	.002	.006	.015	.036	.073
	10						.000	.001	.003	.008	.019
	11							.000	.000	.001	.003
	12									.000	.000
13	**1**	.487	.746	.879	.945	.976	.990	.996	.999	1.000	1.000
	2	.135	.379	.602	.766	.873	.936	.970	.987	.995	.999
	3	.025	.134	.270	.498	.667	.798	.887	.942	.973	.989
	4	.003	.034	.097	.253	.416	.579	.722	.831	.907	.954
	5	.000	.007	.026	.009	.206	.346	.500	.647	.772	.867
	6		.001	.005	.030	.080	.165	.284	.426	.573	.710
	7		.000	.001	.007	.024	.062	.130	.229	.356	.500
	8			.000	.001	.006	.018	.046	.098	.179	.291
	9				.000	.001	.004	.013	.032	.070	.133
	10					.000	.001	.003	.008	.020	.046
	11						.000	.000	.001	.004	.011
	12								.000	.001	.002
	13									.000	.000

Table F

(*Continued*)

		π									
n	**n_0**	**.05**	**.10**	**.15**	**.20**	**.25**	**.30**	**.35**	**.40**	**.45**	**.50**
14	**1**	.512	.771	.897	.956	.982	.993	.998	.999	1.000	1.000
	2	.153	.415	.643	.802	.899	.953	.980	.992	.997	.999
	3	.030	.158	.352	.552	.719	.839	.916	.960	.983	.993
	4	.004	.044	.147	.302	.479	.645	.780	.876	.937	.971
	5	.000	.009	.047	.130	.259	.416	.577	.721	.833	.910
	6		.002	.012	.044	.112	.220	.360	.514	.663	.788
	7		.000	.002	.012	.038	.093	.184	.308	.454	.605
	8			.000	.002	.010	.032	.075	.150	.259	.395
	9				.000	.002	.008	.024	.058	.119	.212
	10					.000	.002	.006	.018	.043	.090
	11						.000	.001	.004	.011	.029
	12							.000	.001	.002	.007
	13								.000	.000	.001
	14										.000
15	**1**	.537	.794	.913	.965	.987	.995	.998	1.000	1.000	1.000
	2	.171	.451	.681	.833	.920	.965	.986	.995	.998	1.000
	3	.036	.184	.396	.602	.764	.873	.938	.973	.989	.996
	4	.006	.056	.177	.352	.539	.703	.827	.910	.958	.982
	5	.001	.013	.062	.164	.314	.485	.648	.783	.880	.941
	6	.000	.002	.017	.061	.148	.278	.436	.597	.739	.849
	7		.000	.004	.018	.057	.131	.245	.390	.548	.696
	8			.001	.004	.017	.050	.113	.213	.347	.500
	9			.000	.001	.004	.015	.042	.095	.182	.304
	10				.000	.001	.004	.012	.034	.077	.151
	11					.000	.001	.003	.009	.026	.059
	12						.000	.001	.002	.006	.018
	13							.000	.000	.001	.004
	14									.000	.001
	15										.000
16	**1**	.560	.815	.926	.972	.990	.997	.999	1.000	1.000	1.000
	2	.189	.485	.716	.859	.937	.974	.990	.997	.999	1.000
	3	.043	.211	.439	.648	.803	.901	.955	.982	.993	.998
	4	.007	.068	.210	.402	.595	.754	.866	.935	.972	.989
	5	.001	.017	.079	.202	.370	.550	.711	.833	.915	.962
	6	.000	.003	.024	.082	.190	.340	.510	.671	.802	.895
	7		.001	.006	.027	.080	.175	.312	.473	.634	.723
	8		.000	.001	.007	.027	.074	.159	.284	.437	.598
	9			.000	.002	.008	.026	.067	.142	.256	.402
	10				.000	.002	.007	.023	.058	.124	.227
	11					.000	.002	.006	.019	.049	.105
	12						.000	.001	.005	.015	.038
	13							.000	.001	.004	.011
	14								.000	.001	.002
	15									.000	.000

[a] Values of cumulative binomial distribution, depending on π (theoretical proportion of occurrences in a random trial), n (sample size), and n_0 (number of occurrences observed). Given π, n, and n_0, the corresponding entry in the table body represents the probability that n_0 or more occurrences (or alternatively that n_0/n proportion observed occurrences) would have been observed by chance alone.

Table G

Poisson Distribution[a]

n_0	λ (= $n\pi$)														
	.1	**.2**	**.3**	**.4**	**.5**	**.6**	**.7**	**.8**	**.9**	**1.0**	**1.1**	**1.2**	**1.3**	**1.4**	**1.5**
1	.095	.181	.259	.330	.394	.451	.503	.551	.593	.632	.667	.699	.728	.753	.777
2	.005	.018	.037	.062	.090	.122	.159	.191	.228	.264	.301	.337	.373	.408	.442
3	.000	.001	.004	.008	.014	.023	.034	.047	.063	.080	.100	.121	.143	.167	.191
4		.000	.000	.001	.002	.003	.006	.009	.014	.019	.026	.034	.043	.054	.066
5				.000	.000	.000	.001	.001	.002	.004	.005	.008	.011	.014	.019
6							.000	.000	.000	.001	.001	.002	.002	.003	.005
7										.000	.000	.000	.000	.001	.001

n_0	λ (= $n\pi$)														
	1.6	**1.7**	**1.8**	**1.9**	**2.0**	**2.1**	**2.2**	**2.3**	**2.4**	**2.5**	**2.6**	**2.7**	**2.8**	**2.9**	**3.0**
1	.798	.817	.835	.850	.865	.878	.889	.900	.909	.918	.926	.933	.939	.945	.950
2	.475	.507	.537	.566	.594	.620	.645	.669	.692	.713	.733	.751	.769	.785	.801
3	.217	.243	.269	.296	.323	.350	.377	.404	.430	.456	.482	.506	.531	.554	.577
4	.079	.093	.109	.125	.143	.161	.181	.201	.221	.242	.264	.286	.308	.330	.353
5	.024	.030	.036	.044	.053	.062	.073	.084	.096	.109	.123	.137	.152	.168	.185
6	.006	.008	.010	.013	.017	.020	.025	.030	.036	.042	.049	.057	.065	.074	.084
7	.001	.002	.003	.003	.005	.006	.008	.009	.012	.014	.017	.021	.024	.029	.034
8	.000	.000	.001	.001	.001	.002	.002	.003	.003	.004	.005	.007	.008	.010	.012
9			.000	.000	.000	.000	.001	.001	.001	.001	.002	.002	.002	.003	.004
10							.000	.000	.000	.000	.000	.001	.001	.001	.001

n_0	λ (= $n\pi$)														
	3.1	**3.2**	**3.3**	**3.4**	**3.5**	**3.6**	**3.7**	**3.8**	**3.9**	**4.0**	**4.1**	**4.2**	**4.3**	**4.4**	**4.5**
1	.955	.959	.963	.967	.970	.973	.975	.978	.980	.982	.983	.985	.986	.988	..989
2	.815	.829	.841	.853	.864	.874	.884	.893	.901	.908	.916	.922	.928	.934	.939
3	.599	.620	.641	.660	.679	.697	.715	.731	.747	.762	.776	.790	.803	.815	.826
4	.375	.398	.420	.442	.463	.485	.506	.527	.547	.567	.586	.605	.623	.641	.658
5	.202	.219	.237	.256	.275	.294	.313	.332	.352	.371	.391	.410	.430	.449	.468
6	.094	.105	.117	.130	.142	.156	.170	.184	.199	.215	.231	.247	.263	.280	.297
7	.039	.045	.051	.058	.065	.073	.082	.091	.101	.111	.121	.133	.144	.156	.169
8	.014	.017	.020	.023	.027	.031	.035	.040	.045	.051	.057	.064	.071	.079	.087
9	.005	.006	.007	.008	.010	.012	.014	.016	.019	.021	.025	.028	.032	.036	.040
10	.001	.002	.002	.003	.003	.004	.005	.006	.007	.008	.010	.011	.013	.015	.017
11	.000	.001	.001	.001	.001	.001	.002	.002	.002	.003	.003	.004	.005	.006	.007
12		.000	.000	.000	.000	.000	.001	.001	.001	.001	.001	.001	.002	.002	.002
13							.000	.000	.000	.000	.000	.000	.001	.001	.001

Table G

(Continued)

n_0	λ (= $n\pi$)														
	4.6	4.7	4.8	4.9	5.0	5.1	5.2	5.3	5.4	5.5	5.6	5.7	5.8	5.9	6.0
1	.990	.991	.992	.993	.993	.994	.995	.995	.996	.996	.996	.997	.997	.997	.998
2	.944	.948	.952	.956	.960	.963	.966	.969	.971	.973	.976	.978	.979	.981	.983
3	.837	.848	.858	.867	.875	.884	.891	.898	.905	.912	.918	.923	.929	.933	.938
4	.674	.690	.706	.721	.735	.749	.762	.775	.787	.798	.809	.820	.830	.840	.849
5	.487	.505	.524	.542	.560	.577	.594	.611	.627	.643	.658	.673	.687	.701	.715
6	.314	.332	.349	.367	.384	.402	.419	.437	.454	.471	.488	.505	.522	.538	.554
7	.182	.195	.209	.223	.238	.253	.268	.283	.298	.314	.330	.346	.362	.378	.394
8	.095	.104	.113	.123	.133	.144	.155	.167	.178	.191	.203	.216	.229	.242	.256
9	.045	.050	.156	.062	.068	.075	.082	.089	.097	.106	.114	.123	.133	.143	.153
10	.020	.022	.025	.028	.032	.036	.040	.044	.049	.054	.059	.065	.071	.077	.084
11	.008	.009	.010	.012	.014	.016	.018	.020	.023	.025	.028	.031	.035	.039	.043
12	.003	.003	.004	.005	.006	.006	.007	.008	.010	.011	.013	.014	.016	.018	.020
13	.001	.001	.001	.002	.002	.002	.003	.003	.004	.005	.005	.006	.007	.008	.009
14	.000	.000	.001	.001	.001	.001	.001	.001	.001	.002	.002	.002	.003	.003	.004
15			.000	.000	.000	.000	.000	.000	.000	.001	.001	.001	.001	.001	.001

n_0	λ (= $n\pi$)														
	6.1	6.2	6.3	6.4	6.5	6.6	6.7	6.8	6.9	7.0	7.1	7.2	7.3	7.4	7.5
1	.998	.998	.998	.998	.999	.999	.999	.999	.999	.999	.999	.999	.999	.999	.999
2	.984	.985	.987	.988	.989	.990	.991	.991	.992	.993	.993	.994	.994	.995	.995
3	.942	.946	.950	.954	.957	.960	.963	.966	.968	.970	.973	.975	.976	.978	.980
4	.858	.866	.874	.881	.888	.895	.901	.907	.913	.918	.923	.928	.933	.937	.941
5	.728	.741	.753	.765	.776	.787	.798	.808	.818	.827	.836	.845	.853	.861	.868
6	.570	.586	.601	.616	.631	.645	.659	.673	.686	.699	.712	.724	.736	.747	.759
7	.410	.426	.442	.458	.474	.489	.505	.520	.535	.550	.565	.580	.594	.608	.622
8	.270	.284	.298	.313	.327	.342	.357	.372	.386	.401	.416	.431	.446	.461	.475
9	.163	.174	.185	.197	.208	.220	.233	.245	.258	.271	.284	.297	.311	.324	.338
10	.091	.098	.106	.114	.123	.131	.140	.150	.151	.170	.180	.190	.201	.212	.223
11	.047	.051	.056	.061	.067	.073	.079	.085	.092	.099	.106	.113	.121	.129	.138
12	.022	.025	.028	.031	.034	.037	.041	.045	.049	.053	.058	.063	.068	.074	.079
13	.010	.011	.013	.014	.016	.018	.020	.022	.025	.027	.030	.033	.036	.039	.043
14	.004	.005	.006	.006	.007	.008	.009	.010	.012	.013	.014	.016	.018	.020	.022
15	.002	.002	.002	.003	.003	.003	.004	.004	.005	.006	.007	.007	.008	.009	.010
16	.001	.001	.001	.001	.001	.001	.002	.002	.002	.002	.003	.003	.004	.004	.005
17	.000	.000	.000	.000	.000	.001	.001	.001	.001	.001	.001	.001	.002	.002	.002
18						.000	.000	.000	.000	.000	.000	.001	.001	.001	.001

(Continued)

Table G

(Continued)

n_0	λ (= $n\pi$)														
	7.6	**7.7**	**7.8**	**7.9**	**8.0**	**8.1**	**8.2**	**8.3**	**8.4**	**8.5**	**8.6**	**8.7**	**8.8**	**8.9**	**9.0**
1	.999	1.00	1.00	1.00	1.00	1.00	1.00	1.00	1.00	1.00	1.00	1.00	1.00	1.00	1.00
2	.996	.996	.996	.997	.997	.997	.998	.998	.998	.998	.998	.998	.999	.999	.999
3	.981	.983	.984	.985	.986	.987	.988	.989	.990	.991	.991	.992	.993	.993	.994
4	.945	.948	.952	.955	.958	.960	.963	.965	.968	.970	.972	.974	.976	.977	.979
5	.875	.882	.888	.895	.900	.906	.911	.916	.921	.926	.930	.934	.938	.942	.945
6	.769	.780	.790	.799	.809	.818	.826	.835	.843	.850	.858	.865	.872	.878	.884
7	.635	.649	.662	.674	.687	.699	.710	.722	.733	.744	.754	.765	.774	.784	.793
8	.490	.504	.519	.533	.547	.561	.575	.588	.601	.614	.627	.640	.652	.664	.676
9	.352	.366	.380	.394	.408	.421	.435	.449	.463	.477	.491	.504	.518	.531	.544
10	.235	.247	.259	.271	.283	.296	.309	.321	.334	.347	.360	.373	.386	.399	.413
11	.147	.156	.165	.174	.184	.194	.204	.215	.226	.237	.248	.259	.271	.282	.294
12	.085	.092	.098	.105	.112	.119	.127	.135	.143	.151	.160	.169	.178	.187	.197
13	.046	.050	.055	.059	.064	.069	.074	.079	.085	.091	.097	.104	.110	.117	.124
14	.024	.026	.029	.031	.034	.037	.041	.044	.048	.051	.056	.060	.064	.069	.074
15	.011	.013	.014	.016	.017	.019	.021	.023	.025	.027	.030	.033	.035	.038	.042
16	.005	.006	.007	.007	.008	.009	.010	.011	.013	.014	.015	.017	.018	.020	.022
17	.002	.003	.003	.003	.004	.004	.005	.005	.006	.007	.007	.008	.009	.010	.011
18	.001	.001	.001	.001	.002	.002	.002	.002	.003	.003	.003	.004	.004	.005	.005
19	.000	.000	.000	.001	.001	.001	.001	.001	.001	.001	.002	.002	.002	.002	.002
20				.000	.000	.000	.000	.000	.001	.001	.001	.001	.001	.001	.001

[a] Values of the cumulative Poisson distribution, depending on $\lambda = n\pi$ (sample size × theoretical proportion of occurrences in random trials) and n_0 (number of occurrences observed). Given λ and n_0, the corresponding entry in the table body represents the probability that n_0 or more occurrences (or alternatively that n_0/n proportion observed occurrences) would have been observed by chance alone. (Probability is always 1.000 for $n_0 = 0$.)

Table H
Signed-Rank Probabilities[a]

T	Sample Size n								
	4	5	6	7	8	9	10	11	12
1	.250	.125	.063	.031	.016	.008	.004	.002	.001
2	.375	.188	.094	.047	.024	.012	.006	.003	.002
3	.625	.313	.156	.078	.039	.020	.010	.005	.003
4	.875	.438	.219	.109	.055	.027	.014	.007	.004
5		.625	.313	.156	.078	.039	.020	.010	.005
6		.801	.438	.219	.109	.055	.027	.014	.007
7		1.000	.563	.297	.149	.074	.037	.019	.009
8			.688	.375	.195	.098	.049	.025	.012
9			.844	.469	.250	.129	.065	.032	.016
10			1.000	.578	.313	.164	.084	.042	.021
11				.688	.383	.203	.106	.054	.027
12				.813	.461	.250	.131	.067	.034
13				.938	.547	.301	.160	.083	.043
14					.641	.359	.193	.102	.052
15					.742	.426	.233	.1123	.064
16					.844	.496	.275	.148	.077
17					.945	.570	.322	.175	.092
18						.652	.375	.206	.110
19						.7344	.432	.240	.129
20						.820	.492	..278	.151
21						.910	.557	.320	.176
22						1.000	.625	.365	.204
23							.695	.413	.233
24							.770	.465	.266
25							.846	.520	.301
26							.922	.577	.339
27							1.000	.638	.380
28								.700	.424
29								.765	.470
30								.831	.519
31								.899	.569
32								.966	.622
33									.677
34									.733
35									.791
36									.850
37									.910
38									.970

[a] Two-tailed probabilities for the distribution of T, the signed-rank statistic. For a sample size n and value of T, the entry gives the p-value. If a one-tailed test is appropriate, halve the entry. If $n > 12$, go to Section 14.6.

Table I

Rank-Sum U Probabilities[a]

	n_2:	3			4				5				
	n_1:	1	2	3	1	2	3	4	1	2	3	4	5
U	0	.500	.200	.100	.400	.133	.056	.028	.333	.094	.036	.016	.008
	1	1.00	.400	.200	.800	.267	.114	.058	.337	.190	.072	.032	.016
	2		.800	.400		.534	.228	.114	1.00	.380	.142	.064	.032
	3			.700		.800	.400	.200		.572	.250	.112	.056
	4			1.00			.628	.342		.858	.392	.190	.096
	5						.858	.486			.572	.286	.150
	6							.686			.786	.412	.222
	7							.886			1.00	.556	.310
	8											.730	.420
	9											.904	.548
	10												.690
	11												.842
	12												1.00

	n_2:	6						7						
	n_1:	1	2	3	4	5	6	1	2	3	4	5	6	7
U	0	.286	.072	.024	.010	.004	.002	.250	.054	.016	.006	.002	.002	.001
	1	.572	.142	.048	.020	.008	.004	.500	.112	.034	.012	.006	.002	.001
	2	.856	.286	.096	.038	.018	.008	.750	.222	.066	.024	.010	.004	.002
	3		.428	.166	.066	.030	.016	1.00	.334	.116	.042	.018	.008	.004
	4		.642	.262	.114	.052	.026		.500	.184	.072	.030	.014	.006
	5		.858	.380	.172	.082	.042		.666	.233	.110	.048	.022	.012
	6			.548	.258	.126	.064		.888	.384	.164	.074	.034	.018
	7			.714	.352	.178	.094			.516	.230	.106	.052	.026
	8			.904	.476	.246	.132			.666	.316	.148	.074	.038
	9				.610	.330	.180			.834	.412	.202	.102	.054
	10				.762	.428	.240			1.00	.528	.268	.138	.072
	11				.914	.536	.310				.648	.344	.180	.098
	12					.662	.394				.788	.432	.134	.128
	13					.792	.484				.928	.530	.296	.164
	14					.930	.588					.638	.366	.208
	15						.700					.756	.446	.260
	16						.818					.876	.534	.318
	17						.938					1.00	.628	.382
	18												.730	.456
	19												.836	.534
	20												.946	.620
	21													.710
	22													.804
	23													.902
	24													1.00

Table I

(Continued)

	n_2:	8							
	n_1:	**1**	**2**	**3**	**4**	**5**	**6**	**7**	**8**
	0	.222	.044	.012	.004	.002	.001	.000	.000
	1	.444	.088	.024	.008	.004	.002	.001	.001
	2	.666	.178	.048	.016	.006	.003	.002	.001
	3	.888	.266	.082	.028	.010	.004	.003	.002
	4		.400	.134	.048	.018	.008	.004	.002
	5		.534	.194	.072	.030	.012	.006	.003
	6		.712	.278	.110	.046	.020	.010	.004
	7		.888	.376	.154	.066	.030	.014	.006
	8			.496	.214	.094	.042	.020	.010
	9			.630	.282	.138	.060	.028	.014
	10			.774	.368	.170	.082	.040	.020
	11			.922	.460	.222	.108	.052	.028
	12				.570	.284	.142	.072	.038
	13				.682	.354	.182	.094	.050
	14				.808	.434	.228	.120	.064
U	**15**				.934	.524	.282	.152	.082
	16					.622	.344	.190	.104
	17					.724	.414	.232	.130
	18					.832	.490	.280	.160
	19					.944	.572	.336	.194
	20						.662	.396	.234
	21						.754	.464	.278
	22						.852	.536	.328
	23						.950	.612	.382
	24							.694	.442
	25							.778	.506
	26							.866	.574
	27							.956	.626
	28								.720
	29								.798
	30								.878
	31								.960

[a] Two-tailed probabilities for the distribution of U, the rank-sum statistic. For two samples of size n_1 and n_2 ($n_2 > n_1$) and the value of U, the entry gives the p-value. If a one-tailed test is appropriate, halve the entry. If $n_2 > 8$, go to Section 14.7. It can be seen from inspection that, if $n_1 + n_2 < 7$, a rejection of H_0 at $\alpha = 0.05$ is not possible.

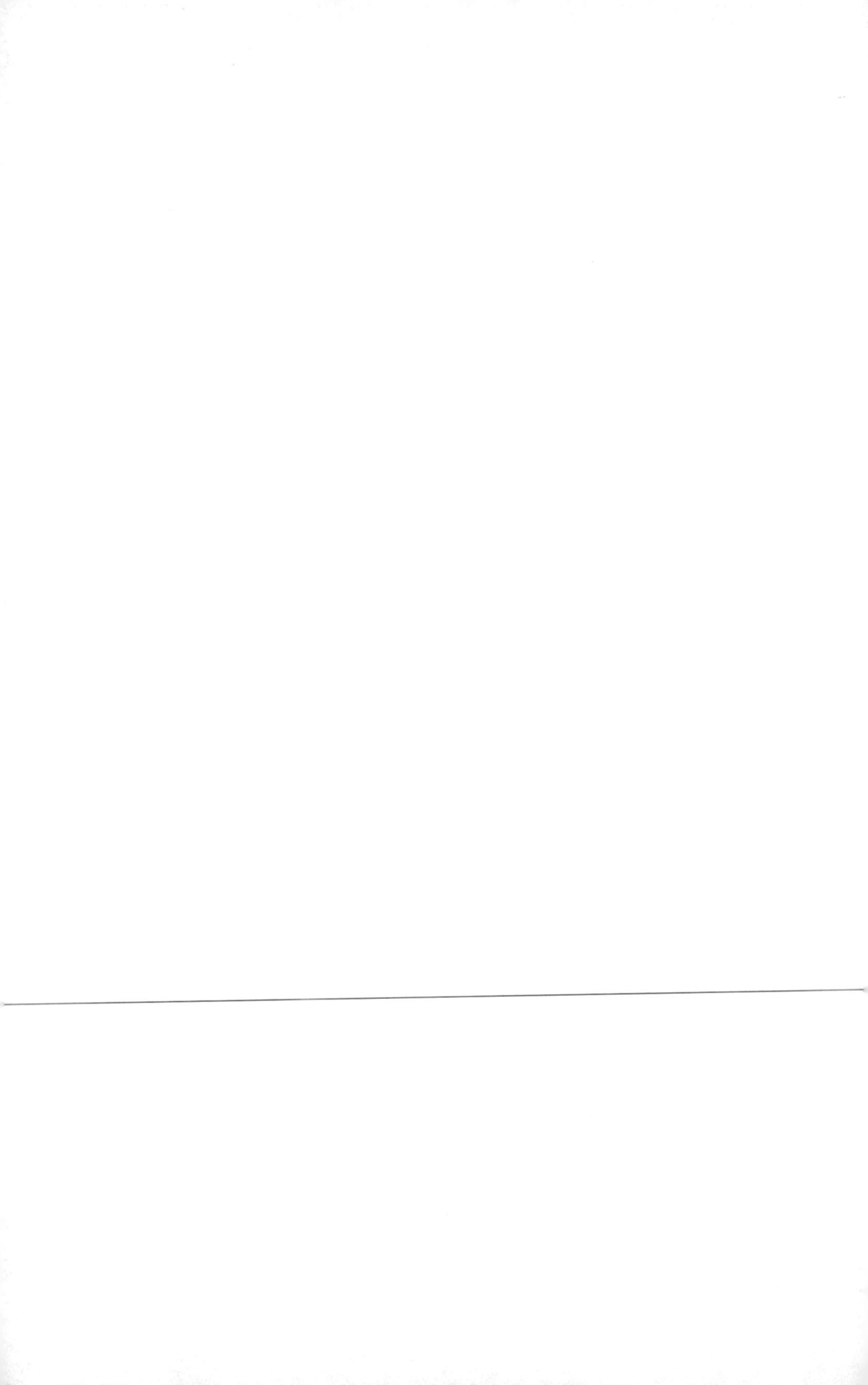

Index

G

H

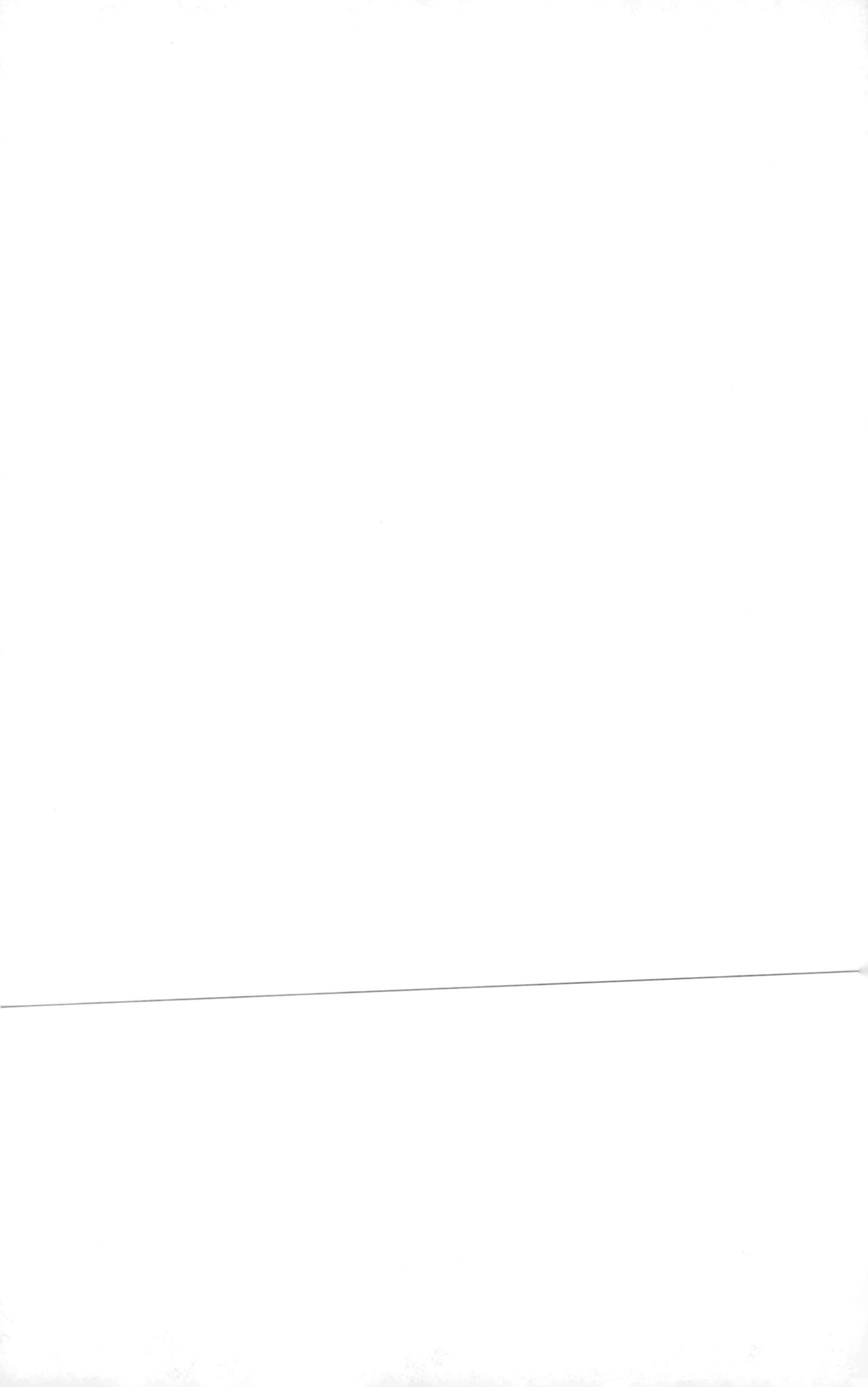

Table 10.1

A First-Step Guide to Choosing Statistical Tests Found in Part II[a]

Type of data:		Counts (nominal)			Ranks	Continuous measurements (including discrete)				
		Proportions								
Questions about:		p not near 0 or 1	p near 0 or 1	Counted quantities	Position in distribution	Averages		Spread	Distribution normality	Distribution equality
Assumed distributions:		Binomial or multinomial			Not required	Normal curve	Far from normal curve	Chi-square	Any	
Small sample	Single or paired sample	Binomial table *13.6*	Poisson table *13.7*	Matched pairs (McNemar) *13.8*	Signed-rank test *14.2*	Normal test if σ; t if s *15.2*	Go to rank methods	Chi-square *16.2*	Shapiro–Wilk or KS test *17.2*	
	Two samples	Form a 2 × 2 contingency table and use Fisher–Irwin or χ^2 *13.2*			Rank-sum test *14.3*	Normal test if σ's; t if s's *15.3*	Go to rank methods	F test *16.3*		Two-sample KS test *17.3*
	Three or more samples	Form an $r \times c$ contingency table and use Fisher–Irwin or χ^2 *13.3*			Kruskal–Wallis/ Friedman paired *14.4/5*	One-way ANOVA with multiple comparisons *15.4*	Go to rank methods	Bartlett's test *16.4*		
Large sample	Single or paired sample	Normal approximation *13.6*	Poisson approximation *13.7*	Matched pairs (McNemar) *13.8*	Signed-rank normal approx *14.6*	Normal test if σ or if large n; t if s *15.2*		Chi-square *16.2*	KS test or test of fit 17.2	
	Two samples	Form a 2 × 2 contingency table and use Fisher–Irwin or χ^2 *13.2*			Rank-sum normal approximation *4.7*	Normal test if σ_1, σ_2 or if large n; t if s_1, s_2 *15.3*		F test *16.3*		Two-sample KS test *17.3*
	Three or more samples	Form an $r \times c$ contingency table and use Fisher–Irwin or χ^2 *13.3*			Kruskal–Wallis/ Friedman paired *14.4/5*	One-way ANOVA with multiple comparisons *15.4*		Bartlett's test *16.4*		

[a] The column is selected by specifying the type of data you have, the question you are asking of these data, and the distribution you are willing to assume. The row is selected by specifying the sample size and the number of samples. The row–column intersection provides the most apparent test fitting these conditions. This selection does not satisfy all requirements and therefore must be taken as only tentative. Italicized numbers indicate the text section in which the item may be found.